HANDBOOK OF THE PSYCHOLOGY
OF RELIGION AND SPIRITUALITY

HANDBOOK OF THE PSYCHOLOGY OF RELIGION AND SPIRITUALITY

Edited by
RAYMOND F. PALOUTZIAN
CRYSTAL L. PARK

THE GUILFORD PRESS
NEW YORK   LONDON

©2005 The Guilford Press
A Division of Guilford Publications, Inc.
72 Spring Street, New York, NY 10012
www.guilford.com

Printed in the United States of America

This book is printed on acid-free paper.

Last digit is print number: 9 8 7 6 5 4 3 2 1

Library of Congress Cataloging-in-Publication Data

Handbook of the psychology of religion and spirituality / edited by Raymond F.
Paloutzian, Crystal L. Park.
    p. cm.
  Includes bibliographical references and index.
  ISBN 1-57230-922-9 (hard cover : alk. paper)
  1. Psychology, Religious. 2. Spirituality—Psychology. I. Paloutzian,
Raymond F., 1945–   II. Park, Crystal L.
  BL53.H288 2005
  200′.1′9—dc22

                                       2005015576

About the Editors

Raymond F. Paloutzian, PhD, is Professor of Experimental and Social Psychology at Westmont College in Santa Barbara, California. Previously, he taught at the University of Idaho and was a visiting professor at Stanford University and a guest professor in the Faculty of Psychology at Katholieke Universiteit in Leuven, Belgium. A Fellow of the American Psychological Association, the American Psychological Society, and the Western Psychological Association, Dr. Paloutzian is a past president of Division 36 of the American Psychological Association (Psychology of Religion). He is the author of *Invitation to the Psychology of Religion, Second Edition,* and the editor of *The International Journal for the Psychology of Religion.*

Crystal L. Park, PhD, is Associate Professor of Psychology at the University of Connecticut. Her research focuses on the roles of religious beliefs and religious coping in response to stressful life events, the phenomenon of stress-related growth, and people's attempts to find meaning in negative life events. She is associate editor of *Psychology and Health* and is on the editorial boards of the *Journal of Clinical and Consulting Psychology* and *The International Journal for the Psychology of Religion.* A past president of Division 36 of the American Psychological Association, Dr. Park is also Principal Investigator on research projects funded by the Lance Armstrong Foundation (examining positive life changes in cancer survivors) and the Fetzer Foundation (examining changes in spirituality and well-being in patients with terminal heart failure).

Contributors

Carolyn M. Aldwin, PhD, is Professor and Chair, Department of Human Development and Family Sciences, Oregon State University, Corvallis, Oregon.

Bob Altemeyer, PhD, is Associate Professor, Department of Psychology, University of Manitoba, Winnipeg, Manitoba, Canada.

Gene G. Ano, MA, is a doctoral student in clinical psychology, Department of Psychology, Bowling Green State University, Bowling Green, Ohio.

Roy F. Baumeister, PhD, is Eppes Eminent Professor, Department of Psychology, Florida State University, Tallahassee, Florida.

Jacob A. Belzen, PhD, is Full Professor of Psychology of Religion, University of Amsterdam, Amsterdam, The Netherlands. He is coeditor of the *Archiv für Religionpsychologie.*

Giacomo Bono, PhD, is a postdoctoral fellow, Department of Psychology, University of Miami, Coral Gables, Florida.

Chris J. Boyatzis, PhD, is Associate Professor, Department of Psychology, Bucknell University, Lewisburg, Pennsylvania.

Jozef Corveleyn, PhD, is Professor and Dean, Faculty of Psychology, Katholieke Universiteit, Leuven, Belgium, and Part-time Professor of Clinical Psychology of Religion, Faculty of Psychology and Educational Sciences, Free University of Amsterdam, The Netherlands.

Michelle D'Mello, MA, is a graduate student, Department of Human and Community Development, University of California, Davis, Davis, California.

Michael J. Donahue, PhD, is Associate Professor, Institute for the Psychological Sciences, Arlington, Virginia.

Robert A. Emmons, PhD, is Professor, Department of Psychology, University of California, Davis, Davis, California.

Julie Juola Exline, PhD, is Assistant Professor, Department of Psychology, Case Western Reserve University, Cleveland, Ohio.

Louis W. Fry, PhD, is in the Department of Management, Tarleton State University–Central Texas, Killeen, Texas.

Anne L. Geyer, MA, is a graduate student, Department of Psychology, Florida State University, Tallahassee, Florida.

Robert A. Giacalone, PhD, is Professor, Department of Human Resource Management, Fox School of Business and Management, Temple University, Philadelphia, Pennsylvania.

Peter C. Hill, PhD, is Professor, Rosemead School of Psychology, Biola University, La Mirada, California. He is editor of the *Journal of Psychology and Christianity*.

Ralph W. Hood, Jr., PhD, is Professor, Department of Psychology, University of Tennessee, Chattanooga, Chattanooga, Tennessee. He is coeditor of the *Archiv für Religionpsychologie*.

Bruce Hunsberger, PhD, was Professor, Department of Psychology, Wilfrid Laurier University, Waterloo, Ontario, Canada, until his death in October 2003.

Carole L. Jurkiewicz, PhD, is John W. Dupuy Endowed Professor and Women's Hospital Distinguished Professor of Healthcare Management, Louisiana State University, Baton Rouge, Louisiana.

Brien S. Kelley, MA, is a doctoral student in clinical psychology, Department of Psychology and Education, Teachers College, Columbia University, New York, New York.

Lee A. Kirkpatrick, PhD, is Associate Professor and Director of Graduate Studies, Department of Psychology, College of William & Mary, Williamsburg, Virginia.

Michael R. Levenson, PhD, is Associate Professor, Department of Human Development and Family Sciences, Oregon State University, Corvallis, Oregon.

Patrick Luyten, PhD, is Postdoctoral Fellow of the Fund for Scientific Research–Flanders (FWO) (Belgium), Department of Psychology, Katholieke Universiteit, Leuven, Belgium.

Annette Mahoney, PhD, is Professor, Department of Psychology, Bowling Green State University, Bowling Green, Ohio.

Michael E. McCullough, PhD, is Associate Professor, Departments of Psychology and Religious Studies, University of Miami, Coral Gables, Florida.

Susan H. McFadden, PhD, is Professor and Chair, Department of Psychology, University of Wisconsin, Oshkosh, Oshkosh, Wisconsin.

Lisa Miller, PhD, is Associate Professor, Department of Psychology and Education, Teachers College, Columbia University, New York, New York.

Andrew B. Newberg, MD, is Assistant Professor, Departments of Radiology and Psychiatry, University of Pennsylvania Health System, Philadelphia, Pennsylvania.

Stephanie K. Newberg, MEd, MSW, is Assistant Director, Council for Relationships, Philadelphia, Pennsylvania.

Michael E. Nielsen, PhD, is Associate Professor, Department of Psychology, Georgia Southern University, Statesboro, Georgia.

Doug Oman, PhD, is Adjunct Assistant Professor, School of Public Health, University of California, Berkeley, Berkeley, California.

Elizabeth Weiss Ozorak, PhD, is Associate Professor, Department of Psychology, and Coordinator of the Values, Ethics and Social Action Program, Allegheny College, Meadville, Pennsylvania.

Raymond F. Paloutzian, PhD, is Professor, Department of Psychology, Westmont College, Santa Barbara, California.

Kenneth I. Pargament, PhD, is Professor, Department of Psychology, Bowling Green State University, Bowling Green, Ohio, and Adjunct Professor, School of Theology, Boston University, Boston, Massachusetts. He is coeditor of *Mental Health, Religion, and Culture*.

Crystal L. Park, PhD, is Associate Professor, Department of Psychology, University of Connecticut, Storrs, Connecticut, and Editor, *The International Journal for the Psychology of Religion*.

Ralph L. Piedmont, PhD, is Director of Research for the Graduate Programs in Pastoral Counseling, Loyola College, Baltimore, Maryland. He is coeditor of *Research in the Social Scientific Study of Religion*.

Lindsey M. Root, BA, is a graduate student, Department of Psychology, University of Miami, Coral Gables, Florida.

Ephraim Rose, BA, is a doctoral student in clinical psychology, Department of Psychology, Case Western Reserve University, Cleveland, Ohio.

Edward P. Shafranske, PhD, is Professor of Psychology and Director of the PsyD Program in Clinical Psychology, Graduate School of Education and Psychology, Pepperdine University, Irvine, California.

Israela Silberman, PhD, is Associate Research Scientist, Department of Psychology, Columbia University, New York, New York.

Bernard Spilka, PhD, is Professor Emeritus, Department of Psychology, University of Denver, Denver, Colorado.

Nalini Tarakeshwar, PhD, is Associate Research Scientist, Department of Epidemiology and Public Health, Yale University, New Haven, Connecticut.

Carl E. Thoresen PhD, is Professor Emeritus, School of Education and Departments of Psychology and Psychiatry/Behavioral Sciences, Stanford University, Stanford, California.

Amy B. Wachholtz, MDiv, is a doctoral student in clinical psychology, Department of Psychology, Bowling Green State University, Bowling Green, Ohio.

Brian J. Zinnbauer, PhD, is Staff Psychologist, Cincinnati Veterans Affairs Medical Center, and in private practice in Cincinnati, Ohio.

Preface

As with any creative work, we had a mix of professional and personal reasons for working together to create this handbook. The compelling scholarly reason was that the time for it had come. From time to time, in any area of inquiry, the accumulated knowledge progresses to such a degree that a new level of maturity becomes identifiable. The psychology of religion is at this stage now. We see it reflected in the nature of the research questions asked, the range of topics investigated, the sophistication of the research methods used, the adequacy of the theoretical advancements to account for and integrate the increasing body of data, and the connections between research in the psychology of religion and scholarship in other areas of psychology and allied fields. Throughout this volume, the contributors document myriad indicators that the psychology of religion as a field has reached this level of maturity. One indicator is that many of our colleagues now call this area of research "the psychology of religion and spirituality." We hope this book firmly documents this maturity and serves to guide research and theory in this field to its next level of development.

Our personal reasons for working on this handbook reflect our commitment to study what we think is of timeless importance: people's quest for and involvement in religion and spirituality. For Ray: My interest goes back to my graduate education, in the heydays of the 1960s, when a new generation of doctoral students in psychology decided to research topics that they considered relevant to the real world. Psychologists began to study every imaginable social issue, including prejudice, racism, sexism, gender, poverty, aggression and violence, and the effects of mass media. But nowhere did I see psychologists tackling one of the biggest issues of all: religion. I figured that if psychology was going to take the challenge to be relevant to real-world issues seriously, it was going to have to deal with religion and its then-budding alternative expression, spirituality. Since that time, the importance of the study of the psychology of religion and spirituality has advanced to a degree that I could not previously have imagined.

For Crystal: My interest in existential issues of dealing with loss and making meaning long preceded my awareness of the discipline of psychology. Early in my graduate career, I was drawn to the study of the influence of religion and spiritual influences on coping with stressful life events, and I have continued to pursue a greater understanding of these fundamental processes of human experience in my life as a scholar, a clinician, and a human being.

It was apparent to us almost immediately that this book had to be comprehensive. Thus the breadth of topics covered ranges from the micro (e.g., neuropsychology of religious experience) to the macro (e.g., the role of religion in international violence and terrorism). In the opening and closing chapters we provide integrative themes on which to anchor this research. These themes enable researchers to pull together diverse material and discuss it within a common framework and with a common language. Two key conceptual devices are especially important: the multilevel interdisciplinary paradigm and the concept of religion as a meaning system. We contend that these two ideas provide a compelling overall framework within which a wide spectrum of research and theory can flourish. We hope these ideas serve as a guide to new ideas and cross-fertilization with other areas, as well as the integration of the ideas that come from this research into newer and better theory.

Recent trends in the research literature have added a new and vibrant area of interest: spirituality. Some scholars draw distinctions between religion and spirituality, while others draw none and see them as functionally equivalent. The contributors present a range of approaches that we think will help future researchers to untangle the important psychological distinctions, while maintaining an integrated view of the psychology of religion research enterprise as a whole.

We wish to highlight some aspects of the development of this handbook. First, all the contributors are paramount scholars in the topic about which they wrote. We made no compromises in selecting the contributors, who constitute a virtual "who's who" in the field of the psychology of religion and spirituality. Second, we designed this book to be highly useful in the service of the "handbook function," so it was important that readers could pick up this book and easily locate material on a particular topic or by a particular author. We chose to include both author and subject indices to facilitate this function, and the book includes extensive cross-referencing among the chapters. Third, we strove to see that the organization of the chapters would accurately reflect the nature of the material. Thus the table of contents evolved in a way that, on the one hand, reflects the larger field of psychology, so that many of our topics correspond with their larger subdisciplinary counterparts (e.g., emotion, health, lifespan development), while, on the other, reflects the topics of particular interest to psychologists of religion and spirituality (e.g., spiritual transformation, struggle, and doubt). Fourth, because it is important to promote new empirical research, we explicitly asked the contributors to suggest the next research steps necessary to advance knowledge in their areas of expertise. Finally, Chapters 1 and 30 are of particular note. In Chapter 1, we present five themes that are currently emerging in the field and through which the material in the other chapters can be viewed and integrated. These themes concern the nature of the research in the field at a certain time, the multilevel interdisciplinary paradigm for the field, the concept of religion as a meaning system, the future expanding and integrating path of the research, and the role of the psychology of religion. In Chapter 30, we again review these themes and use them to describe, in broad strokes, directions that the field might take.

We have many people to acknowledge for their help along the way. Several leaders in the field encouraged and helped us by their own contributions as well as by their willingness to evaluate our book proposal. We are grateful for the contributors' efforts to complete their chapters on time, in spite of personal and professional challenges. In the course of completing this handbook, authors became parents, married, changed jobs, and so forth.

Sadly, one of the contributors, Bruce Hunsberger, died of cancer, which he had been fighting for a number of years. Bruce is already greatly missed.

Although developing and seeing this project through to completion has not always been easy, it has been a very satisfying and pleasurable process. We made a good editorial team, in large part because we complemented each other's strengths in areas of knowledge and diplomatic skills. We began our collaborative relationship as passing acquaintances, but through our intense work together, we have become good friends.

We thank our two institutions, Westmont College and the University of Connecticut, for providing the intellectual home base that each of us needed to complete this project. Thanks also go to the Katholieke Universiteit, Leuven, Belgium, for providing a wonderful intellectual and personal environment, as well as the resources, for one of us (R. F. P.) to do a substantial portion of the work on this book during the summer of 2004. We thank our friends and loved ones for their support and patience while each of us repeatedly chose to keep on task. We owe a special note of gratitude to Jim Nageotte, Senior Editor at The Guilford Press, for his knowledge, guidance, and wisdom. His gentle and calming touch rested our thoughts and refocused our attention at just the right moments.

RAYMOND F. PALOUTZIAN
CRYSTAL L. PARK

Contents

PART I

FOUNDATIONS OF THE PSYCHOLOGY OF RELIGION

Integrative Themes in the Current Science of the Psychology of Religion

RAYMOND F. PALOUTZIAN
CRYSTAL L. PARK

That religion is the greatest force for both good and evil in the history of the world is such a truism that we hesitate to begin the opening chapter of this handbook by saying so. But we highlight it at the outset because, as the chapters unfold, religion, in its vast range of forms and expressions, is shown again and again to relate in positive and negative ways to the whole range of human behaviors, experiences, and emotions. In spite of this, however, the science of psychology has paid only sporadic attention to the psychological processes underlying human religiousness. In fact, for much of the 20th century, academic psychology did not address it (Beit-Hallahmi, 1974; Belzen, 2000; Paloutzian, 1996; Wulff, 1998). There are a variety of reasons for this discrepancy between the undeniable importance of religion to individual people as well as its role in the long, hard march of humans from antiquity to now and this lack of attention. Because these reasons are thoroughly documented elsewhere (e.g., Paloutzian, 1996; Wulff, 1998), we will not reiterate them here. Instead, in this chapter, we condense the history of this field to provide context for the upsurge in interest and research in the psychology of religion that has been occurring during the past approximately 25 years and that continues unabated today. These cutting edges are our focus, and we present a modern five-theme conceptual model for organizing the increasingly rich and complex knowledge that the psychology of religion now comprises.

Although religion shows a history of grand and sometimes awesome display of its powerful role in human affairs—illustrated in a positive way in its provision, to billions of people, of guidance and ultimate reasons to live and endure life's tragedies, and in a negative way by the events of September 11, 2001—the science of the psychology of reli-

---

Chapters 1 and 30 form a collaborative unit, with the authors' names in alternate alphabetical order on each chapter.

gion has no such glorious history. Instead, after a smattering of more or less independent investigations in the first third of the 20th century (Freud, 1927/1961; Hall, 1904; James, 1902/1958; Leuba, 1912, 1925; Pratt, 1920; Starbuck, 1899), systematic scientific research in the psychology of religion was abandoned for over 40 years. However, the 1960s brought a generation of psychologists who insisted on doing research that they perceived spoke directly to human life, and they undertook with great zest the study of a variety of psychological phenomena with real-world personal and social implications. Their topics included racism and prejudice, aggression and violence, poverty, the subordinate status of women and its effects, and religion.

The initial strands of this work in the psychology of religion involved researchers who carried out their studies in a somewhat isolated way, only marginally integrated with mainstream psychology, and certainly few in numbers. In fact, although the American Psychological Association Division 36, Psychology of Religion, was formally established in 1976, as recently as 1980 a scholar who wanted to launch new research or teach a course in this specialty would find that no systematic or comprehensive summaries of research existed. This lack of resources has completely reversed itself in a short period (Emmons & Paloutzian, 2003; Hester & Paloutzian, in press).

THE PAST 25 YEARS

The succeeding two and one-half decades have seen these initial strands grow into a field amazingly vast, with high-level research that uses myriad sophisticated methods and data-analytic techniques, both quantitative and qualitative—a field that spans the entire range of research corresponding to its parent discipline of psychology. Research in the psychology of religion has moved far beyond simple zero-order correlational coefficients and speculation as the only guides for how one variable is related to others in the human mind. Instead, complex and integrative conceptual models have evolved that allow us to tie together threads of research from different areas and to test hypotheses that were until recently unimaginable. Research questions are now posed along a wide range of levels of analysis, from neuropsychological (see Newberg & Newberg, Chapter 11, this volume) to social-psychological and cross-cultural (see Donahue & Nielsen, Chapter 15, and Silberman, Chapter 29, this volume). And because these models are tied directly to the same ideas that come from general psychology, the findings from psychological research on religiousness speak directly back to the parent discipline. Thus, two kinds of integration are occurring at the same time: integration of material within the psychology of religion itself and integration of psychology of religion research within psychology as a whole. As the chapters in this handbook document, the richness of the research is impressive. At the same time, as noted by Emmons and Paloutzian (2003), we regard these recent advances not as the culmination of research but as the starting point from which the psychology of religion can step forward to make its most important contributions to the science of psychology and to human welfare.

One of the perennial concerns of scholars grappling with how best to conceptualize the psychological processes that mediate religiousness, and seeking the best concepts and categories with which to present, talk about, and integrate the various strands of research, has been the cry for theory. Scholars have repeatedly pointed out that the psychology of religion is long on data and short on theory (Dittes, 1969). In fact, in the past, not only was there no single theory to guide work in the field (let alone to promote integration of the available data), there was not even a good conceptual model that could be used as a working tool to help researchers think, integrate material, and develop new and better hypotheses. This lack is apparent when one examines the opening chapters of several of the standard books in the field (e.g., Batson, Schoenrade, & Ventis, 1993; Beit-Hallahmi & Argyle, 1997; Paloutzian, 1996; Pargament, 1997; Spilka, Hood, Hunsberger, & Gorsuch, 2003; Wulff, 1997). All of these books present information that the reader needs to know, such as a sketch of the field's history, a statement about the problem of defining religion, and definitions of key terms or dimensions of religiousness. However, none of these books presents ideas that cut across the range of topics in the field and that can serve as comprehensive integrating devices. It is precisely such integrating themes that the field needs.

INTEGRATIVE THEMES

In an ideal world, the framework that would integrate all aspects of the discipline would be a fully developed theory, well tested and supported by the data, that has stood the test of time and gained acceptance by scholars who hold a wide range of opinions. Of course, no such framework currently exists. However, throughout this handbook there are hints about the direction such theorizing may take, and, in fact, in total, the chapters in this handbook may provide a major impetus for the development of such a framework. We therefore offer the following *integrative themes*, not as a theoretical framework, but as a set of ideas that cut across all or most of the topics. Together, they identify common issues and processes and provide a unifying language that is valid for all of the topics and that allows us to tie the disparate threads of work together, pose new research questions that integrate them, and foster the development of integrative theory. We identify five integrative themes, summarized in general form below. Although presented in parallel sequence in the first and the last chapters of this handbook, the themes are used to integrate past and current knowledge in this chapter, while in Chapter 30 these themes integrate our look at the future.

1. *The paradigm issue.* There has long been a need for a paradigm that would serve as an overall framework to guide research, debate, and thinking. Such a framework would serve as an overarching umbrella within which research studies in various areas and subareas would proceed and be related to each other. It would include the assumptions that enable such interrelationships among diverse lines of research to develop and flourish, and within which theory building about the psychological processes that mediate religiousness would proceed. Researchers in the psychology of religion disagree about many things, but share a consensus that the field has been preparadigmatic for almost all of its history. Where is the field now, and what ideas do we have to guide its future?

2. *Methods and theory.* Scholars who study the psychology of religion disagree about what we can know and how we can know it. Should the field mimic those parts of psychology that rely on the laboratory experiment as the "gold standard" for good science? Because scientific concepts are constructs, should we instead deconstruct all of them and conclude that one narrative about the psychological processes that mediate religiousness is as good as another because there are no bias-free rules by which to evaluate

them? How these issues and their variations are resolved will affect the very basis, or even the very possibility of, this field in the future.

3. *The question of meaning.* Meaning has long been an undercurrent in the work of some scholars in the psychology of religion, but is the concept of meaning powerful enough to accommodate the greatly varied approaches to studying the psychology of religion that have emerged in recent years? Questions of meaning, typically understood as theological questions, are also psychological questions. Finding the answer to the question of meaning's meaning and its role in religion is essential in order to begin creating a theory of the psychological processes in religiousness that captures the heart and soul of its object of study. This involves understanding the psychology of religion through its meaning-related functions.

4. *The path of the psychology of religion.* For a science to flourish, a critical mass of ideas and knowledge must be developed that can serve as the springboard that will stimulate research that either extends one topic or supports cross-topic collaboration. This is how one domain of research expands and how all domains move forward. Each topic addressed in this book shows this development. The pathways ahead are far-reaching in their implications.

5. *The role of the psychology of religion.* To whom and to what is the psychology of religion contributing now, and what should we understand to be its proper and possible goals with respect to general psychology and with respect to overall human well-being? Does this field contribute unique knowledge to psychology, an insight or understanding that is not obtainable by studying other phenomena? And if we do learn about the psychological aspects of religiousness in the manner to which we aspire, should this knowledge be used, and if so, how and how much?

We now describe each of these integrative themes in greater detail and illustrate how they inform the specific topics in the 28 areas covered in this handbook.

IS THERE A PSYCHOLOGY OF RELIGION PARADIGM?

The psychology of religion has come a long way from its nonparadigmatic past to its current position on the edge of expanding and integrating within a paradigm: the *multilevel interdisciplinary paradigm.* This paradigm, as presented by Emmons and Paloutzian (2003), "recognizes the value of data at multiple levels of analysis while making nonreductive assumptions concerning the value of spiritual and religious phenomena" (p. 395). A similar version of this idea is found in Silberman (2005b). The precursors to the present movement into this new paradigm grew out of past calls by scholars for some common ground, combined with the articulation of various key issues that needed to be worked through in order to set the stage for this common ground. One of these issues is the attempt at theory, which we address in the next section of this chapter. The others include (1) a long-enduring preoccupation with the creation of the "right" measure of key religious variables, referred to as the "measurement paradigm" (Gorsuch, 1988), and (2) the question of whether religion is unique among all human behaviors (Dittes, 1969) and/or unique in a way that would preclude its incorporation into the whole of psychology (e.g., due to supernatural or other spiritual forces that can presumably operate outside the realm of a natural order). Let us briefly examine these issues as stepping-stones to the new paradigm.

Going Beyond Measurement

Gorsuch (1984, 1988) observed that the field had spent such a long time attempting to create finer measures that it appeared to be stuck at the starting line. He argued that psychology of religion should advance from measurement as a main focus and instead get on with the task of testing hypotheses derived from models of mental processes and theories that connect the models together, so that the field could finally make progress in the truly scientific task of building incremental, cumulative knowledge within a paradigm and explained by a theory. Fortunately, many researchers in the field heeded his advice: the multilevel interdisciplinary paradigm is a response to his call for change.

In order for us to progress from measuring psychology of religion variables to explaining their relationships, we need a workable degree of common agreement about (1) the range of phenomena that are "in" and "out" of the area of concern, and (2) the wholistic versus reductionistic ways of explaining them. These two concerns are at the heart of what are called the issues of *uniqueness* and *reductionism*, respectively. One's position on them affects one's ability to work within the multidisciplinary paradigm.

Uniqueness and Reductionism

Dittes (1969) highlighted the uniqueness issue and vividly identified a question pivotal to our understanding of the relation between the psychology of religion and the rest of psychology: To what degree can religion be explained by relying only upon more elemental processes and concepts, those that apply to any other behaviors, instead of requiring unique concepts and processes to account for it? At one end of his four-step spectrum is the position that religion is but one instance of behavior-in-general, and that therefore it can be studied by using the same methods that are used to study any other behavior and can be understood by applying the same ideas that apply to other behaviors. At the other end is the perspective that religious behaviors are unique, not found elsewhere in human action, experience, or perception. The "unique" end of this spectrum means that religion cannot be reduced to more elemental processes—that is, religion is no more reducible to "nothing but other known psychological forces" than a hurricane is reducible to "nothing but wind." The argument is that although religion and hurricanes involve other, more elemental processes, each one is something different from "just" the operation of the parts it comprises. If this is so, then special psychological concepts and processes are needed to explain it. The "nonunique" end of this spectrum assumes that because religion is one instance of behavior-in-general, no such special concepts and processes are needed. The unique view obviously lends itself to easy application of nonreductionistic assumptions, and the nonunique view is normally taken to mean that reductionistic explanations are more or less automatically invoked (Pargament, 2002; Pargament, Magyar, & Murray-Swank, 2005).

However, we argue that working within the multilevel interdisciplinary paradigm (which supports nonreductionistic assumptions) does *not* mean that a split somewhere between the unique and nonunique ends of this spectrum is necessary, such that a religious phenomenon that is explained at one level effectively explains away an explanation of that same phenomenon at another level. Instead, the multilevel interdisciplinary paradigm acknowledges that valid explanations of the same religious phenomenon can be stated both within the multiple levels of analysis within psychology itself and across traditional disciplinary boundaries. For example, a valid explanation of religious conversion can in principle be stated at both a neuropsychological level and at a social-psychological level, and the ideas and knowledge of allied sciences can be added to these explanations. The nonunique end of the spectrum is more amenable to reductionistic explanations but does not depend upon them. This means that the multilevel interdisciplinary paradigm is a valid framework to guide research on the psychological processes involved in all aspects of human religiousness, regardless of where they fall on the unique–nonunique spectrum.

Uniqueness and the Role of Psychology of Religion

Is religion unique among human behaviors as such or is it unique because of a belief that supernatural agency has a causal role in it in a way that it does not in other behaviors? We agree with Kirkpatrick (2005 and Chapter 6, this volume) that this latter position is not knowable one way or the other by the methods of science, that it may or may not be so, and that in any case our job as scientific psychologists of religion is to create good theory to explain religiousness in a way that allows the theory to be assessed against evidence. This means ideas about possible causal factors that are not, in principle, capable of being tested against evidence may be interesting, but they do not meet the criteria necessary to bear upon our theory construction process. Scientific explanations about the psychological processes in religiousness are neutral with respect to them.

Why do we care whether religion is a unique human behavior as such? If it is, then the discipline of psychology needs to include religion among its essential foci of study in order to eventually arrive at a comprehensive theory of human behavior. If it is not, then studying religion is useful only because it happens to be so important in comparison to other behaviors in a practical sense (McCrae, 1999). If religion is unique, then human phenomena are found there that are found nowhere else, so that a psychology that does not address religion can never create a valid comprehensive theory (see Piedmont, Chapter 14, this volume). On the other hand, if religion is not unique, then it can be accounted for by the same principles that account for other human behaviors, and there is no compelling reason, on grounds of pure science, for psychologists to give it any special attention. This issue has been hotly debated (Baumeister, 2002) and the answer to it will determine whether the psychology of religion is to be regarded as a core topic within psychology or whether it is to be regarded as important due only to the obvious importance of its subject matter.

Because opinions about religion are often stated as generalities, it is easy to forget that religion is not one thing but is instead a multidimensional variable that is among the most complex properties of the human mind. We believe that all four steps along Dittes (1969) spectrum are valid for one or another religious behavior. Part of religion is unique and part of it is not; more refined research will clarify which is which, and why. One way that religion seems to be unique is that it provides people with ultimate meaning in life (Emmons, 1999; Levenson, Aldwin, & D'Mello, Chapter 8, this volume; Tillich, 1952, 1963), centered on what the individual perceives to be sacred (cf. Pargament, 1997), especially in a way that is nonveridical such that its truth claims or the person's idiosyncratic meanings derived from them can carry the weight of absolute reality without being bound by the rules of evidence (Paloutzian & Silberman, 2003; see Silberman, 2005b, for a partly overlapping and partly complementary discussion of the uniqueness issue). The multilevel interdisciplinary paradigm accommodates these variations and provides the framework within which these issues can be teased apart for all instances of religiousness.

The Multilevel Interdisciplinary Paradigm

The multilevel interdisciplinary paradigm can serve as a framework within which research at all levels of analysis (both within the discipline of psychology and between psychology and allied fields) can advance. Yet there are certain phenomena for which it seems particularly suited or essential. Consider two examples of emergent properties that come from within the discipline of psychology itself. One of them, the phenomenon of emergent leadership in groups, is at the social-psychological level of analysis; the other one, the phenomenon of consciousness as an emergent property of brain function, is at the neuropsychological level of analysis. The chapters in this book illustrate others. Using these two simple examples of emergent properties (leadership, consciousness), however, highlights the principle that for certain phenomena the sum of the elements that are known to operate at a lower level of analysis does not equal the phenomenon at the higher level. Leadership and consciousness are not reducible to nothing but the elements and processes that constitute them, and they exert control over as well as are controlled by those elements and processes. The multilevel interdisciplinary paradigm is particularly well suited to accommodate research on such phenomena.

If the multilevel interdisciplinary paradigm has even a small ability to accommodate fairly narrow-band topics within a subdiscipline of psychology, then it has an even greater ability to serve as an overall umbrella that can help us in our efforts to think of multilevel *intra*disciplinary research within the discipline of psychology itself. Further, this paradigm can be expanded to promote *inter*disciplinary research into the workings of religion, and even further to integrate theory that surrounds this research around a set of common ideas. The psychology of religion is poised to reach out to evolutionary biology, neuroscience, anthropology, cognitive science, and allied sciences generally, and to philosophy in a generalized cross-disciplinary approach to critiquing and sharpening the assumptions of science. Thus the multilevel interdisciplinary paradigm allows for the linking of subfields within psychology as the core discipline in a broader effort, and, when the notions of reductionism and nonreductionism are properly understood, also allows the cross-fertilization of allied areas of science in a way that fosters integrative lines of research, findings, and theories.

In its most visionary form, the multilevel disciplinary paradigm would be able to accommodate whatever knowledge is necessary in pursuit of the ultimate goal: the full understanding of human beings. This means that we should understand human beings not as amazing creatures unique unto themselves as the most complex or intelligent endpoint of the phylogenetic scale, but as beings that are the most advanced example of an emergent property. Whatever else the human being is, it is an emergent property of the interaction of nature and nurture, whose ability to function has gone far beyond the more narrow survival needs that prevailed whenever human nature as we know it came about. Although we came from our environment, we also control it. The being that emerged from the interaction of nature and nurture is now in the process of changing that very nature and nurture to make them fundamentally different. This means that more singular ways of explaining how humans and how human religiousness work, such as a direct causal model and a single-level explanation, are inadequate. Instead, satisfactory explanations will require the application of principles such as reciprocal determinism (Bandura, 1986) and multilevel approaches that are beginning to emerge, illustrated by social-cognitive neuroscience (Ochsner & Lieberman, 2001). Regarding the human being as an emergent property makes explicit that just as the environment controls people, people exercise control over their environments in ways that change how the environment in turn controls people. Because understanding how this works requires application of the principle of reciprocal determinism and multilevel theory, it means that human behavior and its religiousness are not reducible to their elements or the forces from which they emerged, and that the multilevel interdisciplinary paradigm would be the framework within which their understanding can be obtained.

To move steadily forward in these directions will require the most engaging, mind-stretching, and collaborative work that has been done in the history of the psychology of religion. Accomplishing it in the next generation is the task ahead of us.

METHODS AND THEORIES

In the normal progress of science, there is a relation between research methods, the data that derive from them, and the theoretical ideas that prevail in the field, such that advances in one lead to advances in the others. But in the psychology of religion this self-corrective and growth-inducing feedback process has rarely functioned until recent times. It is precisely this self-corrective feedback loop that is required for the science of the psychology of religion to develop.

The most important historical example of this lack becomes evident when one examines the relationship between the grand theories of religion proposed during the first third of the 20th century and the empirical research conducted during the first 75 or so years of the 20th century. For a generation, the variations of psychodynamic theory about religion that were proposed during the early part of the century dominated the psychology of religion "theory" landscape. However, for the most part the empirical data that were collected had no role as a test of the theories, and the research was neither directly derived from these theories nor typically had much relevance to them. Until very recently, as was the case when Dittes (1969) pointed out this glaring gap, the field of psychology of religion included both comprehensive theories and growing amounts of data, but neither had much bearing upon the other. In effect, while the early theories about religion developed by Freud (1927/1961) and Jung (1938/1969) were well known, new empirical studies came into being mostly as single studies that were not part of a systematic research program. The result was two independent psychologies of religion, one of ideas and one of numbers. The two continued as if they were on two separate tracks, with neither helping the other to become more refined.

Fortunately, these trends have recently changed dramatically. Recent developments include (1) advances in psychoanalytic theorizing (see Corveleyn & Luyten, Chapter 5, this volume); (2) a proliferation of models of more narrow-range processes such as religious attributions (Spilka et al., 2003; Spilka, Shaver, & Kirkpatrick, 1985), spiritual intelligence (Emmons, 1999, 2000), conversion as spiritual transformation (see Paloutzian, Chapter 18, this volume), religious orientation (see Donahue & Nielsen, Chapter 15, this volume), spirituality as a personality factor (see Piedmont, Chapter 14, this volume), and religion as schema (McIntosh, 1995) or schemas (Ozorak, 1997); and (3) efforts at integrating large swaths of biological and psychological science within the theory of evolution (see Kirkpatrick, 2005, and Chapter 6, this volume). These developments provide promise for integrating the psychology of religion at the multiple levels within psychological boundaries and connecting it across disciplinary boundaries as this material gradually becomes integrated into the larger orbit of the life sciences.

Methodological Developments

Along with an expansive list of ideas to research comes a need for methods adequate to study them. An increasing amount of research is being done with novel, creative methods, both quantitative and qualitative, that are well equipped to do the field good service in the next generation. Their application promises to refine and broaden these theoretical advances (see Hood & Belzen, Chapter 4, this volume).

The methodological advance that has occurred in recent times is truly impressive to anyone who has watched how empirical studies were conducted for the past 30 years. In 1975, the field was at a point of methodological infancy, with most studies conducted by distributing questionnaires assessing theoretically weak aspects of religion. The results were not impressive. In summarizing the level of sophistication at that time, Hunsberger (1991) wrote, "Countless studies report thousands of weak correlational relationships between many aspects of religion and almost every other variable imaginable" (p. 498).

Today the menu is vastly expanded. The keynote chapter on methods by Hood and Belzen (Chapter 4, this volume) presents clear examples, prototypes of a technique, and exemplars of ways to adapt a particular method to the unique problems in studying human religiousness. It also illustrates the puzzles that arise when different studies that purport to test the same idea with different methods yield opposite results (such as with a laboratory experiment and an attempted field study replication, or with a quantitative study and a parallel qualitative study).

The remaining substantive chapters document the creativity, cleverness, and thoroughness with which researchers in all areas of specialization within the field have invented new techniques in order to find out the answers to key questions. These include neuroimaging (Newberg & Newberg, Chapter 11, this volume); interview, observational, and qualitative methodologies adapted for use with children (Boyatzis, Chapter 7, this volume); specialized adaptations of the tools from the cognitive psychology laboratory (Ozarak, Chapter 12, this volume); and the inclusion of real-world physical and mental health outcome variables (Oman & Thoresen, Chapter 24, and Miller & Kelley, Chapter 25, this volume).

It is especially promising that this large number of new methods has come into use in addition to, but not in place of, questionnaires. Questionnaire measures have shown much improvement in the precision with which they capture a meaningful dimension of religion (Hill, Chapter 3, this volume; Hill & Hood, 1999). Add to this the recent advances in the application of qualitative methods to the study of religious experience (Hood, Chapter 19, this volume), as a complement to traditional quantitative methods, and it begins to look as though all the methodological tools that we could hope for are in place for us to use and extend into new territory. By researching questions in diverse and complementary ways, we will gather the data we need to feed the development of integrative theory.

Modernism and Postmodernism

Recent scholarship in the philosophy of science requires us to address the issue of a modernist versus postmodernist approach to scientific knowledge in general, and its expression in the psychology of religion in particular. The traditional modernist approach led to those methods that have prevailed until recently. Valid knowledge was gained by using methods that conformed to the prototype, or gold standard, of the conduct of good science: the laboratory experiment. It would be against this model that data from other, less-controlled methods would be compared. As recently as 30 years ago, psychologists of religion debated whether they should strive to do controlled laboratory experiments (Batson, 1977, 1979; Gorsuch, 1982). Today the methodological discussion is about whether psychologists of religion should use quantitative methods versus qualitative methods. Those favoring quantitative methods emphasize the objectivity of the data and the requirement that there be public agreement about what the data are, although not necessarily about what the data mean. Others endorse qualitative methods, especially hermeneutical interpretations of personal texts (Belzen, 1997) and methods based on the principle that data are culturally relative and that their interpretation must be culturally sensitive (Belzen, 1999, 2003). These researchers point out that the meaning attributed to data, including those obtained by traditional quantitative methods, cannot be divorced from the cultural context of the subjects and the culture-bound biases of the researcher, and that therefore it is essential that those judgments define the data categories in a unique way from study to study. At one level, this distinction is based upon variations in understanding what precisely "empirical" data are.

At another level, this issue of modernism versus postmodernism concerns operationalism, deconstruction, and the confrontation between these two derived from positivistic modernism, on the one hand, and postmodernism, on the other. It is agreed that scientific advances have occurred because of the power of empirical science, and especially because of the use of the pure experiment to discover cause-and-effect relations. This approach emphasizes operational definitions of both independent variable categories and dependent variable measures. An unnecessary and sometimes unspecified assumption is that these operations represent true categories or real dimensions that exist in ontological reality. This may or may not be so. But in either case the correspondence between an operational definition of a variable and the psychological category that it is purported to represent can always be a matter of debate. Because of this, scholars who reason from a postmodernist orientation point out that our categories are actually constructed by us. If this is so, then the correspondence between them and whatever their counterparts in ontological reality are is either something that should be questioned (in soft versions of postmodernism) or is not knowable (in more extreme versions of postmodernism). The most extreme variant of this presupposition states that all such categories are inherently meaningless and unknowable. For such reasons, it is the task of critics of traditional empirical science to deconstruct them. It is based upon such reasoning that those who extend the argument of postmodernist orientation to psychology of religion research argue for qualitative, hermeneutical, and cultural approaches (Belzen, 1999, 2003). They assume that the proper categories of study are those that come from the subject him- or herself, not those imposed by research design or measured by a preexisting tool external to the person.

Fortunately, Corveleyn and Luyten (Chapter 5, this volume) have stated the ideal way for us to establish integrative progress even with the cogency of this dilemma. They have called for peaceful and collaborative coexistence between the opposing camps, as has evolved over the same dilemma in the allied fields of sociology and anthropology. There is no need for those on either side to argue as if the other approach had nothing to offer. They point out that those emphasizing operationalistic, quantitative methods do so with categories and measures based upon already existing ideas about what processes are important, and that those emphasizing qualitative and hermeneutical methods neverthe-less use operations and measures in the course of interpreting their texts. These two approaches are complementary, not competitive, and in the end may not be as far apart as arguments narrowly endorsing one side or the other would make it appear.

Theory and Definition

Allowing quantitative and qualitative methods to complement each other holds promise for the development of exceptionally rich theory, so long as we can validly blend the knowledge gained from the combined approaches. It also refutes the idea that the developments today are so fatally flawed, narrowly positivistic, closed to enrichment by alternative methods, and fraught with bias that the psychology of religion should start over (Wulff, 2003). The field is so ripe with good ideas and good methods that it is poised to make contributions that could not be imagined in the past. As stated by Emmons and Paloutzian (2003) when they introduced the multilevel interdisciplinary paradigm, "The field has made great strides in its effort to say something important to the rest of psychology . . . what has come before is only a platform and the field is now poised, ready to begin" (p. 395). Going forward from this platform enriches the field in a way that trying to reconstitute itself with an adherence to the definition of religion stated by James (1902/1958) cannot (Wulff, 2003). Because our theories and our definitions promote the development of each other, a new picture of the psychology of religion will evolve that will do far greater service than James could have hoped for.

How do we get from here to there? At least three things need to be in place for integrative development of the psychology of religion to occur:

1. The extensive exploitation of the range of methods noted above.
2. A common language that can be applied across the specialized topics in the field.
3. An overarching framework that is powerful and flexible enough to contain a variety of midlevel theories about religious phenomena and that connects psychology of religion theory to the rest of the life sciences more generally.

As part of our five integrative themes, we believe that the latter two needs may be met by construing religion as a meaning system (Park, Chapter 16, this volume; Silberman, 2005b) and by an evolutionary approach to the psychology of religion (Kirkpatrick, Chapter 6, this volume), and that the first need is met by knowing the status of the field, understanding a wide range of methods and the unique benefits of each, and by conducting programmatic research that connects them.

Can methods, theory, and application converge? If so, around what common themes might they come together? The multilevel interdisciplinary paradigm describes an overarching idea for how fields and subfields can be seen in relation to each other and productively cross-fertilize. But what about within the psychology of religion itself? All of these ideas can be fruitfully discussed as an expression of the question of meaning.

MEANING AND THE PSYCHOLOGY OF RELIGION

Meaning holds much promise as a unifying construct in psychology. The notion of meaning-related constructs as an approach to many phenomena within the psychology of religion is very new, but seems to be rapidly gaining momentum. For example, in the third edition of their classic text on the psychology of religion, Spilka et al. (2003) broadened their framework for organizing the material from an emphasis on attributions to a more comprehensive emphasis on meaning. Similarly, Hood, Hill, and Williamson (2005) centered their discussion of religious fundamentalism on the concept of religion as a meaning system. An issue of the *Journal of Social Issues* is devoted to the topic of religion as a meaning system, highlighting the centrality of meaning for the psychology of religion (Silberman, 2005a).

Like most words, there is a great deal that can be said regarding the meaning of the term "meaning," which spans the domains of purpose, intent, order, sense, interpretation, signification, and denotation (Janoff-Bulman & Frantz, 1997). In his book on meaning, Baumeister (1991) noted that "the term meaning is used here in its ordinary, conventional sense, as when one speaks of the meaning of a word, a sentence, a story, or an event. Meaning cannot be easily defined, perhaps because to define meaning is already to use meaning. A rough definition would be that meaning is shared mental representations of possible relationships among things, events, and relationships. Thus, meaning connects things" (p. 16). As with the concept of value, something has meaning insofar as it stands for or represents something else.

Although existential psychologists have promoted the centrality of meaning for many years (e.g., Frankl, 1969; Yalom, 1980), mainstream psychology has been slow to come around. Recent developments in areas as diverse as evolutionary psychology, developmental psychology, and cognitive psychology have brought meaning to the forefront (Baumeister, 1991). A growing body of research supports the idea that people's meaning systems are central to their everyday patterns of life and may be of particular importance in coping with adversity (Park, 2005; Silberman, 2005b). In their everyday lives, individuals operate on the basis of personal beliefs or theories that they have about themselves, other people, the world at large, and their place in it. These beliefs and the goals and purposes they engender constitute idiosyncratic meaning systems that allow individuals to organize and comprehend the world around them and their experiences, as well as to plan and direct their behavior (Silberman, 2005a, 2005b, and Chapter 29, this volume).

While many areas of psychology would benefit from embracing meaning as a focus, the psychology of religion seems especially well positioned to embrace a meaning-centered approach. After all, all religion concerns meaning in one sense or another. Spilka et al. (2003) noted that "for all religious people, religion is indeed a struggle to comprehend their place in the scheme of things and what this entails for their relations with the world and others" (p. 15). In fact, while Baumeister, quoted above, notes that meaning "connects things," *that which connects* is the literal meaning of the term "religion." Thus, religion and meaning appear to be intimately related. As a meaning system, religion is unique in that it centers on what is perceived to be sacred (Pargament, 1997, 2002; Silberman, 2005b).

While one chapter in this handbook is specifically devoted to the topic of meaning and religion (Park, Chapter 16, this volume), most of the topics covered in this handbook explicitly discuss or implicitly incorporate meaning-related concepts. Thus, meaning concepts are integral to the development of religiousness (e.g., how children come to understand the world and their roles in it; see Boyatzis, Chapter 7, this volume), adult religious experiences (such as forming life goals; see Levenson & Aldwin, Chapter 8, this volume), and beliefs about aging and life after death (McFadden, Chapter 9, this volume); coping with stressful experiences, which often pull for more religious responses (Pargament, Ano, & Wacholtz, Chapter 26, this volume), including attributions and coping strategies as well as negative responses such as struggle and doubt (Exline & Rose, Chapter 17, this volume); spiritual transformation (Paloutzian, Chapter 18, this volume); cognitive aspects of psychology (Ozorak, Chapter 12, this volume); emotional and motivational aspects (Emmons, Chapter 13, this volume); and fundamentalism (Altemeyer & Hunsberger, Chapter 21, this volume). Further, the chapters on religion and physical and mental health touch on how religious meaning can have pervasive influences on well-being (Oman & Thoresen, Chapter 24, and Miller & Kelley, Chapter 25, this volume). The chapters dealing with applications of the psychology of religion also inherently involve meaning, including topics such as religion and psychotherapy (Shafranske, Chapter 27, this volume) and religious violence and terrorism versus peace (Silberman, Chapter 29, this volume).

CONTEMPORARY RESEARCH

The interest in religion among psychologists tends to be consistent over time (given that it was one of William James's enduring contributions), but also somewhat uncomfortable for many people and therefore somewhat marginalized and out of the mainstream (Emmons & Paloutzian, 2003). Thus, the psychology of religion as a field of endeavor has a pulse—albeit a weak pulse!—always coursing, but beyond the awareness of most psychologists. Most mainstream researchers paid scant attention to the enterprise of the psychology of religion, but the research plodded along, advancing slowly, hampered by the samples used, the isolated thinking and theorizing that characterized the area, the limited measurement and methodological strategies, and even the biased agendas of many in the field (i.e., researchers who set out to "prove" their points of view, especially that religion is positive and helpful).

As noted above, this bleak situation changed rapidly over the past quarter of a century (see Emmons & Paloutzian, 2003, for a review of recent historical developments). As the chapters in this handbook show, this new era of burgeoning research in the psychology of religion has seen an increasing diversity of areas that have been explored (e.g., ranging from neurobiology to terrorism). At the same time, there are nascent hints of convergence in the development of some broader theories and attempts at definition that may help tie this research together. We note a few points relevant to all this here and expand upon them in the corresponding sections of Chapter 30.

Definitions

A great deal of attention has been paid in the recent past to defining religion and related constructs. Researchers have been concerned not only with defining religion, but in particular have been attempting to differentiate the constructs of religion and spirituality. "Spirituality" as a term and as a construct in scientific discussion is a relatively new kid on the block. Its appearance reflects the shifts within Western culture occurring in the past decade or so, wherein religion, which previously connoted both organizational and personal aspects of religion, has increasingly been assigned to denote only the organizational aspects, while the construct of spirituality has increasingly been used to denote the personal aspects. Along with this shift has come a shift in cultural assignations of desirability. Among many groups, religion is considered to denote dogmatism and rigidity, while spirituality is viewed as positive and growth-oriented. Yet, this relatively recent distinction is open to question (Zinnbauer & Pargament, Chapter 2, this volume) and criticism (Silberman, 2003).

The issue of definition is obviously critically important for developing conceptual understandings and for proceeding with empirical work, which requires operationalization of conceptual constructs into measurable ones. In their chapter on definition, Zinnbauer and Pargament (Chapter 2, this volume) grapple with the issues involved in definition. They conclude that there is at present no consensus on these definitional issues, and it does not appear that any such general consensus is on the horizon. One is left to agree, then, with the observation made many years ago by Yinger (1967) that "any definition of religion is likely to be satisfactory only to its author" (p. 18).

Part of the confusion over how to define religion may center on whether attempts to define it are intended to represent cultural categories or a psychological process operative within the individual. Defining religion (and its newer counterpart, spirituality) in ways that reflect people's usages of those concepts in a culture is good for certain purposes, especially when that distinction is critical to the theoretical question posed. On the other hand, religion and spirituality may largely service the same psychological function and the different terms that people use themselves may be a matter of personal preference or style. Thus people call themselves religious *and* spiritual, religious *but not* spiritual, spiritual *but not* religious, *neither* spiritual *nor* religious, and, very interestingly, a hairsplitting blend of religious spirituality plus nonreligion (e.g., as one of our students said, "I am a spiritual Christian *but not* religious").

Overall, it seems that various definitions may be useful when it is necessary to focus on cultural or subgroup religious meanings, although a purely psychological functional definition would not need to draw such distinctions. Thus a purely psychological approach would emphasize that "whatever does it" (i.e., serves a religious function) for someone, is it. Thus we look back at Batson's (Batson et al., 1993) encompassing attempt at writing a functional definition stated in terms of the need to answer existential questions. That and other definitions did good service for a time. We believe, however, that future functional definitions of religion are more likely to be stated in terms of a human need for meaning and to invoke the model of religion as a meaning system.

Definitional issues do not need to impede progress in the field. Taking a functional approach, it may be that there is no meaningful distinction between the positions presented by Zinnabauer and Pargament (Chapter 2, this volume), or perhaps not only between those two positions but even among the whole set of definitions. At this point in the development of the field, it appears that breadth is to be preferred over narrowness.

Participants

The vast bulk of existing research in the psychology of religion has been conducted with samples of Western Judeo-Christians, primarily white college students. However, within this research body, there is some variation and some attention to group differences, such as studies of religion in African Americans and Latinos and studies of differences in affiliation or denomination (e.g., comparisons of Catholic, Protestant, and Jewish participants). However, much remains to be learned about other religious groups. For example, there is very little psychological research on Islam in spite of its recent prominence in the world. Hunsberger and Jackson (2005) and Roccas (2005) review cross-cultural and cross-religion research on religion and prejudice and on religion and values, respectively.

Methods

In addition to the methodological issues noted above, even in light of the creative advances in methods (Hood & Belzen, Chapter 4, this volume), questionnaires will remain a primary assessment technique in the psychology of religion. This is partly because the psychometrics of these measures have improved dramatically in recent times (see Hill, Chapter 3, this volume). Also, a primary focus of the psychology of religion is the study of religious meaning and its expressions, and one obvious way to capture part of that is through paper-and-pencil measures. Questionnaires remain necessary because many aspects of religiousness, such as beliefs or motivation, are interior processes that cannot be inferred but must be reported by the subject. However, many nonquestionnaire measures have been employed as both dependent and independent variables in studies of the psychology of religion. For example, studies of religiousness and health have included assessments of mortality and physiological indices (e.g., interleukin-6, blood pressure), while other studies have employed neurophysiological indices (see Newberg & Newberg, Chapter 11, this volume).

Mini-Models

Another relatively recent development in research in the psychology of religion is that of mini-models that help to guide theory and research in circumscribed areas and for particular phenomena. For example, spiritual intelligence is an idea about a hypothetical dimension of personality/intelligence that is concerned with the sustaining of behavior in the pursuit of goals, and the regulation of subgoal behavior under the umbrella of more global goals; the overarching one (or *suprameaning*, in Frankl's [1969] terms, or *ultimate concern*, in Tillich's [1952, 1963] terms) is what is of ultimate concern to the person (Emmons, 1999). In contrast, religion as schema (McIntosh, 1995) or a constellation of schemas (Ozorak, 1997) proposes a structure of religious ideas, teachings, behavioral scripts, and other knowledge in the information storage system. Religion and coping describes how the use of different types of religious coping strategies differentially influence health and well-being (Pargament, 1997). Right now, each of these lines of research is relatively independent of the others. Thus, they can be described as mini-models whose work runs in parallel but has yet to be integrated within psychology (thus, intra-disciplinary development), let alone across disciplinary boundaries (thus, multilevel and interdisciplinary).

THE ROLE OF THE PSYCHOLOGY OF RELIGION

What role does the psychology of religion now play in the broader field of psychology? Perhaps its most immediate disciplinary contributions are the publication of research that has put the topic of religion in front of the rest of the psychological community. Psychology of religion articles are now published in leading journals, psychology of religion books are published by leading publishers and the American Psychological Association, and a comfortable amount of program time for this topic is evident at professional meetings. Applied contributions are also current. For example, training in the application of some of this knowledge is more likely than in prior years to be available as part of doctoral programs in clinical and counseling psychology. Therefore, an overview of the field of psychology shows that the psychology of religion is present, contributing, and engaging other areas in dialogue.

One way to identify the potential contributions of the psychology of religion is to assume that they parallel those of the larger discipline of psychology. When people are introduced to psychology, they typically learn that its goals are to describe, predict, understand, and control behavior. In general psychology, the pursuit of these goals has resulted in a discipline with a self-evident expanse. Its contributions to myriad lines of intellectual work and applications to a broad array of human problems are far-reaching. It would be proper, therefore, for advances in the psychology of religion to fill a similar role. Scholars in the field would agree upon the first three goals (describe, predict, understand). Understanding all of the psychological mechanisms underlying human religiousness is an aim inherent in the process. There may be differences of opinion, however, about the fourth goal, control. Following the next 28 topical chapters, we return to this issue in Chapter 30.

Also in Chapter 30, we discuss the material in these 28 topical chapters in light of the integrative themes identified above. These 28 chapters describe the various mini-theories, conceptual frameworks, and empirical work that are on the cutting edge of the psychology of religion. They make it clear that the psychology of religion is becoming ever more sophisticated and integrative while also pushing the boundaries of relevant subject matter in very exciting ways. We think that the multilevel interdisciplinary paradigm and the model of religion as a meaning system will emerge as intellectual tools that contribute to these developments in significant ways.

ACKNOWLEDGMENTS

We thank the contributors in this handbook for providing a number of good suggestions for the preparation of these chapters, and Adam Cohen, Ralph Hood, Jr., and Ralph Piedmont for helpful critical comments on the rough drafts.

REFERENCES

Bandura, A. (1986). *The social foundations of thought and action: A social cognitive theory.* Englewood Cliffs, NJ: Prentice Hall.

Batson, C. D. (1977). Experimentation in psychology of religion: An impossible dream. *Journal for the Scientific Study of Religion, 16,* 413–418.

Batson, C. D. (1979). Experimentation in psychology of religion: Living with or in a dream? *Journal for the Scientific Study of Religion, 18,* 90–93.

Batson, C. D., Schoenrade, P., & Ventis, W. L. (1993). *Religion and the individual: A social psychological perspective.* London: Oxford University Press.

Baumeister, R. F. (1991). *Meanings of life.* New York: Guilford Press.

Baumeister, R. F. (Ed.). (2002). Religion and psychology. *Psychological Inquiry: An International Journal of Peer Commentary and Review* [Special issue], *12*(3).

Beit-Hallahmi, B. (1974). Psychology of religion 1880–1930: The rise and fall of a psychological movement. *Journal of the History of the Behavioral Sciences, 10,* 84–90.

Beit-Hallahmi, B., & Argyle, M. (1997). *The psychology of religious behaviour, belief and experience.* New York: Routledge.

Belzen, J. A. (Ed.). (1997). *Hermeneutical approaches in psychology of religion.* Amsterdam, The Netherlands: Rodoi B. V.

Belzen, J. A. (1999). Religion as embodiment: Cultural–psychological concepts and methods in the study of conversion among "Bevindelijken." *Journal for the Scientific Study of Religion*, 38(2), 236–253.

Belzen, J. A. (Ed.). (2000). *Aspects in contexts: Studies in the history of psychology of religion*. Amsterdam, The Netherlands: Rodoi B. V.

Belzen, J. A. (2003). Culture, religion and the "dialogical self": Roots and character of a secular cultural psychology of religion. *Archiv für Religionspsychologie*, 25, 7–24.

Dittes, J. E. (1969). Psychology of religion. In G. Lindzey & E. Aronson (Eds.), *The handbook of social psychology* (2nd ed., Vol. 5, pp. 602–659). Reading, MA: Addison-Wesley.

Emmons, R. A. (1999). *The psychology of ultimate concerns: Motivation and spirituality in personality*. New York: Guilford Press.

Emmons, R. A. (2000). Is spirituality an intelligence?: Motivation, cognition, and the psychology of ultimate concern. *The International Journal for the Psychology of Religion*, 10, 3–26.

Emmons, R. A., & Paloutzian, R. F. (2003). The psychology of religion. *Annual Review of Psychology*, 54, 377–402.

Frankl, V. E. (1969). *The will to meaning*. New York: New American Library.

Freud, S. (1961). *The future of an illusion* (J. Strachey, trans.). New York: Norton. (Original work published 1927)

Gorsuch, R. L. (1982). Practicality and ethics of experimental research when studying religion. *Journal for the Scientific Study of Religion*, 21, 370–372.

Gorsuch, R. L. (1984). Measurement: The boon and bane of investigating religion. *American Psychologist*, 39, 228–236.

Gorsuch, R. L. (1988). Psychology of religion. *Annual Review of Psychology*, 39, 201–221.

Hall, G. S. (1904). *Adolescence: Its psychology and its relations to physiology, anthropology, sociology, sex, crime, religion, and educations* (2 vols.). New York: Appleton.

Hester, M. P., & Paloutzian, R. F. (in press). Teaching psychology of religion: Teaching for today's world. In W. Buskist & S. F. Davis (Eds.), *Handbook of the teaching of psychology*. Oxford, UK: Blackwell.

Hill, P. C., & Hood, R. W., Jr. (1999). *Measures of religiosity*. Birmingham, AL: Religious Education Press.

Hood, R. W., Jr., Hill, P. C., & Williamson, W. P. (2005). *The psychology of religious fundamentalism: An intratextual model*. New York: Guilford Press.

Hunsberger, B. (1991). Empirical work in the psychology of religion. *Canadian Psychology*, 32, 497–504.

Hunsberger, B., & Jackson, L. M. (2005). Religion, meaning and prejudice. *Journal of Social Issues*, 61(4).

James, W. (1958). *The varieties of religious experience*. New York: New American Library. (Original work published 1902)

Janoff-Bulman, R., & Frantz, C. M. (1997). The impact of trauma on meaning: From meaningless world to meaningful life. In M. Power & C. R. Brewin (Eds.), *The transformation of meaning in psychological therapies* (pp. 91–106). New York: Wiley.

Jung, C. G. (1969). Psychology and religion. In *Collected works* (2nd ed., Vol. 11, pp. 3–105). (Original work published in English 1938)

Kirkpatrick, L. A. (2005). *Attachment, evolution, and the psychology of religion*. New York: Guilford Press.

Leuba, J. H. (1912). *A psychological study of religion: Its origin, function, and future*. New York: Macmillan.

Leuba, J. H. (1925). *The psychology of religious mysticism*. New York: Harcourt, Brace.

McCrae, R. R. (1999). Mainstream personality psychology and the study of religion. *Journal of Personality*, 67, 1209–1218.

McIntosh, D. N. (1995). Religion-as-schema, with implications for the relation between religion and coping. *The International Journal for the Psychology of Religion*, 5, 1–16.

Ochsner, K. E., & Lieberman, M. D. (2001). The emergence of social cognitive neuroscience. *American Psychologist, 56,* 717–734.

Ozorak, E. W. (1997). In the eye of the beholder: A social-cognitive model of religious belief. In B. Spilka & D. McIntosh (Eds.), *The psychology of religion: Theoretical approaches* (pp. 194–203). Boulder, CO: Westview.

Paloutzian, R. F. (1996). *Invitation to the psychology of religion* (2nd ed.). Boston: Allyn & Bacon.

Paloutzian, R. F., & Silberman, I. (2003). Religion and the meaning of social behavior: Concepts and issues. In P. Roelofsma, J. Corveleyn, & J. van Saane (Eds.), *One hundred years of psychology and religion: Issues and trends in a century long quest* (pp. 155–167). Amsterdam, The Netherlands: VU University Press.

Pargament, K. I. (1997). *The psychology of religion and coping.* New York: Guilford Press.

Pargament, K. I. (2002). Is religion nothing but . . . ?: Explaining religion versus explaining religion away. *Psychological Inquiry, 13*(3), 239–244.

Pargament, K. I., Magyar, G. M., & Murray-Swank, N. (2005). The sacred and the search for significance: Religion as a unique process. *Journal of Social Issues, 61*(4).

Park, C. L. (2005). Religion as a meaning-making framework in coping with life stress. *Journal of Social Issues, 61*(4).

Pratt, J. B. (1920). *The religious consciousness: A psychological study.* New York: Macmillan.

Roccas, S. (2005). Religion and value systems. *Journal of Social Issues, 61*(4).

Silberman, I. (2003). Spiritual modeling: The teaching of meaning systems. *The International Journal for the Psychology of Religion, 13*(3), 175–195.

Silberman, I. (Ed.) (2005a). Religion as meaning system. *Journal of Social Issues* [special issue], *61*(4).

Silberman, I. (2005b). Religion as a meaning system: Implications for the new millennium. *Journal of Social Issues, 61*(4).

Spilka, B., Hood, R. W., Jr., Hunsberger, B., & Gorsuch, R. (2003). *The psychology of religion: An empirical approach* (3rd ed.). New York: Guilford Press.

Spilka, B., Shaver, P., & Kirkpatrick, L. A. (1985). A general attribution theory for the psychology of religion. *Journal for the Scientific Study of Religion, 24,* 1–20.

Starbuck, E. D. (1899). *The psychology of religion.* London: Walter Scott.

Tillich, P. J. (1952). *The courage to be.* New Haven, CT: Yale University Press.

Tillich, P. J. (1963). *Systematic theology.* Chicago: University of Chicago Press. (See also Tillich, P. [1965], *Ultimate concern: Tillich in dialogue* [D. Brown, Ed.]. New York: Harper.)

Wulff, D. M. (1997). *Psychology of religion: Classic and contemporary* (2nd ed.). New York: Wiley.

Wulff, D. M. (1998). Rethinking the rise and fall of the psychology of religion. In A. L. Molendijk & P. Pels (Eds.), *Religion in the making: The emergence of the sciences of religion* (pp. 181–202). Boston: Brill.

Wulff, D. M. (2003). A field in crisis: Is it time for the psychology of religion to start over? In P. Roelofsma, J. Corveleyn, & J. van Saane (Eds.), *One hundred years of psychology and religion: Issues and trends in a century long quest* (pp. 155–167). Amsterdam, The Netherlands: VU University Press.

Yalom, I. D. (1980). *Existential therapy.* New York: Basic Books.

Yinger, J. M. (1967). Pluralism, religion, and secularism. *Journal for the Scientific Study of Religion, 6,* 17–28.

2

Religiousness and Spirituality

BRIAN J. ZINNBAUER
KENNETH I. PARGAMENT

Religiousness and spirituality have been a part of human experience throughout the length and breadth of human history. Crossing every category of human endeavor, they have been the subject and object of art, music, poetry, culture, warfare, inspiration, aspiration, sacrifice, morality, devotion, contemplation, conflict, and multitudes of other human activities. For the past 100 years these phenomena have been examined though the lens of social science. Early inquiries within the field of psychology were undertaken by scholars such as William James (1902/1961), Edwin Starbuck (1899), G. Stanley Hall (1904, 1917), and George Coe (1900). And despite a lull in such research during the mid-20th century (Hill et al., 2000), there has been an upsurge in attention to religion and spirituality among psychologists at the turn of the 21st century.

This increase in interest has been well documented by a number of researchers (e.g., Emmons & Paloutzian, 2003; Hill et al., 2000; Miller & Thoresen, 2003; Shafranske, 2002; Zinnbauer, Pargament, & Scott, 1999). In particular, the relationship between religiousness, spirituality, and health has received a great deal of attention and was the focus of the January 2003 edition of the *American Psychologist*. As noted by Mills (2002, cited in Shafranske, 2002), citations including the keywords *religion and health* or *spirituality and health* in databases such as PsychINFO and Medline quintupled from 1994 to 2001. Also currently prevalent are articles and books describing the integration of religiousness and spirituality with psychological treatment (e.g., Miller, 1999; Richards & Bergin, 1997, 2000; Shafranske, 1996; Zinnbauer & Pargament, 2000).

This scholarly and scientific inquiry has generated a considerable amount of theory, data, and information about religiousness and spirituality. Indeed, this *Handbook of the Psychology of Religion* is itself a culmination of the fruitful theoretical and empirical efforts of numerous scientists and scholars, past and present. Given this increasing knowledge base, one might assume that there exists a clear consensus among psychologists about the nature and definition of religiousness and spirituality. Alas, this is not the case. The psychology of religion is presently in the midst of flux about the meaning of its key constructs. Previous research has documented the diversity of definitions of religiousness and spirituality among researchers and adherents (see Zinnbauer, Pargament, & Scott, 1999, for a summary). From the earliest studies by Coe (1900) and Clark (1958), through more recent studies by McReady and Greeley (1976) and Scott (1997), the terms have been associated with various beliefs, behaviors, feelings, attributes, relationships, and experiences. Similarly, the content analysis of Zinnbauer et al. (1997), as well as the policy-capturing studies of Pargament, Sullivan, Balzer, Van Haitsma, and Raymark (1995) and Zinnbauer and Pargament (2002), suggest that individuals have clear ideas about the meaning of these terms, are able to describe their beliefs in a reliable fashion, and are able to distinguish religiousness and spirituality from other constructs and phenomena. What has been missing, though, is agreement within the psychology of religion community itself. Some positive signs are finally appearing in the literature, but definitions of religiousness and spirituality remain relatively inconsistent across researchers.

This lack of consensus presents a critical challenge for the psychology of religion. Progress within the field rests on a certain degree of agreement about the identity and meaning of its key constructs, and the nature of the most relevant phenomena of interest (Emmons & Paloutzian, 2003; Hill et al., 2000; Moberg, 2002; Shafranske, 2002). Without such agreement, the field loses focus, its boundaries become diffuse, and it produces findings that do not generalize across studies (Zinnbauer et al., 1997).

This chapter begins with an examination of historical trends and current challenges faced by psychologists who seek to define religiousness and spirituality. Modern tendencies to differentiate and polarize religiousness and spirituality are then examined and evaluated, and some of the challenges and possibilities for the conceptualization and measurement of these constructs are considered. The chapter concludes with the presentation of definitions of religiousness and spirituality that avoid past and present pitfalls, and incorporate the concepts of multilevel-multidimensional analysis and developmental change.

DEFINING RELIGIOUSNESS AND SPIRITUALITY THROUGH THE TRADITIONAL LENS

Although the terms "religiousness" and "spirituality" have been defined by psychologists in a number of different ways over the past century (see Zinnbauer et al., 1997; Zinnbauer et al., 1999; Zinnbauer & Pargament, 2002), there has been general agreement that both concepts are multidimensional (Hill et al., 2000; Moberg, 2002). Furthermore, psychologists have traditionally regarded religion as a "broad-band" construct, not explicitly differentiated from spirituality (Hill et al., 2000; Pargament, 1999; Zinnbauer et al., 1997, 1999). From this perspective, religious and spiritual phenomena have been subsumed beneath the broad umbrella of the construct religion, or the terms *religion* and *spirituality* have been used interchangeably (Spilka & McIntosh, 1996). A selection of several past and present definitions of religiousness and spirituality can be seen in Tables 2.1 and 2.2.

A feature of traditional approaches is the understanding of religious phenomena from both substantive and functional perspectives. Substantive approaches define religion by its substance: the sacred. Research thus investigates those emotions, thoughts, behaviors, relationships, and the like that are explicitly related to a transcendent or imminent power (Bruce, 1996), or that have acquired sacred qualities themselves (Pargament & Mahoney, 2002; Emmons, 1999). One example of this is the definition of religion by

TABLE 2.1. Past and Present Definitions of Religion

Argyle and Beit-Hallahmi (1975, p. 1): A system of beliefs in a divine or superhuman power, and practices of worship or other rituals directed towards such a power.

Batson, Schoenrade, and Ventis (1993, p. 8): Whatever we as individuals do to come to grips personally with the questions that confront us because we are aware that we and others like us are alive and that we will die.

Bellah (1970, p. 21): A set of symbolic forms and acts that relate man to the ultimate conditions of his existence.

Clark (1958, p. 22): The inner experience of the individual when he senses a Beyond, especially as evidenced by the effect of this experience on his behavior when he actively attempts to harmonize his life with the Beyond.

Dollahite (1998, p. 5): A covenant faith community with teachings and narratives that enhance the search for the sacred.

James (1902/1961, p. 42): The feelings, acts, and experiences of individual men in their solitude, so far as they apprehend themselves to stand in relation to whatever they may consider the divine.

O'Collins and Farrugia (1991, p. 203): Systems of belief in and response to the divine, including the sacred books, cultic rituals, and ethical practices of the adherents.

Peteet (1994, p. 237): Commitments to beliefs and practices characteristic of particular traditions.

Argyle and Beit-Hallahmi (1975) as "a system of beliefs in a divine or superhuman power, and practices of worship or other rituals directed towards such a power" (p. 1).

Functional approaches examine the purposes religiousness serves in an individual's life. Beliefs, emotions, practices, and experiences are investigated as functional mechanisms that are used to deal with fundamental existential issues, such as meaning, death, suffering, isolation, and injustice (Bruce, 1996; Pargament, 1997). The definition of religiousness by Batson, Schoenrade, and Ventis (1993) captures the functional approach: "whatever we as individuals do to come to grips personally with the questions that confront us because we are aware that we and others like us are alive and that we will die" (p. 8).

Traditional psychological research has also emphasized the personal aspects of religiousness (Miller & Thoresen, 2003). Although sociologists of religion have typically in-

---

TABLE 2.2. Past and Present Definitions of Spirituality

Armstrong (1995, p. 3): The presence of a relationship with a Higher Power that affects the way in which one operates in the world.

Benner (1989, p. 20): The human response to God's gracious call to a relationship with himself.

Doyle (1992, p. 302): The search for existential meaning.

Elkins, Henderson, Hughes, Leaf, and Saunders (1988, p. 10): A way of being and experiencing that comes about through awareness of a transcendent dimension and that is characterized by certain identifiable values in regard to self, life, and whatever one considers to be the Ultimate.

Fahlberg and Fahlberg (1991, p. 274): That which is involved in contacting the divine within the Self or self.

Hart (1994, p. 23): The way one lives out one's faith in daily life, the way a person relates to the ultimate conditions of existence.

Shafranske and Gorsuch (1984, p. 231): A transcendent dimension within human experience . . . discovered in moments in which the individual questions the meaning of personal existence and attempts to place the self within a broader ontological context.

Tart (1975, p. 4): That vast realm of human potential dealing with ultimate purposes, with higher entities, with God, with love, with compassion, with purpose.

Vaughan (1991, p. 105): A subjective experience of the sacred.

cluded social or communal aspects of religious life in their conceptualizations, psychologists of religion have traditionally focused on individuals' beliefs, emotion, behavior, motivations, and so on (Pargament, 1997). The definition of religiousness by William James (1902/1961) illustrates this individual focus: "the feelings, acts, and experiences of individual men in their solitude, so far as they apprehend themselves to stand in relation to whatever they may consider the divine" (p. 42).

Traditional research also rests on the understanding that religiousness and spirituality can have both positive and negative forms (Hill et al., 2000; Hood, Spilka, Hunsberger, & Gorsuch, 1996; Zinnbauer et al., 1999). Despite the efforts of a few writers to paint religion as illusory or pathological (e.g., Ellis, 1980; Freud, 1927/1961), most investigators have provided balanced depictions. For example, Fromm (1950) contrasted *authoritarian religion* in which people demean themselves in relation to a greater power with a *humanistic religion* in which God represents and empowers individuals' strength and self-realization. There is also Allport's (1966) famous contrast of *intrinsic religion* with *extrinsic religion*. The intrinsic believer "lives" his or her religion and views faith as an ultimate value in itself. In contrast, the extrinsic believer "uses" religion in a strictly utilitarian sense to gain safety, social standing, or other secular or antireligious goals.

Whereas traditional approaches have been marked by their use of substantive and functional frames, an individual level of analysis, and depiction of positive and negative forms, the picture has changed. The most notable shift has occurred with the rise in popularity and recognition of the construct spirituality.

SPIRITUALITY AND THE RISE OF OPPOSITES

As outlined in several sources (Hill et al., 2000; Hood, 2003; Wulff, 1997; Zinnbauer et al., 1999), spirituality has emerged as a distinct construct and focus of research in the past several decades. Previously undifferentiated from religiousness, numerous forms of faith under the label "spirituality" have risen in popularity from the 1980s to the present. References to spirituality in the Religion Index increased substantially from the 1940s and 1950s to the present (Scott, 1997), and spirituality has received increasing attention within psychology in terms of measurement and scale development. These changes have occurred against a background of decline in traditional religious institutions, an increase in individualized forms of faith expression, movement from an emphasis on belief toward direct experience of the sacred, and a U.S. culture of religious pluralism (see Hill et al., 2000; Hood, 2003; Roof, 1993; Zinnbauer et al., 1999). Spirituality has also replaced religiousness in popular usage, as illustrated by the increasing number of mass-market books on spiritually related topics.

With the emergence of spirituality, a tension appears to have risen between the constructs of religiousness and spirituality. In its most extreme form, the two terms are defined in a rigidly dualistic framework. The most egregious examples are those that place a substantive, static, institutional, objective, belief-based, "bad" religiousness in opposition to a functional, dynamic, personal, subjective, experience-based, "good" spirituality.

Substantive Religion versus Functional Spirituality

Functional descriptions that were once applied to religion are now becoming the province of spirituality. Spirituality has come to represent individuals' efforts at reaching a variety of sacred or existential goals in life, such as finding meaning, wholeness, inner potential, and interconnections with others. For example, spirituality is now being depicted as a search for universal truth (Goldberg, 1990) and as a form of belief that relates the individual to the world and gives meaning and definition to existence (Soeken & Carson, 1987). In contrast, religiousness is substantively associated with formal belief, group practice, and institutions. As such, it is often portrayed as peripheral to these existential functions (Pargament, 1999).

This polarity is also becoming evident in the reports of adherents. In an interview study of faith among the seriously ill, Woods and Ironson (1999) found that those identifying themselves as "religious" tended to link their beliefs to institutional, traditional, ritualized, and social expressions of faith. In contrast, those who identified themselves as "spiritual" presented their beliefs and practices as mechanisms for transcendence and connectedness.

Static Religion versus Dynamic Spirituality

Speaking to this contrast, Wulff (1997) notes that, traditionally, religion was conceptualized as a verb. More recently, however, it has been transformed into a noun. In the process it has become a static entity to many people (Pargament, 1997), reduced to its elements and stripped of its function. Static depictions of religion portray "what religion is, not what it does or how it works" (Zinnbauer et al., 1999, p. 904). In contrast, spirituality is associated with dynamic verbs and adjectives (Emmons & Paloutzian, 2003). As discussed by Hill et al. (2000), it is often used in modern discourse as a substitute for words such as *fulfilling*, *moving*, or *important*.

Institutional Objective Religion versus Personal Subjective Spirituality

Departing from traditional analyses of individual beliefs, emotions, and experiences, many writers are now contrasting the "institutional," "organized," and "social" aspects of religion with the "personal," "transcendent," and "relatedness" qualities of spirituality (e.g., Miller & Thoresen, 2003). Peteet's (1994) conceptualization of the terms within psychotherapy illustrates this contrast. *Religiousness* is defined as "[reflecting] commitments to beliefs and practices characteristic of particular traditions," and *spirituality* is characterized as "[viewing] the human condition in a larger and or transcendent context and [being] therefore concerned with the meaning and purpose of life and with unseen realities, such as one's relationship to a supreme being" (p. 237).

This contrast is evident among researchers and adherents alike. For example, Emblen (1992) conducted a content analysis of references to religiousness and spirituality that appeared in the last 30 years of the nursing literature. After compiling lists of the key words identified with the two constructs, definitions of each were derived from the most common associations. *Religiousness* was thus defined as "a system of organized beliefs and worship which a person practices," and *spirituality* was defined as "a personal life principle which animates a transcendent quality of relationship with God" (p. 45).

In a well-regarded examination of trends in the conceptualization of the terms, Hill et al. (2000) have also used the individual–institutional dimension to distinguish between spirituality and religiousness. Whereas they propose that the sacred lies at the core of both constructs, religion also includes "the means and methods of [a] search [for the sacred] that receive validation and support from within an identifiable group of people" (p. 66).

This contrast is becoming more evident in the general culture. Walker and Pitts's

(1998) study of moral maturity included a section of questions that asked participants to rate a number of descriptors in terms of the degree to which they represented a prototypically moral, religious, or spiritual person. Results indicated that manifesting moral character and believing in a higher power were central descriptors of both religious and spiritual people. However, spirituality was seen as a "personal affirmation of the transcendent" in contrast to religion which was seen as "the creedal and ritual expression of spirituality that is associated with institutional church organizations" (p. 409).

Similarly, in a content analysis of religious and spiritual definitions by Zinnbauer et al. (1997), personal beliefs in the sacred were common to definitions of both constructs. However, definitions of religiousness often included references to organizational practices or activities, attendance at services, performance of rituals, church membership or allegiance, commitment to organizational beliefs, or adherence to institutionally based belief systems. In contrast, definitions of spirituality often referred to feelings or experiences of connectedness or relationship with sacred beings or forces. Also, from the policy-capturing study of Zinnbauer and Pargament (2002), the participant group comprised of nurses tended to characterize religiousness in terms of formal/organizational religion, and spirituality in terms of a closeness with God or feelings of interconnectedness with the world and living things.

Belief-Based Religion versus Emotional/Experiential-Based Spirituality

This polarity can be seen in both theoretical writings and empirical research. Elkins (1995), for example, defines *religion* as institutional, dogmatic, and theological. In contrast, *spirituality* "is a way of being that comes about through awareness of a transcendent dimension and that is characterized by certain identifiable values in regard to self, others, nature, life, and whatever one considers to be the Ultimate" (Elkins, Hedstrom, Hughes, Leaf, & Saunders, 1988, p. 10).

The research literature also contains this contrast. In an interview study of 42 African American and 37 European American elderly participants, Nelson-Becker (2003) gathered personal definitions of the terms and found that religion was more often associated with beliefs, and spirituality more often associated with connection or a feeling in the heart. The two constructs were not always sharply distinguished from each other, but the unique descriptors of religion included elements such as heritage, basic principles, a way of thinking, and duty. In contrast, unique descriptors of spirituality included connection with God, relationships with others, and choice.

Negative Religion versus Positive Spirituality

Another contrast is the valence attached to the terms. In many writings, spirituality is credited with the positive: the loftier side of life, the highest in human potential, and pleasurable affective states. Religiousness gets slapped with the negative: mundane faith, outdated doctrine, or institutional hindrances to human potentials. For example, writing during a time of countercultural upheaval, Tart (1975) stated that religiousness implies "too strongly the enormous social structures that embrace so many more things than direct spiritual experience." Religion is associated with "priests, dogmas, doctrines, churches, institutions, political meddling, and social organizations" (p. 4). In contrast, "the term 'spiritual' . . . implies more directly the experience that people have about the meaning of life, God, ways to live, etc." Spirituality, for Tart, is "that vast realm of human potential dealing with ultimate purposes, with higher entities, with God, with life, with compassion, with purpose" (p. 4).

CRITICISMS OF POLARIZATION

In general, the usefulness of polarizing religiousness and spirituality is unclear. Certainly, the constructs will evolve in professional and popular usage over time, and differences between the two will continue to be identified. But narrow definitions of the terms or polarizations of the two as incompatible opposites are likely to hinder inquiry within the psychology of religion for several reasons.

First, the polarization of substantive static religion and functional dynamic spirituality is unnecessarily constrictive. Solely substantive definitions of religiousness reduce the construct to rigid entities that do not address the way religion works and evolves in the life of the individual. The result is an impersonal religion frozen in time (Pargament, 1997). Likewise, purely functional definitions of spirituality can leave the construct with weak boundaries (Bruce, 1996). Lacking a substantive sacred core, there is little to distinguish spirituality from other responses to existential issues, and little to distinguish the psychology of religion from other disciplines such as philosophy, the humanities, and other areas of psychology (e.g., community, humanistic). At worst, to identify spirituality with innumerable secular experiences, existential quests, and personal values is to render it fuzzy (Spilka, 1993; Spilka & McIntosh, 1996), if not meaningless.

The polarization of institutional religiousness and personal spirituality as incompatible opposites is also problematic. Although psychological inquiry has expanded from a traditional focus on the individual to include social, political, historical, and economic contexts (Chatters & Taylor, 2003; American Psychological Association, 2003), this expansion of inquiry has not been evenly adopted within the psychology of religion. By limiting religiousness only to social context and disconnecting it from the individual, we lose sight of the fact that every major religious institution is fundamentally concerned with personal belief, emotion, behavior, and experiences. Some have written that the primary objective of religious organizations is to bring individuals closer to God (Carroll, Dudley, & McKinney, 1986). Likewise, to conceptualize spirituality as a solely personal phenomenon is to ignore the cultural context in which this construct has emerged. Spirituality as an individual expression is not culture-free; it is neither interpreted nor expressed in a social vacuum. As a movement toward individualism (see Hood, 2003; Roof, 1993, 1998), a rebellion against tradition, or a reaction to hierarchically arranged social organizations, spirituality is still embedded within a cultural context.

It is no coincidence that the popularity of spirituality has grown in a culture that values individualism, and has risen during a historical period in which traditional authority and cultural norms were being rejected (Berger, 1967; Hood, 2003; Roof, 1993). Interestingly, in spite of the anti-institutional rhetoric surrounding this construct, spiritual organizations and groups have emerged and gained in popularity (Hood et al., 1996). Those who leave traditional religions for spiritual pursuits often join others of like mind. Thus, there are established spiritual organizations that differ from established religions only in their novelty and in the content of their beliefs—not on the basis of a personal versus an organizational level of analysis.

This polarization also appears related to an errant choice of words. There appear to be four terms relevant to the previous discussion rather than two: religion, religiousness, spirit, and spirituality. As discussed by Miller and Thoresen (2003), *religion* is commonly characterized as an institutional, material phenomenon, and *religiousness* is often depicted in terms of individual belief or practice. Likewise, *spirit* as an external transcendent or internal animating force can be differentiated from *spirituality*, a sacred human activity. More appropriately, religion should be compared to spirit and religiousness to spirituality. However, in a dualism reminiscent of Descartes, religion is often distinguished from spirituality; that is, religion as an objective external entity (matter) is contrasted with spirituality, a subjective internal human attribute or process (mind). Thus, "findings" that differentiate the constructs on the basis of the social–personal and objective–subjective dimensions may be related to an a priori choice of words. To minimize confusion, investigators may do well to recognize when they are comparing constructs at the same level of analysis (e.g., religiousness and spirituality) or when they are comparing across levels of analysis (e.g., religion and spirituality).

The distinction between cognitive religion and emotional spirituality is fraught with limitations. It is difficult to imagine a religious adherent attracted to his or her faith solely through an idea, concept, or belief. It is also difficult to imagine a spiritual person whose devotion is bereft of beliefs or cognitive activity. Thoughts and feelings occur together and influence one another. Passionless religious belief and thoughtless spiritual experience are indeed possible, but are not representative of the rich ways thoughts, feelings, behavior, motivation, and experiences come together to mark both religiousness and spirituality.

Finally, the bifurcation of spirituality as "good" and religion as "bad" recalls criticisms already leveled against other theories: evaluation has been confounded with description (Hood et al., 1996). The determination of whether a set of beliefs or practices leads to positive or negative outcomes is an empirical question. To define the constructs as inherently good or bad severely limits psychological inquiry and may reflect simple prejudice rather than informed analysis.

A growing literature on religiousness and health also contradicts the characterization of religious involvement as pathological or malevolent (see Hill et al., 2000; Miller & Thoresen, 2003; Pargament, 1997; Powell, Shahabi, & Thoresen, 2003; Seeman, Dubin, & Seeman, 2003). A sizable body of research has documented the supportive effects of involvement in religious institutions, especially for the disenfranchised (e.g., Hill et al., 2000; Pargament, 1997). The naïve notion of "good" spirituality may also lead investigators to ignore the potentially destructive side of spiritual life. In addition to seeking closeness with God through altruism and compassion, there are all-too-many examples of spiritual seekers who have used extreme self-punishing asceticism, suicide bombings, and mass suicides to achieve their sacred goals. To overlook the dark side of spirituality by definition is to leave an incomplete or distorted picture of this phenomenon.

It is also important to note that the splitting of religiousness and spirituality into incompatible opposites does not reflect the perspectives of all respondents. In a recent empirical study, Zinnbauer et al. (1997) found that most of their respondents identified themselves as both spiritual and religious (74%); in contrast, 19% identified themselves as spiritual but not religious, and 4% labeled themselves as religious but not spiritual. Similarly, in a large-scale study conducted by Corrigan, McCorkle, Schell, and Kidder (2003), 63% of respondents identified themselves as spiritual and religious, 22% identified themselves as spiritual but not religious, and 4% identified themselves as religious but not spiritual. According to another large-scale survey with a representative U.S. sample (Shahabi et al., 2002), 52% of respondents identified themselves as very or moderately religious and spiritual, 10% identified themselves as very or moderately spiritual but slightly or not at all religious, 9% identified themselves as very or moderately religious but slightly or not at all spiritual, and 29% identified themselves as slightly or not at all religious or spiritual. Self-perceptions of religiousness and spirituality were also significantly correlated in the studies by Zinnbauer et al. (1997) and Shahabi et al. (2002). From these studies it appears that most people view themselves as both religious and spiritual (see also Cook, Borman, Moore, & Kunkel, 2000), and that spiritual development for most may occur within the context of a supportive religious environment.

Of note is the finding discussed by Hood (2003) and Roof (1993, 1998), and reported in studies by Zinnbauer et al. (1997) and Shahabi et al. (2002), that the subgroup of believers who characterize themselves as "spiritual but not religious" do indeed hold a negative opinion of religiousness and may maintain some of the polarized opinions of religiousness and spirituality. This group does report more mystical experiences and group experiences related to spiritual growth, and less religious involvement than those who identify themselves as both religious and spiritual. For these "spiritual mystics" (Hood, 2003), it may be the separation from religion that defines their spiritual identity. However, it is important to keep in mind that this is a subgroup rather than a majority of people in the United States.

From previous critical summaries and research efforts, several general conclusions about the meanings of religiousness and spirituality can be offered (see Emmons & Paloutzian, 2003; Hill et al., 2000; Hood, 2003; Shafranske, 2002; Shafranske & Bier, 1999):

1. Religiousness and spirituality are cultural "facts" not reducible to other processes or phenomena.
2. Most people define themselves as both religious and spiritual.
3. An identifiable minority identify themselves as spiritual but not religious, and they use spirituality as a means of rejecting religion.
4. Religiousness and spirituality overlap considerably in the U.S. population, and the constructs are generally regarded as "related but not identical."
5. Religiousness and spirituality are multidimensional, complex constructs.
6. Religiousness and spirituality can be associated with both mental health and emotional distress.
7. There are substantive and functional aspects of both religiousness and spirituality.
8. Religiousness and spirituality are multilevel constructs—that is, they are related to biological, affective, cognitive, moral, relational, personality or self-identity, social, cultural, and global phenomena.
9. Religiousness and spirituality can develop and change over time for individuals and groups.
10. Religiousness and spirituality are acquiring different denotations as their use evolves. Religiousness is often associated with a social or group level of analysis, and spirituality is often associated with an individual level of analysis.

CHALLENGES AND POSSIBILITIES

The above historical and lexical trends point to vital challenges for the psychology of religion as the field moves into the 21st century. In this section a number of these challenges are highlighted, followed by the presentation of definitions and a framework for psychological inquiry.

Consensus

One obvious challenge for the field is to generate some degree of professional consensus about the definitions of religiousness and spirituality while remaining sensitive to the various phenomenological nuances of the terms. Whereas a plethora of popular definitions may honor a diversity of groups and voices (Moberg, 2002), within the realm of psychological research a lack of consistency can be problematic. As suggested by Emmons and Paloutzian (2003, p. 381), "in order for progress to occur in a scientific discipline, there must be a minimum of consensus concerning the meaning of core constructs and their measurement." This commonsense reminder has also been advanced by Hill et al. (2000), Moberg (2002), and Shafranske (2002), and speaks to the need for a certain degree of intragroup reliability in definitions in order to build a cumulative knowledge base. Lacking such consistency, communication within the field is impaired, as is the ability to generalize research findings across studies (Zinnbauer et al., 1997).

On the other hand, should researchers define the terms in ways that are fully removed from popular uses, or in ways that narrowly exclude great sections of the religious and spiritual landscape, the legitimacy or relevance of the field may be questioned. The varieties of religious and spiritual experiences provide remarkable examples of human diversity. Universalist assumptions about the religiousness or spirituality of *all* people obscure important variations in the belief and practice of some people (Moberg, 2002). At worst, they have the potential to insult or oppress minority groups. Accordingly, there have been numerous calls for increased attention to religious and spiritual differences among various groups, and cautions that existing research and theory overrepresent white Protestants (Hill & Pargament, 2003; Moberg, 2002).

It should be noted that psychology is neither the first nor the only discipline to wrestle with issues of definition. For example, in an anthropological discussion of the term "shamanism," Bourguignon (1989) discusses the long history of efforts to refine conceptualizations that bridge emic and etic vocabularies. *Emic descriptions* are culture-specific and recognizable by cultural insiders. *Etic descriptions* are supracultural, and as such they permit comparative research. By using native concepts and terminology, emic conceptualizations can capture the essence of meaning within a given group or culture. Etic descriptions, on the other hand, allow for the identification of commonalities across different groups. Both approaches are important. A solely emic science can produce little more than accumulations of unique cases (Bourguignon, 1989): a solely etic science can minimize or distort important cultural differences.

It may be tempting to stay in the shallow waters to avoid tackling these deep issues. Limiting the study of religiousness and spirituality to simple quantitative behaviors, such as the number of church services attended in the week or the number of praying behaviors completed each day, has the great advantage of being observable and countable, but this approach falls far short of the depth of human experience touched by religiousness and spirituality. If we agree that these concepts can encompass core sacred elements that orient, motivate, and shape central aspects of the human psyche, we must not limit investigations based on the ease of measurement. The challenge is to produce studies that can capture the richness and diversity of religiousness and spirituality while striving for the precision required by scientific inquiry.

It may also be tempting to sidestep these issues through the development of new measures of spirituality. However, in some instances, the new measures overlap with old measures of religion. For instance, one purportedly new index of spiritual experiences, INSPIRIT, consists of items that tap into closeness to God and mystical experiences, constructs that have been measured previously in the psychology of religion (Kass, Freidman, Lesserman, Zuttermeister, & Benson, 1991). Other spiritual measures contain items that could just as easily be found on secular measures of life satisfaction, happiness, and well-being. For example, the spiritual well-being measure developed by Brady, Peterman, Fitchet, Mo, and Cella (1999) includes items that assess meaning and peace in life without any explicit reference to God or a faith tradition. Thus, it is doubtful that more scale development will solve the problems of definition in the field in and of itself. The community of researchers may be better served by focusing on definition and theory development as a prelude to the next wave of measures (see also Hill, Chapter 3, this volume).

Reductionism and Levels of Analysis

A controversy that often is raised in discussions of measurement and definition is that of *reductionism*, the process of understanding a phenomenon at one level of analysis by reducing it to presumably more fundamental processes (see discussions in Idinopulos & Yonan, 1994, and Wilber, 1995). In some sense this process is unavoidable in scientific study (Moberg, 2002; Segal, 1994). However, reductionism is often accompanied by a loss of information. For example, the reduction of mystical experiences of oneness with the universe to a change in neurotransmitter levels eliminates information at all other levels (e.g., the cultural, social, familial, affective, cognitive, and behavioral). There may indeed be important physical correlates of such an experience, but to deny the relevance or value of other modes of interpretation and understanding is to commit the error of reductionism.

One way to avoid reductive investigations is to be mindful of the concept of levels of analysis. As used here, this presupposes different interconnected planes of information, ranging from the subatomic level up through the global level. Wilber (1995) presents this idea in the following progression from the microscopic to the macroscopic: subatomic particles, atoms, molecules, organelles, cells, tissues, organ systems, person, family, community, culture/subculture, society/nation, biosphere. Referring to the "great chain of being" concept from the philosophical tradition (Huxley, 1944; see also Wilber, 1995, 1999), each increasing level includes and transcends the previous level, and displays emergent phenomenon appearing at each novel level that are nonreducible to previous levels. Fundamental levels are necessary but not sufficient for the organization of higher levels. Thus, organ systems are composed of cells, but the function of the organs is not fully captured at the cellular level, and having cells does not guarantee the development of organ systems. Groups are composed of individuals, but group processes and behavior are not captured in the study of any single person in the group. Causality can move up and down the levels of analysis, and a phenomenon at one level may have correlates at different levels.

Confusion within the study of religiousness and spirituality may arise when different researchers define the constructs from different levels of analysis, but do not identify their definitions as such. Identifying religiousness as a social phenomenon and spirituality as an individual phenomenon, and then casting them as incompatible opposites illustrates this kind of mistake. For example, the phenomenon of religious conversion can be understood at multiple levels: cellular changes, brain system changes, cognitive–affect–behavioral changes, social changes, cultural changes, and global changes. A narrow focus on one level to the exclusion of others can distort the picture or fall into a reductionist trap. Even people who define themselves as "spiritual but not religious," rejecting religion and embracing spiritual individualism, can be understood through a social/institutional level of analysis (albeit one that is defined as a polemic). This is not to say that all levels are equally salient at all times. The important point is that different levels are not necessarily incompatible. A glance at Tables 2.1 and 2.2 reveals that many of the current definitions encompass only a single level of analysis or fail to address the range of information planes.

The process of defining religiousness and spirituality, in itself, can be viewed at individual, social, cultural, and global levels. In the above discussion it has been argued that social changes have produced a new emphasis on personal spirituality (see also Hood, 2003). One could also state that the intense personal mystical experiences of Jesus, Mohammed, and the Buddha led to changes in the social, cultural, and global consciousness of religiousness and spirituality. Social pressures inside and outside of the academic community of psychology can also direct the definitions of the terms religiousness and spirituality. Adequate theories in the psychology of religion such as the multilevel interdisciplinary paradigm (Emmons & Paloutzian, 2003) will allow for research to be undertaken at various levels of analysis, examining the interactions between levels, determining the salience of different levels to a given phenomenon, and avoiding the pitfalls of reductionism.

Multidimensional Religiousness and Spirituality

The dimensions of religiousness and spirituality include different levels of analysis and different strands of human activity and experiences. The cross-disciplinary character and reach of these phenomena have been appreciated within the psychology of religion in two ways. First, there is increasing emphasis on collaboration with other sciences (Belzen, 2002; Emmons & Paloutzian, 2003; Shafranske, 2002). Second, there are calls for more complex and far-reaching models that recognize the multiple levels of reality and psychological phenomena in ways relevant to the applied clinician (Vande Kemp, 2003). As noted by Emmons and Paloutzian (2003), new developments for the investigation of religion in cognitive science, neurobiology, evolutionary psychology, and behavioral genetics are part of the leading edge of research in a "multilevel interdisciplinary paradigm" (p. 395). Hall and Gorman's (2003) presentation of a relational metapsychology that includes elements of object relations, attachment theory, and interpersonal neurobiology and Reich's (1998) discussion of pluralistic religious theory are steps in this direction. A quick glance at the chapter titles within this volume can provide a sense of the breadth of research on religiousness and spirituality. Single-strand definitions are inadequate to the current demands for theoretical sophistication. Religiousness is not just beliefs about God. Spirituality is not just oneness with life. Both constructs contain multiple dimensions including, but not limited to, biology, sensation, affect, cognition, behavior, identity, meaning, morality, relationships, roles, creativity, personality, self-awareness, and salience.

Developmental Changes

Another source of confusion is the failure to provide room within definitions of religiousness and spirituality for the concept of developmental changes. The means and ends of religious and spiritual belief, behavior, perception, and so on are reflective of and change with different stages of development for individuals and groups (Worthington, 1989). Religiousness and spirituality have their own developmental trajectory (and are not reducible to other developmental strands), but are also impacted by other changes, such as developments in cognition, affect, and morality (see McFadden, Chapter 9, this volume). Thus, religiousness is not a lower level of development than spirituality (or vice versa). As stated by Hill et al. (2002) religiousness and spirituality develop across the lifespan. They also reflect, and are interdependent with, other strands of human development. For example, a child at a magical thinking level of development may hold certain beliefs about the nature of God. As she grows and matures cognitively, her beliefs will likely become more sophisticated even if she remains within the same religious tradition, rates herself at the same level of religiousness, and attends the same number of church services each year. An adequate understanding of religiousness and spirituality must account for the process of development and change over time. Likewise, it must recognize the mutual impacts of religiousness and spirituality with other developmental strands.

Thus, several elements of an adequate approach to religiousness and spirituality have been offered. First, the field must move toward greater consensus in defining its terms. Second, definitions must be broad enough to account for the varieties of religious and spiritual experience, while allowing for differences of culture and context. Etic and emic concerns must be mindfully addressed, and reductionism that distorts the essence of religious and spiritual phenomenon must be avoided. Third, the perspectives of levels of analysis and developmental changes must be included.

TWO PROPOSED WAYS TO DEFINE RELIGIOUSNESS AND SPIRITUALITY

In this section, we suggest several terms and characteristics that we believe are critical to definitions of religiousness and spirituality. Building on these common concepts, we then offer two different ways religiousness and spirituality can be defined that reflect contrasting trends in the field, one in which spirituality is viewed as the overarching construct and the other in which religiousness represents the more encompassing process.

Critical Terms

The first construct that is critical to both spirituality and religiousness is "significance." As explained by Pargament (1997), significance is, in part, a phenomenological construct that involves the experience of caring, attraction, or attachment. We can speak of a sense of or feelings of significance. Significance also refers to a particular set of valued, meaningful, or ultimate concerns. These concerns may be psychological (e.g., growth, self-esteem, comfort), social (e.g., intimacy, social justice), physical (e.g., health, fitness), material (e.g., money, food, cars), or related to the divine (e.g., closeness with God, religious experience).

The concept of "search" is a second critical feature of both religiousness and spirituality (see Pargament, 1997, for a review). By search, we are underscoring the fact that people are goal-directed beings engaged in the pursuit of whatever they hold significant. The process of search involves the attempt to discover significance. But the searching process does not end with discovery. Once people find something significant in their lives, they attempt to hold on to or conserve that significance. Although people are often successful in their efforts to sustain significance, pressures within the individual or within the individual's world may prompt the need for fundamental change. At times, then, the process of search involves a transformation of the individual's understanding of or relationship to significance (see also Paloutzian, Chapter 18, this volume). The searching process then shifts back once again to the attempt to conserve this newly transformed significance. In this fashion, the search for significance—discovery, conservation, and transformation—unfolds throughout the lifespan.

Finally, the concept of the sacred is the substantive core of both religiousness and spirituality, the construct that distinguishes these phenomena from all others. The *sacred* refers to concepts of God, higher powers, transcendent beings, or other aspects of life that have been sanctified (see Idinopulos & Yonan, 1996, for a discussion). Virtually any dimension can be perceived as holy, worthy of veneration or reverence. As stated by Durkheim (1915), "by sacred things one must not understand simply those personal beings which are called Gods or spirits; a rock, a tree, a spring, a pebble, a piece of wood, a house, in a word, anything can be sacred" (p. 52). Thus, the designation is not limited to higher powers or imminent forces, but includes others aspects of life that take on divine character and meaning through their association with or representation of the holy (Pargament & Mahoney, 2002).

Sacred aspects of life can be found at multiple levels of analysis: health (vegetarianism, body as temple), psychological attributes (self, meaning), people (saints, cult leaders), roles (marriage, parenting, work), social attributes or relationships (compassion, patriotism, community), cultural products (music, literature), and global concerns (Gaia, world peace). They also cross levels of analysis, such as the quality of relationship between an individual and God or congregation, or the nature of conflict between one's religious beliefs and the social or political order. One may view a relationship to others of the same faith as a sacred connection, or view the holding of religious tenets against the tide of popular opinion as a holy, noble charge. These objects or processes can change in status in two ways: they can move from secular to sacred through the process of sanctification (Pargament & Mahoney, 2002), or they can move from sacred to secular through the process of desanctification. There is already mounting evidence that people regard, react, and pursue those things sacred to them in ways different from secular objects and processes (see Pargament & Mahoney, 2002; Emmons, 1999).

There are a few other common features to the definitions of religiousness and spirituality that follow. First, in contrast to approaches that distinguish the terms by level of analysis, this view maintains that both religiousness and spirituality can be pursued by individuals and groups. Further, they have their own developmental trajectories, are influenced by related developments of phenomena at other levels, and can have both substantive and functional elements.

Second, it is the religious or spiritual adherents' perspective that is privileged when determining whether a given search for significance is sacred or secular. This avoids imposing a certain value perspective on adherents, but does not place constraints on the ways in which investigators may approach or evaluate the constructs. In this sense, the definitions are sensitive to emic concerns but do not preclude etic characterizations or force investigators to make ontological assumptions about whether "holy" or "divine" realities exist. Recognizing multiple perspectives and multiple levels of analysis is vital to a progressive research program. The means and ends of significance, as well as the substance and function of religiousness and spirituality, have been and will continue to be examined through various sacred and secular lenses by investigators. Regardless of the interpretive frame used by investigators, it is suggested that the essential feature of both religiousness and spirituality is that religious and spiritual adherents take paths and/or seek goals that are related to what they perceive as sacred.

Third, neither religiousness nor spirituality is inherently good or bad, effective or ineffective. Pathological forms of both constructs may exist along all levels of analysis and all strands of development. Extreme spiritual asceticism or self-denial can damage the physical body, exaggerated spiritual beliefs of specialness can lead to narcissism, spiritual groups can engage in self-destructive behaviors, and sanctified cultural beliefs of superiority can lead to civil wars and genocide. Religiously justified abuse under the guise of "discipline," systematic religious oppression of one gender or group, and manipulation of mass media for monetary purposes can also be seen as the seedy side of religiousness.

Finally, religiousness and spirituality may involve both unique and universal phenomenon. They may include local truths, such as particular aspects of sacred belief or worship among identified cultural groups, or single unique experiences of the sacred. They may also involve supracultural truths such as the identification of core mystical experiences (see Hood, 2003), worldviews such as the great chain of being (Huxley, 1944; see also Wilber, 1995, 1999), and metagroup developmental processes (e.g., Beck & Cowan, 1996). Therefore, in order to understand and integrate wide-ranging currents such as biological components of spiritual experience and global trends in defining religiousness, multiple forms of investigation from multiple perspectives are needed. Accordingly, the use of a variety of methods, qualitative and quantitative, is unavoidable (Moberg, 2002).

Keeping in mind these points of commonality, we now present two sets of definitions of spirituality and religiousness that reflect two trends that are now visible in the field.

Spirituality as the Broader Construct

According to the first author (Zinnbauer), *spirituality is defined as a personal or group search for the sacred. Religiousness is defined as a personal or group search for the sacred that unfolds within a traditional sacred context.* From the perspective of these definitions, religiousness and spirituality are both embedded within context, and the nature of that context can be used to discriminate between the constructs. Both constructs are directed toward the search for one particular type of significant concern: the sacred. However, religiousness specifically represents the personal or communal search for the sacred that occurs within a traditional context or organized faith tradition. This context includes systems of belief, practices, and values that center around sacred matters and are explicitly embedded within or flow from institutions, traditions, or cultures. For instance, a believer's religiousness may involve pondering scriptural passages, cultivating religious virtues, performing rituals, listening to the experiences of other believers, achieving formal status as a member of a religious congregation, and connecting with others of the tradition from different parts of the world. Of note is the interest that religious settings (e.g., churches, synagogues, temples, denominations) have in teaching people to sanctify their lives, and to imbue seemingly secular pursuits with sacred value and meaning (Pargament & Mahoney, 2002). Through religious services, systems of belief, rituals, and educational programs, people are encouraged to perceive many aspects of life (e.g., physical health, personal identity, relationships, work, etc.) within a greater transcendent perspective.

Whereas some spiritual adherents describe spirituality solely in terms of individualistic belief or practice, spirituality always manifests within a context. That is, culture, community, society, family, and tradition exist as the crucible within which spirituality unfolds, or the background from which it differentiates. As with religiousness, spirituality may occur within a traditional context. When it does, adherents may be less likely to draw strong distinctions between the terms. Spirituality may also occur within nontraditional, novel, or emergent contexts. Such spiritual adherents, like the "spiritual mystics" discussed by Hood (2003) and the "spiritual but not religious" adherents identified by Zinnbauer et al. (1997), may make a greater distinction between religiousness and spirituality, and define their search for the sacred in part as a rejection of tradition.

Thus, according to these definitions, spirituality is a broader term than religiousness. Spirituality includes a range of phenomena that extends from the well-worn paths associated with traditional religions to the experiences of individuals or groups who seek the sacred outside of socially or culturally defined systems. For example, an individual's spirituality may include feelings of devotion, memories of a mystical experience, gatherings with other seekers, rebellion against a culture antagonistic to such a search, and a sense of unity with all sentient life. Significant changes in any of these levels or developmental strands may change the search itself. Development of a serious illness, for example, may change feelings of devotion to confusion or anger, make gatherings more difficult to attend, and cause psychological isolation from a sacred connection to others.

It is particularly important to recognize that the primary mission of organized religions is the individual and communal search for the sacred. Additional objectives such as social connection, community service, education, healthy lifestyle promotion, or financial assistance may also be pursued by religious organizations, families, and cultures in order to support the spiritual development of its members. As opposed to some contentions that organized religion exists by definition as a barrier or hindrance to personal experiences of the sacred, it is maintained here that the search for the sacred is in fact the core function of both spirituality and religiousness, and that most individuals seek the sacred within existing traditions. The success or failure of different organized religions to nurture this search is a question open for investigation.

Religiousness as the Broader Construct

According to the second author (Pargament), *spirituality is a search for the sacred. Religiousness refers to a search for significance in ways related to the sacred.* In contrast to the first set of definitions that differentiates religiousness and spirituality according to their contexts, this set of definitions distinguishes the two constructs by the place of the sacred in the means and ends of the searching process. Every search consists of an ultimate destination, a significance, and a pathway to reach that destination. Spirituality refers to a search in which the sacred is the ultimate destination. In search of the sacred, people may take any number of traditional or nontraditional pathways, from prayer; meditation; participation in churches, synagogues, and mosques; fasting; study of Scriptures; and the monastic life to a walk in the woods, quilting, sexuality, social action, psychotherapy, and listening to a symphony. What these diverse pathways may share is a common endpoint: the sacred.

Spirituality is the heart and soul of religiousness, the core function of religious life. Psychologist Paul Johnson (1959) once wrote: "It is the ultimate Thou, whom the religious person seeks most of all" (p. 70). However, religiousness in this second set of definitions has a broader set of ends than spirituality. Certainly, many people take sacred pathways in search of a relationship with the sacred, but they may be seeking other destinations as well, such as physical health, emotional well-being, intimacy with others, self-development, and participation in a larger community. In this sense, religiousness addresses a wider range of goals, needs, and values than spirituality—the material as well as the immaterial, the basic as well as the elevated, and the secular as well as the sacred. Admittedly, this definition is less consistent with the popular shift toward a more narrow view of religiousness (Zinnbauer et al., 1997). It is, however, consistent with the large and growing body of literature in the psychology of religion that has focused on the implications of various religious beliefs and practices for physical health, mental health, and social functioning (e.g., Wulff, 1997).

It is important to note that, within the psychology of religion literature, a number of theorists and investigators have labeled these "extrinsic" forms of religiousness as immature (e.g., Allport & Ross, 1967). Yet there is nothing necessarily tawdry or inappropriate about the pursuit of secular ends through sacred means. Allport himself noted that the satisfaction of basic human needs through sacred pathways sets the stage for the pursuit of more elevated spiritual destinations. In fact, the process of religious socialization is largely concerned with both facilitating the shift among adherents from immediate goals and values to more ultimate concerns and teaching people to see the sacredness in even mundane aspects of life.

In short, spirituality is highlighted as a distinctive dimension of human functioning in the second set of definitions. Spirituality alone addresses the discovery, conservation, and transformation of the most ultimate of all concerns, the sacred. Yet religiousness is not viewed as inconsistent with or an impediment to spirituality. In fact, spirituality is the core function of religion. Indeed, considerable religious energy is dedicated to helping people integrate the sacred more fully into their pathways and destinations of living. But to succeed at this task, religion accepts and attempts to address the full range of human strivings. Thus, as defined here, religiousness represents a broader phenomenon than spirituality, one that is concerned with all aspects of human functioning, sacred and profane.

Implications of the Different Definitions

As we have argued throughout the chapter, the ways in which religiousness and spirituality are defined have implications for psychological inquiry. Accordingly, the definitions presented above each have different strengths.

Presenting spirituality as a broader construct than religiousness has the advantage of following recent trends by believers and psychologists who also characterize the terms in this manner. This facilitates communication with the general public and within the discipline. Its also has the potential to provide a link with other developments within psychology (e.g., positive psychology, wellness, spirituality and medicine, the study of virtues) that have begun to investigate spiritual phenomena without acknowledging the long history of scholarship within the psychology of religion (Park, 2003).

Presenting religiousness as the broader process has the advantage of maintaining continuity with a century of research and scholarship within the psychology of religion. It also allows for the study of extrinsic religiousness and thus maintains breadth within the field. By defining religiousness in a broad and inclusive manner, sacred paths taken toward secular goals are explicitly included as phenomena of psychological inquiry.

Finally, presenting any scholarly definition of religiousness or spirituality runs the risk of contradicting a given individual's self-definition. For example, in contrast to the first of the above definitions, a believer could describe her spirituality as membership in a church, or her religion as taking personal time to pursue a hobby. Clearly, as alluded to previously in the discussion of etic and emic definitions, the tension between a diversity of definitions and a cumulative science must be mindfully addressed. There may well be times when scholars define these terms differently from believers. It becomes necessary in these cases to be explicit about the meanings of the terms, to explicate and operationalize the constructs clearly in research and writing, and to remain aware that over time the constructs may continue to change or evolve.

RECOMMENDATIONS AND FUTURE DIRECTIONS

Over the past century, religiousness and spirituality have been investigated in a number of different ways and from a number of different perspectives. Modern investigations make clearer demarcations between the terms than traditional ones, sometimes with mixed results. Unfortunately, many recent characterizations polarize religiousness and spirituality in ways that fail to reflect the length and breadth of religious and spiritual experience.

It is clear that religiousness and spirituality are fundamental human processes and phenomena. As such, they cannot be reduced to other processes, or limited to a single level of analysis. Instead, investigations must account for the micro and the macro, the individual and the social, the particular and the universal, the subjective and the objective, and the meaning and the manifestations of religiousness and spirituality.

Religiousness and spirituality both involve the sacred. The notion of the sacred offers some much-needed boundaries for the psychology of religion and spirituality, yet is broad enough to incorporate both traditional and nontraditional expressions. Both constructs are also best understood as active processes of search that involve efforts to discover, conserve, and transform whatever may be held of greatest significance. Furthermore, both constructs extend up and down the various levels of analysis, and have developmental trajectories that reflect and influence other strands of human development.

We have not tried to resolve all of the definitional questions in this chapter. For instance, we have presented two sets of definitions of religiousness and spirituality that reflect two competing trends in the field: the belief that spirituality is broader than religiousness and the belief that religiousness is broader than spirituality.

Based upon the ongoing evolution of these terms, the following general recommendations are given regarding the meaning and measurement of these constructs. First, context must be accounted for when studying the religiousness or spirituality of individuals or groups. The search for the sacred can take place within and outside organized faith traditions, and can be impacted by sacred and secular elements at all levels of analysis. Second, the term religiousness has changed in popular use from a broad construct to a narrowly defined one. Measures of both religiousness and spirituality need to be included by researchers in their investigations of the sacred. Studies that link self-rated religiousness to various outcomes may yield different results today than in the past based upon these changes in definition. And finally, the meanings attributed to the terms religiousness and spirituality by individuals and groups must be assessed on an ongoing basis to ensure that researchers and participants are in agreement. A shared understanding cannot be assumed.

The field is poised to enter a new phase of investigation that welcomes multidimensional/multilevel models and characterizations of its two core constructs. Thus, today, psychologists investigating religiousness and spirituality have the opportunity to bridge barriers that have limited inquiry in the past. Etic and emic differences, objective and subjective truths, research and clinical practice relevancy, local and universal truths, and science and hermeneutics may begin to be reconciled. There is much work to be done, but many to share it, and a great deal of interest and enthusiasm to energize the process.

Within the next several decades one thing is certain. Social and technological changes will continue to alter human culture and communication dramatically, leading to changes in all spheres of life. We stand at the edge of tomorrow, curious about some of the most fundamental human beliefs, feelings, and experiences. And whereas the field may evolve in due time to use methods and means currently undreamt of, current movements toward multidimensional/multilevel paradigms appear to hold great promise.

REFERENCES

Allport, G. W. (1966). The religious context of prejudice. *Journal for the Scientific Study of Religion, 5*, 447–457.

Allport, G .W., & Ross, J. M. (1967). Personal religious orientation and prejudice. *Journal of Personality and Social Psychology, 5*, 432–443.

American Psychological Association. (2003). Guidelines on multicultural education, training, research, practice, and organizational change for psychologists. *American Psychologist, 58*, 377–402.

Argyle, M., & Beit-Hallahmi, B. (1975). *The social psychology of religion*. London: Routledge.

Armstrong, T. D. (1995, August). *Exploring spirituality: The development of the Armstrong Measure of Spirituality*. Paper presented at the annual convention of the American Psychological Association, New York, NY.

Batson, C. D., Schoenrade, P., & Ventis, W. L. (1993). *Religion and the individual: A social- psychological perspective*. New York: Oxford University Press.

Beck, D. E., & Cowan, C. C. (1996). *Spiral dynamics: Mastering values, leadership, and change*. Malden, MA: Blackwell.

Bellah, R. N. (1970). *Beyond belief*. New York: Harper & Row.

Belzen, J. A. (2002, Spring). Developing science infrastructure: The International Association for Psychology of Religion after its reconstitution. *Newsletter of the Psychology of Religion, 27*, 1–12.

Benner, D. G. (1989). Toward a psychology of spirituality: Implications for personality and psychotherapy. *Journal of Psychology and Christianity, 5*, 19–30.

Berger, P. (1967). *The sacred canopy: Elements of a sociological theory of religion*. New York: Doubleday.

Bourguignon, E. (1989). Trance and shamanism: What's in a name? *Journal of Psychoactive Drugs, 21*, 9–15.

Brady, M. J., Peterman, A. H., Fitchett, G., Mo, M., & Cella, D. (1999). A case for including spirituality in quality of life measurement in oncology. *Psycho-Oncology, 8*, 417–428.

Bruce, S. (1996). *Religion in the modern world: From cathedrals to cults*. Oxford, UK: Oxford University Press.

Carroll, J., Dudley, C., & McKinney, W. (1986). *Handbook for congregational studies*. Nashville, TN: Abingdon Press.

Chatters, L. M., & Taylor, R. J. (2003). The role of social context in religion. *Journal of Religious Gerontology, 14*, 139–152.

Clark, W. H. (1958). How do social scientists define religion? *Journal of Social Psychology, 47*, 143–147.

Coe, G. A. (1900). *The spiritual life: Studies in the science of religion*. New York: Eaton & Mains.

Cook, S. W., Borman, P. D., Moore, M. A., & Kunkel, M. A. (2000). College students' perceptions of spiritual people and religious people. *Journal of Psychology and Theology, 28,* 125–137.

Corrigan, P., McCorkle, B., Schell, B., & Kidder, K. (2003). *Religion and spirituality in the lives of people with serious mental illness.* Manuscript submitted for publication.

Dollahite, D. C. (1998). Fathering, faith, and spirituality. *Journal of Men's Studies, 7,* 3–15.

Doyle, D. (1992). Have we looked beyond the physical and psychosocial? *Journal of Pain and Symptom Management, 7,* 302–311.

Durkheim, E. (1915). *The elementary forms of religious life.* New York: Free Press.

Elkins, D. N. (1995). Psychotherapy and spirituality: Toward a theory of the soul. *Journal of Humanistic Psychology, 35,* 78–98.

Elkins, D. N., Hedstrom, L. J., Hughes, L. L., Leaf, J. A., & Saunders, C. (1988). Toward a humanistic-phenomenological spirituality: Definition, description, and measurement. *Journal of Humanistic Psychology, 28,* 5–18.

Ellis, A. (1980). Psychotherapy and atheistic values: A response to A. E. Bergin's "Psychotherapy and Religious Values." *Journal of Consulting and Clinical Psychology, 48,* 635–639.

Emblen, J. D. (1992). Religion and spirituality defined according to current use in nursing literature. *Journal of Professional Nursing, 8,* 41–47.

Emmons, R. A. (1999). *The psychology of ultimate concerns: Motivation and spirituality in personality.* New York: Guilford Press.

Emmons, R. A., & Paloutzian, R. F. (2003). The psychology of religion. *Annual Review of Psychology, 54,* 377–402.

Fahlberg, L. L., & Fahlberg, L. A. (1991). Exploring spirituality and consciousness with an expanded science: Beyond the ego with empiricism, phenomenology, and contemplation. *American Journal of Health Promotion, 5,* 273–281.

Freud, S. (1961). The future of an illusion. In J. Strachey (Ed. and Trans.), *The standard edition of the complete psychological works of Sigmund Freud* (Vol. 11, pp. 5–56). London: Hogarth Press. (Original work published 1927)

Fromm, E. (1950). *Psychoanalysis and religion.* New Haven, CT: Yale University Press.

Goldberg, R. S. (1990). The transpersonal element in spirituality and psychiatry. *Psychiatric Residents Newsletter, 10,* 9.

Gorsuch, R. (1984). Measurement: The boon and bane of investigating religion. *American Psychologist, 39,* 228–236.

Hall, G. S. (1904). *Adolescence: Its psychology and its relations to physiology, anthropology, sociology, sex, crime, religion, and education* (2 Vols.). New York: Appleton.

Hall, G. S. (1917). *Jesus, the Christ, in light of psychology.* New York: Doubleday.

Hall, T. W., & Gorman, M. (2003, Spring). Relational spirituality: Implications of the convergence of attachment theory, interpersonal neurobiology, and emotional information processing. *Newsletter of the Psychology of Religion, 28,* 1–12.

Hart, T. (1994). *The hidden spring: The spiritual dimension of therapy.* New York: Paulist Press.

Hill, P. C., & Pargament, K. I (2003). Advances in the conceptualization and measurement of religion and spirituality: Implications for physical and mental health research. *American Psychologist, 58,* 64–74.

Hill, P. C., Pargament, K. I., Hood, R. W., McCullough, M. E., Swyers, J. P., Larson, D. B., & Zinnbauer, B. J. (2000). Conceptualizing religion and spirituality: Points of commonality, points of departure. *Journal for the Theory of Social Behavior, 30,* 51–77.

Hood, R. W. (2003). The relationship between religion and spirituality. *Defining Religion: Investigating the Boundaries between the Sacred and Secular Religion and the Social Order, 10,* 241–265.

Hood, R. W., Spilka, B., Hunsberger, B., & Gorsuch, R. L. (1996). *The psychology of religion: An empirical approach.* New York: Guilford Press.

Hunt, R. A. (1972). Mythological-symbolic religious commitment: The LAM Scales. *Journal for the Scientific Study of Religion, 11,* 42–52.

Huxley, A. (1944). *The perennial philosophy*. New York: Harper & Row.

Idinopulos, T. A., & Yonan E. A. (Eds.). (1994). *Religion and reductionism*. Leiden: Brill.

Idinopulos, T. A., & Yonan, E. A. (Eds.). (1996). *The sacred and its scholars*. Leiden: Brill.

James, W. (1961). *The varieties of religious experience*. New York: Collier Books. (Original work published 1902)

Johnson, P. E. (1959). *Psychology of religion*. Nashville, TN: Abingdon Press.

Kass, J. D., Friedman, R., Lesserman, J., Zuttermeister, P., & Benson, H. (1991). Health outcomes and a new index of spiritual experience. *Journal for the Scientific Study of Religion, 30,* 203–211.

McReady, W. C., & Greeley, A. M. (1976). *The ultimate values of the American population* (Vol. 23). Beverly Hills, CA: Sage.

Miller, W. R. (Ed.). (1999). *Integrating spirituality into treatment*. Washington DC: American Psychological Association.

Miller, W. R., & Thoresen, C. E. (2003). Spirituality, religion, and health: An emerging research field. *American Psychologist, 58,* 24–35.

Moberg, D. O. (2002). Assessing and measuring spirituality: Confronting dilemmas of universal and particular evaluative criteria. *Journal of Adult Development, 9,* 47–60.

Nelson-Becker, H. (2003). Practical philosophies: Interpretations of religion and spirituality by African American and European American elders. *Journal of Religious Gerontology, 14,* 85–100.

O'Collins, G., & Farrugia, E. G. (1991). *A concise dictionary of theology*. New York: Paulist Press.

Pargament, K. I. (1997). *The psychology of religion and coping*. New York: Guilford Press.

Pargament, K. I. (1999). The psychology of religion and spirituality?: Yes and no. *The International Journal for the Psychology of Religion, 9,* 3–16.

Pargament, K. I., & Mahoney, A. (2002). Spirituality: Discovering and conserving the sacred. In C. R. Synder & S. J. Lopez (Eds.), *Handbook of positive psychology* (pp. 646–659). Oxford, UK: Oxford University Press.

Pargament, K. I., Sullivan, M. S., Balzer, W. K., Van Haitsma, K. S., & Raymark, P. H. (1995). The many meanings of religiousness: A policy capturing approach. *Journal of Personality, 63,* 953–983.

Park, C. (2003, Fall). The psychology of religion and positive psychology. *Psychology of Religion Newsletter, 28,* 1–8.

Peteet, J. R. (1994). Approaching spiritual problems in psychotherapy: A conceptual framework. *Journal of Psychotherapy Practice and Research, 3,* 237–245.

Powell, L. H., Shahabi, L., & Thoresen, C. E. (2003). Religion and spirituality: Linkages to physical health. *American Psychologist, 58,* 36–52.

Reich, K. H. (1998, Winter). Psychology of religion and the coordination of two or more views: From William James to present day approaches (Part I). *Psychology of Religion Newsletter, 23,* 1–5, 8.

Richards, P. S., & Bergin, A. E. (1997). *A spiritual strategy for counseling and psychotherapy*. Washington, DC: American Psychological Association.

Richards, P. S., & Bergin, A. E. (Eds.). (2000). *Handbook of psychotherapy and religious diversity*. Washington, DC: American Psychological Association.

Roof, W. C. (1993). *A generation of seekers: The spiritual journeys of the baby-boomer generation*. San Francisco: HarperCollins.

Roof, W. C. (1998). Modernity, the religious, and the spiritual. In W. C. Roof (Ed.), *Americans and religions in the twenty-first century*. Thousand Oaks, CA: Sage.

Scott, A. B. (1997). *Categorizing definitions of religion and spirituality in the psychological literature: A content analytic approach*. Unpublished manuscript. Bowling Green State University, Bowling Green, OH.

Seeman, T. E., Dubin, L. F., & Seeman, M. (2003). Religiosity/spirituality and health. *American Psychologist, 58,* 53–63.

Segal, R. A. (1994). Reductionism in the study of religion. In T. A. Idinopulos & E. A. Yonan (Eds.), *Religion and reductionism* (pp. 4–14). Leiden: Brill.

Shafranske, E. P. (Ed.). (1996). *Religion and the clinical practice of psychology*. Washington, DC: American Psychological Association.

Shafranske, E. P. (2002). The necessary and sufficient conditions for an applied psychology of religion. *Psychology of Religion Newsletter, 27,* 1–12.

Shafranske, E. P., & Bier, W. C. (1999, Spring). Religion and the clinical practice: A continuing discussion. *Psychology of Religion Newsletter, 24,* 4–8.

Shafranske, E. P., & Gorsuch, R. L. (1984). Factors associated with the perception of spirituality in psychotherapy. *Journal of Transpersonal Psychology, 16,* 231–241.

Shahabi, L., Powell, L. H., Musick, M. A., Pargament, K. I., Thoresen, C. E., Williams, D., Underwood, L., & Ory, M. A. (2002). Correlates of self-perceptions of spirituality in American adults. *Annals of Behavioral Medicine, 24,* 59–68.

Soeken, K. L., & Carson, V. J. (1987). Responding to the spiritual needs of the chronically ill. *Nursing Clinics of North America, 22,* 603–611.

Spilka, B. (1993, August). *Spirituality: Problems and directions in operationalizing a fuzzy concept.* Paper presented at the annual conference of the American Psychological Association, Toronto, Canada.

Spilka, B., & McIntosh, D. N. (1996, August). *Religion and spirituality: The known and the unknown.* Paper presented at the annual conference of the American Psychological Association, Toronto, Canada.

Starbuck, E. D. (1899). *The psychology of religion.* New York: Scribner.

Tart, C. (1975). Introduction. In C. T. Tart (Ed.), *Transpersonal psychologies* (pp. 3–7). New York: Harper & Row.

Vande Kemp, H. (2003, Summer). Interpersonal psychologies for a religion of encounter and reconnection. *Newsletter of the Psychology of Religion, 28,* 9–11.

Vaughan, F. (1991). Spiritual issues in psychotherapy. *Journal of Transpersonal Psychology, 23,* 105–119.

Walker, L. J., & Pitts, R. C. (1998). Naturalistic conceptions of moral maturity. *Developmental Psychology, 34,* 403–419.

Wilber, K. (1995). *Sex, ecology, spirituality: The spirit of evolution.* Boston: Shambhala Press.

Wilber, K. (1999). Integral psychology. In *The collected works of Ken Wilber* (Vol. 4, pp. 423–717). Boston: Shambhala Press.

Woods, T. E., & Ironson, G. H. (1999). Religion and spirituality in the face of illness. *Journal of Health Psychology, 4,* 393–412.

Worthington, E. L. (1989). Religious faith across the lifespan: Implications for counseling and research. *Counseling Psychologist, 17,* 555–612.

Wulff, D. (1997). *Psychology of religion: Classical and contemporary.* New York: Wiley.

Zinnbauer, B. J., & Pargament, K. I. (2000). Working with the sacred: Four approaches to working with religious and spiritual issues in counseling. *Journal of Counseling and Development, 78,* 162–171.

Zinnbauer, B. J., & Pargament, K. I. (2002). Capturing the meanings of religiousness and spirituality: One way down from a definitional Tower of Babel. *Research in the Social Scientific Study of Religion, 13,* 23–54.

Zinnbauer, B. J., Pargament, K. I., Cole, B., Rye, M. S., Butter, E. M., Belavich, T. G., Hipp, K. M., Scott, A. B., & Kadar, J. L. (1997). Religion and spirituality: Unfuzzying the fuzzy. *Journal for the Scientific Study of Religion, 36,* 549–564.

Zinnbauer, B. J., Pargament, K. I., & Scott, A. B. (1999). The emerging meanings of religiousness and spirituality: Problems and prospects. *Journal of Personality, 67,* 889–919.

3

Measurement in the Psychology of Religion and Spirituality

Current Status and Evaluation

PETER C. HILL

Emmons and Paloutzian (2003) suggest that the psychology of religion is now entering what they call a *multilevel interdisciplinary paradigm* that "recognizes the value of data at multiple levels of analysis while making nonreductive assumptions concerning the value of spiritual and religious phenomena" (p. 395). Indeed, Emmons and Palotuzian have identified the contemporary pulse of religious and spiritual research and rightfully claim this to be a dominant constellation of values and techniques. However, paradigmatic change suggests that some existing paradigm had to serve the field well until its useful value was fulfilled (Kuhn, 1970). Gorsuch (1984), in a highly influential *American Psychologist* article, claimed that the then current paradigm in the scientific study of religion was one of measurement.

ASSESSING THE CURRENT STATE OF RELIGIOUS AND SPIRITUAL MEASUREMENT

Measurement's Boon and Bane

The success of the measurement paradigm, Gorsuch (1984) argued, was both a boon and a bane to the psychology of religion. It is clear that the ability to reliably measure is a key indicator of a developing field's health and maturity. Moreover, instruments produced during the psychology of religion's age of measurement were in Gorsuch's words "reasonably effective" and "available in sufficient variety for most any task in the psychology of religion" (p. 234). At the least, the fact that psychologists of religion had a long-standing concern with measurement issues suggests that continued attention will (and should) be devoted to measurement issues, as noted in several chapters within this volume (e.g., Paloutzian & Park, Chapter 1, this volume; Zinnbauer & Pargament, Chapter 2, this volume; see also Hill & Pargament, 2003). To this extent, the measurement paradigm has been good to the psychology of religion.

Gorsuch (1984), however, also reminded us that measurement success can be a bane in that such success can reinforce an interest in measurement itself, and not the objects of measurement. In fact, Gorsuch later (1988) appeared to suggest that it was now time for the psychology of religion to move beyond the measurement paradigm's search for the elusive conceptually pure measure. Perhaps such warnings helped set the stage for the paradigm shift to today's multilevel interdisciplinary focus.

In yet another article, Gorsuch (1990) contended that researchers should not develop new scales until a clear need can be established on one of four bases: (1) existing measures are not psychometrically adequate to the task; (2) conceptual or theoretical issues demand modification of existing measures; (3) no existing measures appear useful within a specific clinical population; or (4) there are no measures available for particular constructs. Indeed, modification of existing measures, the second criterion listed above, is sometimes necessary in this young and developing field, especially since people's understanding of religion appears, as noted earlier, to be undergoing change. Furthermore, religious and spiritual measures designed for clinical populations (the third criterion above) are rare, and new or revised measures for such populations may be necessary. And, surely, with regard to the fourth criterion, there are specific functional or operational relationships that religion and spirituality may have with other variables that call for specific new measures (e.g., religious coping with stressful agents). All too often, however, Gorsuch's advice has been largely ignored and many new measures, some unnecessarily duplicating other measures, have been constructed. In fact, since Hill and Hood's (1999) edited volume reviewing 125 scales, many new scales (some of which are discussed in this chapter) have been developed, perhaps in some cases unnecessarily so.

This is all to say that the study of religion and spirituality is now largely beyond the point of just focusing on measurement issues and is ready to apply many already existing instruments to various research domains. Therefore, while one cannot say with authority that no new religious or spiritual measures should be developed, it is safe to say that many existing measures have been underutilized and researchers can find adequate measures for religious and spiritual constructs of substantial variety. Researchers are thus encouraged to refrain from constructing new measures and instead to utilize and, if necessary, modify existing assessment instruments. As Miller (1998) stated when addressing the rarity of empirical studies involving religious and spiritual constructs in addictions research, "it is not for lack of reliable instrumentation" (p. 980).

Measurement Hurdles and Advances

If what has been said is indicative of measurement success, it is not uncritically so. While it is true that the variety of scales do a respectably good job of measuring religiousness, collectively they are not without limits and deficiencies. Some of these limitations are due to the inherently complex nature of religious and spiritual constructs; other deficiencies are the responsibility of the scientific community. Fortunately, researchers have made systematic strides in addressing many of these shortcomings.

Conceptual Clarity

What was missing from the measurement paradigm was a conceptual or theoretical focus that provides coherence to the field, resulting in a call for more systematic programs of research with stronger conceptual bases (Hill & Pargament, 2003; Kirkpatrick & Hood, 1990). Consider the case of the foremost research framework in the psychology of religion to date: Allport's (1950) intrinsic–extrinsic (I–E) religious orientation model. Driven by puzzling findings relating religion to prejudice, Allport provided a theoretical framework to the study of religious motivation by positing *intrinsic faith* as a master motive in life, an end in itself, a religion to be lived and not just used. In contrast, an *extrinsic faith* motivation, Allport maintained, tends to use religion for one's own self-interest, a means to some other end, a religion to be used rather than lived. What may have been a good theoretical beginning did not develop further and, by 1990, Kirkpatrick and Hood claimed that the I–E model was "theoretically impoverished and has really taught us little about the psychology of religion" (p. 442). The problem was that much subsequent scientific effort was spent wholly on issues of measurement despite the fact that the underlying theory had not been sufficiently developed to warrant this effort.

One cannot stress enough the foundational importance of theory-driven research to good measurement. Despite the wide variety of religious and spiritual research, little has been drawn from well-established theoretical models in mainstream psychology. Fortunately, we are beginning to see greater application to the religion and spirituality variable from such mainstream literature as the psychology of coping (Pargament, 1997; Pargament, Koenig, & Perez, 2000), attachment theory (Kirkpatrick, 1992, 1995), developmental psychology (Fowler, 1981), motivation theory (Emmons, 1999), personality theory (Paloutzian, Richardson, & Rambo, 1999), and the study of both emotion (Hill, 1995, 2002) and cognition (McIntosh, 1995). Some of these developments (e.g., religion-as-coping and religion-as-attachment) have already yielded empirically fruitful programs of research. Other research programs are in earlier stages of development. However, the key to the success of these programs is the sophistication of the theories and ideas that generated them, without which measurement is barren.

Sample Representativeness

Research in psychology has long been afflicted with unrepresentative samples, most notably convenience samples of college students who are generally younger and better educated (two variables strongly implicated in religious experience) than the population as a whole. Sampling in the psychology of religion, including samples with whom instrumentation has been developed, is not immune to this affliction. This problem of representation is further complicated by the fact that Protestantism dominates the samples found in much of the literature investigating religiousness (Gorsuch, 1988, 1990; Hill & Hood, 1999). While such domination is understandable demographically (at least historically in the United States), it is nonetheless problematic when desiring to use a scale with a more pluralistic population. In contrast, if one is interested in developing measures of spirituality (especially nontheistic or transpersonal spirituality), it is important that the "traditionally" religious (e.g., people who identify with such designations as Protestants, Catholics, Jews, Greek Orthodox, etc.) not be *under*represented which, if the researcher needs a scale representing a broad population (e.g., North Americans), is equally problematic as Protestant *over*representation.

Cultural Sensitivity

Measures of religiousness also sometimes do not reflect sensitivity to cultural variables (Chatters, Taylor, & Lincoln, 2002), a deficiency clearly related to the problem of adequate sample representation (for a review of cultural issues in testing, see Sandoval, Frisby, Geisinger, Ramos-Grenier, & Scheuneman, 1998). Of course, differences in religious and spiritual perspectives, affiliations, and practices are often related to cultural factors, and thus the representation problem is not just one of Protestant overrepresentation, but also one of white, middle-class, U.S., and sometimes male overrepresentation as well. Hill and Pargament (2003) have noted that, even within U.S. Protestantism, cultural insensitivity has been demonstrated when measuring African Americans— perhaps the most Protestant of all ethnic groups. While some scale items may be directly offensive, perhaps a more common deficiency is either to emphasize irrelevant issues (or issues of secondary importance) or to deemphasize issues of great importance (e.g., a strong ethos of community service [Ellison & Taylor, 1996] and the notion of reciprocal blessings with God [Black, 1999]) to the African American church. When attempting to create or modify existing measures to generalize research to non-Western religious traditions, the need for cultural sensitivity is even further magnified (Hill & Pargament, 2003).

It is not uncommon for researchers to attempt to develop a measure of spirituality that is not linked to specific religious traditions. Of course, the idea is that such a measure can be used across religious traditions and may also be of value in assessing those who see themselves as spiritual but not religious. Such an approach assumes that one can validly assess a generic spiritual experience without focusing on substantive and perhaps functional issues associated with specific traditions, and may thus demonstrate a pluralistic ignorance not unlike other cultural insensitivities. Still, however, certain religious and spiritual functional characteristics likely generalize across traditions (and perhaps to the spiritual but nonreligious population as well), and the identification of such generalized functions is of value to the field. One skeptic regarding the generic approach (Moberg, 2002) suggests that constructing such a measure "that will be recognized as ontologically authentic in every religious and philosophical sphere may be as elusive as capturing the mythical pot of gold at the foot of the rainbow" (p. 58), but still admits that it may "serendipitously yield vastly increased understanding of the spiritual nature of humanity and of the means by which to enhance spiritual well-being and maturity" (p. 58). Clearly, one solution is to create general (or tradition-specific) measures from which parallel tradition-specific (or general) measures can be further developed.

Sustained Research Programs

A major problem in the area has been the failure to develop sustained research programs using standardized measures. While notable exceptions exist, such as Batson's (Batson, Schoenrade, & Ventis, 1993) extensive research program on religious questing, Hood's (1975, 1995, 1997) research with his *Mysticism Scale*, Pargament's (1997) programmatic use of his religious coping measures, and perhaps most notably the extensive and diverse tradition of research with varieties of intrinsic–extrinsic religious orientation scales (see Donahue, 1985, and Hood, Spilka, Hunsberger, & Gorsuch, 1996, for reviews), many measures have been utilized in only a few (if any) studies beyond their original development.

At least three reasons for the lack of continuing systematic research can be proffered. First, without a clear conceptual understanding of religion and spirituality, it is difficult to generate and maintain sustained research programs. As pointed out earlier, the study of religion has not had strong theoretical underpinnings. Second, funding for research on religion has until recently been virtually nonexistent. Third, because of this lack of funding, much religious research has been conducted within the context of other research agendas, often with religion, in particular, as an "add-on" variable only. As a result, measures of religion have often been imprecise, frequently involving single-item measures of general religious identification or church attendance (see Larson, Swyers, & McCullough, 1998). Of course, single-item measures are less reliable and contain more measurement error, are vulnerable to small wording changes, are especially problematic for cross-cultural adaptation or comparisons (Braithwaite & Scott, 1991), and should therefore be used only as a last resort.

Measurement in the psychology of religion has paid a price for this lack of systematic research. First, issues of scale validity are difficult to assess. Second, there is an absence and inutility of normative data for many of the scales. Though clearly defined norms are not necessary for scales used solely for research purposes, it is important to consider the samples upon which instruments have been used to establish psychometric adequacy. Many scales, especially those published before the 1980s, have not been used beyond their initial introduction (see Hill & Hood, 1999), so in such cases any validity assessments or normative data are usually based upon a single sample. Fortunately, however, given the recent proliferation of research in the field, we are beginning to see repeated usage of some measures, particularly those more recently developed (e.g., in the past 20 years).

Alternatives to Self-Report Measures

As in many other research domains, measures of religion and spirituality tend to rely primarily on paper-and-pencil self-reports. As Hill and Pargament (2003) point out, the well-documented limitations of self-reports in other domains of study apply equally well to investigating religiousness: (1) some aspects of religion and spirituality may be inadequately measured because they are difficult to articulate through closed-ended questions; (2) religion and spirituality may be especially susceptible to a social desirability bias (Batson et al., 1993); (3) such scales may require reading levels beyond the ability of children, poorly educated adults, and some clinical populations; and (4) some paper-and-pencil measures may be boring or disengaging, thereby fostering a potential response set bias. Several alternative methodologies are currently being explored by religious researchers: attitude accessibility (measured by response time) as an implicit indicator of the importance or centrality of religion (Hill, 1994); pictures to assess religious understandings (Bassett et al., 1990) or religious coping (Pendleton, Cavilli, Pargament, & Nasr, 2002); and physiological indicators such as computerized tomography and positron-emission tomography scans (Newberg, d'Aquili, & Rause, 2001).

APPROACH TO THE REVIEW OF INDIVIDUAL SCALES

To discuss all available measures is beyond the scope of this chapter and would be redundant in light of the reviews already completed in Hill and Hood (1999). Instead, a number of promising scales that demonstrate reasonably strong psychometric properties (based on four criteria identified and discussed below) are highlighted through use of a two-level hierarchical model to the construct organization of religion and spirituality recommended by Tsang and McCullough (2003). Within each level, many of the categories recommended by the Fetzer Institute/National Institute of Aging Working Group (1999) on religion and spirituality are used. Space prohibits even a brief discussion of promising measures from each domain. Instead, recommended measures of each domain are listed in Appendix 3.1, with an attempt to minimize listing and discussion of scales with considerable overlap. The scales listed are therefore not a complete listing but stand as examples of the more sophisticated scales designed to assess each domain.

A Hierarchical Approach

Tsang and McCullough (2003) propose that religion be viewed as a hierarchically structured psychological domain with "higher levels of organization reflecting broad individual differences among persons in highly abstracted, trait-like qualities," whereby "the goal of measurement is to assess broad dispositional differences in religious tendencies or traits so that one might draw conclusions about how 'religious' a person is" (p. 349). This superordinate dispositional level of organization (what they call "Level I") can be used to measure a general religious factor that may predict many other variables (Gorsuch, 1984).

The subordinate level in the hierarchy proposed by Tsang and McCullough (2003) is what they call the "operational level" in that "people manifest tremendous diversity in how they experience religious (and spiritual) realities, their motivations for being religious, and their deployment of their religion to solve problems in the world" (pp. 349–350). This lower functional level of organization (what they call "Level II") often assesses subdimensions of the general religiousness factor and is useful in predicting more specific variables to see a complete relationship. Hence, highly religious people may use religion in different ways to help cope with specific stressors. Recognizing that the two levels of the hierarchy do not function independently, Tsang and McCullough correctly maintain that the general nature and functional operations of religiousness are complex and propose that before researchers explore Level II functional or operational variables, they should first control for the more general Level I religiousness factor to disentangle the operational variable from the more general trait-like quality. Tsang and McCullough's hierarchical approach provides a helpful distinction that will be useful in reviewing a number of measures used in the psychology of religion. Their terminology of Level I and Level II measures for dispositional and operational (or functional) levels of organization, respectively, is borrowed for the remaining part of this chapter.

Given that there is surely a finite number of ways to conceptualize general religiousness, it seems that Gorsuch's (1984) claim of a sufficient availability of measures is especially true for Level I measures. However, as we discover more ways in which religion is individually experienced and deployed, further precise measures at the functional Level II may yet need to be constructed.

Four Criteria

Four criteria for evaluating scales were used and are summarized in Table 3.1: theoretical structure, representative sampling/generalization, measures of reliability, and measures of validity. Four levels of each criterion ranging from "exemplary" to "none or minimal" are presented in the table. These levels are not meant to be absolute and could surely be refuted, especially when such descriptors as "exemplary" or "minimally acceptable" are used. Also, the purpose here is not to grade each measure listed in Appendix 3.1 on each of the four criteria. Rather, the purpose is simply to demonstrate how measurement suc-

TABLE 3.1. General Rating Criteria for Evaluating Measures of Religion or Spirituality

Criterion	Criterion rating			
	Exemplary (rating = 3)	Good (2)	Acceptable (1)	Minimal or None (0)
Theoretical basis	Clearly grounded in well-established (perhaps dominant) theoretical framework	Clearly grounded in a plausible but not necessarily consensual theoretical framework	Only partially well connected to theory	Theory is posed but connection to theory is unclear or the theory is suspect; no theory discussed
Sample representativeness/ generalization	Clearly represents a broadly conceived population, not limited by a religious tradition or narrow spirituality	Clearly represents by design a less broadly conceived population (e.g., Christians, people in treatment, etc.)	Clearly represents by design a narrowly conceived population (e.g., Evangelicals, Mormons) or a less clear representation of a broader population	Limited to a restrictive sample in one study only; clearly not representative of population or sample not identified
Reliability (coefficient alpha or test–retest at minimum 2 weeks)	Excellent ($r > .80$) across two or more studies	Good ($r = .70$ to $.80$) across two or more studies	Excellent ($r > .80$) or good ($r = .70$ to $.80$) in one study only; moderate ($r = .60$ to $.70$) in two or more studies	Moderate ($r = .60$ to $.70$) or low ($r < .60$) in one study only; no reliability reported
Validity	Highly significant correlations across multiple (diverse) samples from different studies on at least two types of validity	Significant correlations across multiple samples (from one study or multiple studies) on at least two types of validity	Significant correlations on at least two types of validity on only one sample or one type of validity on multiple samples	Significant correlations on only one measure of validity on only one sample; no significant correlations found

cess is defined in the psychology of religion and also to communicate a basis for how the scales included for review here were selected. Specifically, only scales that would achieve at least "acceptable" ratings on all four criteria were selected for review. Most of the scales reviewed here, however, clearly exceed the acceptable rating on more than one criterion.

Theoretical Basis

Consideration of the theoretical basis of a measure involves two criteria: (1) the scale itself should have a theoretical underpinning and (2) the researcher should also have a clear theoretical basis for the research at hand. Unfortunately, for reasons already discussed (e.g., complex multidimensional constructs, religion or spirituality as an "add-on" variable only, lack of sustained research programs), empirical research on the religion variable, including that which has involved the development of instruments, has often lacked a strong theoretical basis. Preference for inclusion here was given to scales developed in the context of larger theoretical programs.

Representative Sampling and Generalization

As already discussed, deficiencies in sampling are common and researchers are cautioned to recognize that, for example, scales that measure non-Protestant religion are frequently underrepresented, and that as one moves to non-Western religious traditions relevant scales are quite rare (though such scales are beginning to be developed). Somewhat related is the subtle, but significant, problem that many measures of religion likely reflect Christian religious biases, even when not explicitly identified as measures of Christian religion (Heelas, 1985).

Ideally, then, what we would have is a measure that clearly represents a broadly conceived population that is limited neither by a religious tradition (hence, a measure of religion that cuts across all religions) nor by a narrow spirituality (e.g., one that is defined by only one dimension). At the opposite extreme is a nonrepresentative sample or a representative sample of such a narrow population (e.g., members of a local church school class or students at a particular denominational college) that renders the sample meaningless for research purposes. Thus, for the broader research community, there are two dimensions to consider: the representation of the sample to its population and the breadth of the population for generalization.

Reliability

Scale reliability when measuring religiousness or spirituality is typically assessed through two techniques: (1) internal consistency describing the internal structure of the scale, and (2) test–retest reliability. The majority of scales rely on internal consistency reliability, the most common of which is Cronbach's (1951) coefficient alpha, while the test–retest measure of reliability is used less frequently. The use of parallel forms for reliability testing of instruments in psychology of religion research is exceedingly rare.

There is a practical issue to consider with regard to reliability. Though the statistical reliability of a scale suffers when there are relatively few items that comprise the scale, short scales are appealing because they are generally more feasible, especially when the measure of religion or spirituality is part of a larger battery of research or clinical instruments. Also, short scales are attractive and sometimes necessary for research involving large samples, which, in turn, allows researchers to retain the scale's statistical power. Many of these same trade-offs are involved in validity issues as well.

Validity

Validity, of course, is the question of whether the instrument measures what in fact it claims to be measuring. Issues regarding validity have been interspersed throughout this chapter and have usually been alluded to in the context of two concerns: problems of validity due to nonrepresentative samples (usually where a U.S. Protestant orientation is overrepresented) and problems of validity due to a lack of sustained research programs across different samples. Nevertheless, the scales reviewed here are not without some validity claims.

Whereas reliability of religiousness measures tends to be assessed primarily by internal consistency, validity assessment is more heterogeneous. At least one of the four following methods (with each method well represented among the scales discussed here) of determining validity is used in most scales: (1) convergent validity, (2) factorial validity, (3) criterion-related validity (either "known-groups" or discriminant validity), and (4) content validity. Determining content validity is quite subjective and is therefore not included as a validity criterion in Table 3.1.

DISCUSSION OF SELECTED SCALES

Many of the scales listed in Appendix 3.1 could be included in categories other than the one listed. Representative scales from selected domains are now briefly discussed.

Level 1: Measures of Dispositional Religiousness

Scales That Assess General Religiousness or Spirituality

The attempt here is to assess religious or spiritual differences between people, perhaps as broadly as a personality trait that may be independent of the Big Five personality dimensions. Tsang and McCullough (2003) cite evidence from three sources that suggests indirect support for the existence of such a broad characteristic: (1) conceptually meaningful correlations among distinct aspects of religiousness (e.g., church attendance, engagement in private religious practices, self-rated importance of religion) found especially in homogenous cultural groups; (2) factors found within multiple-item measures that are frequently intercorrelated, suggesting some higher order factor; and (3) evidence that religiousness may be partially heritable (see D'Onofrio, Eaves, Murrelle, Maes, & Spilka, 1999). Piedmont's (1999) *Spiritual Transcendence Scale* and Hood's (1975) *Mysticism Scale* are examples that measure general spiritual orientations (transcendent or mystical orientations in these cases) without reference to a specific religious tradition. Though the Rohrbaugh and Jessor (1975) eight-item unidimensional measure of general religiousness is heavily influenced by a general Western religious perspective, it too attempts to measure an orientation toward a transcendent reality independent of a particular religious creed.

Paloutzian and Ellison's (1982) 20-item *Spiritual Well-Being Scale* (SWBS) has become a standard-bearer in the religious and spiritual well-being literature and has been used in hundreds of studies. (A far more extensive but time-consuming and less-used measure of religious and spiritual well-being is Moberg's [1984] *Spiritual Well-Being Questionnaire.*) The SWBS has three dimensions: a religious well-being (RWB) dimension, an existential well-being (EWB) dimension, and an overall spiritual well-being (SWB) dimension that is the combined RWB and EWB scores. The RWB items cluster together as one factor, thus suggesting a general religiousness measure. Through its frequent use, the SWBS has well-established convergent and discriminant validity, though it is subject to ceiling effects among conservative religious populations (Ledbetter, Smith, Vosler-Hunter, & Fischer, 1991).

Scales That Assess Religious or Spiritual Commitment

One way of defining a general dispositional measure is to assess the degree to which a person is religiously committed. Though some measures of religious commitment might better assess a functional element of religious experience (e.g., the motivating force of an intrinsic religious orientation), the measures listed here clearly identify a reliable assessment of general religiousness.

The *Religious Commitment Inventory* (RCI-10; Worthington et al., 2003) is a 10-item measure of religious commitment that has been tested on individuals from a variety of religious traditions (Christians, Buddhists, Muslims, Hindus). Though a two-factor structure was supported, the two factors are highly intercorrelated, suggesting that this measure best be used as a full-scale assessment of general religious commitment. The RCI-10 shows good internal consistency, 3-week and 5-month test–retest reliability, and construct as well as discriminant validity.

The *Santa Clara Strength of Religious Faith Questionnaire* (SCSRFQ; Plante & Boccaccini, 1997) is a 10-item scale designed to measure the strength of religious faith in the general population, not just among people who rate themselves as religious. If brevity of assessment is necessary, a five-item short form (SCSRFQ-SF) has also been developed (Plante, Vallaeys, Sherman, & Wallston, 2002) with a single-factor structure that includes all five items with good internal consistency and convergent validity (Storch et al., 2004).

Scales That Assess Religious or Spiritual Development

The *Faith Maturity Scale* by Benson, Donahue, and Erickson (1993) is a 38-item scale, the purpose of which is to measure "the degree to which a person embodies the priorities, commitments, and perspectives characteristic of vibrant and life transforming faith, as these have been understood in 'mainline' Protestant traditions" (p. 3). Thus, the focus of this measure tends to emphasize values or behavioral manifestations of faith rather than belief content (Tisdale, 1999).

The *Spiritual Assessment Inventory* (Hall & Edwards, 1996) measures spiritual development or maturity from both an object relations and a contemplative spirituality perspective. The scale is limited to a Western Christian context (e.g., it stresses an individual relationship with God), and most of the initial testing of the scale has been conducted among religious college students. However, the scale has a strong theoretical base and is currently used in numerous research programs involving more general populations.

Leak and his colleagues have recently created two promising measures of religious development. The first is a 59-item 5-point Likert scale of *religious maturity* (Leak &

Fish, 1999) based on Allport's (1950) conceptualization of mature religion as a combination of commitment and doubt. The second is an eight-item forced-choice questionnaire of *faith development* (Leak, Loucks, & Bowlin, 1999) rooted in Fowler's (1981) theory. Both measures are well grounded in theory, both are reasonably reliable, and both demonstrate strong content, predictive, and construct validity.

Level II: Measures of Functional Religiousness

Understanding the varieties of *how* a person's religious or spiritual life is experienced is often an issue of utmost importance to psychologists of religion, especially when they are trying to uncover the mechanisms that link religion to some other phenomena. For example, when discussing the relationship of religion to physical and mental health, Hill and Pargament (2003) identified recent advances in conceptualizing and measuring religion that may be functionally relevant: perceived closeness to God, religion and spirituality as orienting or motivating forces, religious support, and religious or spiritual struggle. Below is a brief discussion of representative measures of several key religious operations or functions.

Scales That Assess Religious Social Participation

Research indicates that one of the benefits of religion and perhaps of spirituality is that it often provides a basis for social support. Measures of social participation have typically utilized single items centering around church attendance or, less frequently, financial contributions. Multi-item measures of perceived social support from one's religion are rare and, when used, are frequently included as part of a larger measure. For example, the *Religious Involvement Inventory* (Hilty & Morgan, 1985) is a multidimensional measure that demonstrates reasonably good psychometric qualities and includes a 14-item church involvement subscale. The church involvement subscale maintains comparable psychometric qualities to the entire scale and appears to be a useful measure of church participation. Thurstone and Chave's (1929) *Attitude toward the Church Scale*, whose dated wording may require modest revision, has been used in more than 30 studies (Wulff, 1999).

Scales That Assess Religious or Spiritual Private Practices

Measures of private practices are well represented in multidimensional measures including, for example, such subscales as the *religious practice dimension* of DeJong, Faulkner, and Warland's (1976) measure of religiosity, the *Christian Behavior and Home Religious Observance* subscales of the *Dimensions of Religiosity Scale* (Cornwall, Albrecht, Cunningham, & Pitcher, 1986), the *Christian Walk* subscale of Bassett's *Shepherd Scale* (Bassett et al., 1981), or the *Jewish Religious Observance* subscale of Katz's (1988) *Student Religiosity Questionnaire*. Other subscales that tend to emphasize ritualistic behavior, prayer or meditation, or reading of sacred documents are fairly common as parts of larger multidimensional measures.

The *Buddhist Beliefs and Practices Scale* (Emavardhana & Tori, 1997) is an 11-item scale with reasonably strong psychometric qualities that assesses agreement with Buddhist teachings regarding specific beliefs (e.g., the theory of karma and rebirth, the doctrine of *anatta* or no soul, etc.) and practices (e.g., observing the five precepts, practice of meditation, etc.). The *Religious Background and Behavior Scale* (Connors, Tonigan, & Miller, 1996) has good psychometric qualities, is devoted primarily to measuring private religious and spiritual practices, is less exclusively Christian in focus than many other scales, was developed for use with a clinical population, and is increasingly being used in various research programs.

Scales That Assess Religion as a Motivating Force

Though measurement issues differentiating the "flagrantly utilitarian motivation" (Burris, 1999, p. 144) underlying the extrinsic (E) religious orientation versus the " 'otherly,' nonmundane, even self-denying quality" (p. 144) of the intrinsic (I) religious orientation have been mired in methodological and theoretical debate, religious orientation remains a potentially important construct for research employing religious constructs. Gorsuch and McPherson's (1989) *Revised Religious Orientation Scale* (I–E/R) modifies the original Allport and Ross (1967) scale along the lines of Kirkpatrick's (1989) reanalysis of results from several studies of religious orientation, namely, that the extrinsic scale subdivides into two categories (personally oriented [Ep] and socially oriented [Es] extrinsicness). This brief 14-item scale, with its strong psychometric qualities, is probably the single best current measure of religious orientation, if for no other reason than its advantageous position of utilizing two decades of research findings on the I–E construct. There are a number of other measures of religious orientation (11 measures of religious orientation are reviewed in Hill & Hood, 1999) including three items from the five-item *Duke Religion Index* (Koenig, Patterson, & Meador, 1997) which, despite its brevity (an appeal if only a limited number of items can be afforded), maintains reasonably strong psychometric qualities.

There is, however, an important challenge, posited by Batson and his colleagues, suggesting that a thorough understanding of Allport's notion of a mature religious sentiment must include "the degree to which an individual's religion involves an open-ended, responsive dialogue with existential questions raised by the contradictions and tragedies of life" (Batson, Schoenrade, & Ventis, 1993, p. 169). Batson and Schoenrade's (1991a, 1991b) *Quest Scale* is an operationalization of this approach to religion that emphasizes the positive role of doubt and an appreciation for the complexities of issues when approaching life through one's religious or spiritual framework.

Scales That Assess Religious or Spiritual Experiences

Many measures of religion and spirituality stress their experiential nature. Underwood's (1999) *Daily Spiritual Experiences Scale* is "intended to measure the individual's perception of the transcendent (God, the divine) in daily life and the perception of interaction with, or involvement of, the transcendent in life . . . this domain makes spirituality its central focus and can be used effectively across many religious boundaries" (Underwood, 1999, p. 11).

Of course, religious or spiritual experiences are not necessarily positive. Many researchers are interested in documenting liabilities that may accompany religious experience. One example would be the various types of religious and spiritual struggles such as struggles with God, with others (such as family members), or within one's self. Exline's (Exline, Yali, & Sanderson, 2000) measure of *religious strain* is a psychometrically sound measure that may be useful for research on religious or spiritual struggles.

Multidimensional Measures

Many measures attempt to tap the multidimensionality of the religious or spiritual experience. The Fetzer Institute/National Institute of Aging Working Group (1999) has produced a 38-item *multidimensional measure of religion and spirituality* that cuts across their 10 conceptual domains. This measure was embedded in the 1997–1998 General Social Survey (GSS), a random national survey of the National Data Program for the Social Sciences. Initial psychometric analyses from the GSS data "support the theoretical basis of the measure and indicate it has the appropriate reliability and validity to facilitate further research" (p. 89). If a general, multidimensional measure of both religion and spirituality is needed, then this measure is clearly worthy of consideration.

CONCLUSION

The results of this analysis support Gorsuch's (1984) claim 20 years ago that the measurement paradigm in the scientific study of religion and spirituality has been largely successful and that we now have a sufficient arsenal of measurement instruments. The rise of interest among scientific researchers in religion and spirituality, much of which has occurred since Gorsuch's influential article, has triggered a further proliferation of measures—a source of concern given the complexity and conceptual confusion surrounding particularly the spirituality variable. Still, however, what has developed in this short period of time is an impressive array of measures of religious and spiritual experience for the numerous domains of the religious and spiritual experience.

APPENDIX 3.1. SPECIFIC MEASURES OF RELIGION AND SPIRITUALITY BY 12 DOMAINS

The following list of scales are grouped by nine domains of religion and spirituality as outlined by the Fetzer Institute/National Institute of Aging (1999) Working Group. Three domains (General Religiousness or Spirituality, Spiritual Development, and Religion or Spirituality as a Motivating Force) were added. Also see Hill and Hood (1999).

Level I: Measures of Dispositional Religiousness or Spirituality

1. Scales That Assess General Religiousness or Spirituality
   Mysticism Scale (Hood, 1975)
   Religiosity Measure (Rohrbaugh & Jessor, 1975)
   Spiritual Transcendence Scale (Piedmont, 1999)
   Spiritual Well-Being Scale (Paloutzian & Ellison, 1982)

2. Scales That Assess Religious or Spiritual Commitment
   Dimensions of Religious Commitment Scale (Glock & Stark, 1966)
   Religious Commitment Scale (Pfeifer & Waelty, 1995)
   Religious Commitment Inventory—10 (Worthington et al., 2003)
   Santa Clara Strength of Religious Faith Questionnaire (Plante & Boccaccini, 1997)

3. Scales That Assess Religious or Spiritual Development
   Faith Development Interview Guide (Fowler, 1981)
   Faith Development Scale (Leak, Loucks, & Bowlin, 1999)
   Faith Maturity Scale (Benson, Donahue, & Erickson, 1993)
   Religious Maturity Scale (Leak & Fish, 1999)
   Spiritual Assessment Inventory (Hall & Edwards, 1996)

4. Scales That Assess Religious or Spiritual History
   The SPIRITual History (Maugans, 1996)
   Spiritual History Scale (Hays, Meador, Branch, & George, 2001)

Level II: Measures of Functional Religiousness or Spirituality

5. Scales That Assess Religious or Spiritual Social Participation
   Attitude Toward the Church Scale (Thurstone & Chave, 1929)
   Attitude Toward Church and Religious Practices (Dynes, 1955)
   Religious Involvement Inventory (Hilty & Morgan, 1985)

6. Scales That Assess Religious or Spiritual Private Practices
   Buddhist Beliefs and Practices Scale (Emavardhana & Tori, 1997)
   Religious Background and Behavior (Connors, Tonigan, & Miller, 1996)
   Types of Prayer Scale (Poloma & Pendleton, 1989)

7. Scales That Assess Religious or Spiritual Support
   Religious Pressures Scale (Altemeyer, 1988)
   Religious Support (Krause, 1999)
   Religious Support Scale (Fiala, Bjorck, & Gorsuch, 2002)

8. Scales That Assess Religious or Spiritual Coping
   Religious Coping Scale (RCOPE) (Pargament, Koenig, & Perez, 2000)
   Religious Coping Activities Scale (Pargament et al., 1990)
   Religious Problem-Solving Scale (Pargament et al., 1988)

9. Scales That Assess Religious or Spiritual Beliefs and Values
   Christian Orthodoxy Scale (Fullerton & Hunsberger, 1982)
   Love and Guilt Oriented Dimensions of Christian Belief (McConahay & Hough, 1973)
   Loving and Controlling God Scale (Benson & Spilka, 1973)
   Religious Fundamentalism Scale (Altemeyer & Hunsberger, 1992)
   Spiritual Belief Inventory (Holland et al., 1998)
   Spiritual Belief Scale (Schaler, 1996)

10. Scales That Assess Religion or Spirituality as Motivating Forces
    Intrinsic–Extrinsic Scale—Revised (Gorsuch & McPherson, 1989)
    Quest Scale (Batson, Schoenrade, & Ventis, 1993)
    Religious Orientation Scale (Allport & Ross, 1967)
    Religious Internalization Scale (Ryan, Rigby, & King, 1993)

11. Scales That Assess Religious or Spiritual Techniques for Regulating and Reconciling Relationships

Forgiveness Scale (Brown, Gorsuch, Rosik, & Ridley, 2001)

Tendency to Forgive Measure (Brown, 2003)

Transgression-Related Interpersonal Motivations Inventory (McCullough et al., 1998)

12. Scales That Assess Religious or Spiritual Experiences

Daily Spiritual Experiences Scale (Underwood, 1999)

Index of Core Spiritual Experiences (INSPIRIT) (Kass, Friedman, Leserman, Zuttermeister, & Benson, 1991)

Religious Experiences Episode Measure (REEM) (Hood, 1970)

Religious Strain (Exline, Yali, & Sanderson, 2000)

Spiritual Experience Index-Revised (Genia, 1997)

Spiritual Orientation Inventory (Elkins, Hedstrom, Hughes, Leaf, & Saunders, 1988)

REFERENCES

Allport, G. W. (1950). *The individual and his religion.* New York: Macmillan.

Allport, G. W., & Ross, J. M. (1967). Personal religious orientation and prejudice. *Journal of Personality and Social Psychology, 5*, 432–443.

Altemeyer, B. (1988). *Enemies of freedom: Understanding right-wing authoritarianism.* San Francisco: Jossey-Bass.

Altemeyer, B., & Hunsberger, B. (1992). Authoritarianism, religious fundamentalism, quest, and prejudice. *The International Journal for the Psychology of Religion, 2*, 113–133.

Bassett, R. L., Miller, S., Anstey, K., Crafts, K., Harmon, J., Lee, Y., Parks, J., Robinson, M., Smid, H., Sterner, W., Stevens, C., Wheeler, B., & Stevenson, D. H. (1990). Picturing God: A nonverbal measure of God concept for conservative Protestants. *Journal of Psychology and Christianity, 9*(2), 73–81.

Bassett, R. L., Sadler, R. D., Kobischen, E. E., Skiff, D. M., Merrill, I. J., Atwater, B. J., & Livermore, P. W. (1981). The Shepherd Scale: Separating the sheep from the goats. *Journal of Psychology and Theology, 9*, 335–351.

Batson, C. D., & Schoenrade, P. A. (1991a). Measuring religion as quest: 1. Validity concerns. *Journal for the Scientific Study of Religion, 30*, 416–429.

Batson, C. D., & Schoenrade, P. A. (1991b). Measuring religion as quest: 2. Reliability concerns. *Journal for the Scientific Study of Religion, 30*, 430–447.

Batson, C. D., Schoenrade, P., & Ventis, W. L. (1993). *Religion and the individual: A social-psychological perspective* (rev. ed.). New York: Oxford University Press.

Benson, P. L., Donahue, M. J., & Erickson, J. A. (1993). The Faith Maturity Scale: Conceptualization, measurement, and empirical validation. In M. L. Lynn & D. O. Moberg (Eds.), *Research in the social scientific study of religion* (Vol. 5, pp. 1–26). Greenwich, CT: JAI Press.

Benson, P., & Spilka, B. (1973). God-image as a function of self-esteem and locus of control. *Journal for the Scientific Study of Religion, 12*, 297–310.

Black, H. K. (1999). Poverty and prayer: Spiritual narratives of elderly African-American women. *Review of Religious Research, 40*, 359–374.

Braithwaite, V. A., & Scott, W. A. (1991). Values. In J. P. Robinson, P. R. Shaver, & L. S. Wrightsman (Eds.), *Measures of personality and social psychological attitudes* (pp. 661–753). New York: Academic Press.

Brown, R. P. (2003). Measuring individual differences in the tendency to forgive: Construct validity and links with depression. *Personality and Social Psychology Bulletin, 29,* 759–771.

Brown, S. W., Gorsuch, R. L., Rosik, C. H., & Ridley, C. R. (2001). The development of a scale to measure forgiveness. *Journal of Psychology and Christianity, 20,* 40–52.

Burris, C. T. (1999). Religious Orientation Scale. In P. C. Hill & R. W. Hood, Jr. (Eds.), *Measures of religiosity* (pp. 144–154). Birmingham, AL: Religious Education Press.

Chatters, L. M., Taylor, R. J., & Lincoln, K. D. (2002). Advances in the measurement of religiosity among older African Americans: Implications for health and mental health researchers. In J. H. Skinner & J. A. Teresi (Eds.), *Multicultural measurement in older populations* (pp. 199–220). New York: Springer.

Connors, G. J., Tonigan, J. S., & Miller, W. R. (1996). A measure of religious background and behavior for use in behavior change research. *Psychology of Addictive Behaviors, 10,* 90–96.

Cornwall, M., Albrecht, S. L., Cunningham, P. H., & Pitcher, B. L. (1986). The dimensions of religiosity: A conceptual model with an empirical test. *Review of Religious Research, 27,* 226–244.

Cronbach, L. (1951). Coefficient alpha and the internal structure of tests. *Psychometrika, 31,* 93–96.

DeJong, G. F., Faulkner, J. E., & Warland, R. H. (1976). Dimensions of religiosity reconsidered: Evidence from a cross-cultural study. *Social Forces, 54,* 866–889.

Donahue, M. J. (1985). Intrinsic and extrinsic religiousness: Review and meta-analysis. *Journal of Personality and Social Psychology, 48,* 400–419.

D'Onofrio, B. M., Eaves, L. J., Murrelle, L., Maes, H. H., & Spilka, B. (1999). Understanding biological and social influences on religious affiliation, attitudes, and behaviors: A behavior genetic perspective. *Journal of Personality, 67,* 953–984.

Dynes, R. R. (1955). Church-sect typology and socio-economic status. *American Sociological Review, 20,* 555–660.

Elkins, D. N., Hedstrom, L. J., Hughes, L. L., Leaf, J. A., & Saunders, C. (1988). Toward phenomenological spirituality: Definition, description and measurement. *Journal of Humanistic Psychology, 28*(4), 5–18.

Ellison, C. G., & Taylor, R. J. (1996). Turning to prayer: Social and situational antecedents of religious coping among African-Americans. *Review of Religious Research, 38,* 111–131.

Emavardhana, T., & Tori, C. D. (1997). Changes in self-concept, ego defense mechanisms, and religiosity following seven-day Vipassana meditation retreats. *Journal for the Scientific Study of Religion, 36,* 194–206.

Emmons, R. A. (1999). *The psychology of ultimate concerns: Motivation and spirituality in personality.* New York: Guilford Press.

Emmons, R. A., & Paloutzian, R. F. (2003). The psychology of religion. *Annual Review of Psychology, 54,* 377–402.

Exline, J. J., Yali, A. M., & Sanderson, W. C. (2000). Guilt, discord, and alienation: The role of religious strain in depression and suicidality. *Journal of Clinical Psychology, 56,* 1481–1496.

Fetzer Institute/National Institute of Aging Working Group. (1999, October). *Multidimensional measurement of religiousness/spirituality for use in health research: A report of the Fetzer Institute/ National Institute on Aging Working Group.* Kalamazoo, MI: John E. Fetzer Institute.

Fiala, W. E., Bjorck, J. P., & Gorsuch, R. L. (2002). The Religious Support Scale: Construction, validation, and cross-validation. *American Journal of Community Psychology, 30,* 761–786.

Fowler, J. (1981). *Stages of faith.* San Francisco: Harper & Row.

Fullerton, J. T., & Hunsberger, B. (1982). A unidimensional measure of Christian orthodoxy. *Journal for the Scientific Study of Religion, 21,* 317–326.

Genia, V. (1997). The Spiritual Experience Index: Revision and reformulation. *Review of Religious Research, 38,* 344–361.

Glock, C., & Stark, R. (1966). *Christian beliefs and anti-Semitism.* New York: Harper & Row.

Gorsuch, R. L. (1984). Measurement: The boon and bane of investigating religion. *American Psychologist, 39,* 228–236.

Gorsuch, R. L. (1988). Psychology of religion. *Annual Review of Psychology, 39,* 201–221.

Gorsuch, R. L. (1990). Measurement in psychology of religion revisited. *Journal of Psychology and Christianity, 9*(2), 82–92.

Gorsuch, R. L., & McPherson, S. E. (1989). Intrinsic/extrinsic measurement: I/E-revised and single-item scales. *Journal for the Scientific Study of Religion, 28,* 348–354.

Hall, T. W., & Edwards, K. J. (1996). The initial development and factor analysis of the Spiritual Assessment Inventory. *Journal of Psychology and Theology, 24,* 233–246.

Hays, J. C., Meador, K. G., Branch, P. S., & George, L. K. (2001). The Spirituality History Scale in Four Dimensions (SHS-4): Validity and reliability. *The Gerontologist, 41,* 239–249.

Heelas, P. (1985). Social anthropology and the psychology of religion. In L. B. Brown (Ed.), *Advances in the psychology of religion* (pp. 34–51). Oxford, UK: Pergamon Press.

Hill, P. C. (1994). Toward an attitude process model of religious experience. *Journal for the Scientific Study of Religion, 33,* 303–314.

Hill, P. C. (1995). Affective theory and religious experience. In R. W. Hood, Jr. (Ed.), *Handbook of religious experience: Theory and practice* (pp. 353–377). Birmingham, AL: Religious Education Press.

Hill, P. C. (2002). Spiritual transformation: Forming the habitual center of personal energy. *Research in the Social Scientific Study of Religion, 13,* 87–108.

Hill, P. C., & Hood, R. W., Jr. (1999). *Measures of religiosity.* Birmingham, AL: Religious Education Press.

Hill, P. C., & Pargament, K. I. (2003). Advances in the conceptualization and measurement of religion and spirituality. *American Psychologist, 58,* 64–74.

Hill, P. C., Pargament, K. I., Hood, R. W., Jr., McCullough, M. E., Swyers, J. P., Larson, D. B., & Zinnbauer, B. J. (2000). Conceptualizing religion and spirituality: Points of commonality, points of departure. *Journal for the Theory of Social Behaviour, 30,* 51–77.

Hilty, D. M., & Morgan, R. L. (1985). Construct validation for the Religious Involvement Inventory: Replication. *Journal for the Scientific Study of Religion, 24,* 75–86.

Holland, J. C., Kash, K. M., Passik, S., Gronert, M. K., Sison, A., Lederberg, M., Russak, S. M., Baider, L., & Fox, B. (1998). A brief spiritual beliefs inventory for use in quality of life research in life-threatening illness. *Psycho-Oncology, 7,* 460–469.

Hood, R. W., Jr. (1970). Religious orientation and the report of religious experience. *Journal for the Scientific Study of Religion, 9,* 285–291.

Hood, R. W., Jr. (1975). The construction and preliminary validation of a measure of reported mystical experience. *Journal for the Scientific Study of Religion, 14,* 29–41.

Hood, R. W., Jr. (1995). The facilitation of religious experience. In R. W. Hood, Jr. (Ed.), *Handbook of religious experience* (pp. 568–597). Birmingham, AL: Religious Education Press.

Hood, R. W., Jr. (1997). The empirical study of mysticism. In B. Spilka & D. N. McIntosh (Eds.), *The psychology of religion: Theoretical approaches* (pp. 222–232). Boulder, CO: Westview Press.

Hood, R. W., Jr., Spilka, B., Hunsberger, B., & Gorsuch, R. (1996). *The psychology of religion: An empirical approach* (2nd ed.). New York: Guilford Press.

Kass, J. D., Friedman, R., Leserman, J., Zuttermeister, P. C., & Benson, H. (1991). Health outcomes and a new index of spiritual experience. *Journal for the Scientific Study of Religion, 30,* 203–211.

Katz, Y. J. (1988). A validation of the Social–Religious–Political Scale. *Educational and Psychological Measurement, 48,* 1025–1028.

Kirkpatrick, L. A. (1989). A psychometric analysis of the Allport–Ross and Feagin measures of intrinsic–extrinsic religious orientation. In D. O. Moberg & M. L. Lynn (Eds.), *Research in the social scientific study of religion* (Vol. 1, pp. 1–31). Greenwich, CT: JAI Press.

Kirkpatrick, L. A. (1992). An attachment-theory approach to the psychology of religion. *The International Journal for the Psychology of Religion, 2,* 3–28.

Kirkpatrick, L. A. (1995). Attachment theory and religious experience. In R. W. Hood, Jr. (Ed.), *Handbook of religious experience* (pp. 446–475). Birmingham, AL: Religious Education Press.

Kirkpatrick, L. A., & Hood, R. W., Jr. (1990). Intrinsic–extrinsic religious orientation: The boon or bane of contemporary psychology of religion. *Journal for the Scientific Study of Religion, 29,* 442–462.

Koenig, H., Patterson, G. R., & Meador, K. G. (1997). Religion Index for Psychiatric Research: A 5-item measure for use in health outcome studies. *American Journal of Psychiatry, 154,* 885.

Krause, N. (1999). Religious support. In *Multidimensional measurement of religiousness/spirituality for use in health research: A report of the Fetzer Institute/National Institute on Aging Working Group* (pp. 57–64). Kalamazoo, MI: John E. Fetzer Institute.

Kuhn, T. S. (1970). *The structure of scientific revolutions* (2nd ed.). Chicago: University of Chicago Press.

Larson, D. B., Swyers, J. P., & McCullough, M. E. (1998). *Scientific research on spirituality and health: A consensus report.* Bethesda, MD: National Institute for Healthcare Research.

Leak, G. K., & Fish, S. B. (1999). Development and initial validation of a measure of religious maturity. *The International Journal for the Psychology of Religion, 9,* 83–103.

Leak, G. K., Loucks, A. A., & Bowlin, P. (1999). Development and initial validation of an objective measure of faith development. *The International Journal for the Psychology of Religion, 9,* 105–124.

Ledbetter, M. F., Smith, L. A., Vosler-Hunter, W. L., & Fischer, J. D. (1991). An evaluation of the research and clinical usefulness of the Spiritual Well-Being Scale. *Journal of Psychology and Theology, 19,* 49–55.

Maugans, T. A. (1996). The SPIRITual history. *Archives of Family Medicine, 5,* 11–16.

McConahay, J. B., & Hough, J. C., Jr. (1973). Love and guilt-oriented dimensions of Christian belief. *Journal for the Scientific Study of Religion, 12,* 53–64.

McCullough, M. E., Rachal, K. C., Sandage, S. J., Worthington, E. L., Brown, S. W., & Hight, T. (1998). Interpersonal forgiving in close relationships: II. Theoretical elaboration and measurement. *Journal of Personality and Social Psychology, 75,* 1586–1603.

McIntosh, D. N. (1995). Religion as schema, with implications for the relation between religion and coping. *The International Journal for the Psychology of Religion, 5,* 1–16.

Miller, W. R. (1998). Researching the spiritual dimensions of alcohol and other drug problems. *Addiction, 93,* 979–990.

Moberg, D. O. (1984). Subjective measures of spiritual well-being. *Review of Religious Research, 25,* 351–359.

Moberg, D. O. (2002). Assessing and measuring spirituality: Confronting dilemmas of universal and particular evaluative criteria. *Journal of Adult Development, 9,* 47–60.

Newberg, A., d'Aquili, E. G., & Rause, V. (2001). *Why God won't go away: Brain science and the biology of belief.* New York: Ballantine Books.

Paloutzian, R. F., & Ellison, C. W. (1982). Loneliness, spiritual well-being, and quality of life. In L. A. Peplau & D. Perlman (Eds.), *Loneliness: A sourcebook of current theory, research and therapy* (pp. 224–237). New York: Wiley Interscience.

Paloutzian, R. F., Richardson, J. T., & Rambo, L. R. (1999). Religious conversion and personality change. *Journal of Personality, 67,* 1047–1079.

Pargament, K. I. (1997). *The psychology of religion and coping.* New York: Guilford Press.

Pargament, K. I., Ensing, D. S., Falgout, K., Olsen, H., Reilly, B., Van Haitsma, K., & Warren, R. (1990). God help me: I. Religious coping efforts as predictors of the outcomes to significant life events. *American Journal of Community Psychology, 18,* 793–824.

Pargament, K. I., Kennell, J., Hathaway, W., Grevengoed, N., Newman, J., & Jones, W. (1988). Religion and the problem-solving process: Three styles of coping. *Journal for the Scientific Study of Religon, 27,* 90–104.

Pargament, K. I., Koenig, H. G., & Perez, L. M. (2000). The many methods of religious coping: Development and initial validation of the RCOPE. *Journal of Clinical Psychology, 56,* 519–543.

Pendleton, S., Cavilli, K. S., Pargament, K. I., & Nasr, S. (2002). Spirituality in children with cystic fibrosis: A qualitative study. *Pediatrics, 109,* 1–11.

Pfeifer, S., & Waelty, U. (1995). Psychopathology and religious commitment: A controlled study. *Psychopathology, 28,* 70–77.

Piedmont, R. L. (1999). Does spirituality represent the sixth factor of personality?: Spiritual transcendence and the five-factor model. *Journal of Personality, 67,* 985–1013.

Plante, T. G., & Boccaccini, M. T. (1997). The Santa Clara Strength of Religious Faith Questionnaire. *Pastoral Psychology, 45,* 375–387.

Poloma, M. M., & Pendleton, B. F. (1989). Exploring types of prayer and quality of life: A research note. *Review of Religious Research, 31,* 46–53.

Rohrbaugh, J., & Jessor, R. (1975). Religiosity in youth: A personal control against deviant behavior. *Journal of Personality, 43,* 136–155.

Ryan, R. M., Rigby, S., & King, K. (1993). Two types of religious internalization and their relations to religious orientations and mental health. *Journal of Personality and Social Psychology, 65,* 586–596.

Sandoval, J. H., Frisby, C. L., Geisinger, K. F., Ramos-Grenier, J., & Scheuneman, J. D. (1998). *Test interpretation and diversity: Achieving equity in assessment.* Washington, DC: American Psychological Association.

Schaler, J. A. (1996). Spiritual thinking in addiction-treatment providers: The Spiritual Belief Scale. *Alcoholism Treatment Quarterly, 14*(3), 7–33.

Storch, E. A., Roberti, J. W., Bagner, D. M., Lewin, A. B., Baumeister, A. L., & Geffken, G. R. (2004). Further psychometric properties of the Santa Clara Strength of Religious Faith Questionnaire—Short-Form. *Journal of Psychology and Christianity, 23,* 51–53.

Thurstone, L. L., & Chave, E. J. (1929). *The measurement of attitude: A psychophysical method and some experiments with a scale for measuring attitude toward the church.* Chicago: University of Chicago Press.

Tisdale, T. C. (1999). Faith Maturity Scale. In P. C. Hill & R. W. Hood, Jr. (Eds.), *Measures of religiosity* (pp. 171–174). Birmingham, AL: Religious Education Press.

Tsang, J., & McCullough, M. E. (2003). Measuring religious constructs: A hierarchical approach to construct organization and scale selection. In S. J. Lopez & C. R. Snyder (Eds.), *Positive psychological assessment: A handbook of models and measures* (pp. 345–360). Washington, DC: American Psychological Association.

Underwood, L. G. (1999). Daily spiritual experiences. In *Multidimensional measurement of religiousness/spirituality for use in health research: A report of the Fetzer Institute/National Institute of Aging Working Group* (pp. 11–17). Kalamazoo, MI: John E. Fetzer Institute.

Worthington, E. L., Jr., Wade, N. G., Hight, T. L., Ripley, J. S., McCullough, M. E., Berry, J. W., Schmitt, M. M., Berry, J. T., Bursley, K. H., & O'Connor, L. (2003). The Religious Commitment Inventory—10: Development, refinement, and validation of a brief scale for research and counseling. *Journal of Counseling Psychology, 50,* 84–96.

Wulff, D. M. (1999). Attitude Toward the Church Scale. In P. C. Hill & R. W. Hood, Jr. (Eds.), *Measures of religiosity* (pp. 467–471). Birmingham, AL: Religious Education Press.

4

Research Methods in the Psychology of Religion

RALPH W. HOOD, JR.
JACOB A. BELZEN

The *Annual Review of Psychology* has published only two reviews of the psychology of religion. While both reviews focused upon empirical research, the contents of those reviews, separated by 15 years, are strikingly different. The first review emphasized correlational (Gorsuch, 1988), the second experimental research (Emmons & Paloutzian, 2003). In the decade prior to Gorsuch's (1984) identification of a measurement paradigm, Capps, Ransohoff, and Rambo (1976) noted that out of a total of almost 2,800 articles in the psychology of religion to that date only 150 were empirical studies and of these 90% were correlational. The shift toward an experimental paradigm has become for many the ideal for the field. It does not abandon the measurement/correlational paradigm; rather, it embeds it in research methods exhibiting the characteristic of mainstream psychology.[1] However, it is worth noting that as the criticisms of laboratory-based research were most intense (in the decades of the 1960s and 1970s), the percent of experimental studies in the *Journal of Personality and Social Psychology* increased (Moghadam, Taylor, & Wright, 1993, p. 26). Thus, the call by Emmons and Paloutzian (2003) for a new *multilevel interdisciplinary paradigm* (p. 395; emphasis in original) is most welcome. It is accompanied by the assertion of the value of using data at multiple levels of analysis as well as the value of nonreductive assumptions regarding the nature of religious and spiritual phenomena (p. 395). Our discussion of methodology in this chapter will affirm these ideals and suggest areas in which multiple methods have already been profitably used in the psychology of religion. In the process we show how different methods compliment one another and provide a more complete understanding of religious and spiritual phenomena than can be achieved by any single method. We will not concentrate on research in a more hermeneutical vein (Belzen, 1997) insofar as it has not yet been incorporated into mainstream psychology, although we hope that the new paradigm will alter this situation in the future.

CHEMICAL FACILITATION OF RELIGIOUS OR SPIRITUAL EXPERIENCES

"Entheogen" is becoming the preferred term, replacing the older term "psychedelic," for a class of chemicals that facilitate religious or spiritual experiences. An often-cited study in the psychology of religion and one of the few truly experimental designs is the Good Friday experiment of Pahnke (1969). Pahnke administered either psilocybin or a placebo (nicotinic acid) to 20 volunteer graduate students at Andover–Newton Theological Seminary. Participants met in groups of four, with two experimental subjects and two controls matched for compatibility. Each group had two leaders, one of whom had been given psilocybin. The participants met to hear a Good Friday service so that religious set and setting were maximized for all participants. Immediately after the service and in a 6-month follow-up all participants filled out a questionnaire largely consisting of Stace's (1960) criteria of mysticism. Results for the immediate and long-term follow-up indicated that the controls responded to the criteria of mysticism at a significantly lower percentage than did the experimentals. Doblin (1991) used Pahnke's original questionnaire to assess nine of the original controls and seven of the experimentals nearly 25 years after their participation in the original study. The follow-up results indicated similar difference between controls and experimentals found in the original study.

Pahnke's study is significant for three reasons. First, it is a true experimental design with participants randomly assigned to experimental and control conditions. Second, by having seminary students participate in a religious service on a significant day, religious/spiritual set and setting were maximized. Third, there was an immediate posttest, followed by a longer term posttest (and with Dublin's assessment, a very long-term assessment of the effects of this experience). However, despite this being a true experimental design, it had several flaws. Among them are the likelihood that in psilocybin studies, placebo controls are readily identified so that the double-blind fails and the participants were only rated on Stace's (1960) criteria of mysticism so that the diversity of the experiences could not be expressed.[2]

Complementary Research Methods Employing Entheogens

Pahnke's study is often cited as exemplary in use of a true experimental design to assess the spiritual significance of chemically triggered experiences under appropriate set and setting conditions. Shanon's (2002) extensive study of ayahuasca provides a complementary methodological approach to the study of chemically triggered religious/spiritual experiences. Ayahuasca is a hallucinogenic drink prepared from the bark of a South American vine that is widely used throughout the upper Amazon. Shanon, a cognitive psychologist, has extensively studied experiences elicited by ayahuasca in a variety of religious and nonreligious settings. He has also drunk ayahuasca himself more than a hundred times across many years. He was able to compare his own experiences with those of other participants he has interviewed. Shanon's primary method is phenomenological and he has provided the best cartography of mental states elicited by ayahuasca. He also provides quantitative analyses based upon the first 67 of his own sessions and structured interviews with others who have taken ayahuasca for moderate or extensive periods of time in both religious and nonreligious settings. He then compares this material to reports in the anthropological literature. Shanon's work is exemplary in that it suggests an analogue to quasi-experimental methods. By carefully comparing the use of ayahuasca in various settings in an $N = 1$ study as well as by comparing his own experiences to reports by others who concurrently drink this brew with reports from anthropologists Shanon can study the effects of dosage, experiences over time, and the effects of set and setting in an analogue to a quasi-experimental design. The very subjectivity that some might suggest contaminates single-person reports becomes a necessary source of objectivity in charting the phenomenology of the ayahuasca experience.

In a 5-year series (1990–1995) of U.S. Drug Enforcement Administration-approved studies, Strassman and his colleagues used quasi-experimental methods to explore experiences facilitated by N-dimethyltryptamine (DMT), an active ingredient in ayahuasca. Most controversial is the claim than DMT-facilitated states of consciousness are similar to naturally occurring states of consciousness that occur in near-death, mystical, and even alien abduction encounters—perhaps due to the natural occurrence of DMT in the pineal gland that also is implicated in all these experiences. Strassman (2002, Chap. 22) provides suggestions for research with DMT employing not only experimental and quasi-experimental methods but also other innovative methods consistent with a multilevel interdisciplinary paradigm. Shanon argues for actually making ayahuasca from natural ingredients while Strassman argues for utilizing chemically pure DMT. Interesting differences in the experiences are apparent when one compares experiences under the naturally concocted brew with those under pharmaceutically pure DMT. It would be useful to compare ayahuasca under the quasi-experimental settings and other conditions under which DMT is taken in clinical studies.

A final example of a novel methodological twist is the use of multidimensional scaling on autobiographical material. Oxman, Rosenberg, Schnurr, Tucker, and Gala (1988) obtained 94 autobiographical accounts of personal experiences that fulfilled four criteria: (1) the passage was from a published source, (2) it was written in English, (3) it contained at least several hundred words to provide data for textual analysis, and (4) the passage was written after an acute episode or important experience. The accounts were divided into four categories: 19 schizophrenic experiences, 26 experiences triggered by psychoactive substances, 21 mystical/ecstatic experiences, and 26 autobiographical experiences. The texts were coded into 83 thematic categories using a specialized computer program (see Stone, Dunphy, Smith, & Ogilvie, 1966). The researchers then used multidimensional scaling to provide cartography of the key words that differentiated these groups from one another. Results showed that discriminant functional analysis could correctly identify 84% of the experiences based upon the language used to express the experience. The most important difference between groups was that experiences facilitated by psychoactive chemicals were dominated by words referring to sense impressions, while mystical/ecstatic experiences were associated with words referring to ideal values and life-altering "religious" encounters (see Hood, Chapter19, this volume).

Research on entheogens is one of the best exemplars of the multilevel interdisciplinary paradigm.[3] The range of studies includes qualitative and quantitative work, longitudinal and N = 1 research, experimental and quasi-experimental field analogies. It is instructive that when researchers themselves serve as subjects, despite breaking a cardinal rule of objectivity that obtains in true experimental designs, the result is a strong plea for the objective nature of what is experienced. In this sense, research on psychoactive substances parallels early research in U.S. psychology in which introspection was a respected method and the researcher was the subject (Danziger, 1990). Staal (1971) has proposed this procedure for the study of mysticism from a phenomenological perspective. Researchers in both experimental and complementary research methodologies provide nonreductive interpretation of chemically facilitated experiences, especially when they have taken these chemicals themselves.

COGNITIVE DISSONANCE

When participants cannot be randomly assigned to groups one can use quasi-experimental designs that often exceed experimental designs in contextual realism and still allow internal validity (Campbell & Stanley, 1963). For example, Batson (1975) took advantage of a church retreat to divide junior-high females into those who did and those who did not believe that Jesus was the Son of God. He then had these naturally occurring nonequivalent groups read a contrived newspaper article in which Christianity was presented as a hoax. While most girls in both groups did not believe the article, those who did (about one-third) indicated a greater intensity of religious belief if they were in the believers group. The apparently paradoxical finding was interpreted as supporting cognitive dissonance theory. Batson and his colleagues reviewed other quasi-experimental studies on cognitive dissonance as well as historical and field studies to support the claim that faced with belief-disconfirming information, devout believers are likely to hold firmer to rather than abandon their beliefs (Batson, Schoenrade, & Ventis, 1993, pp. 210–216).

Complementary Research on Cognitive Dissonance and Failed Prophecy

In light of the call for a multilevel interdisciplinary paradigm, it is worth noting that field research methods reveal a different pattern of results than laboratory-based experimental methods. This is especially the case when beliefs are assumed to have been disconfirmed. Melton (1985) notes that beliefs are seldom perceived as disconfirmed by the believer. Melton denies what Festinger's theory requires, that one can identify "unequivocal and undeniable disconfirmation of a prophecy" (Festinger, Riecken, & Schachter, 1956, p. 3). Melton (1985) notes that "within religious groups prophecy seldom fails" (p. 20). To understand why within religious groups prophecy is seldom perceived to fail requires researchers to move from laboratory studies to a consideration of field research.

Using interview-, ethnomethodological-, and phenomenological-oriented methods to understand how the participants reason within a real-life situation suggests that belief disconfirmation or failed prophecy are negotiated terms and cannot be simply operationalized by experimenters (Pollner, 1987). One common assumption is that people are driven by the need to reduce dissonance, and hence refuse to accept disconfirmation. The strongest support for this assumption is provided by quasi-experimental laboratory research. However, participant observation, interview, and ethnomethodological studies indicate that the most common response of members within groups is to deny the failure of prophecy and to seek an interpretative frame within which their beliefs continue to make sense (Dein, 1997, 2001; Tumminia, 1998). Reviewing studies of actual groups in which prophecies presumably failed (including his own research), Bader (1999, p. 120) notes that "no study of a failed prophecy, the current research included, has provided support for the cognitive dissonance hypothesis."

Understanding that different methods yield differing views illustrates the value of the call for a new multilevel interdisciplinary paradigm. While laboratory experiments often provide evidence for experimentally induced dissonance reduction, participant observation and field studies suggest that what constitutes evidence of disconfirmation for the researcher is not what constitutes evidence of disconfirmation for participants in religious groups. The laboratory context is itself a social construction in which dissonance reduction perhaps functions more precisely than in actual life contexts where individuals in prophetic groups seldom acknowledge that prophecy fails. The failure to acknowledge prophetic failure is an inconsistency likely to be perceived by outsiders but not by members inside the religious group.

Natural "Manipulations" in Quasi-Experimental Field Studies

Neither experimental nor quasi-experimental designs need to be restricted to the laboratory (Aronson, Wilson, & Brewer, 1998, p. 106). Field studies can have the advantage of being more consistent with "real life" and thus maximizing contextual realism while maintaining the internal validity of an experiment. Also, sometimes one can take advantage of naturally occurring events to approximate a "manipulation."

The use of natural conditions as a "manipulation" is illustrated by researchers who took advantage of a nature program consisting of a mandatory 5-day wilderness experience for seniors at an all-male private school (Hood, 1977). The focus of the research was the elicitation of mystical experiences, which are often reported in nature settings. Researchers predicted that anticipatory stress and activity stress incongruity would elicit reports of mystical experience. The researchers identified three high-stress activities (white-water rafting, a solitary evening in the woods with minimal equipment, and rock climbing). A control condition, smooth-water canoeing, was identified as a low-stress event. Immediately before each activity, participants were assessed for anticipatory stress on an objective measure. In all cases, those who had low anticipatory stress for the high-stress activities reported higher mysticism scores than those anticipating high-stress for the high stress activities. In addition, because none of the boys regarded the canoe activity as a high-stress activity, each individual could serve as his own control, indicating that anticipatory stress/setting stress incongruity accounted for the higher reports of mystical experience. However, within the field study, because no one anticipated the low-stress activity as highly stressful, researchers could not test the other possible incongruity, low anticipatory stress/high setting stress.

Researchers used the same school and program in a subsequent year to attempt to test the incongruity between the anticipatory stress and the setting stress hypothesis (Hood, 1978a). The researchers focused upon the solo experience in which small groups of individuals were led into the woods by the researcher. Each individual was dropped off at an isolated place such that no one could see or be seen by anyone else. Just prior to being dropped off each individual was assessed on an objective measure of anticipatory stress. Since different groups participated in the solo experience over five separate evenings, the researchers took advantage of the likelihood of thunderstorms occurring on at least some of the nights. (The researchers had informed consent to leave participants out even in storm conditions.) Fortunately, storms occurred on three of the five nights. Storm versus no storm became the naturally occurring "manipulation" of setting stress. Given that the evening was spent alone, without a tent (only a tarp was provided), the researchers identified the storm evenings as a higher setting stress relative to the non-storm evenings. (Unobtrusive measures provided confirmation of the stress when several individuals "broke solo" during the storm nights and returned to base camp because they were unable or unwilling to complete the solo experience.) As predicted, both low anticipatory stress/high setting stress and high anticipatory stress/low setting stress elicited a greater magnitude of religious experience than the stress congruity conditions. Thus, the anticipatory stress and setting stress incongruity hypothesis was both replicated for high-stress experiences and extended to support the incongruity hypothesis for low-stress experiences anticipated as stressful. These studies indicate the possibility of quasi-experimental studies in field situations as well as the possibility of using anticipated natural events as experimental "manipulations."

The extension of quasi-experimental studies to field conditions adds psychological realism to experimental realism while maintaining internal validity. In their review of quasi-experimental research in the social psychology of religion, Batson et al. (1993) bemoaned the paucity of studies and stated; "We hope quasi-experimental designs will soon become the research method of choice in the social psychology of religion" (p. 385). The Emmons and Paloutzian (2003) review of the field indicates that this hope is being rapidly fulfilled. Quasi-experimental methodologies need not be restricted to the laboratory. Field research not only compliments laboratory research but can often be done with assurance of both experimental realism and internal validity at minimal expense, especially if researchers can take advantage of existing programs in which to embed their research.

CORRELATIONAL AND SURVEY STUDIES

We have already noted above that much of the empirical literature in the psychology of religion has been correlational. While correlation studies are far from useless, their limitations are obvious. Correlated variables are notoriously subject to a variety of interpretations so that the adage "correlation is not causation" has become a mantra for the experimental psychologist. However, despite this fact, correlational studies remain common and complement experimental studies for a variety of reasons. Often they permit the study of noncollege populations. Sears (1986) noted that since the 1960s over 80% of experimental laboratory studies had been conducted on undergraduate college students; little has changed in the last quarter of a century. Survey studies, while correlational, can use random samples and thus study a more representative range of persons. Thus, surveys complement laboratory and field studies.

Surveys of Religious and Spiritual Experience

Numerous survey studies in both the United States and Europe have demonstrated the normalcy of reports of religious experience, including mystical experience (see Spilka, Hood, Hunsberger, & Gorsuch, 2003, pp. 307–312). Depending on the specific wording of the questions asked, anywhere from a third to a half of the populations affirm such experiences. Furthermore, the report of such experiences is correlated with gender (stronger for females), education (more common with higher education), and social class (more common in higher social classes). While this correlational data does not provide evidence of what causes such reports, it does establish the normalcy of such reports and indicates that social scientists have until recently ignored a *common* phenomenon.

Studies of social scientists and mental health professionals have established what Coyle (2001) refers to as the "religious gap" between professionals who treat and study people and the people they study. The religious population studied and treated is more religious at least by a ratio of 2:1. For instance, while 72% of Americans affirm the single best intrinsic item, "My whole approach to life is based upon my religion," only 33% of psychologists endorse this item. In addition, while only 9% of the general population identifies itself as nonreligious, 31% of psychologists identify themselves as nonreligious (Coyle, 2001, p. 550). Belief differences between researchers and those they study have been identified as sources of confusion in both the way studies are conducted and in how they are interpreted. This is especially the case when researchers study those distant from their own beliefs, such as religious fundamentalists (Hood, 1983). For instance, researchers who are not fundamentalists tend to identify intense religious commitments that are intratextually based as "closed-mindedness" even though the process of fundamentalist thought privileges a single scared text above the use of multiple texts as the authoritative basis for belief and practice (Hood, Hill, & Williamson, 2005).

Authoritarianism, Dogmatism, and Religion

Correlational studies can be especially useful in comparing sampling with college undergraduates with predictions made from "real-life" data. Since the days of the original authoritarian personality research (Adorno, Frenkel-Brunswik, Levinson, & Sanford, 1950) authoritarianism, first as a personality construct, then as a learned social behavior (Altemeyer, 1988) has been correlated with religious fundamentalism. Authoritarianism measures are more strongly linked with a "right-wing" or conservative political stance. Rokeach's (1960) dogmatism theory ranges across the entire political spectrum, while Altemeyer (1988) focuses only upon "right-wing authoritarianism" (RWA). However both Rokeach (1960) and Altemeyer (Alteymer & Hunbsberger, 1992) focus upon the process rather than the content of belief. The massive literature on authoritarianism, dogmatism, and religious fundamentalism has led to the persistent claim of a relationship between these two constructs (see reviews in Spilka et al., 2003, pp. 467–479, and Paloutzian, 1996, pp. 229–231, 241–244). While this claim is supported by laboratory studies, field studies reveal a different result. It has been over a quarter of a century since one prominent empirical researcher noted that "the widespread belief that there is a strong relationship between religious orthodoxy and authoritarianism appears to be a prominent instance of [the] tendency to transform suspicions and speculations into certainties" (Stark, 1971, p. 172). Given that most measures of fundamentalism are belief-oriented, "orthodoxy" is often but a synonym for "fundamentalism" in empirical studies, such that strong correlations are built in between orthodoxy, authoritarianism, and RWA (Altemeyer, 1988; Gorsuch & Alshire, 1974), and thus Stark's (1971) criticism applies doubly. However, not only can fundamentalism as a *process* of belief be separated from orthodoxy as *content* of belief, correlation methods such as regression can be used to identify the differential relationship of authoritarianism and orthodoxy to measures of authoritarianism (Hood et al., 2005; Kirkpatrick, 1993; Kirkpatrick, Hood, & Hartz, 1991). That field studies do not find the consistent relationships between authoritarianism and fundamentalism that are reported by laboratory studies suggests that it would be useful for each to use the measures common to the other to see if it is the context (survey vs. questionnaire studies), the samples (college undergraduate samples vs. national samples), or the measures that reflect such startling differences. In addition, common measures of authoritarianism and fundamentalism can be included in interview studies to compare persons who deconvert from fundamentalist religions with controls in the same groups who stay (Streib & Keller, 2004). This permits the identification of individual differences that lead some persons within the same religious group to exit while others remain in the group. Identifying these differences within a real-life context of differential religious engagement and disengagement requires the use of complimentary methods.

As a final note with respect to the ongoing study of fundamentalism and authoritarianism (and their relationship to prejudice with various targeted and nontargeted groups), it is worth noting two contributions that correlational studies have made. First, it is unlikely that personality variables contribute much to the variance. The strongest relationship between authoritarianism as a personality construct is between dogmatism and fundamentalism, and this suggest only a weak relationship between personality and authoritarianism. An exception is RWA and fundamentalism. However, RWA was not developed as a personality construct (Altemeyer, 1988), and empirical measures of RWA and fundamentalism correlate consistently so high (in the range of .6–.8) as to be essentially redundant measures of one construct (see Altemeyer & Hunsberger, Chapter 21, this volume). Thus, as with conversion research, basic personality traits seem to explain little of the variance in authoritarianism (Paloutzian, Richardson, & Rambo, 1999). This is supported by a study of authoritarianism in "real-life" contexts. Neither in mass hatred (Kressel, 1996, pp. 211–246) nor in genocide (Waller, 2002, pp. 5–87) have basic personality traits been found to distinguish the perpetrators of such acts. Finally, in an extremely provocative study, Browder (1996) used the actual personnel files of 526 men who joined the SS, the Nazi internal security service, in the period 1932–1934. Bowder found that when using sociocultural factors supposedly predictive of an authoritarian personality, SS volunteers were *less* likely to have the precursors of an authoritarian personality than those in the general population. Bowder's data is especially valuable as it included virtually all SS officers and 62% of the total SS membership by 1934, all of whom were volunteers.

Mystical Experience

Surveys, questionnaires, and interviews continue to play a prominent role in the psychology of religion. Survey data can be used to provide a backdrop for experimental and quasi-experimental studies. For instance, numerous surveys over the last decade in both the United States and Europe have assessed the report of mystical experiences (see Spilka et al., 2003, pp. 307–312). Given that at least one-third of appropriately sampled populations report such experiences is consistent with the ease by which persons scoring high on measures of mysticism can be identified and studied in quasi-experimental conditions. Furthermore, the worry that self-reports of religious experience may not be truthful can be methodologically approached from a variety of means. For instance, Hood and Morris (1981a) demonstrated that when using criteria of mysticism common in the empirical literature, persons equally knowledgeable about these criteria reported different experiences. This suggests that persons refuse to report experiences they do not have and do not simply affirm having experiences that they are knowledgeable about. In addition, Hood (1978b) used a voice stress analysis to measure microtremors in the voices of persons reporting or denying that they had had mystical experiences. As predicted, intrinsic subjects reported mystical experience and extrinsic subjects denied having such experiences—and both indicated stress in their voice response. However, indiscriminately pro-religious subjects tended both to report mystical experiences and to indicate stress, suggesting that they are false positives. Even more intriguing was the fact of indiscriminately antireligious subjects who denied having mystical experiences but showed stress patterns in their voice. This suggests false negatives, or those denying experiences they might in fact have had.

Thus, self-report data can be approached in ways that allow some assessment of their veracity. Another approach not yet widely used in the psychology of religion is to identify the emotional states of respondents by distinctive facial expressions (Keltner, 1995). These various methods permit researchers to provide evidence regarding whether or not the assertion that one has had an experience is truthful.

Triggers of Mystical Experience: Prayer and Isolation Tanks

Another use of survey data for quasi-experimental research is to identify commonly reported triggers of religious and spiritual experiences that can then be studied in the laboratory. For instance, the nature and frequency of varieties of prayer is well documented in major surveys (Poloma & Gallup, 1991). Furthermore, independent factor analytic studies yield similar types of prayers (Spilka et al., 2003, p. 281). Suggestions from survey studies indicating that meditative or contemplative prayer were especially significant in terms of subjective consequences led Hood and his colleagues to use an isolation tank in two quasi-experimental studies of prayer. In one study, Hood and Morris (1981b) used a double-blind procedure to have either intrinsic or extrinsic participants try to imagine either religious or cartoon figures while floating in a hydrated magnesium sulfate solution, heated to external body temperature, in a totally sound-proofed and dark isolation tank. As predicted, religious types did not differ in their ability to image figures in the cartoon condition, but did differ in the religious condition, with the intrinsics reporting more religious imagery than the extrinsics. Intrinsics even reported more religious imagery under the cartoon set than extrinsics did under the religious set.

In a second double-blind study, Hood, Morris, and Watson (1990) placed intrinsics, extrinsics, and indiscriminately pro-religious participants in the isolation tank under either a neutral or a specific religious set condition. The most relevant finding was that intrinsics reported religious experiences whether prompted or not. However, as hypothesized, indiscriminately pro-religious participants reported religious experiences only when prompted (religious set). Extrinsics did not report religious experiences under either set.

This study relates to one discussed above in which indiscriminately pro-religious persons (but not intrinsics) exhibit stress while reporting religious experiences. Hood interpreted these studies to support Allport's original contention that indiscriminately pro-religious types are conflicted with respect to religion and tend to attempt to appear religious under appropriate religious sets. Together these two studies show that quasi-experimental studies under laboratory conditions are not only possible but can, as in the case of isolation tanks, use laboratory environments that are especially relevant to religious traditions that seek solitude as a meaningful context for prayer.

Survey studies of the subjective consequences of prayer compliment quasi-experimental studies of the subjective effects of prayer and the religious set effects on experiences during prayer. It is important to note that the focus is upon subjective effects of prayer. It is unclear what efforts to determine objective effects of prayer would be insofar as one looks for experimental evidence of single acts of transcendent interventions (see Spilka, Chapter 20, this volume). As Gorsuch (2002, pp. 64–66) notes, the methodology of science would seem to be inert in the face of the claim that one has a control group whose members are certain God is not acting. Thus, as we shall shortly discuss, a nonreductive approach advocated by the new paradigm may exclude claims to identify causal factors associated with transcendence. The focus of research must remain psychological (Belzen & Uleyn, 1992).

Paranormal Experiences

A parallel issue from survey research closely related to prayer is the widely documented but ignored fact that one of the most consistent correlates of religious experience is paranormal experiences (see Spilka et al., 2003, pp. 312–315). As with prayer, experimental and quasi-experimental studies can best identify the subjective consequences of claims to have had paranormal experiences, and perhaps could be useful to explore the phenomenology of such experiences (Targ, Schlitz, & Irwin, 2000, pp. 223–224). Thalbourne and Delin (1994, 1999) have proposed the concept of *transliminality* as a common factor underlying both mystical and paranormal experiences. McDonald (2000) found paranormal beliefs to be one of the five dimensions that underlie 11 measures of spirituality. However, as with prayer, experimental psychology has no meaningful methods to falsify the occurrence of paranormal phenomenon. Psychologists are better served by shying away from objective claims about or experimental studies of what is nevertheless a powerful correlate of the report of religious and spiritual experiences (Hood, 2003).

However, multiple methods reveal a strong relationship between belief in God and belief in paranormal phenomena and how both intervene to have real perceived effects in believers' lives. It is the perception of such effects that psychologists can study.

SPIRITUALITY, RELIGION, ATTACHMENT, AND ILLUSION

Another place where quantitative and qualitative methodologies compliment one another is in the continuing concern over distinctions between religion and spirituality (Belzen, 2004; Ričan, 2004). In many instances, spirituality measures function the same as religiosity measures. However, this is confounded by the fact that most people in the United States who identify themselves as "religious" also identify themselves as "spiritual" (Zinnbauer et al., 1997). However, a significant minority (typically less than a third) identify themselves as "spiritual but not religious." Interview studies are useful in indicating that these individuals are often antireligious and opposed not only to institutionalized practices but also to dogmatic (in the positive religious sense) constructions or interpretations of religious experiences (Hood, 2003). Spirituality is constructed and clarified within the "religious and spiritual" types by their faith tradition (see Zinnbauer & Pargament, Chapter 2, this volume).

As narrative studies reveal (Hovi, 2004; Lindgren, 2004), rather than spirituality being a "fuzzy" concept for those outside religion, it is fluid and flexible and relates to what psychoanalytic theorists see as an expanded and mature use of illusion (Sorensen, 2004, Chap. 1). It remains controversial within feminist psychology, which sees Freud's abandonment of the seduction theory as an abandonment of the search for objective truth (Hood, 1992, 1997). However, insofar as an expanded theory of illusion in psychoanalysis focuses upon the psychological recollection and reconstruction of events, ontological claims to objectivity are bracketed in the same way they are in narrative analyses.

Surveys and questionnaires can also be useful in longitudinal research. For instance, Kirkpatrick (1997) solicited responses from female readers of the *Denver Post* to a variety of measures of religiosity as well as indicators of attachment style. He was able to assess the same 146 women at a 4-year interval. When statistically controlling for religion at the first assessment, he found that insecure–anxious persons were more likely to report having had a religious experience or a religious conversion than either secure or ambivalent attachment types. He replicated these findings with a sample of college students in a much shorter (4-month) longitudinal study (Kirkpatrick, 1998). Thus, survey and questionnaire studies can yield meaningful data, even though they cannot establish causation directly.

Studies with Children and Adolescents

Survey and interviews have also proven useful with children and adolescents. A useful technique has been to ask people whether they ever had an experience like one described for them. The technique is similar to Hood's Religious Experience Episodes Measure, which has people respond to experiences adapted from James's *Varieties of Religious Experiences* (see Burris, 1999, pp. 220–224). For instance, Pafford (1973) had both university and grammar-school students respond to a written text from W. H. Hudson's autobiography, *Far Away and Long Ago* (1939). Participants were asked to describe any experience of their own like the one they had read. He found that 40% of male and 61% of female grammar-school students reported such experiences compared to 56% and 65% respectively, for university students (1973, p. 91). Pafford also had participants mark all those words in a checklist of 15 words that applied to their experience. The most frequently endorsed word across all subjects (54%) was "awesome" (Pafford, 1973, p. 26). Pafford concluded that transcendent experiences are most common in the middle teens, under conditions of solitude. Such experiences are positively emotionally satisfying and individuals wish to have more of them. Jannsen, de Hart, and den Draak (1990) did a content analysis of the responses of 192 Dutch high-school students to open-ended interviews regarding prayer. From these data they developed a sequential model for prayer. Most typically a personal problem leads to a monologue addressed to God in which the individual seeks help while alone in bed in the evening.

Survey items have been used in longitudinal studies with children. Most significant is Tamminen's (1991) work with Scandinavian youth followed from grade 1 through 11 at 2-year intervals. His large sample ($N = 1,336$) responded to an item widely used with adults in survey studies ("Have you at times felt that God is particularly close to you?"). Tamminen's work indicates not only that experiences of nearness to God can be identified in young children, but also that the percentage reporting this experience declines with age. Cross-cultural research is needed to explore various trajectories of increase and decrease in religion with age. Such trajectories are likely to vary in different cultures and within cultures with different types of social support (see Boyatzis, Chapter 7, this volume).

Narrative Psychology and Psychoanalysis

The focus upon narrative psychology has been useful in studies of conversion. The earlier paradigm of a sudden change elicited by a crisis situation leading to a permanent conversion has been overshadowed by the gradual seeker model (see Spilka et al., 2003, pp. 343–356). In this model, the individual actively searches for meaning and is involved in a gradual process of spiritual transformation that may continue throughout his or her life. How one narrates this transformation is part of the linguistic turn in psychology in which narrative history is more crucial than factual history. Narrative analysis focuses upon the means by which individuals utilize the language of their culture and tradition to construct the story of their own spiritual or religious transformation.

Psychoanalytic theory continues to be a rich source for hypotheses that can be empirically studied by a variety of means (see Corveleyn & Luyten, Chapter 5, this volume).

One example is the provocative work done by Carroll (1983) who empirically tested psychological factors involved in historical apparitions (hallucinations) of the Virgin Mary. One of Carroll's hypotheses regarding the psychological origin of the cult of the Virgin Mary was tested in a laboratory setting and supported. Protestant males (unfamiliar with Catholic tradition) who had strong recollected attachment to their mothers preferred an ambivalent (nurturing/erotic) image of the Virgin Mary and also preferred a suffering Christ figure as predicted by Carroll's theory (Carroll, 1986; Hood. Morris, & Watson, 1991).

An appropriate psychological method to explore psychoanalytic theories and psychological narrative is to use archive-taped interviews so that other researchers can evaluate the original material from which such constructions are made. Examples are Hovi's (2004) study of the Word of Life congregation in Turku, Finland, or the studies by Hood and his colleagues of a serpent-handling sect in Appalachia (Hood, 1998). These investigators have archived their original videos at their respective universities. Thus, unlike the private data associated with the psychoanalytic "couch," the taped or videotaped open interview is public data.

Even nonpsychoanalytically oriented narrative psychologists have returned to $N = 1$ studies as exemplified by Lindgren's (2004) study of the conversion of the former Swedish ambassador Mohammed Knut Bernstrom to Islam at the age of 67. Narrative psychology also interfaces with reflexive ethnography in which the investigators' own commitments are acknowledged and used in illustrating how narration plays a significant role in structuring our experience and life histories (Gergen & Gergen, 1988; McAdams & Bowman, 2002). Consistent with the call for a new paradigm, narrative analyses are nonreductive relative to the religions and spiritualities encoded in the narration. This parallels the contemporary psychoanalytic expanded use of illusion (Sorenson, 2004, Chap. 1).

Narrative studies can compliment measurement and correlational studies. Many religious phenomena seem most related to second-order or higher order personality dimensions such as a search for meaning or finding a sense of purpose in life (Hood et al., 2005; Paloutzian et al., 1999). It will be useful for quasi-experimental, measurement, and narrative methods to converge. For instance, insofar as spirituality may be an additional sixth factor to be added to the five-factor model of personality, scales to measure spirituality should be used in quasi-experimental and correlational studies to see if they add incremental variance over and above the "Big Five" (Piedmont, 1999b). Research suggests this may be the case, and thus there is a need for mainstream psychologists to add such measures in empirical work that seeks to maximize the variance explained (McDonald, 2000; Piedmont, 1999a).

SERPENT HANDLERS AND THE MULTILEVEL INTERDISCIPLINARY PARADIGM

As a final example, it might be useful to look at a research example that fits well within the call for a new paradigm. Hood and his colleagues have focused upon the serpent-handling sect of Appalachia using a variety of methods. For a decade Hood and his colleague have documented entire services and have archived this material for use by other researchers (Hood–Williamson Research Archives on the Serpent Handlers of Southern Appalachia). Williamson, Polio, and Hood (2000) employed an opened-ended interview process and used phenomenological methods to identify the experience of snake handling from the handler's perspective. Part of their technique was to articulate the phenomenology of handling and then have handlers who did not participate in the original interviews read the analysis and concur that it captured as best words can the experience. The phenomenology of anointing compliments electrophysical physiological data of an actually handler "under the anointing" recorded in a laboratory setting (Burton, 1993, pp. 141–144). These data in turn compliment actual samples taken from handlers before a service and immediately after handling a serpent in a regular church service that same evening (Schwartz, 1999, pp. 61–65).

The experience of anointing has been incorporated into explanatory models derived from psychoanalytic theory (Hood & Kimbrough, 1995). Serpent-handling sermons have been analyzed for their narrative form (Williamson & Polio, 1999) and the social history of the movement has been empirically documented in terms of the Church of God's initial support and subsequent abandonment of the practice (Williamson & Hood, 2004). An oral history of the tradition by a handler has recently been compiled (Hood, 2005). Finally, two quasi-experimental studies have explored prejudice toward serpent handlers. In the first study, participants evaluated hypothetical conversion narratives based upon each of the five signs in Mark 16. As predicted, conversion attributed to experiences in churches where serpents were handled were judged less positively than conversions attributed to participation in churches that practiced healing, speaking in tongues, or casting out of demons. Furthermore, even among persons rationally opposed to serpent handling (and poison drinking), partial correlations indicated a residual prejudice effect (Hood, Williamson, & Morris, 1999). A second quasi-experimental study was designed not to change rational rejection of serpent handling but prejudice toward handlers (Hood, Williamson, & Morris, 2000). Using a modified Solomon four-groups design, researchers demonstrated that when viewing actual field tapes in which handlers express their faith in the ritual of serpent handling as opposed to viewing a tape of a Pentecostal service without handling, individuals in the experimental group changed their prejudicial attitudes toward handlers without changing their rational rejection of the practice. Pretest- and posttest-only experimental groups came to see handling as a sincere expression of faith and a practice that ought not to be outlawed for consenting adults. However, they still rejected the practice for themselves. Finally, extensive taping of individuals and services over 10 years (all archived) allows longitudinal studies of persons who have been bitten, and what effects this had on subsequent participation in the tradition. It also permits actual studies of persons who have been bit and who sought medical aid versus those who were bit and suffered the bite, including maiming and even loss of life, all documented on archived video. Thus, the study of these sects has used a variety of methods, in the field and in the lab, both quantitative and qualitative, to document a living tradition that many have stereotyped but whose dynamic history continues. No single method could capture the variety of interesting questions that can be asked of this unique U.S. religious tradition.

CONCLUSION

The psychology of religion is enriched by the use of multiple methods and will profit from opening itself up to interdisciplinary approaches. This includes experimental and quasi-experimental methods under laboratory conditions and in the field as well where contextual realism is often enhanced (and where collaboration with anthropologists and historians of religion is desirable (cf. Kripall, 1995). Experimental and quasi-experimental paradigms will benefit from the utilization of additional complimentary methods if a truly multilevel interdisciplinary paradigm is to be actualized. This is not only desirable, but can be empirically assessed. Here empirical psychology can take a lesson from psychoanalysis. A multilevel interdisciplinary paradigm will also make applications of psychology more attractive to researchers on religion from other disciplines (e.g., by enabling fruitful collaboration with narrative, personality, and social psychology to broaden the psychohistorical approaches that have been employed in research on religious personalities and phenomena primarily from a psychoanalytically perspective; see Belzen, 2001, 2005).

Hood et al. (2005) have proposed an intratextual model of fundamentalism that can be applied to nonreligious, quasi-fundamentalist groups. Here "intratextual" refers to reliance upon a single scared text, not the multiple authoritative sources that are more familiar to academics, who rely on an "intertextual" model for knowledge. Sorenson (2004) has suggested that the intratextual model creates a cohesive group of isolated disciplines or schools. His interest as a relational psychoanalyst (and clinical psychologist) is to compare the literature citations of three psychoanalytic schools (Kleinian psychology, self psychology, and relational psychoanalysis). Using multidimensional scaling for the authors cited in the schools' respective journals revealed that the more "fundamentalist" schools (Klein and Kohut) each cited a very restrictive range of their own authorities, while relational psychoanalysts cited a broader range (Sorenson, 2004, pp. 1–17). It would be useful to use a similar method to assess the progress toward a multilevel interdisciplinary paradigm for the psychology of religion. Not only could such a method be applied to disciplines and levels of analysis within mainstream journals, but to methods as well. By this process we can assess progress toward realizing the new paradigm.

NOTES

1. Emmons and Paloutzian (2003) identify the new paradigm as multilevel and interdisciplinary (p. 395); while we applaud this call, the field is far from realizing this ideal (Belzen, 2005; Belzen & Hood, in press; Wulff, 2003).
2. In an indefensible breach of research ethics, a psychological disruptive experience that occurred to one of the experimental participants was not reported in any of the write-ups of this widely cited study (see Doblin, 1991; Smith, 2000, pp. 99–105).
3. Another example is research on meditation (see Newberg & Newberg, Chapter 11, this volume).

REFERENCES

Adorno, T. W., Frenkel-Brunswik, E., Levinson, D. J., & Sanford, R. N. (1950). *The authoritarian personality.* New York: Harper & Row.

Altemyer, B. (1988). *Enemies of freedom: Understanding right-wing authoritarianism.* San Francisco: Jossey-Bass,

Alteymer, B., & Hunsberger, B. (1992). Authoritarianism, religious fundamentalism, quest, and prejudice. *The International Journal for the Psychology of Religion, 13,* 17–28.

Aronson, E., Wilson, T. D., & Brewer, M. B. (1998). Experimentation in social psychology. In D. T. Gilbert, S. T. Fiske, & G. Lindzey (Eds.), *The handbook of social psychology* (Vol. 1, pp. 99–142). New York: Oxford University Press.

Bader, C. (1999). New perspectives on failed prophecy. *Journal for the Scientific Study of Religion, 38,* 119–131.

Batson, C. D. (1975). Rational processing or rationalization?: The effect of disconfirmining information on a stated religious belief. *Journal of Personality and Social Psychology, 32,* 176–184.

Batson, C. D., Schoenrade, P., & Ventis, W. L. (1993). *Religion and the individual: A social-psychological perspective.* New York: Oxford University Press.

Belzen, J. A. (Ed.). (1997). *Hermeneutical approaches in psychology of religion.* Atlanta, GA: Rodopi.

Belzen, J. A. (2001). *Psychohistory in psychology of religion: Interdisciplinary studies.* Atlanta, GA: Rodopi.

Belzen, J. A. (2004). *Religie, melancholie en zelf. Een historische en psychologische studie over een psychiatrisch ego-document uit de negentiende eeuw.* Kampen, The Netherlands: Kok.

Belzen, J. A. (2005). In defense of the object: On trends and directions in the psychology of religion. *The International Journal for the Psychology of Religion, 15,* 1–16.

Belzen, J. A., & Hood, R. W., Jr. (in press). Methodological issues in the psychology of religion. *Journal of Psychology.*

Belzen, J. A., & Uleyn, A. J. R. (1992). What is real?: Speculations on Hood's implicit epistemology and theology. *The International Journal for the Psychology of Religion, 2,* 165–169.

Browder, G. C. (1996). *Hitler's enforcers: The Gestapo and SS security services in the Nazi revolution.* New York: Oxford University Press.

Burris, C. T. (1999). The Mysticism Scale: Research form D (M Scale). In P. C. Hill & R. W. Hood, Jr. (Eds.), *Measure of religiosity* (pp. 363–367). Birmingham, AL: Religious Education Press.

Burton, T. (1993). *Serpent-handling believers.* Knoxville: University of Tennessee Press.

Campbell, D. T., & Stanley, J. C. (1963). *Experimental and quasi-experimental designs for research.* Chicago: Rand McNally.

Capps, D., Ransohoff, R., & Rambo, L. (1976). Publication trends in the psychology of religion to 1974. *Journal for the Scientific Study of Religion, 15,* 15–28.

Carroll, M. P. (1983). Visions of the Virgin Mary: The effect of family structures on Marian apparitions. *Journal for the Scientific Study of Religion, 22,* 205–221.

Carroll, M. P. (1986). *The cult of the Virgin Mary: Psychological origins.* Princeton, NJ: Princeton University Press.

Coyle, B. R. (2001). Twelve myths of religion and psychiatry: Lessons for training psychiatrists in spiritual sensitive treatments. *Mental Health, Religion, and Culture, 4,* 147–174.

Danziger, K. (1990). *Constructing the subject: Historical origins of psychological research.* Cambridge, UK: Cambridge University Press.

Dein, S. (1997). Lubavitch: A contemporary messianic movement. *Journal of Contemporary Religion, 12,* 191–204.

Dein, S. (2001). What really happens when prophecy fails: The case of Lubavitch. *Sociology of Religion, 62,* 383–401.

Doblin, R. (1991). Panke's "Good Friday" experiment: A long-term follow-up and methodological critique. *Journal of Transpersonal Psychology, 23,* 1–28.

Emmons, R. A., & Paloutzian, R. F. (2003). The psychology of religion. *Annual Review of Psychology, 54,* 377–402.

Festinger, L., Riecken, H. W., & Schachter, S. (1953). *When prophecy fails.* Minneapolis: University of Minnesota Press.

Gergen, K. J., & Gergen, M. M. (1988). Narrative and the self as relationship. *Advances in Experimental Psychology, 21,* 17–56.

Gorsuch, R. L. (1984). Measurement: The boon and bane of investigating the psychology of religion. *American Psychologist, 39,* 228–236.

Gorsuch, R. L. (1988). The psychology of religion. *Annual Review of Psychology, 39,* 201–221.

Gorsuch, R. L. (2002). *Integrating psychology and spirituality.* Westport, CT: Praeger.

Gorsuch, R. L., & Alshire, D. (1974). Christian faith and ethnic prejudice: A review and interpretation of research. *Journal for the Scientific Study of Religion, 13,* 281–307.

Hood, R. W., Jr. (1977). Eliciting mystical states of consciousness with semi-structured nature experiences. *Journal for the Scientific Study of Religion, 15,* 155–163.

Hood, R. W., Jr. (1978a). Anticipatory set and setting stress incongruity as elicitors of mystical experience in solitary nature situations. *Journal for the Scientific Study of Religion, 17,* 278–287.

Hood, R. W., Jr. (1978b). The usefulness of the indiscriminitively pro and anti categories of religious orientation. *Journal for the Scientific Study of Religion, 17,* 278–287.

Hood, R. W., Jr. (1983). Social psychology and religious fundamentalism. In A. W. Childs & G. B. Melton (Eds.), *Rural psychology* (pp. 169–198). New York: Plenum Press.

Hood, R. W., Jr. (1992). Mysticism, reality, illusion and the Freudian critique of religion. *The International Journal for Psychology of Religion, 2,* 141–159.

Hood, R. W., Jr. (1997). Psychoanalysis and fundamentalism: Lessons from a feminist critique of Freud. In J. L. Jacobs & D. Capps (Eds.), *Religion, society and psychoanalysis* (pp. 42–67). Boulder, CO: Westview Press.

Hood, R. W., Jr. (1998). When the spirit maims and kills: Social psychological considerations of the history of serpent handling and the narrative of handlers. *The International Journal for the Psychology of Religion, 8,* 71–96.

Hood, R. W., Jr. (2003). The relationship between religion and spirituality. In D. Bromley (Series Ed.) & A. L. Greil & D. Bromley (Vol. Eds.), *Defining religion: Investigating the boundaries between the sacred and the secular: Vol. 10. Religion and the social order* (pp. 241–265). Amsterdam, The Netherlands: Elsevier Science.

Hood, R. W., Jr. (Ed.). (2005). *Handling serpents: Pastor Jimmy Morrow's narrative history of his Appalachian Jesus' name tradition.* Mercer, GA: Mercer University Press.

Hood, R. W., Jr., Hill, P. C., & Williamson, W. P. (2005). *The psychology of religious fundamentalism.* New York: Guilford Press.

Hood, R. W., Jr., & Kimbrough, D. (1995). Serpent-handling holiness sects: Theoretical considerations. *Journal for the Scientific Study of Religion, 34,* 311–322.

Hood, R. W., Jr. & Morris, R. J. (1981a). Knowledge and experience criteria in the report of mystical experience. *Review of Religious Research, 23,* 76–84.

Hood, R. W., Jr. & Morris, R. J. (1981b). Sensory isolation and the differential elicitation of the report of visual imagery in intrinsic and extrinsic subjects. *Journal for the Scientific Study of Religion, 20,* 261–273.

Hood, R. W., Jr., Morris, R. J., & Watson, P. J. (1990). Quasi-elicitation of the differential report of mystical experience among intrinsic and indiscriminately pro-religious types. *Journal for the Scientific Study of Religion, 29,* 164–172.

Hood, R. W., Jr., Morris, R. J., & Watson, P. J. (1991). Male commitment to the cult of the Virgin Mary and the Passion of Christ as a function of early maternal bonding. *The International Journal for the Psychology of Religion, 1,* 221–231.

Hood, R. W., Jr., Williamson, W. P., & Morris, R. J. (1999). Evaluation of the legitimacy of conversion experience as a function of the five signs of Mark 16. *Review of Religious Research, 41,* 96–109.

Hood, R. W., Jr., Williamson, W. P., & Morris, R. J. (2000). Changing views of serpent handling: A quasi-experimental study. *Journal for the Scientific Study of Religion, 39,* 531–544.

Hood–Williamson research archives on the serpent-handlers of southern Appalachia. Lupton Library, University of Tennessee at Chattanooga.

Hovi, T. (2004). Religious conviction shaped and maintained by narration. *Archiv für Religionspsychologie, 26,* 35–50.

Janssen, J., de Hart, J., & den Draak, C. (1990). A content analysis of the praying practices of Dutch youth. *Journal for the Scientific Study of Religion, 29,* 99–107.

Keltner, D. (1995). Signs of appeasement: Evidence for the distinct displays of embarassment, amusement, and shame. *Journal of Personality and Social Psychology, 68,* 441–454.

Kirkpatrick, L. A. (1993). Fundamentalism, Christian orthodoxy, and intrinsic religious orientation. *Journal for the Scientific Study of Religion, 32*, 256–268.

Kirkpatrick, L. A. (1997). A longitudinal study of changes in religious belief and behavior as a function of individual differences in adult attachment styles. *Journal for the Scientific Study of Religion, 36*, 207–217.

Kirkpatrick, L. A. (1998). God as substitute attachment figure: A longitudinal study of adult attachment style and religious changes in college. *Personality and Social Psychology Bulletin, 24*, 961–973.

Kirkpatrick, L. A., Hood, R. W., Jr., & Hartz, G. (1991). Fundamentalist religion conceptualized in terms of Rokeach's theory of the open and closed mind: New perspectives on some old ideas. *Research in the Social Scientific Study of Religion, 3*, 157–170.

Kressel, N. J. (1996). *Mass hate: The global rise of genocide and terrorism*. New York: Plenum Press.

Kripall, J. J. (1995). *Kali's child: The mystical and the erotic in the life and teaching of Ramakrishna*. Chicago: University of Chicago Press.

Lindgren, T. (2004). The narrative construction of Muslim identity: A case study. *Archiv für Religionspsychologie, 26*, 51–73.

McAdams, D. P., & Bowman, P. J. (2002). Narrating life's turning points: redemption and contamination. In D. P. McAdams, R. Josselson, & A. Lieblich (Eds.), *Turns in the road: Narrative studies of lives in transition* (pp. 3–34). Washington, DC: American Psychological Association.

McDonald, D. A. (2000). Spirituality: Description and measurement, and relation to the five-factor model of personality. *Journal of Personality, 68*, 153–197.

Melton, J. G. (1985). Spiritualization and reaffirmation: What really happens when prophecy fails? *American Studies, 26*, 17–29.

Moghadam, F. M., Taylor, D. M., & Wright, S. C. (1993). *Social psychology in cross cultural perspective*. New York: Freeman.

Oxman, T. E., Rosenberg, S. D., Schnurr, P. P., Tucker, G. J., & Gala, G. G. (1988). The language of altered states. *Journal of Nervous and Mental Disease, 176*, 401–408.

Pafford, M. (1973). *Inglorious Wordsworths: A study of some transcendent experiences in childhood and adolescence*. London: Hodder & Stoughton.

Paloutzian, R. F. (1996). *Invitation to the psychology of religion* (2nd ed.). Needham Heights, MA: Allyn & Bacon.

Paloutzian, R. F., Richardson, J. T., & Rambo, L. R. (1999). Religious conversion and personality change. *Journal of Personality, 67*, 1047–1079.

Pahnke, W. N. (1969). Psychedelic drugs and mystical experience. In E. M. Pattison (Ed.), *Clinical psychiatry and religion* (pp. 149–162). Boston: Little, Brown.

Piedmont, R. L. (1999a). Does spirituality represent the sixth factor of personality?: Spiritual transcendences and the five-factor model. *Journal of Personality, 67*, 985–1014.

Piedmont, R. L. (1999b). Strategies for using the five-factor model of personality in religious research. *Journal of Psychology and Theology, 27*, 338–350.

Pollner, M. (1987). *Mundane reason: Reason in everyday and sociological discourse*. Cambridge, UK: Cambridge University Press.

Poloma, M. M., & Gallup, G. H., Jr. (1991). *Varieties of prayer: A survey report*. Philadelphia: Trinity Press International.

Ričan, P. (2004). Spirituality: The story of a concept in the psychology of religion. *Archiv für Religionspsychologie, 26*, 135–156.

Rokeach, M. (1960). *The open and closed mind*. New York: Basic Books.

Schwartz, S. (1999). *Faith, serpents, and fire: Images of Kentucky holiness believers*. Jackson: University Press of Mississippi.

Sears, D. (1986). College sophomores in the laboratory: Influence of a narrow data base on social psychology's view of human nature. *Journal of Personality and Social Psychology, 51*, 515–530.

Shanon, B. (2002). *The antipodes of the mind*. New York: Oxford University Press.

Smith, H. (2000). *Cleansing the doors of perception: The religious significance of ethegeonic plants and chemicals.* New York: Tarcher/Putman.

Sorenson, R. L. (2004). *Minding spirituality.* Hillsdale, NJ: Analytic Press.

Spilka, B., Hood, R. W., Jr., Hunsberger, B., & Gorsuch, R. (2003). *The psychology of religion: An empirical approach* (3rd ed.). New York: Guilford Press.

Staal, F. (1971). *Exploring mysticism.* Harmondsworth, UK: Penguin Books.

Stace, W. T. (1960). *Mysticism and philosophical analysis.* Philadelphia: Lippincott.

Stark, R. (1971). Psychopathology and religious commitment. *Review of Religious Research, 12,* 165–176.

Stone, P. J., Dunphy, D. C., Smith, M. S., & Ogilvie, D. M. (1966). *The general inquirer: A computer approach to content analysis.* Cambridge, MA: MIT press.

Strassman, R. (2001). *DMT: The spirit molecule.* Rochester, VT: Park Street Press.

Streib, H., & Keller, B. (2004). The variety of deconversion experiences: Contours of a concept and emerging research results. *Archiv für Religionspsychologie, 26,* 181–200.

Targ, E., Schlitz, M., & Irwin, H. J. (2000). Psi-related experiences. In E. Cardena, S. J. Lynn, & S. Krippner (Eds.), *Varieties of anomalous experience: Examining the scientific evidence* (pp. 219–252). Washington, DC: American Psychological Association.

Tamminen, K. (1991). *Religious development in childhood and youth: An empirical study.* Helsinki, Finland: Suomalinen Tiedeakatemia.

Thalbourne, M. A., & Delin, P. S. (1994). A common thread underlying belief in the paranormal, creative personality, mystical experience and psychopathology. *Journal of Parapsychology, 58,* 3–38.

Thalbourne, M. A., & Delin, P. S. (1999). Transliminality: Its relation to dream life, religiosity, and mystical experience. *The International Journal for the Psychology of Religion, 9,* 35–43.

Tumminia, D. (1998). How prophecy never fails: Interpretative reason in a flying saucer group. *Sociology of Religion, 59,* 157–170.

Waller, J. (2002). *Becoming evil: How ordinary people commit genocide and mass killing.* New York: Oxford University Press.

Williamson, P. W., & Hood, R. W., Jr. (2004). Differential maintenance and growth of religious organizations based upon high-cost behaviors: Serpent-handling within the Church of God. *Review of Religious Research, 45,* 150–168.

Williamson, P. W., & Polio, H. R. (1999). The phenomenology of religious serpent handling: A rational and thematic study of extemporaneous sermons. *Journal for the Scientific Study of Religion, 38,* 203–218.

Williamson, P. W., Polio, H. R., & Hood, R. W., Jr. (2000). A phenomenological analysis of anointing among serpent handlers. *Journal for the Scientific Study of Religion, 10,* 221–240.

Wulff, D. (2003). A field in crisis: Is it time to start over? In H. M. P. Roelofsma, J. M. T. Corveleyn, & J. W. van Saane (Eds.), *One hundred years of psychology of religion* (pp. 11–32). Amsterdam, The Netherlands: VU University Press.

Zinnbauer, B. J., Pargament, K. I., Cole, B., Rye, M. S., Butter, E. M., & Belavich, T. G. (1997). Religion and spirituality: Unfuzzying the fuzzy. *Journal for the Scientific Study of Religion, 36,* 549–564.

5

Psychodynamic Psychologies and Religion

Past, Present, and Future

JOZEF CORVELEYN
PATRICK LUYTEN

Faced with the task of writing a chapter offering an overview of psychodynamic or psychoanalytic approaches to religion, one feels both hesitation and trepidation. Psychoanalytic approaches have been considered by some to have "clearly led to a revolution in the study of religion in general and in the psychology of religion in particular" (Beit-Hallahmi, 1996, p. 12). There would be "no substitute and no theoretical alternative to psychoanalysis, as the most, and the only, comprehensive theoretical approach to the psychology of religion" (Beit-Hallahmi, 1996, p. 12). Others, however, have concluded that psychoanalytic theorizing concerning religion, although not without merit, is sometimes overly simplistic, often reductionistic, and generally not empirically supported (e.g., Hood, Spilka, Hunsberger, & Gorsuch, 1996; Wulff, 1997). Hence, whereas the psychoanalytic literature on religion continues to be vast, at the same time many contemporary overviews of the psychology of religion only devote a small and mostly historical sketch of psychoanalytic thinking concerning religion (e.g., Emmons & Paloutzian, 2003; Paloutzian, 1996; Spilka, Hood, Hunsberger, & Gorsuch, 2003).

Given these conflicting conclusions concerning the value of psychoanalytic approaches to religion, it is not our intention to give in this chapter a complete overview of all psychoanalytic research efforts of the past century. This would be an almost impossible task. Moreover, several extensive older (e.g., Meissner, 1984; Saffady, 1976) as well as more recent (e.g., Beit-Hallahmi, 1996; Wulff, 1997) reviews exist.

Thus, rather than attempting to present a complete overview, we will try to address and clarify both the strengths and limitations of psychoanalytically inspired approaches to religion. In order to be able to provide a balanced review of strengths and limitations, following Freud (1923/1961b, 1924/1961d), we distinguish between psychoanalysis as (1) an encompassing theory concerning both "normal" and "pathological" psychological functioning, (2) a method of investigation, and (3) a form of treatment. First, we address what we consider to be one of the most central theoretical propositions of a psychoanalytic approach toward religion, namely, the distinction between religion as a cultural phenomenon, on the one hand, and personal religion, on the other. Next, we outline some main lines of Freud's theoretical views on religion, which allows us to provide a balanced discussion of the critique that is most often leveled against psychoanalytic approaches to religion, namely, that they are overly reductionistic. In a third section, we provide a brief sketch of developments in psychoanalytic theorizing since Freud and its contribution to the study of religion. Strengths and limitations of psychodynamically inspired empirical research concerning religion are discussed in a fourth section in the context of recent theoretical and methodological developments in psychoanalysis. Subsequently, we discuss clinical implications of psychoanalytic theorizing and research in the context of the debate concerning the integration of religion and spirituality in psychotherapy and counseling. We close this chapter with some conclusions and directions for further research.

THE TWO SIDES OF "RELIGION": RELIGION AS A CULTURAL PHENOMENON AND RELIGION AS A PERSONAL EXPERIENCE

Any psychoanalytic—and for that matter any psychological—approach to religion should distinguish between religion as a general *cultural* and *social* fact, on the one hand, and *personal* religion, on the other hand. As a cultural phenomenon, religion is always a "given" that cannot be explained, let alone explained away, by psychology. Following Vergote (1996), who draws on Geertz (1973), religion can be defined as a system of symbols that acts to establish powerful, pervasive, and long-lasting moods and motivations. Although religions in this sense of the term are subject to changes over time and within a particular culture, they nevertheless consist of rather stable theological principles and a more or less established and stable organization.[1] Hence, the term "religion" refers to a number of organized forms of belief, first, to the "great" religions (e.g., Christianity, Islam, Judaism, etc.), and second, to some so-called new religious movements. Personal religion, on the other hand, or religion as it is lived, is made up of a mix of these theological principles with psychological (personal) and sociological influences. Or better: it is the result of a continuous confrontation of the individual with the preexisting culture, including religion, in which he or she is born and living. Personal religion is thus colored by one's own personal, idiosyncratic history.

This distinction between personal religion and religion as a cultural phenomenon finds an important parallel in psychoanalysis between psychoanalysis "proper" and so-called applied psychoanalysis. Although the distinction is to some extent artificial, the former is mainly occupied with explaining the psychological functioning of the individual, whereas the latter is broadly aimed at explaining sociocultural processes and phenomena. It was Freud who initiated this latter approach, and applied it to religion in his now classic work *The Future of an Illusion* (Freud, 1927/1961c). His purpose was not only to understand (*Verstehen*) religion, but also to explain (*Erklären*) it. However, this "psychoanalytic archeology" (Beit-Hallahmi, 1996, p. 11) has often been criticized for being overly reductionistic. Despite this, the application of psychoanalytic theories and hypotheses to religion has been and continues to be very popular, not only among psychoanalytic authors, but also among many philosophers and sociologists (e.g., Devereux, 1953/1974).

The distinction between personal religion and religion as a cultural phenomenon also overlaps with Freud's so-called ontogenetic and phylogenetic theories of religion (Wulff, 1997). Interestingly, whereas Freud did show interest in the development of personal religion (ontogenetic perspective), as is for instance shown in his famous case study of the Wolf Man (Freud, 1918/1955a), he was nevertheless mainly interested in the phylogenetic perspective, that is, in explaining the origin and development of religion as such (e.g., Freud, 1913/1953). Again, Freud's preference for theories concerning the origin of religion as a cultural phenomenon influenced many studies after him. It has only been relatively recently, with the growing popularity of object relations theory and self psychology, that personal religion has become the center of attention of psychoanalytic studies of religion (see Kernberg, 2000). Moreover, as Blass (2004) has convincingly argued, this growing attention within psychoanalysis for personal religion is also partly due to a shift in religion itself, away from organized religion and religion as a quest for truth, toward religion as deeply held, personal beliefs and experiences that are not necessarily linked to organized forms of religion (see Zinnbauer & Pargament, Chapter 2, this volume).

FREUD AND RELIGION

From his early experiences with the Judaic faith and traditions of his family and with the Catholic tradition of his nanny (Blatt, 1988; Gay, 1987; Rice, 1990; Rizzuto, 1998) to his final work *Moses and Monotheism* (Freud, 1939/1964a), his ultimate attempt to understand the historical origins of Jewish religion and (monotheistic) religion in general, religion was always an important aspect in Freud's life. Although Freud is often depicted as a rationalistic and atheistic thinker, and although many of his works can be read from that perspective, he was not at all fundamentally antireligious. For example, he did count religion, together with art, as one of the most impressive accomplishments of humanity (Freud, 1930/1961a).

Freud's influence on the psychoanalytic study of religion can be particularly discerned among his contemporaries. Some of them have applied, "in the shadow of the master" (Meissner, 2000, p. 55), his theories to other aspects of religion or to religions other than those in the Judeo-Christian tradition, which was Freud's major focus (e.g., Jones, 1916/1967; Reik, 1931). On the other hand, it is interesting to note that the major "dissidents" in the psychoanalytic movement of the first decades, such as Carl Gustav Jung and Alfred Adler (Nuttin, 1950/1962) were very interested in religion and disagreed in many respects with Freud about religion (e.g., Vandermeersch, 1991). In fact, the only real opponent of Freud's perspective on religion who did not become a dissident during his lifetime was the Lutheran pastor and psychoanalyst Oskar Pfister. In his virulent criticism *The Illusion of a Future* (Pfister, 1928)—the title itself mocks Freud's *The Future of an Illusion*—he argued that Freud's view of religion was itself a tribute to the ideology of rational progress and of the triumphs of rationalistic science, and thus—according to Freud's own definition—an illusion (see Goossens, 1990). Pfister's critique can be seen as the starting point of a series of critiques of Freud's views on religion.

First and foremost is the criticism of reductionism, which concerns Freud's philosophical rationalistic background. According to this criticism, Freud completely reduces religion to an irrational prephase in the evolution of humankind toward a more realistic, rationalistic, and scientific civilization (cf. Meissner, 2000; Vergote, 1998). This reductionism criticism is nowadays often the major and frequently the only criticism leveled at Freud and psychoanalytic approaches to religion in general. And, in fact, if it is not taken as a final judgment on Freud's approach to religion, one must say that this criticism is valid. Freud did consider religion to be essentially an illusion, a fulfillment of personal desires, such as a deep longing for protection against the perils of nature, preferably by an exalted father figure. With Vergote (1998), we agree that it is clear that Freud should not have made this attempt of *explaining* religion as such. His attempts to explain religion are not based on any detailed or systematic observations, clinical or otherwise. To the contrary, he seems to have been driven by a rationalistic Enlightenment philosophy which pushed him to tackle religion in its entirety. Remarkably, this is in strong contrast with his repeated affirmation that psychoanalysis is not a worldview, not even a complete anthropology (Freud, 1933/1964b). In his opinion, psychoanalysis always should be, both as a science and as a method of treatment, neutral toward religion. It is also in contrast to his otherwise great effort to observe and understand phenomena in great detail and depth (Vergote, 1998).

Nevertheless, it would also be incorrect to reduce Freud's approach to religion to one completely biased by a rationalistic ideology (see Vergote, 1998). His approach did raise fundamental psychological questions about religion and about individual religious faith. More concretely, Freud did ask important questions about the part that is played in personal religion by personal desires, fantasies, and conflicts linked to the individual's personal history and his or her encounters with significant others.

A second criticism of Freud's views on religion, which is mostly leveled by more "interpersonally" oriented authors (e.g., Jones, 1991), is that Freud reduces religion to a one-person motivational matter, and neglects the interpersonal and, more generally, sociocultural components of religion. And again, indeed, many of his theories can be read from such a perspective, although, as mentioned above, it would also be too simplistic to reduce Freud's approach to religion as being completely a "one-person" psychology.

Hence, although both variants of the reductionism criticism may be essentially correct, Freud's contribution to the study of religion contains more than his easy rationalistic reduction of religion to an irrational temporary phase of human evolution, or to a purely individual issue. Indeed, he did raise some fundamental questions about the interaction between personal history and religion as a social fact, as we illustrate further on in this chapter.

THERE IS MORE THAN ONE PSYCHOLOGY IN THE FAMILY OF PSYCHOANALYSIS

Psychoanalysis is not, as some critics of psychoanalysis often want us to believe, limited to the eternal rephrasing of Freud, nor is it limited to the exegetical rereading and rediscussion of the *n*-th interpretation of some of his not-so-clear sentences. Freud's work is not the "gold standard" of a metric system. Psychoanalysis, and psychoanalytic approaches to religion in particular, did not stop to evolve after Freud's death—quite the contrary. With Pine (1990), one can currently distinguish somewhat schematically "four psychologies of psychoanalysis": drive psychology, ego psychology, object relations psychology, and self psychology. Although somewhat overlapping, each of these perspectives focuses on different aspects of psychological functioning, and thus should not be seen as competing perspectives, but as complementary views of the same, complex, psychological reality (Wallerstein, 1992). The first three of these approaches have inspired most of the psychodynamically oriented research in the field of the psychology of religion. In addition, especially with the advent of object relations theories, psychoanalysis has become less reductionistic and less hostile toward religion than Freud's original formulations and those of many of his contemporaries (Blass, 2004).

Drive Psychology

This was Freud's primary approach to human behavior. It looks at human behavior from the perspective of personal motives or tendencies and wishes, which are formulated in terms of "pulsions" (drives) and their vicissitudes. It is hypothesized that some wishes give rise to inner conflicts because they are experienced as unacceptable by the inner moral and ethical standards of the individual, and/or dangerous in relation to the requirements of the outside world. A central role is allocated to defense or transmutation mechanisms to deal with unacceptable wishes (drives). These defense mechanisms are, of course, largely influenced by social, cultural, and educational factors. In that sense, Freud was not an unrealistic "monadist" (Leibniz), as some of his critics suppose. He did not consider the individual as a self-sufficient being. To the contrary, from the early beginnings of his work he took into account the interaction of the individual with the surrounding environment, although it must be admitted that he mainly focused on intrapsychic factors. This "classical" approach inspired much of the older psychoanalytic literature on religion (Capps, 2001), and focused, as Freud himself did, mostly on the "hidden" personal desires and conflicts in religion (e.g., Daim, 1951; Zilboorg, 1955).

According to Pine (1990), the work of the influential French psychoanalyst Jacques Lacan and of his followers should also be situated in the drive psychology tradition. Although regularly referring to religion, Lacan in fact never wrote a single work devoted solely to religion. His views, however, have inspired several important approaches to religion (e.g., Dolto & Sévérin, 1977; Maître, 1997). For example, Vasse (1991) has applied Lacanian concepts and theories to study the main authobiographical works of the creative religious Theresa of Avila. Michel de Certeau, in turn, has provided interesting insights and hypotheses concerning the raise of mysticism in the 17th century in general and the possession of Sister Jeanne des Anges of Loudun and her exorcist Surin in particular (de Certeau, 1963, 1980; see also Lietaer & Corveleyn, 1995). Also, the seminal work of Vergote (1988, 1996, 1998) on religion has to be mentioned here because it has been heavily influenced by both "classical" Freudian and Lacanian psychoanalysis. In fact, Vergote has always emphasized the intrinsic and reciprocal influence between the individual psyche and the cultural and symbolic environment, which in turn results from a continuous encounter between the individual and the given cultural environment. His research on topics such as the image of God (Vergote & Tamayo, 1980), religious experience (Vergote, 1996), and pathological forms of religion (Vergote, 1988, 1996), testifies of this deep awareness of the reciprocity between individual desires and conflicts and given cultural environments.

Ego Psychology

Ego psychology mainly focuses on the "other side" of the psychic conflict, namely, the capacity of the ego to defend against personal drives and to adapt to reality (Pine, 1990). Erik Erikson (e.g., 1950, 1958, 1968, 1969) is probably the most well-known representative of this perspective in the psychology of religion, not only because of his works on identity formation in great religious leaders, such as Martin Luther (Erikson, 1958) and Mahatma Gandhi (Erikson, 1969), but also because of his seminal work in the area of developmental psychology (see Zock, 1990, for an overview). Together with the structuralistic approach to child development of Jean Piaget, Erikson's developmental theories have heavily influenced research on religious development in childhood and adolescence as well as on religious education (see also Boyatzis, Chapter 7, and Levenson, Aldwin, & D'Mello, Chapter 8, this volume).

Another good example of the ego psychology approach can be found in the work of William Meissner (1992) on Ignatius of Loyola, the founder of the Jesuits. In this psychobiographical study, Meissner convincingly shows that Ignatius, despite considerable psychopathological problems in his young adulthood, was able to overcome these problems to a great extent, as is evidenced by his great creativity and religious leadership, even in religiously and politically very troubled times. In particular, Meissner shows that Ignatius was able to successfully mobilize constructive ego capacities and defense mechanisms to compensate for certain ego defects. Moreover, with this work, Meissner also shows that sanctity (in religious terms) is not the result of a "supernatural" transformation of personality, but is constructed with the ordinary building blocks of human personality, including pathological ones (Corveleyn, 1997).

Psychology of Object Relations

In this approach, the focus is on the individual's representations of self and others, the development of these representations, and the influence they exert on current perceptions, experiences, and behaviors.

Rizzuto's (1979) work on the representation of God is a good example of this approach, because she mainly attempts to show how representations from significant others influence and shape, in interaction with the sociocultural environment, an individual's representation of God (see also McDargh, 1983; Spero, 1992). Object relational theories have also played an important role in broadening the scope of psychoanalytic studies of religion in that they provided new theoretical tools to study the role of early object relations in particular religious phenomena, such as religious experiences and Eastern religions (Wulff, 1997), where "classical" drive and ego psychological theories seemed to be less applicable. Moreover, Winnicott's notion of the transitional space has not only led to a recognition of creative processes in religion, but has also resulted in a more positive regard within psychoanalysis toward religious beliefs, as is for instance exemplified in the work of Paul W. Pruyser (Malony & Spilka, 1991).

CURRENT EMPIRICAL RESEARCH IN PSYCHOANALYSIS AND ITS RELEVANCE FOR A PSYCHOANALYTIC PSYCHOLOGY OF RELIGION

Recent Developments within Psychoanalysis: A Growing Research Culture

Empirical research on personal religion from a psychodynamic perspective has mainly focused on the detailed study of individual lives, mostly by means of the traditional case study method. This research method has been, without a doubt, psychoanalysis's preferred method of investigation, and has undeniably resulted in a wide variety of valuable insights and theoretical hypotheses about human beings, including their religious beliefs, experiences, and behaviors (e.g., Beit-Hallahmi, 1996; Spilka et al., 2003; Wulff, 1997).

However, at the same time, it has become increasingly clear, also within the psychoanalytic community, that the traditional case study method has serious methodological flaws (e.g., Spence, 1994). One of the most important pitfalls is related to the selective release of data that is typical of case studies, if any data are included at all. For example, Klumpner and Frank (1991) found that not a single study of the 15 most cited papers in psychoanalysis included a substantial amount of (clinical) data. There is little reason to believe that psychoanalytic studies of religion would fare any better. This makes it hard to judge to which extent theoretical prejudices might have played a role in the selection and interpretation of material, or to which extent alternative, and perhaps more parsimonious, explanations are possible. Because of this selective release and virtual absence of data, not surprisingly, psychoanalysis as a whole has shown a remarkable resistance against falsification. This is also true for the psychoanalytic study of religion. If one reviews the history of psychoanalytic approaches to religion, time and time again the same religious phenomena were interpreted and reinterpreted, depending on the "fashion of the day." When the Oedipus complex was the shibboleth of psychoanalysis, almost every religious behavior or belief was considered to be an expression of Oedipal conflicts or tendencies. When ego psychology started to take off, these same conflicts and tendencies were suddenly seen as an expression of the adaptation of the ego to reality. And when object relation theories were in their heyday, studies linking religious phenomena to the development, structure, and/or content of object relations mushroomed.

Although the influence of trends and new discoveries on scientific research is inevitable, and the meaning of psychological phenomena is often if not always overdetermined, there has been little progress in the empirical study of religion from a psychodynamic point of view precisely because of this overreliance on anecdote, authority, and selectively released case material.[2] This has led to a proliferation of theories and hypotheses, without the necessary correlate of discarding "older" theories or hypotheses. Hence, "old" and "new" psychoanalytic theories concerning religion stand side by side, even if they contradict each other. Debates concerning the value of a theory or hypothesis are mostly settled by relying on anecdote, authority, and the selective release of data that confirm each author's beloved theory. Because psychoanalysis continued to rely on an outdated research methodology, which was no longer accepted as scientific by the larger scientific community, once its boon, the traditional case study method was rapidly becoming psychoanalysis's bane.

However, the waning influence of psychoanalysis in mainstream psychology and psychiatry, in combination with the advent of evidence-based medicine and managed care, finally led to a growing awareness in some psychoanalytic circles toward the end of the 1980s that if psychoanalysis was to survive, it had to use other research methods than the traditional case study method (Luyten, Blatt, & Corveleyn, 2004). The result was not only a boom in psychodynamically inspired empirical research, but also an increasing dialogue and integration between psychoanalysis and various branches of mainstream psychology, as well as the development of new methods that are specifically designed to test often complex psychodynamic hypotheses (e.g., Westen, 1998). This was paralleled by a growing move within mainstream psychology toward more idiographic research and toward the study of private experiences in general (e.g., Singer & Kolligian, 1987).

The Need for Good Theory and the Promise of Psychoanalysis

Even a quick perusal of the psychological literature in general and research in the field of the psychology of religion in particular demonstrates the need for comprehensive theories. Empirical studies abound, but they are widely scattered, poorly integrated, and more often than not lack an overarching theoretical framework. In fact, many of these studies are, as Spence (1994, p. 23) noted in another context, "impeccable 'studies of nothing very much,' " a situation that reinforces the belief of many that the systematic empirical study of religion has little to offer (see also Hood & Belzen, Chapter 4, this volume). However, in our opinion, the fact that the quality of many of these studies is poor appears to be due more to the poor quality of the research questions asked than to the methods used as such. Yet this only further reinforces the need for good theory.

In fact, this same concern is echoed by Spilka et al. (2003, p. 542, emphasis added): "What appears the *clearest* need in social-scientific work that will assure the vigor, relevance, and compatibility of the psychology of religion with mainstream psychology is theory." In line with Batson (1997), we would like to add that what the psychology of religion needs is not so much theory per se, because there is in fact an abundance of theories, but *good* theories—that is, theories that are not only capable of providing an overarching view of human nature, including humanity's relationship with religion, but that are also able to generate a coherent, theoretically based research program. Here, we believe that psychoanalytic theories, in conjunction with recent methodological developments both within psychoanalysis and within mainstream psychology, have much to offer.

Briefly, we believe that a psychoanalytic approach to religion can transform the traditional "hit-and-run" research into a more detailed study of individual lives. From a theoretical point of view, psychoanalysis provides a wide variety of theories and hypotheses that have been based on the detailed study of individual lives. As is the case in much research in mainstream psychology, research in the psychology of religion has shown an overreliance on broad and abstract notions, which tell us little about what role religion plays in the concrete daily life of people. Hence, most research has been unable to bridge the gap between the nomothetic and idiographic level (for an exception, see Emmons, 1999). This same dissatisfaction with "grand theories" can be observed in mainstream psychology, and has led to a rapidly increasing number of microlevel theories and subsequent studies of very concrete behaviors and attitudes. On a methodological level, this has resulted in a move away from more traditional methods, such as self-report questionnaires and cross-sectional designs, to the use of methods that are able to tap in more detail and more depth psychological processes in real-life (e.g., experience sampling, diary methods, etc.). In addition, instead of relying on cross-sectional designs, which are of limited value to investigate causal relationships, longitudinal studies are increasingly used in combination with more sophisticated statistical methods such as structural equation modeling (SEM), growth curve modeling, and survival analysis (e.g., Willett, Singer, & Martin, 1998). These latter two statistical methods are particularly interesting because they enable data to be analyzed on both the idiographic and the nomothetic levels. As stated earlier, these developments have also led to a growing methodological sophistication in empirical research in psychoanalysis. Psychoanalytically oriented researchers have adapted and adopted these methods because they do more justice to the complexity of psychodynamic hypotheses, which often imply interactive, recursive models (see further below) rather than more traditional linear models and statistical methods (e.g., Westen & Shedler, 1999).

Yet these developments within psychoanalysis have, with very few exceptions, not been applied to the domain of the psychoanalytic study of religion. Here lies an important task for the future for psychodynamically oriented researchers. In this regard, we also would like to make a strong plea for methodological pluralism because we believe that the existing divide within the psychology of religion between a hermeneutic, interpretive approach that focuses on understanding (*Verstehen*) and meaning, on the one hand, and a (neo-)positivistic approach that focuses on explanation (*Erklären*) and general laws, on the other hand, is not only to a large extent artificial, but also unfruitful (Luyten et al., 2004). Any scientific endeavor involves interpretation and meaning, just as all scientific research includes a process of systematic testing and falsification. There is no (quasi-)experimental research without previous theorizing and subsequent interpretation. Likewise, interpretations can and should be empirically tested. Hence, whereas (quasi-)experimental research in the psychology of religion should be more aware of the complexity and overdetermination of phenomena, interpretive approaches should develop clear criteria to judge the probability of interpretations and, more in general, develop more rigorous research methodologies. Whereas it can be said that much (quasi-)experimental research in the psychology of religion concerns "impeccable studies of nothing very much," many interpretive studies are vulnerable to the critique that "anything goes" in such studies. Hence, instead of seeing these approaches as conflicting, they should rather be seen as completing each other, with much possibility of mutual enrichment.

We also believe that this does not mean that the case study method as such has outlived its usefulness. Controlled case study research, and more rigorous qualitative research in general (Denzin & Lincoln, 2002; Elliott, Fisher, & Rennie, 1999), involving a clear set of hypotheses, careful selection of cases, and explicit rules for analysis and interpretation of data, are increasingly used in mainstream psychology (Camic, Rhodes, & Yardley, 2003). These new methodologies provide an excellent opportunity for psychoanalytically oriented scholars in the psychology of religion because they are—like the traditional "uncontrolled" case study method—able to capture the uniqueness of each individual, but this time in a methodologically rigorous manner.

In sum, the recent theoretical and methodological developments just reviewed, within both psychoanalysis and mainstream psychology, may not only lead to significant contributions to the psychoanalytic study of religion, but they may also have much to offer to the psychology of religion in general. In the next section, we illustrate this point with a short review of research on religious experience, the representation of God, and the relationship between mental health and religion.

Some Illustrations

Religious Experience

The topic of religious experience has attracted a lot of research attention (see Hood, Chapter 19, this volume). However, despite this attention, we are far from even reaching a consensus on the meaning of such terms as "religious," "mystical," and "spiritual experience." In addition, comprehensive theories that are able to explain the wide variety of such experiences are lacking (Luyten & Corveleyn, 2003). As Vergote (1996) has pointed out, one of the reasons for this confusion is that there is a lack of a good comprehensive theory. Inspired by psychoanalytic theory, Vergote (1996) has convincingly shown in several studies that one must carefully distinguish between various forms of religious experience based on a thorough historical and sociocultural analysis, as well as by considering at least three interrelated factors that determine whether or not an experience is interpreted by an individual as religious. These factors are (1) the perception of an event or situation (e.g., standing on top of a mountain), (2) the affective endowment of this event by the individual, and (3) the preexisting religious/spiritual belief (or the absence of such beliefs) of the individual. For instance, Vergote and his associates found that only those subjects that were religious were likely to interpret certain experiences (e.g., concerning love, nature, etc.) as *religious*. This was further substantiated by their finding that those who believed in a personal God (religious individuals) believed that these experiences showed the hand of God, whereas those who believed in an impersonal higher power (spiritual individuals) saw a confirmation of their belief in a higher impersonal power in these experiences. Hence, people tend to interpret certain experiences congruent with their preexisting beliefs. For some, such experiences are "only" beautiful, "peak" experiences, for others they are the reflection of a higher power or a personal God. Thus, experiences as such are not religious, nor spiritual, nor mystical. They are endowed with such meanings by human beings.

Hence, these findings point to the importance of taking into account the preexisting personal belief structure of the individual, which in turn is intimately associated with the person's personal history. Traditionally, however, there is a tendency to study religious experiences in complete isolation, as if such experiences exist isolated from historical, sociocultural, and personal factors. However, as the differentiations between different forms and determinants of religious experiences show, it appears that such experiences are only one aspect or phase of a long—sometimes very long—process or history. For instance, religious experiences can be one phase in the process of mourning or in the search for meaning during or after a depressive episode (see Park, Chapter 16, this volume). Hence, carefully designed and detailed longitudinal studies are needed to investigate the complex and often recursive interactions between the life history of the individual, including his religious/spiritual socialization, personality factors, and recent life experiences. Measuring these factors, as is mostly the case in existing studies, at one point in time (or even at two or three points in time), appears to be a rather crude way to investigate a dynamic process that develops over time. As noted before, growth curve modeling could provide one tool to study such complex interactions over time both at the idiographic and the nomothetic levels.

Representation of God

A second example where recent trends in the interface between psychoanalysis and mainstream psychology may lead to important advances in our understanding concerns research on the representation of God. By and large, most systematic empirical research from a psychodynamic point of view in the psychology of religion has focused on the representation of God and more particularly on the relationship between this representation and representations of significant others (e.g., mother, father). These studies have undoubtedly led to significant insights in the development of religiosity in individuals. The studies of Rizzuto (1979) and McDargh (1983), mentioned earlier, are two cases in point. Both authors have made a compelling case for the complex interaction and interweaving of sociocultural images of God and the personal life history of individuals.

However, typically, these studies have been limited to very few subjects, rely heavily on reconstruction with all the difficulties associated with such an approach, and/or are for the most part cross-sectional in nature (e.g., Cecero, Marmon, Beitel,

Hutz, & Jones, 2004; Gerard, Jobes, Cimbolic, Ritzler, & Montana, 2003; Schaap-Jonker, Eurelings-Bontekoe, Verhagen, & Zock, 2002). In addition, these studies have tended to focus on the actual representation of God. However, rigorous cross-cultural research by Vergote and collaborators (e.g., Vergote & Tamayo, 1980) with a specially constructed Semantic Differential Parental Scale (SDPS), has shown, in line with psychoanalytic theorizing, the importance of distinguishing between the symbolic and the actual representation of God. In contrast to the actual representation, which is based on the concrete developmental history of the individual, the symbolic representation refers to the more stable cultural representation of God. It was found that the symbolic representation of God is, in general, across cultures, a function of both paternal and maternal qualities, with maternal qualities being more important. From this perspective, many interesting questions arise, such as: What is the relationship between the actual and symbolic representation of God?; Have the large sociocultural changes in our Western society made maternal aspects more important in the actual and/or symbolic representation of God?; If so, are these changes less clear in more patriarchal cultures and/or specific religious groups? Hence, because representations of God are not static entities, neither on an individual level, nor on the cultural level (McDargh, 1983; Rizzuto, 1979), but dynamic concepts that continue to evolve over time, longitudinal research is needed to answer such questions (see also Granqvist, 2002). As McDargh (1983, p. 148) has so eloquently put it, methods that do not take into account these highly complex, recursive interactions "tend to isolate out a static configuration labelled the God image or God representation which is then impaled inert on a point of nosology like a lifeless butterfly." Unfortunately, however, currently such research is virtually nonexistent, and most studies continue to focus on the actual representation of God using cross-sectional designs.

Yet the methodological tools for such studies are now available. Research methods such as growth curve modeling and controlled case study research appear to be particularly promising in this regard to investigate the complex and recursive interactions between symbolic and actual representations of God over time. A dozen or more reliable and valid measures of object relations are available that could be used in such studies (Huprich & Greenberg, 2003). Some of these can be scored on different kinds of data, including self-report data, (clinical) interviews, narratives, projective measures (such as the Rorschach test and the Thematic Apperception Test; TAT), stories based on the picture arrangement subtest of the Wechsler Adult Intelligence Scale—Revised (WAIS-R), early memories, transcripts from psychotherapy sessions, and responses to experimental stimuli. Westen and his collaborators, for instance, developed the Social Cognition and Object Relations Scale (SCORS; Westen, 2002), which includes scales for rating the Complexity of Representations of Others, Affective Quality of Representations, Emotional Investment in Relationships, and Understanding of Social Causality. Blatt and his collaborators developed several measures that tap various aspects of both content and structural characteristics of object representations (Blatt & Auerbach, 2003). Already, some studies have used these instruments to investigate the representation of God (e.g., Brokaw & Edwards, 1994; Hall & Fletcher-Brokaw, 1995; Hall, Fletcher-Brokaw, Edwards, & Pike, 1998). But more research is needed.

Additionally, research inspired by object relations theories provides ample opportunity for integration between psychodynamic theory and research and developmental psychopathology (Fonagy & Target, 2002), social cognition (Westen, 1991), cognitive psychology (Blatt & Auerbach, 2003), attachment theory (Fonagy, 1999; Granqvist,

2002), and schema theories (Cecero et al., 2004), and is immediately relevant for clinical practice (e.g., Blatt, Auerbach, & Levy, 1997).

Religion and Mental Health

A third and final area where psychoanalytic theory and research might lead to significant advances in our knowledge concerns the relationship between religion and mental health. Psychodynamic theory and research clearly suggests that religion and mental health are intrinsically interwoven. However, again, most research in this area is cross-sectional, thereby neglecting the fact that religion and mental health most probably reciprocally interact. Even longitudinal studies in this area assume that the relationship between religion and mental health is linear and nonrecursive. Notwithstanding this, often sweeping conclusions are made regarding the relationship between religion and mental health based on such studies. In addition, current research tends to reify the constructs of religiosity and mental health, as if they are completely independent things. Of course, theoretically and for research purposes, one can define and operationalize religiosity and mental health separately, but this does not mean that the individual should be seen as the "host" of two "guests," namely religiosity, on the one hand, and mental health, on the other. If one takes the above-mentioned definition of personal religion seriously, it must be clear that personal religiosity and mental health are intrinsically interwoven. From infancy on, people are drawn toward certain aspects of religion or particular religions as a whole. Or, depending on their personal history, they may become indifferent or may start to hate certain aspects of religion or religion in general, but nevertheless they are influenced by it. The reason for this is that (particular aspects of) religion, as a symbolic system, appeals on certain—often universal—human issues. Hence, one should always consider two directions of causality, one going from religion to the individual psyche, the other from the individual psyche to religion (Vergote, 1996). Take, for instance, the example of Christian religion and the issue of guilt, sin, repentance, and forgiveness. Christian teachings concerning these issues attract many people precisely because these are almost universal issues that every human being sooner or later has to deal with. However, the other way around, it is well known that individuals in which obsessive–compulsive traits predominate are often particularly attracted to and occupied with these issues (and particular to sin and punishment). Hence, unraveling the relationship between religiosity and mental health is often like the familiar chicken-and-egg problem. Only longitudinal studies, including recursive influences, can do justice to the complexity of this relationship. Hence, while many have acknowledged, precisely because of the many possible interactions among religion and mental health, that religion may be an expression of a mental disorder, a socializing and suppressing agent, a haven for those under stress, a risk factor for psychopathology, or may have therapeutic value for some (Spilka et al., 2003), research tends to blur these essential distinctions. Moreover, there clearly is a lack of an encompassing theory to explain these various relationships.

In this context, we believe that the psychodynamic distinction between various levels of personality development and functioning may provide a starting point for such a comprehensive theory, and is especially useful for clinical practice when confronted with (alleged) religious psychopathology. From a psychodynamic point of view, one can distinguish between three levels of psychopathology: the psychotic, the borderline, and the neurotic (e.g., McWilliams, 1994). Somewhat schematically, it can be said that at the psychotic level individuals are mainly characterized by a severe disturbance in reality testing, which puts them at increased risk for manifest psychotic symptoms (e.g., delusions and/or hallucinations). The most characteristic disturbances at the borderline level concern low impulse control and identity diffusion, in combination with the use of primitive defense mechanisms (e.g., splitting). On these two levels of personality functioning, one often is able to make a more or less accurate distinction between pathological variants of religion (e.g., the individual who believes that he is God vs. someone whose representation of God is either very cruel, much idealized, or both) and "normal" religiosity. On the neurotic level, however, which is characterized by good reality testing, more differentiated images of self and other, and the use of more mature defense mechanisms (e.g., reaction formation, rationalization), the distinction between normal "lived religiosity" and religious psychopathology is often very difficult to make, precisely because religion at this level of personality functioning is deeply woven in and interwoven with the fabric of the individual's personality.

Other criteria than those traditionally used in research, such as the deviation from a cultural or statistical norm, are needed here to make a judgment concerning the nature of religiosity. Vergote (1988) proposes the following intrinsically psychological criteria: (1) the ability of someone to speak a common (religious) language, (2) the extent to which an individual is still able to work in the broad sense of the term (i.e., to actively exert an influence on his or her *Umwelt*), (3) the extent to which someone is still able to love others in a way that recognizes their autonomy, and (4) the extent to which an individual can enjoy his or her activities. This is not to deny the importance of cultural norms. In fact, many studies of the relationship between religiosity and mental health appear to ignore in whole or in part the importance of cultural norms and only consider a statistical norm to distinguish between normal and "pathological" religiosity. Instead, we propose to speak of the *relative relativity* of the distinction between "normal" and "pathological" religiosity. This distinction is often relative because it is frequently difficult to judge to which extent religion is normal or pathological, especially in individuals functioning at a neurotic level. However, at the same time, this relativity is itself relative, because in some instances individuals within a certain (sub)culture can easily make this distinction, particularly concerning those individuals functioning at the psychotic level. For instance, while there would be much disagreement in Western societies concerning the nature of the belief of a housewife who somewhat neglects her other duties and others around her because she spends most of her day praying in front of an altar at home, most if not many would agree that an individual with a Messiah delusion who completely isolates him- or herself and is not able to communicate anymore with others shows signs of pathological religiosity.

The clinical implications of such a psychodynamic perspective often differ in important respects from clinical approaches inspired by other theoretical frameworks. First, there is no clear distinction between "normal" and "pathological" religiosity, particularly at the neurotic level. Meissner (1991) has provided in this context a very useful distinction between various religious modi depending on the underlying personality structure, such as the hysterical, the obsessional, the depressive-masochistic, the narcissistic, and the paranoid modus. Each of these modi reflect a particular religious faith that is the result of a particular developmental history in which religiosity, mental health, and personal history are intrinsically interwoven. A second clinical implication concerns the attitude toward religious issues in counseling and psychotherapy. Because this issue is part of a wider discussion, we address it in the next section.

PSYCHOANALYSIS AND THE CURRENT DEBATE ON THE INTEGRATION OF PSYCHOTHERAPY AND RELIGION OR SPIRITUALITY

Corveleyn and Lietaer (1994, p. 203) observed already in 1994 a "change in the attitudes of psychologists" toward religiosity and spirituality in general and in their psychotherapeutic work more specifically. Their attitudes had been changing in the 1980s from "anti" or "indifferent" toward religion to openness and positive attention. However, these conclusions were based on mainly, if not exclusively, North American research and review articles. In general, European psychologists and psychotherapists of all kinds of theoretical families have approached the problem of the relationship between psychotherapy and religiosity or spirituality in a different way than their North American colleagues in the past two decades. In several recent North American publications (see Miller & Kelley, Chapter 25, and Shafranske, Chapter 27, this volume), several, often far-reaching, proposals have been made to integrate religion and/or spirituality and psychotherapy. These proposals vary from the integration of traditional Christian (e.g., prayer, bible exegesis) or Eastern (e.g., meditation, yoga) elements in existing forms of counseling and psychotherapy, to the development of explicitly religious and/or spiritually inspired psychotherapy. The fact that religion and spirituality are often positive for (mental) health (see Part V, this volume), and the finding that integrating such religious and/or spiritual elements often leads to increased effectiveness of clinical interventions, especially among strongly religious clients (Worthington, Kurusu, McCullough, & Sandage, 1996), has convinced many, even ardent opponents of religion such as Ellis (Nielsen, Johnson, & Ellis, 2001), of the need and value of integrating religion and/or spirituality with psychotherapy. Hence, psychotherapists are encouraged to be more active in stimulating patients not only to explore, but also to rediscover, the religious and/or spiritual dimension in their lives. In Europe, in contrast, one hardly finds such standpoints in scientific publications. It is not our intention to speculate about the possible interpretations of this difference, nor will we try to develop a representative "European" standpoint. This is quite impossible because there is not such a generalized integration movement, nor a "general" interest in spiritual matters in the European psychotherapy world. However, perhaps in Europe there is a much more keen awareness of the fact that the positive association between (mental) health and religion and/or spirituality does not as such and itself buttress such a "spiritual strategy." This would be a naïve functionalistic "use" of religion and spirituality as an "insurance" for better (mental) health. To use an analogy: since we know that married people live longer, should we advise all our patients to marry (Sloan, Bagiella, VandeCreek, Hover, & Casalona, 2000)?

In contrast to this "spiritual strategy," we would therefore like to argue in favor of a variant of the classical Freudian attitude of the psychotherapist toward the ethical and religious values of the patient, namely, *benevolent neutrality* (Corveleyn, 2000). The classical Freudian standpoint is generally believed to be actively hostile toward religion, or at least simply areligious. In our view, this is based on a misinterpretation of Freud. Although he personally was atheistic, and his theoretical writings describe religion as an illusion, in his clinical writings he actively promoted benevolent neutrality toward religious issues. We believe that this benevolent or sympathetic neutrality can be considered to be the basic attitude of most of the European psychotherapists, not only of those that have received psychoanalytic training, but of all therapists, regardless of their theoretical orientation.

The term "neutrality" implies that the psychotherapist is not a pastoral worker whose task it is to engage actively in a discussion on the truth or falsity of faith (beliefs, attitudes, and emotions). Of course, the psychotherapist must not be too cautious in refraining from directing the dialogue into the religious or spiritual domain. The therapist's tact (Poland, 1975) should not be the alibi for his personal resistance toward religion. The resistance of many clients to speak about religious and/or spiritual issues is often already high because of the intimate character of these issues (Rümke, 1952). The therapist should thus not add his or her personal resistance to that of the client.

Traditionally, the "received view" of neutrality stresses the necessity of a *strict* neutrality (Strean, 1986). In that view, neutrality is defined as impersonal. Relying on some of Freud's rare technical writings, the attitude of the analyst is described in metaphors like "being a perfect mirror" or "being like an unemotional surgeon" (e.g., see Freud, 1912/1958, p. 115). Remarkably, in reference to this so-called classical standard, Freud himself was not a classical psychoanalyst. For instance, already in 1895, explaining what should, in his view, basically characterize the attitude of the analyst, Freud (Freud, 1895/ 1955b) explains how a therapist must counter the resistance of the patient with gentle attempts to *influence* him or her. The analyst must *elicit* the (intellectual) interest of the patient and try to *stimulate* therapist–patient collaboration. Only then, Freud asserts, does it become possible to overcome the affectively based resistance. He stresses that the therapist must try to do "something human" for the patient, based on real sympathy (Freud, 1895/1955b, pp. 282–283, see also p. 265). Thus, *neutrality is not indifference* and acting without human interest for the real concerns of the patient. It implies neutrality toward the *content* about which the patient speaks, but sympathy and compassion for the *person* who is going through the therapeutic process.

But is all this applicable to the domain of spirituality and religion? Freud's repeated negative judgments about religious matters are well known. Is Freud's critical position not automatically leading to the idea that psychoanalytic therapy only can aim at the deconstruction of the personal religious attitude of the patient? Because psychoanalysis is directed toward the demolition of the imaginary illusions of the patient insofar as they inhibit further personal development, psychoanalysis should also cure his or her "illusory" religious beliefs. This simple transposition of Freud's rationalistic explanation of religion as a cultural phenomenon to the level of therapeutic action has de facto seduced more than one psychoanalyst. In our opinion, this is not a correct transposition. Freud, as a person and as a psychotherapist, was much more humble in these matters. For example, in his correspondence with the Protestant pastor Oskar Pfister, Freud wrote, "In itself psycho-analysis is neither religious nor non-religious, but an impartial [*sans parti*] tool which both priest and layman can use in the service of the sufferer" (Meng & Freud, 1963, p. 17).

The psychotherapist must thus take a position *sans parti*. His or her only task is to pay attention to all kinds of things the patient says about him- or herself with the aim of obtaining a greater personal freedom toward inner inhibitions and deformations. It is the therapist's role to promote a greater freedom that enhances the patient's psychological well-being, and in this way opens and improves his or her further personal development. This liberating action in therapy *can* possibly foster the development of a personal religious experience, or it can set the person free from oppressing religious representations or practices. But, intrinsically, this liberation "for" or "from" religion is not the primary goal of the therapeutic action. The psychotherapist should not hinder the (believing or nonbelieving) client's spiritual discovery by indicating to her or him the direction toward a prefabricated spiritual or religious pathway.

One thus could say that the prescription of neutrality mainly concerns the *content* aspect of the therapeutic process. The *relational* aspect that carries the therapeutic process is not well described by only referring to abstinence, the narrow interpretation of neutrality. Therefore, Freud spoke in relation to this aspect of the therapeutic commitment about "sympathy" and "interest," for which he coined the notion of "benevolent neutrality" (*wohlwollende Neutralität*). With this interpretation of the concept of neutrality in relation to religion and spirituality, we feel in good company with the object relations and interpersonal approach of the group of psychoanalytic therapists headed by Ana-Maria Rizzuto (1993; see also McDargh, 1993; Meissner, 2000).

CONCLUSIONS

Although not without limitations and pitfalls, the psychoanalytic study of religion has much to offer to the theoretician, researcher, and clinician. Not surprisingly, therefore, psychoanalysis had and still has an important impact on the field.

However, it appears to be imperative for the future of the psychoanalytic study of religion that more attention is devoted to the empirical testing of theories and hypotheses. In fact, as we suggested, instead of being described in the near future as a once interesting, though long passé, approach, psychoanalysis could play an important role in furthering the field of the psychology of religion, both theoretically and methodologically. Theoretically, psychoanalysis has a wealth of insights and theories to offer that are based on the detailed study of individual lives. The increasing dialogue between psychoanalysis and other social sciences and the neurosciences is likely to open up many interesting research vistas. Methodologically, these complex theories ask for complex designs and analysis methods—both quantitative and qualitative—and thus may lead not only to bridging the gap between "interpretive" and "positivistic" research traditions within the psychology of religion, but ultimately also to a more complete understanding of what fascinates all researchers in the field: the relationship between humanity and what transcends it.

NOTES

1. Although the distinction is not always easy to make, this more or less stable theological and organizational component also distinguishes religion from less traditional forms of belief (e.g., some cults or sects), and from belief(s) in a higher power that transcends humanity, for which we like to reserve the term "spirituality."

2. Readers may find this depiction of the empirical status of psychodynamic hypotheses concerning religion somewhat unfair. We would partially agree with this critique. Indeed, much systematic empirical research in mainstream psychology of religion has either implicitly or explicitly been inspired by psychoanalytic theories and hypotheses (e.g., Beit-Hallahmi & Argyle, 1997; Corveleyn, 1996). However, our point is that psychoanalytic researchers themselves have, with few exceptions, *not* used methods other than anecdote or case material. For instance, a review of the more than 2,000 studies included in Beit-Hallahmi's (1996) authoritative overview of psychoanalytic studies of religion shows that, even when liberal criteria are used, less than 5% used a methodology other than historical sources, anecdote, or traditional case studies. In addition,

with some important exceptions, a considerable number of these studies show a variety of theoretical and methodological flaws, such as the testing of clearly oversimplified psychoanalytic hypotheses and small samples sizes.

REFERENCES

Batson, C. D. (1997). An agenda item for psychology of religion: Getting respect. In B. Spilka & D. N. McIntosh (Eds.), *The psychology of religion: Theoretical approaches* (pp. 3–8). Boulder, CO: Westview Press.

Beit-Hallahmi, B. (1996). *Psychoanalytic studies of religion: A critical assessment and annotated bibliography.* Westport, CT: Greenwood Press.

Beit-Hallahmi, B., & Argyle, M. (1997). *The psychology of religious behaviour, belief and experience.* New York: Routledge.

Blass, R. B. (2004). Beyond illusion: Psychoanalysis and the question of religious truth. *International Journal of Psychoanalysis, 85,* 615–634.

Blatt, D. S. (1988). The development of the hero: Sigmund Freud and the reformation of the Jewish tradition. *Psychoanalysis and Contemporary Thought, 11,* 639–703.

Blatt, S. J., & Auerbach, J. S. (2003). Psychodynamic measures of therapeutic change. *Psychoanalytic Inquiry, 23,* 268–307.

Blatt, S. J., Auerbach, J. S., & Levy, K. N. (1997). Mental representation in personality development, psychopathology, and the therapeutic process. *Review of General Psychology, 1,* 351–374.

Brokaw, B. F., & Edwards, K. J. (1994). The relationship of God image to level of object relations development. *Journal of Psychology and Theology, 22,* 352–371.

Camic, P. M., Rhodes, J. E., & Yardley, L. (Eds.). (2003). *Qualitative research in psychology: Expanding perspectives in methodology and design.* Washington, DC: American Psychological Association.

Capps, D. (Ed.). (2001). *Freud and Freudians on religion: A reader.* New Haven, CT: Yale University Press.

Cecero, J. C., Marmon, T. S., Beitel, M., Hutz, A., & Jones, C. (2004). Images of mother, self, and God as predictors of dysphoria in non-clinical samples. *Personality and Individual Differences, 36,* 1669–1680.

Corveleyn, J. (1996). The psychological explanation of religion as wish-fulfilment. A test-case: The belief in immortality. In H. Grzymala-Moszczynska & B. Beit-Hallahmi (Eds.), *Religion, psychopathology and coping* (pp. 57–70). Atlanta, GA: Rodopi Press.

Corveleyn, J. (1997). The obsessional episode in the conversion experience of Ignatius of Loyola: A psychobiographical contribution. In J. A. Belzen (Ed.), *Hermeneutical approaches in psychology of religion* (pp. 155–172). Atlanta, GA: Rodopi Press.

Corveleyn, J. (2000). In defense of benevolent neutrality: Against a "spiritual strategy." *Journal of Individual Psychology, 56,* 343–352.

Corveleyn, J., & Lietaer, H. (1994). A critical review of current psychological research on the interaction between religion and mental health. In D. Hutsebaut & J. Corveleyn (Eds.), *Belief and unbelief: Psychological perspectives* (pp. 203–218). Atlanta, GA: Rodopi Press.

Daim, W. (1951). *Umwertung der Psychoanalyse* [Transvaluation of psychoanalysis]. Vienna: Verlag Herold.

de Certeau, M. (1963). *Surin: Guide spirituel pour la perfection* [Surin: Spiritual guide toward perfection]. Paris: Desclée de Brouwer.

de Certeau, M. (1980). *La possession de Loudun* [The possession of Loudun] (2nd ed.). Paris: Gallimard/Julliard.

Denzin, N. K., & Lincoln, Y. S. (Eds.). (2002). *Handbook of qualitative research* (2nd ed.). London: Sage.

Devereux, G. (Ed.). (1974). *Psychoanalysis and the occult.* London: Souvenir Press. (Original work published 1953)

Dolto, F., & Séverin, G. (1977). *L'évangile au risque de la psychanalyse* [The New Testament in confrontation with psychoanalysis] (2 vols.). Paris: Jean-Pierre Delarge/Seuil.

Elliott, R., Fischer, C. T., & Rennie, D. L. (1999). Evolving guidelines for publication of qualitative research studies in psychology and related fields. *British Journal of Clinical Psychology, 38,* 215–229.

Emmons, R. A. (1999). *The psychology of ultimate concerns: Motivation and spirituality in personality.* New York: Guilford Press.

Emmons, R. A., & Paloutzian, R. (2003). The psychology of religion. *Annual Review of Psychology, 54,* 377–402.

Erikson, E. H. (1950). *Childhood and society.* New York: Norton.

Erikson, E. H. (1958). *Young man Luther: A study in psychoanalysis and history.* New York: Norton.

Erikson, E. H. (1968). *Identity, youth and crisis.* London: Faber & Faber.

Erikson, E. H. (1969). *Gandhi's truth: On the origin of militant nonviolence.* New York: Norton.

Fonagy, P. (1999). Psychoanalytic theory from the viewpoint of attachment theory and research. In J. Cassidy & P. R. Shaver (Eds.), *Handbook of attachment: Theory, research, and clinical applications* (pp. 595–624). New York: Guilford Press.

Fonagy, P., & Target, M. (2002). *Psychoanalytic theories: Perspectives from developmental psychopathology.* London: Whurr.

Freud, S. (1953). Totem and taboo. In J. Strachey (Ed. and Trans.), *The standard edition of the complete psychological works of Sigmund Freud* (Vol. 13, pp. 1–161). London: Hogarth Press. (Original work published 1913)

Freud, S. (1955a). From the history of an infantile neurosis. In J. Strachey (Ed. and Trans.), *The standard edition of the complete psychological works of Sigmund Freud* (Vol. 17, pp. 1–123). London: Hogarth Press. (Original work published 1918)

Freud, S. (1955b). Studies on hysteria. In J. Strachey (Ed. and Trans.), *The standard edition of the complete psychological works of Sigmund Freud* (Vol. 2). London: Hogarth Press. (Original work published 1895)

Freud, S. (1958). Recommendations to physicians practising psycho-analysis. In J. Strachey (Ed. and Trans.), *The standard edition of the complete psychological works of Sigmund Freud* (Vol. 12, pp. 109–120). London: Hogarth Press. (Original work published 1912)

Freud, S. (1961a). Civilization and its discontents. In J. Strachey (Ed. and Trans.), *The standard edition of the complete psychological works of Sigmund Freud* (Vol. 21, pp. 64–145). London: Hogarth Press. (Original work published 1930)

Freud, S. (1961b). The ego and the id. In J. Strachey (Ed. and Trans.), *The standard edition of the complete psychological works of Sigmund Freud* (Vol. 19, pp. 1–66). London: Hogarth Press. (Original work published 1923)

Freud, S. (1961c). The future of an illusion. In J. Strachey (Ed. and Trans.), *The standard edition of the complete psychological works of Sigmund Freud* (Vol. 21, pp. 5–56). London: Hogarth Press. (Original work published 1927)

Freud, S. (1961d). A short account of psycho-analysis. In J. Strachey (Ed. and Trans.), *The standard edition of the complete psychological works of Sigmund Freud* (Vol. 19, pp. 191–209). London: Hogarth Press. (Original work published 1924)

Freud, S. (1964a). *Moses and monotheism.* In J. Strachey (Ed. and Trans.), *The standard edition of the complete psychological works of Sigmund Freud* (Vol. 23, pp. 7–137). London: Hogarth Press. (Original work published 1939)

Freud, S. (1964b). *New introductory lectures on psycho-analysis.* In J. Strachey (Ed. and Trans.), *The standard edition of the complete psychological works of Sigmund Freud* (Vol. 22, pp. 1–182). London: Hogarth Press. (Original work published 1933)

Gay, P. (1987). *A godless Jew: Freud, atheism, and the making of psychoanalysis.* New Haven, CT/Cincinatti, OH: Yale University Press/Hebrew Union College Press.

Geertz, C. (1973). *The interpretation of cultures.* New York: Basic Books.

Gerard, S. M., Jobes, D., Cimbolic, P., Ritzler, B. A., & Montana, S. (2003). A Rorschach study of interpersonal disturbance in priest child molesters. *Sexual Addiction and Compulsivity, 10,* 53–66.

Goossens, M. A. (1990). *De bijdrage van Oskar Pfister tot het psychoanalytisch denken omtrent religie en religieuze opvoeding* [The contribution of Oskar Pfister to the psychoanalytic approach of religion and religious education]. Unpublished master's thesis, University of Leuven, Leuven, Belgium.

Granqvist, P. (2002). *Attachment and religion: An integrative developmental framework.* Unpublished doctoral dissertation, Department of Psychology, University of Uppsala. Retrieved April 12, 2004, from http://publications.uu.se/theses/abstract.xsql?dbid=1904.

Hall, T. W., & Fletcher-Brokaw, B. (1995). The relationship of spiritual maturity to level of object relations development and God image. *Pastoral Psychology, 43,* 373–391.

Hall, T. W., Fletcher-Brokaw, B., Edwards, K. J., & Pike, P. (1998). An empirical exploration of psychoanalysis and religion: Spiritual maturity and object relations development. *Journal for the Scientific Study of Religion, 37,* 303–313.

Hood, R. W., Jr., Spilka, B., Hunsberger, B., & Gorsuch, R. (1996). *The psychology of religion: An empirical approach* (2nd ed.). New York: Guilford Press.

Huprich, S. K., & Greenberg, R. P. (2003). Advances in the assessment of object relations in the 1990s. *Clinical Psychology Review, 23,* 665–698.

Jones, E. (1967). The theory of symbolism. In E. Jones (Ed.), *Papers on psycho-analysis* (pp. 87–144). Boston: Beacon Press. (Original work published 1916)

Jones, J. W. (1991). *Contemporary psychoanalysis and religion: Transference and transcendence.* New Haven, CT: Yale University Press.

Kernberg, O. F. (2000). Psychoanalytic perspectives on the religious experience. *American Journal of Psychotherapy, 54,* 452–476.

Klumpner, G. H., & Frank, A. (1991). On methods of reporting clinical material. *Journal of the American Psychoanalytic Association, 39,* 537–551.

Lietaer, H., & Corveleyn, J. (1995). Psychoanalytical interpretation of the demoniacal possession and the mystical development of Sister Jeanne des Anges from Loudun. *The International Journal for the Psychology of Religion, 5,* 259–276.

Luyten, P., Blatt, S. J., & Corveleyn, J. (2004). *Mind the gap: Psychoanalytic research caught between the Scylla of positivism and the Charybdis of hermeneutics: A critical overview and a plea for methodological pluralism.* Manuscript submitted for publication.

Luyten, P., & Corveleyn, J. (2003). Mysticism, creativity, and psychoanalysis: Still crazy after all these years? *The International Journal for the Psychology of Religion, 13,* 97–109.

Maître, J. (1997). *Mystique et féminité: Essai de psychanalyse sociohistorique* [Mysticism and femininity: A sociohistorical psychoanalytic essay]. Paris: Editions du Cerf.

Malony, H. N., & Spilka, B. (Eds.). (1991). *Religion in psychodynamic perspective: The contributions of Paul W. Pruyser.* New York: Oxford University Press.

McDargh, J. (1983). *Psychoanalytic object relations theory and the study of religion: On faith and the imaging of God.* Lanham, MD: University Press of America.

McDargh, J. (1993). On developing a psychotheological perspective. In M. L. Randour (Ed.), *Exploring sacred landscapes: Religious and spiritual experiences in psychotherapy* (pp. 172–193). New York: Columbia University Press.

McWilliams, N. (1994). *Psychoanalytic diagnosis: Understanding personality structure in the clinical process.* New York: Guilford Press.

Meissner, W. W. (1984). *Psychoanalysis and religious experience.* New Haven, CT: Yale University Press.

Meissner, W. W. (1991). Religious psychopathology. *Bulletin of the Menninger Clinic, 55,* 281–298.

Meissner, W. W. (1992). *Ignatius of Loyola: The psychology of a saint.* New Haven, CT: Yale University Press.

Meissner, W. W. (2000). Psychoanalysis and religion: Current perspectives. In J. K. Boehnlein (Ed.),

Psychiatry and religion: The convergence of mind and spirit (pp. 53–69). Washington, DC: American Psychiatric Press.

Meng, H., & Freud, E. L. (Eds.). (1963). *Psychoanalysis and faith: The letters of Sigmund Freud and Oskar Pfister*. New York: Basic Books.

Nielsen, S. L., Johnson, W. B., & Ellis, A. (2001). *Counseling and psychotherapy with religious persons: A rational emotive behavior therapy approach*. Mahwah, NJ: Erlbaum.

Nuttin, J. R. (1962). *Psychoanalysis and personality: A dynamic theory of normal personality*. New York: New American Library. (Original work published 1950)

Paloutzian, R. F. (1996). *Invitation to the psychology of religion* (2nd ed.). Boston: Allyn & Bacon.

Pfister, O. (1928). Die Illusion einer Zukunft: Eine freundschaftliche Auseinandersetzung mit Sigmund Freud [The illusion of a future: A friendly discussion with Sigmund Freud]. *Imago, 14*, 149–184.

Pine, F. (1990). *Drive, ego, object and self: A synthesis for clinical work*. New York: Basic Books.

Poland, W. S. (1975). Tact as a psychoanalytic function. *International Journal of Psychoanalysis, 56*, 155–162.

Reik, T. (1931). *Ritual: Psychoanalytic studies*. London: Hogarth Press.

Rice, E. (1990). *Freud and Moses: The long journey home*. Albany: State University of New York Press.

Rizzuto, A.-M. (1979). *The birth of the living God: A psychoanalytic study*. Chicago: University of Chicago Press.

Rizzuto, A.-M. (1993). Exploring sacred landscapes. In M. L. Randour (Ed.), *Exploring sacred landscapes: Religious and spiritual experiences in psychotherapy* (pp. 16–33). New York: Columbia University Press.

Rizzuto, A.-M. (1998). *Why did Freud reject God?: A psychodynamic interpretation*. New Haven, CT: Yale University Press.

Rümke, H. C. (1952). *The psychology of unbelief: Character and temperament in relation to unbelief*. London: Rockliff.

Saffady, W. (1976). New developments in the psychoanalytic study of religion: A bibliographic survey of the literature since 1960. *Psychoanalytic Review, 63*, 291–299.

Schaap-Jonker, H., Eurelings-Bontekoe, E., Verhagen, P. J., & Zock, H. (2002). Image of God and personality pathology: An exploratory study among psychiatric patients. *Mental Health, Religion and Culture, 5*, 55–71.

Singer, J. L., & Kolligian, J. (1987). Personality: Developments in the study of private experience. *Annual Review of Psychology, 38*, 533–574.

Sloan, R., Bagiella, E., VandeCreek, L., Hover, M., & Casalone, C. (2000). Should physicians prescribe religious activities? *New England Journal of Medicine, 342*, 1913–1916.

Spence, D. P. (1994). The failure to ask the hard questions. In P. F. Talley, H. H. Strupp, & S. F. Butler (Eds.), *Psychotherapy research and practice: Bridging the gap* (pp. 19–38). New York: Basic Books.

Spero, M. H. (1992). *Religious objects as psychological structures: A critical integration of object relations theory, psychotherapy, and Judaism*. Chicago: University of Chicago Press.

Spilka, B., Hood, R. W., Jr., Hunsberger, B., & Gorsuch, R. (2003). *The psychology of religion: An empirical approach* (3rd ed.). New York: Guilford Press.

Strean, H. S. (Ed.). (1986). *Countertransference: Current issues in psychoanalytic practice*. New York: Haworth Press

Vandermeersch, P. (1991). *Unresolved questions in the Freud/Jung debate: On psychosis, sexual identity and religion*. Leuven, Belgium: Leuven University Press.

Vasse, D. (1991). *L'autre du désir et le dieu de la foi: Lire aujourd'hui Thérèse d'Avila* [The other of desire and the god of faith: Reading Theresa of Avila today]. Paris: Seuil.

Vergote, A. (1988). *Guilt and desire: Religious attitudes and their pathological derivatives*. New Haven, CT: Yale University Press.

Vergote, A. (1996). *Religion, belief and unbelief: A psychological study*. Leuven, Belgium/Atlanta, GA: Leuven University Press/Rodopi Press.

Vergote, A. (1998). Religion after the critique of psychoanalysis. In J. Corveleyn & D. Hutsebaut (Eds.), *Antoon Vergote: Psychoanalysis, phenomenological anthropology and religion* (pp. 17–37). Leuven, Belgium/Atlanta, GA: Leuven University Press/Rodopi Press.

Vergote, A., & Tamayo, A. (1980). *The parental figures and the representation of God: A psychological and cross-cultural study*. The Hague, The Netherlands: Mouton.

Wallerstein, R. S. (1992). *The common ground of psychoanalysis*. Northvale, NJ: Aronson.

Westen, D. (1991). Social cognition and object relations. *Psychological Bulletin, 109*, 429–455.

Westen, D. (1998). The scientific legacy of Sigmund Freud: Toward a psychodynamically informed psychological science. *Psychological Bulletin, 124*, 333–371.

Westen, D. (2002). *Manual for the Social Cognition and Object Relations Scales (SCORS)*. Unpublished manuscript, Emory University, Atlanta, GA.

Westen, D., & Shedler, J. (1999). Revising and assessing Axis II, Part II: Toward an empirically based and clinically useful classification of personality disorders. *American Journal of Psychiatry, 156*, 273–285.

Willett, J. B., Singer, J. D., & Martin, N. C. (1998). The design and analysis of longitudinal studies of development and psychopathology in context: Statistical models and methodological recommendations. *Development and Psychopathology, 10*, 395–426.

Worthington, E. L., Jr., Kurusu, T. A., McCullough, M. E., & Sandage, S. J. (1996). Empirical research on religion and psychotherapeutic processes and outcomes: A 10-year review and research prospectus. *Psychological Bulletin, 119*, 448–487.

Wulff, D. M. (1997). *Psychology of religion: Classic and contemporary* (2nd ed.). New York: Wiley.

Zilboorg, G. (1955). *Faith, reason and modern psychiatry: Sources for a synthesis*. New York: Kenedy.

Zock, H. (1990). *A psychology of ultimate concern: Erik H. Erikson's contribution to the psychology of religion*. Atlanta, GA: Rodopi Press.

6

Evolutionary Psychology

An Emerging New Foundation
for the Psychology of Religion

LEE A. KIRKPATRICK

> Psychology, if not allowed to be contaminated with too much
> biology, can accommodate endless numbers of theoreticians
> in the future.
>
> —E. O. WILSON (1998, p. 42)

The typical chapter for a handbook provides an overview of a research area, allowing researchers to back away momentarily from their specialized niches to glimpse a bird's-eye view of their larger context. Because progress in science is measured not by any single study but rather the aggregate of many, such essays provide occasion to celebrate the accomplishments within a field or subfield over some period of time.

This is not such a chapter; indeed, its purpose is rather the opposite. I believe that the psychology of religion has made embarrassingly little progress since its inception a century ago. Countless data have been collected, measures developed, and constructs proposed, but the movement has been almost entirely circular rather than progressive. The purpose of this chapter is to offer an explanation for why this has been the case, and to suggest a future course to get things moving forward.

I generally do not blame psychologists of religion for this state of affairs. The problems and weaknesses of the field have by and large been inherited from the field's parent discipline. The psychology of religion, in my opinion, has been wandering aimlessly for decades because psychology generally has done the same, and for the same reasons.

THE PROBLEM WITH PSYCHOLOGY

Psychology has long straddled the fence between Snow's (1959) "two cultures"—between the natural sciences on the one side and humanities and other social sciences on the

101

other—with most subdisciplines leaning one way or the other. Psychology of religion, along with such subfields as personality and social psychology, has generally leaned toward the humanities side. Researchers in these fields might object that their work is more closely allied with science because it employs scientific methods of empirical hypothesis testing, but I think there is a more fundamental issue at stake. The natural sciences begin with the assumption that there is a *real world* out there that has an inherent structure and that operates according to systematic principles that scientists, through a combination of empirical observation and logical reasoning, can *discover*. In contrast, the subject matters of the humanities generally cannot be assumed to have an inherent "reality" to be discovered; scholars instead must *invent* organization and structure. This is why the latter has given rise in recent years to a strong deconstructionist movement claiming that the world presents us nothing but texts to be interpreted, with no interpretation inherently more correct than any other. No definitive external criteria exist to resolve disputes.

In contrast, empirical observation provides a criterion throughout the natural sciences by which hypotheses can be judged, in principle, objectively: theories contradicted by the data can be discarded. This is why, despite claims to the contrary, the deconstructionist critique is not applicable to science (Gross & Levitt, 1994). The Earth really does revolve around the Sun and not the other way around; these two hypotheses are not equally valid because, as adjudicated by an avalanche of empirical data, one is right and the other is wrong.

Subdisciplines of psychology that focus on the brain and other physiological processes have always been the closest to the natural sciences, because such things as the structure of neurons and the electrochemical processes by which they communicate are assumed without controversy to be real things in the world which, like the Earth and the Sun, can be understood through empirical study. These fields makes monotonic progress (at least, on average across time) rather than going in circles because research progressively moves toward more and more accurate understandings of these processes. With the advent of powerful technology such as positron-emission tomography (PET) and magnetic resonance imaging (MRI), the field of neuroscience is today growing by leaps and bounds.

Other areas of psychology have long been confused by their position relative to the two cultures because they have chosen to adopt the empirical research methodology from the natural sciences, but without fully accepting the requisite assumption that the mind has some kind of inherent structure and organization. Psychologists seem to have given up on the idea that there exists, in reality, a "human nature" to be discovered rather than invented. With no a priori constraints imposed by a coherent model of how and why minds work, the generation of theories and hypotheses has been limited only by researchers' imaginations. As suggested in the sardonic quote from E. O. Wilson at the head of this chapter, there is no reason to think that the future will be any different if psychology remains on this course.

However, the brain/mind really does have an inherent structure and functions(s), and psychologists now have at their disposal a strong theoretical basis for discovering them. The emerging discipline of *evolutionary psychology* (hereafter, EP) promises to revolutionize the ways in which psychology approaches the study of human behavior and experience, and consequently the way they approach the psychology of religion as well.

EVOLUTIONARY PSYCHOLOGY AS A SOLUTION

EP begins with the assumption that human beings, like all other living things, are the product of eons of evolution. It further assumes that natural selection—a process of blind variation combined with selective retention operating on genes—has been a major force in shaping the design of organisms. According to the modern view, our genes collectively represent a recipe for building organisms, with mutation and other processes constantly injecting small amounts of variability in the recipes to produce meaningful variability in the structure and functioning of organisms. Those genes whose organisms are more reproductively successful on average than alternative versions—that is, more likely to live long enough to reproduce successfully, and whose offspring and other close kin do the same, and so on—will be disproportionally represented in future generations of organisms. These changes in gene frequencies across time within populations represent *evolution*; the process by which certain genes are probabilistically favored due to their relative effects on the reproductive success of the organisms in which they reside is *natural selection*. Those features that are naturally selected because they function in ways that contribute positively to reproductive success are referred to as *adaptations*. (See Dawkins, 1989, for overviews of how this "selfish gene" perspective on natural selection works and its implications for the evolution of behavior.)

Most people have little trouble seeing how natural selection works in "designing" physical traits of organisms: eyes are useful for seeing, wings are useful for flying, beaks are useful for cracking seeds, and so forth, thereby enhancing the chances of survival to reproductive age (by acquiring adequate nutrition, avoiding predators, etc.), mating, and ensuring the survival of offspring.[1] It is equally obvious to most people how this reasoning applies to physiological traits of humans. Our digestive system, including components such as saliva, the stomach, and the anus, is "designed" to process food in ways that create energy to drive the body's other processes and eliminate waste; the circulatory system, including the heart, arteries, and capillaries, is designed to move oxygen and digestive products to other parts of the body; and so forth.

Less obvious to many people, it seems, is that the same reasoning must apply equally to psychology and behavior. Hardware is useless without software. A digestive system, for example, is valueless unless the right kinds of foods are identified, obtained, and put into it. Thus each species must possess its own unique set of *psychological mechanisms* and systems that have co-evolved with the physical structures required to implement adaptive behavioral strategies. All organisms possess species-specific psychologies for solving adaptive problems such as identifying, evaluating, and obtaining appropriate foods; identifying, evaluating, and attracting quality mates; avoiding predators and other environmental threats; and so forth. In addition, many species possess complex systems for negotiating functionally distinct kinds of relationships with conspecifics, including parental investment in offspring, other kin relations, and intrasexual competition for dominance or rank, to name just a few.

According to the contemporary EP perspective, the human brain/mind (like that of other species) comprises a very large number of highly domain-specific psychological mechanisms organized into functional systems, in much the same way as the rest of the body comprises numerous organs and systems. Each psychological mechanism, like each bodily organ, has been designed to perform one or more adaptive functions; genes encoding recipes for organs designed in this way, rather than alternative ways, were over evolutionary time more successful in propagating themselves in future generations via the successful survival and reproduction of the individuals containing them. *Human nature*— a term that has become virtually extinct from the psychologist's lexicon—represents the totality of this species-universal psychological architecture (Tooby & Cosmides, 1992). Human nature is different in many ways from, though also has much in common with, "chimpanzee nature," "bat nature," and "ant nature." (For overviews of the field, see Buss, 2004, Pinker, 1997, and Tooby & Cosmides, 1992.)

This conceptual model of human psychology contrasts markedly with the prevailing perspective in most of psychology and other social sciences—dubbed the *Standard Social Science Model* (SSSM) by Tooby and Cosmides (1992)—in which the brain/mind is conceptualized as a kind of general, all-purpose computer that operates by a small number of general principles (e.g., symbolic logic, operant conditioning) in the service of a similarly small number of broad motivations (seeking pleasure and avoiding pain, maintaining self-esteem, etc.). Despite lip service routinely paid to the notion that both nature and nurture are important—a debate most researchers claim to have put behind them—the SSSM perspective clearly emphasizes the nurture side of the equation by focusing almost exclusively on such processes as learning, socialization, and culture. The evolutionary history of the human mind, if acknowledged at all, is deemed irrelevant for understanding how we think and behave today. Once cultural evolution took off, it seems widely assumed, the millions of years of biological evolution that preceded and enabled it were relegated to a historical footnote.

However, brains/minds can not be designed as "all-purpose information-processing devices" for the same reasons that computers are not. Computers are capable of performing a wide range of sophisticated tasks precisely because of the existence of numerous functionally specific software programs that are well designed to produce desired outputs in response to particular inputs. A computer without specialized software cannot in fact do anything at all. One needs specialized word-processing programs to write and edit text, statistics programs to analyze data, spreadsheet programs to organize arrays of information, and so forth. To get a computer to behave in more and more complex ways, one needs to add more and more sophisticated, specialized software. As William James (1890) noted more than a century ago, the complexity of human behavior relative to that of other species requires the existence of more instincts, not fewer. Evolution cannot have designed the brain to be a general problem solver, because there is no such thing as a general problem in nature (Symons, 1992).

As seen by evolutionary psychologists, then, the goal of psychology is to discover the design and function of human evolved psychological architecture, by identifying the psychological mechanisms and systems that comprise it and determining how, in interaction with environments, they produce the diverse array of human thought and behavior we observe today. The question for our field therefore becomes, How do the various behaviors and experiences that we refer to as "religion" emerge and take shape from this evolved psychology?

NEW PERSPECTIVES ON OLD QUESTIONS IN THE PSYCHOLOGY OF RELIGION

In some ways, applying EP to religion at the present time risks putting the proverbial cart ahead of the horse. Contemporary EP is a young field, and its promise to emerge as an organizing paradigm for psychology and the social sciences continues to meet stiff resistance from many SSSM researchers. Ideally, a general evolutionary foundation for psychology would be fully in place before we tackle highly complex issues, such as religion, that are up on the roof. Nevertheless, it is possible at this juncture to outline some of the main features such a future psychology of religion is likely to display, and some of the ways in which some of the prevailing, long-standing issues central to psychology of religion might be reconceptualized in such a view.

Nature or Nurture?

Contrary to common misconception, EP does not represent merely another swing of the historical nature–nurture pendulum in the nature direction. Indeed, this perspective provides the only coherent model for what it means to say that human behavior is the product of both. The question of whether nature or nurture (or genes vs. environments, etc.) is more important for explaining religion (or any particular manifestation thereof) is akin to the question, "Which is more important for breathing, lungs or oxygen?" Just as breathing necessarily involves the interaction of specific physiological mechanisms (lungs) with oxygen-rich air, and cannot in principle be understood without reference to both, religion (or any other psychological or behavioral phenomenon) cannot be properly understood except in terms of the interaction of environmental factors with evolved psychological systems.

What about so-called *heritability coefficients*, according to which traits or behavior are parsed in terms of additive proportions of genetic and environmental influences? This (equally valid) approach to the nature–nurture question, associated with the field of *behavioral genetics*, addresses a fundamentally different kind of question than EP. In contrast to EP's approach to explaining why and how a particular trait or behavior exists, behavioral genetics endeavors to explain the observed *variability* in that trait or behavior across individuals. As noted above, explaining the phenomenon of breathing must involve both nature (lungs) and nurture (oxygen) in interaction; it cannot be described as $X\%$ one and 100-minus-$X\%$ the other. Individual differences with respect to breathing, in contrast, *can* be meaningfully parsed into relative and additive contributions of genes (e.g., random genetic variability in lung capacity and efficiency) versus environmental effects (e.g., altitude, smog). Note that although this example involves an unambiguously biological organ and process, the vast majority of variability in breathing across people at a particular point in time is explained not by genetic differences but rather by situational factors. The questions are entirely different, and so can be their answers. In the same way, the degree to which religiosity is heritable (e.g.,Waller, Kojetin, Bouchard, Lykken, & Tellegen, 1990) bears surprisingly little relation to questions about why people are religious and what functions (if any) religion might serve (I return to this topic below).

Another "nature" approach from which EP must be distinguished is *neuroscience*. The two approaches have much in common in their search for an integrated understanding of the structure, organization, and function of the "brain/mind" and how it produces behavior. For example, they have independently converged on the conclusion that the brain/mind must be highly modularized. However, they differ fundamentally with respect to the kinds of questions they ask. In a word, neuroscience provide ways of understanding *how* the brain/mind does these things, in terms of the physical structures and processes involved, whereas EP provides ways of understanding *why* it does these things and not others. To return to the computer metaphor, the brain is analogous to hardware—the hard drives, the wiring, the digital ons and offs—whereas the mind is analogous to software. A comprehensive understanding of computer behavior requires both levels of analysis, with different particular questions associated with different levels. Although answers to the *how* questions can certainly be helpful in some ways for addressing the *why* questions, as well as vice versa, in other ways they are clearly separable.

Evolutionary explanations of behavior are by no means contrary to or inconsistent with explanations in terms of learning, rationality, socialization, or culture. These higher order processes do not represent alternative explanations to biology or adaptation; indeed, they are themselves phenomena to be explained. Learning requires a brain/mind designed to enable it. The valiant attempt of radical behaviorism to establish universal learning principles failed when it was demonstrated in now-classic experiments that in any given species, some associations were learned much more readily than others (e.g., Garcia, Ervin, & Koelling, 1966; Seligman & Hager, 1972), while Chomsky (1957) argued convincingly that the rate and manner in which children learn language could not be explained by simple reinforcement principles and required a dedicated "language organ" to enable and organize language learning.[2] "Culture" not only influences individuals, it is created by and interpreted by them. The effects of culture on individuals, and the processes by which cultures change over time, cannot be understood without reference to the evolved psychology of the individuals interacting with it (Boyd & Richerson, 1985; Sperber, 1996; Tooby & Cosmides, 1992).

Although EP is often grouped for convenience along with other "biological approaches" to psychology—for example, as in opening chapters of psychology of religion texts by Hood, Spilka, Hunsberger, and Gorsuch (1996) and Wulff (1997)—such grouping probably inadvertently fosters the kinds of confusions outlined in this section. At some time in the future, "biological" or "physiological" psychology will no longer be relegated to their own chapters in psychology texts. Evolutionary theory and neuroscience will be intertwined throughout all chapters, with discussions of situational influences on behavior (including religion) integrated with discussion of evolved psychological mechanisms and systems and neurophysiological processes.

Do Humans Possess a Religious Instinct?

Perhaps the most obvious application of evolutionary thinking to religion is the hypothesis that religion, or some particular aspect(s) of religion, represents an *adaptation*—the product(s) of evolved psychological mechanisms or systems designed by natural selection as a solution to one or more adaptive problems. That is, if the mind is like a computer populated by specialized software programs, are one or more of those programs designed specifically to produce religion or some aspect(s) of it? Scholars have long speculated that as *Homo religiosus*, we possess one or more religious "instincts" designed to produce religion for some adaptive purpose. Such claims, whether explicit or implicit, tend to be based on such observations as the apparent universality of religion across time and cultures, neurological evidence for a "God module" in the brain, protoreligious analogs in other species, and so forth. Hypotheses about the *adaptive function* of such religious instincts have ranged from defense against fear of death or other forms of comfort and anxiety reduction to group-level benefits such as promoting cohesion and solidarity or reducing conflict.

As I have argued elsewhere (Kirkpatrick 1999, 2005), however, such arguments for an adaptive function of religion do not stand up to careful examination in light of modern evolutionary theory. For example, natural selection is blind to purely psychological benefits such as anxiety reduction, and it is not a simple matter to demonstrate how such feel-good effects translate into real differences in reproductive success. Simple models of *group selection*, in which natural selection is seen to shape traits in ways that benefit "the species" or groups within it, were rendered obsolete by crucial theoretical developments in the 1960s and 1970s, raising serious questions about the hypothesis that religion reflects adaptations designed to foster group cohesion and related functions that benefit "the species" or "the group." [3] And although it is easy to generate examples in which particular religious beliefs appear consistent with the promotion of reproductive fitness (e.g., "Go forth and multiply"), it is equally easy to generate examples to the contrary (e.g., vows of chastity). In short, the task of identifying a plausible adaptive function of religion, and then specifying the design by which a psychological system performs this function, is far more difficult than has often been appreciated.

Confusion about the relationships among various "biological" approaches, as discussed in the previous section, has contributed to some misguided ideas about religious instincts. For example, it is tempting to infer from the fact that religiosity is (modestly) heritable that there must be genes "for" religion. This does not follow, however, any more than heritability of susceptibility to heart attacks or cancer points to an adaptive design for producing these pathologies. Similarly, the fact that neurological activity in particular brain areas is associated reliably with religious experience (Persinger, 1987; Ramachandran & Blakeslee, 1998) does not establish that the area is designed for the purpose of producing this effect. Religious experiences might be produced, for example, in a manner analogous to the manner in which anxiety attacks represent a hyper- or a misactivation of an otherwise adaptive fear system in the brain (Averill, 1998). Debate about hypothesized adaptive functions of religion will no doubt continue in a future evolutionary psychology of religion, but such debates will be much more fruitful within the context of a shared paradigm that acknowledges and elucidates the importance of evolved psychological architecture for explaining behavior.

Religion (or any other phenomenon) need not be regarded as an adaptation to be understood from an evolutionary perspective, however. Adaptations are only one class of outcomes emerging from evolution. Natural selection also produces various kinds of evolutionary *by-products* as well. *Spandrels* are nonfunctional characteristics that fall incidentally out of adaptive designs, as human chins and navels emerge as by-products of adaptations for eating and language (jaw design) and internal gestation (umbilical cords), respectively. *Exaptations* refer to the use of adaptations for purposes other than those for which they were originally designed, as when (per Pangloss in *Candide*) we use our noses to hold up our spectacles. Particularly in modern environments that differ in countless ways from those in which our ancestors (and our psychological architecture) evolved, much contemporary human behavior is explained better in terms of by-products rather than as direct products of adaptations. This does not render an evolutionary approach any less relevant, but it does shift the task from one of identifying the design and function of an adaptation to specifying those adaptations that are being exapted (or producing a spandrel) and explaining how and why this by-product emerges from the adaptations (Buss, Haselton, Shackelford, Bleske, & Wakefield, 1998).

My own view (Kirkpatrick, 1999, 2005; see also Atran, 2002; Atran & Norenzayan, in press) is that the diverse collection of phenomena we refer to as "religion" represent a collection of by-products of numerous adaptations with other specific, mundane functions. To return to the computer metaphor, explaining religion is analogous to explaining how computers generate some particular class of outputs, such as scientific manuscripts.

Most of us create such products using a diversity of specialized programs for writing and formatting text, computing statistical results, producing graphs, and so forth. Similarly, we do not possess a "basketball instinct," but rather have constructed the game in a way that combines the activity of numerous nonbasketball psychological mechanisms related to such adaptive problems of coalition maintenance and conflict, intrasexual competition for dominance and status, and so forth.

With respect to religion, beliefs about the existence of supernatural forces and beings appear to emerge as a spandrel-like by-product of evolved systems dedicated to understanding the physical, biological, and interpersonal worlds (Boyer, 1994, 2001). For example, an evolved *agency-detector* mechanism, designed to distinguish animate from inanimate objects in the world, can be fooled fairly readily to produce psychological animism and anthropomorphism (Atran, 2002; Atran & Norenzayan, in press; Guthrie, 1993), as when we find ourselves cursing at our aforementioned computer when it crashes. Once these spandrel-like effects enable ideas about gods and other supernatural beings, I have suggested, specific forms of religious belief emerge as by-products of psychological mechanisms dedicated to processing information about functionally distinct kinds of interpersonal relationships—attachments, kinships, dominance and status competitions, social exchange relationships, friendships, coalitions, and so forth—that whir into action to shape specific beliefs and expectations about these beings and guide behavior toward them. Thus, for example, gods might be perceived as attachment figures, dominant or high-status individuals, or social exchange partners, with each possibility leading to a different set of expectations and inferences about those gods' behavior and decisions about how to best interact with them—processes emerging from functionally distinct psychological systems designed to solve such adaptive problems in human relations (Kirkpatrick, 1999, 2005).

Space limitations preclude a fuller discussion here of the details of this or other EP theories of religion. Although the discussion in the remainder of this chapter will more or less assume my own multiple by-product view of religion, all of the issues discussed are applicable to other evolutionary approaches to religion as well.

Types, Dimensions, and Definitions

If there is one activity at which all academics excel, it is conceptually dividing up the world and its contents into categories, types, and dimensions. Psychologists parse their subject matter into emotion versus cognition versus motivation; sensation versus perception; individual/personal versus interpersonal; and the omnipresent positive versus negative. In psychology of religion we find these same distinctions, as well as countless other category systems differentiating ritual, doctrine, emotion, knowledge, ethics, and community components (Verbit, 1970); ideological, ritualistic, experiential, intellectual, and consequential dimensions (Glock, 1962); and committed versus consensual religion (Allen & Spilka, 1967), to name just a few.

One problem with most such approaches is that they are essentially arbitrary. Analogously, the many parts of an automobile might be classified based on color, size and weight, substance or material from which they are constructed, or cost. Certain such systems might be adopted because they are useful for a particular purpose, such as color for painting or weight for choosing a shipping method, but none could claim a privileged status as superior in any broad sense. To humans who rely heavily on their sense of sight and who possess color vision, classification of things by color comes easily and naturally.

However, there is no good reason to think that classifications based on what happens to be salient to our perceptual systems will necessarily be useful for other purposes. Consequently, an infinite number of such schemes are possible, and theorists can (and do) argue fruitlessly about which way is "best," with no possible way of resolving the dispute.

If one's goal, however, is to understand how and why automobiles work—and to provide a useful basis for diagnosing and fixing a problem when one is broken—a conceptual understanding based on *function* is inherently superior to the alternatives. A mechanic or engineer thinks about automobiles in terms of specific components organized into systems (fuel, electrical, etc.) that are designed to perform specific functions. The cause of a car failing to start could be, for example, in the electrical system or the fuel system, each of which consists of particular components designed to do particular things and that therefore can each go wrong in particular ways. Thinking in functional terms immediately leads directly to hypotheses about the possible causes of the problem and procedures for testing them. A function-based system enjoys privileged status because of all the ways in which it is possible to classify car parts, only one of these corresponds to an organization that "really" is inherent in an automobile because it reflects the way in which the automobile "really is" designed to function. To the extent that we, as psychologists, endeavor to understand how and why human brains/minds work, we are in the position of the mechanic or engineer rather than the painter or shipping clerk. We need to carve nature at its joints.

To illustrate, consider the problem of distinguishing types of prayer. The arbitrariness of such schemes is clearly illustrated by the varying numbers and definitions of prayer types proposed by different researchers. Foster (1992) discusses 21 different types, Poloma and Gallup (1991) at least six. Poloma and Pendleton (1989) and Hood, Morris, and Harvey (1993) each have proposed four-category typologies, which overlap considerably in some ways but not others. For example, both include a category labeled *petitionary* prayer, but asking God for material things is categorized here by one scheme but in a separate *material* category in the other. Which way is "better"?

A functional theoretical perspective, in contrast, provides a nonarbitrary basis for making such determinations. To the extent that one's beliefs about God are a product of the attachment system, for example, prayer should reflect efforts to gain proximity to God and to seek comfort and security in the face of stress or perceived danger, and God should not be viewed as expecting something in return. To the extent that one's beliefs about God are a product of a social exchange (reciprocal altruism) system, it should involve asking for material things or specific forms of assistance, in exchange for which one would need to offer something to God in return (e.g., in the form of ritual, sacrifice, or "living right"). To the extent beliefs about God are a product of a dominance competition system, prayers should reflect expressions of fear and awe and requests for mercy and forgiveness. That is, different types of prayer can be distinguished theoretically in terms of the functions they serve and the distinct psychological systems underlying religious beliefs. Such function-based distinctions should prove more useful empirically in examining the relationships between prayer types and other variables because they conform to real functional differences, much as the mechanic's functional approach to automobiles is more likely to lead to correct diagnosis when a car will not start.

The same problem can be seen writ large with respect to defining and distinguishing religion from nonreligion. Scholars have failed for centuries to identify a particular thread or threads common to all things religious, and definitions of religion are as numerous as the researchers studying it. Religion itself is in the category of phenomena that are invented by humans, not an external reality to be discovered. We can define it however we like—and so we do. The history of the psychology of religion has largely been a series of efforts to map a variety of arbitrary conceptualizations of human psychology onto a variety of arbitrary conceptualizations of religion. No wonder little progress has been made!

It might seem to follow from these arguments that an ideal definition of religion (or any particular aspect of it) would be a *functional* one rather than a purely *descriptive* one. Indeed, many scholars have proposed definitions of religion in terms of its presumed functions of ameliorating anxiety or fear of death, answering existential questions, and so forth. It would be foolish to define the heart without reference to its function of pumping blood; the heart's function is central to what it means for something to be a heart. So why not treat religion similarly? Some day I hope that we will be in a position to do so. However, the fact is that at present we simply do not know what "the function" of religion is, if indeed it can meaningfully be said to have one at all. The function(s) of religion is what our theories and empirical research programs should be about, not something to be declared by fiat as part of a definition.

Once it is acknowledged that the human psychology side of the equation is nonarbitrary, and we understand the nature, structure, and function of the human mind as a product of evolutionary processes, we will be able to break out of this unproductive cycle and ask how this universal human psychology produces whichever particular behavioral, cognitive, or emotional phenomenon we wish to explain. Which of these are called "religion" will be unimportant, and we can dispense with endless debate about how to define religion and begin answering real substantive questions about how it works and why.

The Content of Religious Belief

Another undesirable consequence of traditional arbitrary constructs and classification schemes in psychology of religion is that most such approaches tend to be *content-independent*. The eternal quest for a universal definition of religion itself, as well as types or dimensions of religion, has long focused on finding highly abstract distinctions that transcend details of what people actually believe. Religion reflects, for example, one's "ultimate concern" or what one "imbues with sacredness"—entirely independent of what those things actually are. Abstract conceptual dimensions such as *intrinsic* versus *extrinsic* religious orientations are defined, quite deliberately, so as to be equally applicable to any particular religious content—or even beyond religion to contexts such as political ideology or philosophy.

For example, psychologists of religion have gone to considerable effort to define *fundamentalism* as a dimension or type of religiosity independent of belief content—the idea being that such a "way of being religious" is potentially identifiable within any particular belief system. Measured in such a way, fundamentalism has proved to correlate with various forms of prejudice and discrimination more strongly than with other dimensions of religiosity (Hunsberger, 1995) within Western (mostly college) samples. However, once one moves to other religions and cultures, the particular groups against which fundamentalists are prejudiced changes radically (Griffin, Gorsuch, & Davis, 1987). These patterns make sense only in light of the content of the beliefs themselves, in which particular outgroups are explicitly or implicitly disparaged. From a functional perspective, what is at work here is the psychology of coalitions, driven by a system of mechanisms designed by natural selection to monitor ingroup versus outgroup membership and guide behavior differentially as a result of our evolutionary history of intergroup conflict and intragroup cooperation. Allport (1954) saw this connection as an explanation of religion–prejudice relationships long before he (unfortunately) veered off into the much more abstract (and less useful) intrinsic–extrinsic distinction, which has proved of little value in understanding prejudice (Laythe, Finkel, Bringle, & Kirkpatrick, 2002).

Attribution theory, as borrowed from social psychology and applied to religion (see Hood et al., 1996, for a review), suffers from the same limitations. Researchers categorize attributions into abstract categories such as *internal* versus *external*, or *situations* versus *dispositions*, and so forth, and derive hypotheses about which attributions should be made when based on a (usually implicit) model of the mind as a logical analysis-of-variance calculator. But this is not the way the mind is designed to parse the world. Natural selection has not designed human minds to contain general, all-purpose "preference" or "choice" mechanisms, for example, but rather highly content-specific ones relevant to functionally distinct domains: The criteria by which we judge the relative value of foods are qualitatively different from those by which we judge potential mates. In attribution processes, numerous domain-specific inferential mechanisms are at work, each operating on highly content-specific inputs according to highly content-specific inferential rules. When the social-cognitive machinery of the attachment system is at work with respect to God, for example, good fortune is likely to be attributed to protection and support from a loving caregiver. When social exchange mechanisms are activated, ill fortune may be attributed to our own failure to abide by an explicit or implicit social contract with God (to have faith, engage in certain rituals, etc.) and/or God's anger in response to such a failure. (Note, by the way, how poorly a forced-choice measure of internal vs. external attribution would fare in capturing this dual dynamic.) Current approaches to religious attribution provide a skeletal framework that may be useful for some purposes, but an understanding of highly content-specific reasoning mechanisms is what ultimately will put meat on the bones.

One reason that highly abstract dimensions and types are widely preferred is that we generally strive to have only a small number of them. Most conceptual frameworks, including those in psychology of religion, involve between two and five categories or dimensions. (When there are four categories, we generally try to further reduce them to two dimensions!) This approach is generally lauded pursuant to the valued principle of *parsimony*. However, parsimony is often more apparent than real. A theory of the world based on earth, wind, fire, and water is succinct, and one comprising no more than yin and yang even more so, but both are woefully inadequate to actually explain much of anything because the world itself is not that simple. When it comes to human psychology, the evolutionary approach points to the existence of highly numerous, domain-specific mechanisms and systems, each with its own distinct functional organization. A "parsimonious" account that actually explains a substantial amount about human behavior and experience will likely at best involve dozens, and more likely hundreds, of such components. Despite these numbers, this approach reflects real rather than illusory parsimony in that hypotheses and theories about these dozens or hundreds of specific components can be derived from a rather smaller number of principles by which natural selection operates (combined with knowledge about the ancestral conditions in which such evolution took place).

Religious Motivation

One particular problem in psychology of religion for which carving nature at its joints is particularly important is that concerning the widely studied question of religious *motiva-*

tion. Consistent with the discussion above, psychology of religion has tended to follow its parent discipline in attempting to capture human motivation in terms of a small number of highly general fundamental motives, which generally are abstracted conceptually from armchair observation or factor analysis of questionnaire data. In many cases the question of motivation overlaps with that of the ultimate or evolutionary function of religion, as discussed previously; however, it also includes hypotheses about more proximal motives that influence individuals' behavior on a day-to-day basis. Such postulated religious motives have ranged from meaning, control, and self-esteem (Spilka, Shaver, & Kirkpatrick, 1985) to interpersonal relatedness or belongingness (Galanter, 1978), to the resolution of existential concerns (Batson, Schoenrade, & Ventis, 1993), to name just a few examples.

Unfortunately, none of these "basic needs" is likely to exist in such abstract form from an evolutionary perspective. The ability to construct abstract philosophical explanations about the world was almost certainly not directly related to reproductive success in Stone Age environments. A basic motive to "control events" would have been of little value because, like a command line in a chess-playing computer program that says "make good moves," it provides no practical guidance as to how to achieve this goal. Instead, we have inherited domain-specific systems for dealing with particular adaptive problems which require qualitatively different solutions in different domains, such as competing for food, mates, or other resources. For example, when examined carefully from an evolutionary perspective, self-esteem seems much more likely to reflect a collection of highly domain-specific self-evaluative mechanisms related to, for example, mate value, dominance and prestige, and social inclusion in coalitions, rather than a single "global" mechanism (Kirkpatrick & Ellis, 2001). Similarly, an abstract construct such as "relatedness" conflates numerous adaptive domains for which humans surely have evolved highly domain-specific psychological systems, because the adaptive problems (and what constitutes adaptive solutions) differ markedly across functionally distinct kinds of relationships such as kinships, friendships, intrasexual competition, and mating. In short, motivation is an area in which attempts to carve nature into a small number of broad, abstract types or dimensions is inherently misguided, because the design of human psychological architecture necessarily involves a very large number of highly domain-specific motivational systems rather than a few domain-general ones.

Perhaps the most egregious example of this misguided approach in the psychology of religion has been that of lumping together all religious motivations into a catch-all category called "extrinsic"—in contrast, ostensibly, to a somehow motivationless "intrinsic" orientation. My own empirical demonstration (Kirkpatrick, 1989) that the Allport–Ross scales contain at least two distinct "extrinsic" factors—which I referred to as *personal* versus *social*—was barely a step in the right direction. An evolutionary psychological perspective suggests a diversity of specific "personal" or "social" motives reflected in religious involvement, such as gaining comfort and security (i.e., attachment system), feeling socially included in cooperative groups (coalitional psychology), gaining prestige or status (intrasexual competition), and assisting close kin (kinship psychology). Indeed, it should be apparent from this small group of examples that the abstract distinction between "personal" and "social" itself becomes rather murky in the context of a more functional, domain-specific approach.

A future EP of religion, then, will approach the problem of religious motivation from a functional perspective on human motivation in general, which in turn will be organized according to adaptive problems faced by our distant ancestors and the psychological systems evolved to solve them. There exist an infinite number of arbitrary ways in which we could conceptually carve up the domain of human motivation from our armchairs, but only one of these corresponds to the way human psychology is actually designed.

Individual Differences

Another particularly important set of questions in the psychology of religion to which all of these arguments apply with force is that of *individual differences*. In personality psychology generally, researchers have proposed hundreds if not thousands of dimensions and typologies by which to sort differences between people. Researchers eventually managed to determine that the bulk of the variance in all of these dimensions can be captured by five giant factors, the so-called "Big Five" model of individual differences (e.g., Digman, 1990). Unfortunately, this solution is reminiscent of the hilarious sci-fi novel *The Hitchhiker's Guide to the Galaxy* (Adams, 1979), in which an immense supercomputer crunches for millions of years to determine that the answer to "life, the universe, and everything" is precisely "42"—at which time it becomes apparent that an even more immense supercomputer is needed to determine what exactly the question was. Why exactly five personality factors? Why these particular five? Nobody seems to know.

The psychology of religion has very much followed its parent discipline in its quest to determine the dimensionality of religion, with classic factor analysis studies producing large numbers of diverse dimensions (e.g., Broen, 1957; King & Hunt, 1969) and more recent studies focusing more narrowly on dimensions such as intrinsic and extrinsic religiosity (Allport & Ross, 1967), means, ends and quest orientations (Batson et al., 1993), fundamentalism (Hunsberger, 1995), and so forth. A recent addition to the list is *spiritual intelligence* (Emmons, 2000) which, like most other such constructs, is open to criticism for being either too broad or too narrow, glossing over or confounding important differences on the one hand and failing to acknowledge others (e.g., Gardner, 2000). Again the problem is one of arbitrariness: No one way of carving up individual differences can claim superiority over any other because there are no clear criteria for making such decisions.

The issue of individual differences raises interesting questions and problems for an evolutionary perspective: Given the existence of a species-universal psychology, how do stable individual differences emerge? Variability is of course a necessary ingredient for natural selection to occur; however, natural selection tends to reduce variability over time as less adaptive variants are eliminated and more adaptive ones become universal (Tooby & Cosmides, 1990). A discussion of the many ways in which individual differences emerge from this process is beyond the scope of the present chapter; the interested reader is referred to Buss and Greiling (1999) for details. Here I illustrate just two general ways of approaching individual differences in religious belief from the perspective of my multiple by-products theory.

First, given that a diverse collection of numerous domain-specific psychological mechanisms are (hypothesized to be) responsible for religious belief and behavior, people vary in the degree to which different mechanisms underlie their personal religious thinking. Thus, for example, people for whom the attachment system largely drives their religious beliefs will conceptualize God as a personal being who loves them, cares for them, and watches over them. For others, God is conceptualized as a social exchange partner whose provision of benefits is predicated on expectations of some kind of reciprocity. Thus, individual differences in beliefs may reflect the activation of different psychological systems.

Second, many psychological systems give rise to domain-specific patterns of individual differences as they interact with environments and experience across a person's lifetime. For example, a universal attachment system gives rise to well-studied individual differences with respect to the quality and nature of interactions between infants and their primary caregivers and the patterns of thinking and behaving arising from these. These individual differences are thought to originate in particular patterns of parental sensitivity and responsiveness to attachment behaviors across infancy and early childhood (Ainsworth, Blehar, Waters, & Wall, 1978), with parallel styles of individual differences emerging in adulthood in the context of romantic relationships (Hazan & Shaver, 1987). Much research now demonstrates that individual differences in attachment are related empirically, both cross-sectionally and longitudinally, to individual differences in beliefs about God and other religion variables (e.g., Granqvist, 1998, 2002; Granqvist & Hagekull, 1999; Kirkpatrick, 1997, 1998; Kirkpatrick & Shaver, 1990, 1992).

Because some evolved psychological systems are expected to differ between the sexes—particularly those closely related to mating and competition for mates—this line of thinking also provides a framework for examining the surprisingly understudied question of sex differences in religiosity. For example, men more than women compete with one another for status, prestige, and dominance, and thus might be expected (more than women) to conceptualize God with respect to dimensions such as power and dominance. Results consistent with this hypothesis have been reported in both adolescents (Cox, 1967) and adults (Nelsen, Cheek, & Au, 1985).

Finally, these conceptualizations of individual differences can be applied equally well to differences between cultures. Some religions, including most variants of Christianity, appear to be strongly attachment-based, whereas the gods in many other cultures seem to reflect the operation of other psychological systems such as social exchange (e.g., performing sacrifices and rituals in exchange for gods providing various benefits). Questions about cross-cultural variability in religion can be cast in terms of the ways in which particular historical and environmental contexts have led different cultures to develop religions that reflect different aspects of evolved psychology. Alternatively, such variability might be examined in terms of the kinds of domain-specific individual differences that emerge from a given psychological system. For example, predominant beliefs about the benevolence versus malevolence of gods across cultures are correlated empirically with differences in predominant childrearing styles in ways that are theoretically consistent with attachment theory (e.g., Rohner, 1975).

An Integrated Interdisciplinary Science

EP is not another subdiscipline of psychology to be placed alongside developmental, social, and clinical psychology; it is a general conceptual framework and body of theory that provides a coherent perspective from which any of the traditionally defined subdisciplines can be approached. In a field of psychology organized and informed by EP, social psychologists will continue to study situational and interpersonal factors that influence behavior; the effect of EP will be to provide a basis for guiding hypotheses about what factors should influence what behaviors (via interaction with what psychological mechanisms). Personality psychologists will continue to study individual differences, informed by theories about how such differences arise from both genetic and environmental factors in the context of a species-universal design. Developmental psychologists will continue to study how human psychological architecture unfolds via epigenetic processes across time, from a genetic recipe to adult form. Clinical psychologists will continue to study the ways in which human psychology goes awry, an enterprise that will benefit enormously from an understanding of how minds are designed to function and how modern environments differ in many functionally important ways from the ancestral environments to which minds are adapted.

The field of psychology has, for decades, been something of a hodgepodge of barely interconnected subdisciplines, a fact clear to introductory psychology students who struggle to find any meaningful connections between textbook chapters on social psychology, motivation and emotion, and psychopathology. Although most authors struggle mightily to organize themes to provide some integrative structure in their texts, the field is inherently splintered due its lack of a coherent paradigm. Specialists working on narrow questions within increasingly fractured subdisciplines have little concern with what others are doing in other areas and make little effort (nor have much incentive) to find bridges to distant subdisciplines.

For many such researchers this lack of a coherent, large-scale paradigm is a distant concern, but the psychology of religion suffers dramatically as a consequence. Because "religion" refers to such a diverse array of phenomena, and requires explanation across cultures and across historical time, it is a topic that cannot be approached effectively in a piecemeal fashion. A comprehensive psychology of religion must ultimately unite elements of developmental psychology, social psychology, and so forth. In a psychology unified by an evolutionary paradigm, the boundaries between traditional subdisciplines will be much more fluid, and the connections between them much more clear.

Moreover, a comprehensive psychology of religion must ultimately be interconnected with many disciplines beyond psychology, such as (especially) anthropology and biology, to integrate the multiple levels of analysis at which religious processes occur. Again, the evolutionary paradigm provides a powerful framework for doing so. The connection from psychology to biology is obvious, but the implications go far in the other direction as well. The EP approach provides a framework for understanding both cross-cultural consistency and variability, for example, and any theory about how people interact with groups or groups with one another must be firmly rooted in the psychology of individuals who make up those groups. It is crucial to note, however, that such an approach is not necessarily (and should not be) reductionistic in the sense of explaining all group-level phenomena in terms of individual psychology, any more than the principles of chemistry are reducible to the laws of physics or cellular biology is reducible to chemistry. Physics is the foundation of chemistry, and the principles of the latter are constrained by those of the former; however, chemistry involves the study of emergent properties at a level of analysis that emerges from, but is not reducible to, those of physics.

In the same way, the future of psychology hinges on its ability to find its proper place at a level of analysis above biology, rooted firmly within it (but not reducible to it), and providing the foundation for higher level sociological and anthropological approaches (Wilson, 1998). The evolutionary approach I have advocated here has focused mainly on the psychology in the head of each individual, but things get complex quickly when individuals so equipped begin interacting with one another. To understand how religious beliefs spread, and why some become popular and others die out, requires additional levels of analysis beyond (but understood in the context of) that of individual psychology. Many important processes of cultural transmission can be understood only at the population level. For example, which beliefs an individual is likely to adopt depends importantly on which ideas are locally prominent and which individuals are promulgating them (Boyd & Richerson, 1985). Sperber (1996) likens the study of the distribution and transmission of beliefs to epidemiology, requiring an understanding not only of disease processes and effects but also the various ways in which diseases are transmitted. The study of religion at societal and cultural levels by sociologists and anthropologists will be greatly facilitated once psychology provides a clear and well-grounded picture of individual psychology.

In sum, a future evolutionary psychology of religion will integrate the approaches of the traditional subdisciplines within psychology, and between psychology and its neighboring disciplines, in a way that will enable researchers to freely cross such boundaries while maintaining theoretical continuity. For example, a researcher studying prayer will be able to tie together questions about when and how adults pray in the contemporary United States with questions about how these patterns develop across childhood, or with questions about the ways in which such prayer is both similar and different as compared to that in other cultures.

CONCLUSIONS

For most of human history, the field of medicine comprised a motley collection of attempts to understand and repair bodies based on intuition, superstition, and trial and error. Modern medicine did not emerge until it was finally appreciated that the body comprises numerous, functionally specific tissues, organs, and systems, each of which was "designed" to perform particular tasks in concert with other parts. This functional approach to anatomy and physiology not only made sense of the body's structure and organization, but led to testable and practical hypotheses about the kinds of things that can go wrong with bodies and how to fix them. Needless to say, this changed everything. (When was the last time you had a good bloodletting?)

To contemporary evolutionary psychologists, the history of psychology bears a disconcerting resemblance to that of medicine.[4] From this perspective, it seems highly unlikely, if not altogether impossible, to construct a comprehensive and accurate understanding of how the brain and mind work in the absence of a functional approach to its inherent design and organization. The human brain/mind is the product of natural selection processes that have designed it, like the remainder of the body, according to principles that are now well understood. If one wants to ascertain how something works, the most efficient path is to begin with knowledge—or at least strong hypotheses—regarding what it is designed to do. It is just a matter of time before the power and promise of this approach is acknowledged sufficiently widely to produce a paradigm shift in psychology and the social sciences generally.

The revolution, though in its infancy, has begun. The psychology of the future will be guided, shaped, and organized by an evolutionary perspective. The psychology of religion will do well to follow.

NOTES

1. I will freely use the word "designed" to refer to the process by which adaptations evolve; however, it is crucial to avoid misinterpreting this term to imply that natural selection has any purpose, intent, or foresight.
2. Curiously, Chomsky refused to believe that evolution by natural selection could have been the

architect behind such a design, though he was unable to offer a reasonable alternative. Pinker (1994) completed the evolutionary story years later.

3. The idea that selection does occur at the group level, in addition to at the gene level, is still championed by some evolutionary biologists (e.g., Sober & Wilson, 1998) but remains controversial.

4. I do not intend to imply here that practicing clinicians are medieval barbers nor that their techniques are ineffective. However, I have no doubt—and I fully expect that most clinicians would agree—that psychological practice would be much more uniformly effective if based on a strong, comprehensive psychological science.

REFERENCES

Adams, D. (1979). *The hitchhiker's guide to the galaxy.* New York: Pocket Books.

Ainsworth, M. D. S., Blehar, M. C., Waters, E., & Wall, S. (1978). *Patterns of attachment: A psychological study of the Strange Situation.* Hillsdale, NJ: Erlbaum.

Allen, R. O., & Spilka, B. (1967). Committed and consensual religion: A specification of religion-prejudice relationships. *Journal for the Scientific Study of Religion, 6,* 191–206.

Allport, G. W. (1954). *The nature of prejudice.* Reading, MA: Addison-Wesley.

Allport, G. W., & Ross, J. M. (1967). Personal religious orientation and prejudice. *Journal of Personality and Social Psychology, 5,* 432–443.

Atran, S. (2002). *In gods we trust: The evolutionary landscape of religion.* Oxford, UK, and New York: Oxford University Press.

Atran, S., & Norenzayan, A. (in press). Religion's evolutionary landscape: Counterintuition, commitment, compassion, communion. *Behavioral and Brain Sciences.*

Averill, J. (1998). Spirituality: From the mundane to the meaningful—and back. *Journal of Theoretical and Philosophical Psychology, 18,* 101–126.

Batson, C. D., Schoenrade, P., & Ventis, W. L. (1993). *Religion and the individual: A social-psychological perspective.* New York: Oxford University Press.

Boyd, R., & Richerson, P. J. (1985). *Culture and the evolutionary process.* Chicago: University of Chicago Press.

Boyer, P. (1994). *The naturalness of religious ideas: A cognitive theory of religion.* Berkeley: University of California Press.

Boyer, P. (2001). *Religion explained: The evolutionary origins of religious thought.* New York: Basic Books.

Broen, W. E., Jr. (1957). A factor-analytic study of religious attitudes. *Journal of Abnormal and Social Psychology, 54,* 176–179.

Buss, D. M. (2004). *Evolutionary psychology: The new science of the mind* (2nd ed.) Boston: Pearson.

Buss, D. M., & Greiling, H. (1999). Adaptive individual differences. *Journal of Personality, 67,* 209–243.

Buss, D. M., Haselton, M. G., Shackelford, T. K., Bleske, A. L., & Wakefield, J. C. (1998). Adaptations, exaptations, and spandrels. *American Psychologist, 53,* 533–548.

Chomsky, N. (1957). *Syntactic structures.* The Hague: Mouton.

Cox, E. (1967). *Sixth form religion.* London: SCM Press.

Dawkins, R. (1989). *The selfish gene* (New ed.). New York: Oxford University Press.

Digman, J. (1990). Personality structure: The emergence of the five-factor model. *Annual Review of Psychology, 41,* 417–440.

Emmons, R. A. (2000). Is spirituality an intelligence?: Motivation, cognition, and the psychology of ultimate concern. *The International Journal for the Psychology of Religion, 10,* 3–26.

Foster, R. J. (1992). *Prayer: Find the heart's true home.* San Francisco: Harper & Row.

Galanter, M. (1978). The "relief effect": A sociobiological model for neurotic distress and large-group therapy. *American Journal of Psychiatry, 135,* 588–591.

Garcia, J., Ervin, F. R., & Koelling, R. A. (1966). Learning with prolonged delay of reinforcement. *Psychonomic Science, 5,* 121–122.

Gardner, H. (2000). A case against spiritual intelligence. *The International Journal for the Psychology of Religion, 10,* 27–34.

Glock, C. Y. (1962). On the study of religious commitment. *Religious Education, 57,* S98–S110.

Gorsuch, R. L. (1968). The conceptualization of God as seen in adjective ratings. *Journal for the Scientific Study of Religion, 7,* 56–64.

Granqvist, P. (1998). Religiousness and perceived childhood attachment: On the question of compensation or correspondence. *Journal for the Scientific Study of Religion, 37,* 350–367.

Granqvist, P. (2002). Attachment and religiosity in adolescence: Cross-sectional and longitudinal evaluations. *Personality and Social Psychology Bulletin, 28,* 260–270.

Granqvist, P., & Hagekull, B. (1999). Religiousness and perceived childhood attachment: Profiling socialized correspondence and emotional compensation. *Journal for the Scientific Study of Religion, 38,* 254–273.

Griffin, G. A., Gorsuch, R. L., & Davis, A. L. (1987). A cross-cultural investigation of religious orientation, social norms, and prejudice. *Journal for the Scientific Study of Religion, 26,* 358–365.

Gross, P. R., & Levitt, N. (1994). *Higher superstition: The academic left and its quarrel with science.* Baltimore: Johns Hopkins University Press.

Guthrie, S. G. (1993). *Faces in the clouds: A new theory of religion.* New York: Oxford University Press.

Hazan, C., & Shaver, P. (1987). Romantic love conceptualized as an attachment process. *Journal of Personality and Social Psychology, 52,* 511–524.

Hood, R. W., Jr., Morris, R. J., & Harvey, D. K. (1993, October). *Religiosity, prayer, and their relationship to mystical experience.* Paper presented at the annual meeting of the Religious Research Association, Raleigh, NC.

Hood, R. W., Jr., Spilka, B., Hunsberger, B., & Gorsuch, R. (1996). *The psychology of religion: An empirical approach* (2nd ed.). New York: Guilford Press.

Hunsberger, B. (1995). Religion and prejudice: The role of religious fundamentalism, quest and right wing authoritarianism. *Journal of Social Issues, 51*(2), 113–129.

James, W. (1890). *Principles of psychology.* New York: Holt.

King, M. B., & Hunt, R. A. (1969). Measuring the religious variable: Amended findings. *Journal for the Scientific Study of Religion, 8,* 321–323.

Kirkpatrick, L. A. (1989). A psychometric analysis of the Allport–Ross and Feagin measures of intrinsic–extrinsic religiousness. In M. Lynn & D. Moberg (Eds.), *Research in the Social Scientific Study of Religion* (Vol. 1, pp. 1–31). Greenwich, CT: JAI Press.

Kirkpatrick, L. A. (1997). A longitudinal study of changes in religious belief and behavior as a function of individual differences in adult attachment style. *Journal for the Scientific Study of Religion, 36,* 207–217.

Kirkpatrick, L. A. (1998). God as a substitute attachment figure: A longitudinal study of adult attachment style and religious change in college students. *Personality and Social Psychology Bulletin, 24,* 961–973.

Kirkpatrick, L. A. (1999). Toward an evolutionary psychology of religion. *Journal of Personality, 67,* 921–952.

Kirkpatrick, L. A. (2005). *Attachment, evolution, and the psychology of religion.* New York: Guilford Press.

Kirkpatrick, L. A., & Ellis, B. J. (2001). An evolutionary approach to self-esteem: Multiple domains and multiple functions. In G. J. O. Fletcher & M. S. Clark (Eds.), *The Blackwell handbook of social psychology: Vol. 2. Interpersonal processes* (pp. 411–436). Oxford, UK: Blackwell.

Kirkpatrick, L. A., & Shaver, P. R. (1990). Attachment theory and religion: Childhood attachments, religious beliefs, and conversion. *Journal for the Scientific Study of Religion, 29,* 315–334.

Kirkpatrick, L. A., & Shaver, P. R. (1992). An attachment-theoretical approach to romantic love and religious belief. *Personality and Social Psychology Bulletin, 18,* 266–275.

Laythe, B., Finkel, D., Bringle, R., & Kirkpatrick, L. A. (2002). Religious fundamentalism as a predictor of prejudice: A two-component model. *Journal for the Scientific Study of Religion, 41*, 623–635.

Nelsen, H. M., Cheek, N. H., Jr., & Au, P. (1985). Gender differences in images of God. *Journal for the Scientific Study of Religion, 24*, 396–402.

Persinger, M. A. (1987). *The neuropsychological bases of God beliefs*. New York: Praeger.

Pinker, S. (1994). *The language instinct*. New York: Morrow.

Pinker, S. (1997). *How the mind works*. New York: Norton.

Poloma, M. M., & Gallup, G. H., Jr. (1991). *Varieties of prayer: A survey report*. Philadelphia: Trinity Press International.

Poloma, M. M., & Pendleton, B. F. (1989). Exploring types of prayer and quality of life research: A research note. *Review of Religious Research, 31*, 46–53.

Ramachandran, V. S., & Blakeslee, S. (1998). *Phantoms in the brain*. New York: Morrow.

Rohner, R. P. (1975). *They love me, they love me not*. New Haven, CT: HRAF Press.

Seligman, M., & Hager, J. (1972). *Biological boundaries of learning*. New York: Appleton-Century-Crofts.

Snow, C. P. (1959). *The two cultures and the scientific revolution*. New York: Cambridge University Press.

Sober, E., & Wilson, D. S. (1998). *Unto others: The evolution and psychology of unselfish behavior*. Cambridge, MA: Harvard University Press.

Sperber, D. (1996). *Explaining culture: A naturalistic approach*. Oxford, UK: Blackwell.

Spilka, B., Shaver, P. R., & Kirkpatrick, L. A. (1985). General attribution theory for the psychology of religion. *Journal for the Scientific Study of Religion, 24*(1), 1–20.

Symons, D. (1992). On the use and misuse of Darwinism in the study of behavior. In J. H. Barkow, L. Cosmides, & J. Tooby (Eds.), *The adapted mind* (pp. 137–159). New York: Oxford University Press.

Tooby, J., & Cosmides, L. (1990). On the universality of human nature and the uniqueness of the individual: The role of genetics and adaptation. *Journal of Personality, 58*, 17–67.

Tooby, J., & Cosmides, L. (1992). The psychological foundations of culture. In J. H. Barkow, L. Cosmides, & J. Tooby (Eds.), *The adapted mind* (pp. 19–136). New York: Oxford University Press.

Verbit, M. F. (1970). The components and dimensions of religious behavior: Toward a reconceptualization of religiosity. In P. E. Hammond & B. Johnson (Eds.), *American mosaic* (pp. 24–39). New York: Random House.

Waller, N., Kojetin, B., Bouchard, T., Jr., Lykken, D., & Tellegen, A. (1990). Genetic and environmental influences on religious interests, attitudes, and values: A study of twins reared apart and together. *Psychological Science, 1*, 138–142.

Wilson, E. O. (1998). *Consilience: The unity of knowledge*. New York: Knopf.

Wulff, D. M. (1997). *Psychology of religion: Classic and contemporary* (2nd ed.). New York: Wiley.

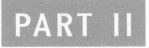

PART II

RELIGION THROUGH THE DEVELOPMENTAL LENS

7

Religious and Spiritual Development in Childhood

CHRIS J. BOYATZIS

This chapter addresses aspects of children's religious development. The discussion is restricted to childhood, as adolescent development is discussed elsewhere (Levenson, Aldwin, & D'Mello, Chapter 8, this volume). This chapter has several major goals: (1) to examine psychologists' historical neglect and recent interest in religious and spiritual development (hereafter RSD); (2) to provide a selective review of advances in research; (3) to examine the hegemony of two paradigms in RSD: (a) cognitive-developmentalism's focus on how children think about religion, and (b) socialization models presuming that children are socialized religiously via unilateral parent → child "transmission"; (4) to encourage work on how children's RSD is affected by parental, contextual, and sociocultural factors; and (5) to recommend new directions in paradigm, theory, methods, and data. A "multilevel interdisciplinary paradigm" (Emmons & Paloutzian, 2003) will be suggested, in which psychologists use multiple measures and multiple theoretical frameworks and draw from multiple disciplines beyond the boundaries of the mainstream academic study of RSD.

PSYCHOLOGISTS' NEGLECT AND RECENT DISCOVERY OF RELIGIOUS AND SPIRITUAL DEVELOPMENT

Spirituality and religion are important, perhaps central, dimensions of human development. Data from American adolescents (Gallup & Bezilla, 1992) show that 95% believe in God and three-quarters try to follow the teachings of their religion. Almost half of U.S. youth say they frequently pray alone and 36% are involved in church youth groups. In a 1999–2000 Search Institute national survey of 6th- to 12th-grade youth, 54% said that "being religious or spiritual" was quite or extremely important (Benson, Roehlkepartain,

& Rude, 2003). Religion is also important to most U.S. families. About 40% attend worship weekly, 95% of U.S. parents have a religious affiliation, and more than 90% want their children to receive some form of religious education (Mahoney, Pargament, Swank, & Tarakeshwar, 2001).

However, database reviews have found that less than 1% of articles on children address spirituality (Benson et al., 2003) and in PsycINFO a mere *two-thirds of one percent* of all records on children (almost 150,000) address children *"and* religion" (Boyatzis, 2003a). The latter search found that children appears with "God" in 90 records, "church" in 76, and "faith" in 43 (or 3 per 10,000 records). In contrast, children "and family" appear in about 16,000 records. Children "and enuresis" (bedwetting) has almost five times more records than children "and faith," and children "and autism" appear about 78 times more often than children "and God." PsycINFO and Sociological Abstracts records are rare on children and Islam, Hinduism, or Buddhism (Boyatzis, 2003a), a neglect incommensurate with the popularity of these religions.

Fortunately, a call has been issued for psychology to "honor spiritual development as a core developmental process that deserves equal standing in the pantheon of universal developmental processes" (Benson, 2004, p. 50). To achieve this goal, scholars must work toward a comprehensive understanding that will require the study of RSD in interaction with many developmental domains (cognition, social relations, emotions, etc.) and disciplines (e.g., anthropology, sociology). Growth will also require advances in paradigm, theory, and method.

RECENT ATTENTION TO RELIGIOUS AND SPIRITUAL DEVELOPMENT

There is a conspicuous surge of interest in RSD. There are many forthcoming volumes and chapters on the topic. Sage Publications will soon release an *Encyclopedia of Religious and Spiritual Development* (Dowling & Scarlett, in press) and *Handbook of Religious and Spiritual Development in Childhood and Adolescence* (Roehlkepartain, King, Wagener, & Benson, 2005). For the first time in its storied history as the "bible" of child development, the next edition of the *Handbook of Child Psychology* will include a chapter on spiritual development. A second growth area is conference meetings, including the International Conference on Children's Spirituality, the inaugural meeting in 2003 of the Children's Spirituality Conference—Christian Perspectives, and a preconference on RSD at the biennial meetings of the Society for Research on Child Development (SRCD; contact the author for information on this SRCD preconference). In addition, many journals are addressing RSD, including the *International Journal of Children's Spirituality* and special issues on RSD in *Review of Religious Research* (Boyatzis, 2003b) and *Applied Developmental Science* (King & Boyatzis, 2004). Another sign of growth is dissertation activity. A PsycINFO search (May, 2004) of truncated subject terms "child* and religio*" found 242 dissertations from 1872 to 2003. Between 1872 and 1959 there were no dissertations on the topic, but there were 11 in the 1960s, 42 in the 1970s, and 58 in the 1980s. This growth exploded in the 1990s, with 102 dissertations. Combining the dissertations from the 1990s and 2000–2003 on children and religion, there were 109, or 45% of all dissertations ever done on the subject.

Thus, at one end of the scholarly pipeline, coverage of RSD in new handbooks by prominent publishers shows that the topic has "made it," and at the other end of the pipeline the surge in dissertation activity promises a large cohort of rising scholars working on RSD. The field of RSD is making inroads into the mainstream of psychology like never before.

DEFINING OUR CONSTRUCTS

Empirical data on definitions of "spiritual" and "religious" are offered elsewhere (Zinnbauer & Pargament, Chapter 2, this volume). Given the terms' overlap, they will be used somewhat interchangeably here. *Religious development* could be defined as the child's growth within an organized community that has shared narratives, practices, teachings, rituals, and symbols in order to bring people closer to the sacred and to enhance one's relationship to community. *Spirituality* has been defined as the search for and relationship with whatever one takes to be a holy or sacred transcendent entity (Pargament, 1999). The concepts of *relationship* and *self-transcendence* permeate definitions of spirituality. In rich qualitative work with children, Nye (Hay & Nye, 1998) and others (Reimer & Furrow, 2001) have identified the core of spirituality as "relational consciousness"—a marked perceptiveness in the child of relation to other people, God, or the self. Others have defined *spiritual development* as "the process of growing the intrinsic human capacity for self-transcendence, in which the self is embedded in something greater than the self, including the sacred" (Benson et al., 2003, p. 205), or as an orientation to self and one's surroundings that involves transcending oneself and developing a commitment to contribute to others (Lerner, Dowling, & Anderson, 2003).

CHILDREN'S RELIGIOUS AND SPIRITUAL DEVELOPMENT

Cognitive-Developmental Approaches

Developmentalists have focused on "religious cognition," or children's thinking about religious concepts. David Elkind was crucial for introducing to U.S. psychologists Piagetian cognitive-developmental models of religious cognition through his studies on children of different faith traditions (e.g., Elkind, 1961, 1963). Elkind's empirical paper on children's prayer concepts (Long, Elkind, & Spilka, 1967) and his broader theoretical explication (Elkind, 1970) are exemplary accounts of that era's cognitive-developmental approach.

Several themes emerged from Elkind's research: Children's religious thinking showed stage-like change from more concrete and egocentric to more abstract and sociocentric thought. The presumption of these trends flavored research on religious cognition for decades, and stage-based cognitive-developmentalism also shaped religious education (e.g., Goldman, 1964). The structural qualities of children's thinking about religious concepts paralleled their thinking about other, nonreligious concepts. Religious cognition was nothing special, merely a specific case of a generic conceptual and representational process. In addition, general constraints in the child's thinking make the child likely to think in particular ways about religious concepts.

A second wave of cognitive-developmentalism ushered in a major revision: the rejection of global stages that characterized, at any one age, all of a child's thinking. In the 1980s, developmentalists endorsed models of domain-specificity in cognitive development, with a view of the child as a builder of naïve theories in specific domains (e.g., Carey, 1985). In the 1990s, theory of mind ascended and the notion of specific domains in religious cognition was largely replaced with the view that religious-cognitive growth is best understood as part of the general growth of understanding of the mind, agency, mental–physical causality, and related concepts. Boyer (1994; Boyer & Walker, 2000) echoed the conclusion offered earlier (Elkind, 1970): children's religious cognitions operate under the same principles and tendencies of children's everyday cognition that has nothing to do with religious ideas.

Despite some fundamental similarities across these waves of cognitive-developmental changes, there were important changes in the array of hypothetical constructs and specific processes at work. In the current zeitgeist, the argot of cognitive-developmentalists has changed to include constructs such as "religious ontologies," or mental representations about the existence and powers of supernatural entities. As Boyer and Walker (2000, p. 152) put it, "the particular way in which religious ontology develops depends on the wider development of ontological categories." These ontologies are marked by several key features. One is the "counterintuitive" nature of religious ontologies (i.e., they violate ordinary expectations, as in the case of spiritual entities who are immortal or omniscient). A second is that counterintuitive religious beliefs operate within the implicit backdrop of theory of mind, which provides children with a prepared set of qualities to extend to the religious agents they think about (e.g., "My supernatural God has wishes and thoughts and worries [just like all beings with minds do]"). Another feature is that the combination of the counterintuitiveness of such agents with the belief that such agents are *real* makes religious beliefs all the more *salient* to those who hold them. This salience enhances their likelihood of being transmitted and shared with others.

Another recent revision is the claim that children and adults may not be altogether different in their thinking. That is, magical thinking and rational thinking, "ordinary reality" and "extraordinary reality," and other thought processes that presumably compete may instead coexist in the minds of children and adults (Subbotsky, 1993; Woolley, 1997). This assertion has engendered a new understanding of children. As Woolley (2000) put it, "children's minds are not inherently one way or another—not inherently magical nor inherently rational" (pp. 126–127). Children *and* adults can chalk up mysterious events to "magic," fear what goes bump in the night, and wrestle with the boundaries between real and imagined. These claims challenge the model of cognitive growth as an invariant, stage-like march away from irrational fantasy (allegedly the stuff of children's, and only children's, thinking) toward the *telos* and adult gold standard of rational logic (allegedly the stuff of adults', and only adults', thinking).

Even if Piaget has fallen from his pedestal, children's religious cognition continues to be the preoccupation of most mainstream child development researchers. Critiques of this fixation on thinking are offered later. Due to space limitations, only a subset of religion concepts are discussed, one that has received ample attention and one that has received little.

Children's Concepts of God

The most established interest in religious development research has been children's concepts of God. This focus is not surprising, for several reasons, including the fact that most research has been done by Westerners in Western settings where monotheism predominates. Children who think about God often do so in anthropomorphic terms. Coles (1990) noted that of his large collection of children's drawings of God, 87% depicted God's face. This anthropomorphizing has been explained by some cognitive-developmentalists as an extension of an intuitive folk psychology to supernatural figures and by attachment, psychoanalytic, or object relations theories (e.g., Rizzuto, 1979; Vergote & Tamayo, 1981) that assert that the child's internal working model of the parents is used as a prototype for a God image.

Empirical work by Barrett calls into question this view of the child's God as a personified God. Barrett and colleagues (Barrett & Keil, 1996; Barrett & Richert, 2003) have conducted a series of studies with young children to test whether children equate God's capabilities with humans' (i.e., think about God anthropomorphically). Preschoolers think rather differently about God's (versus other agents') creative powers, knowledge and perspective, and mortality. Although these observations are not new (see, e.g., Tamminen, Vianello, Jaspard, & Ratcliff, 1988), Barrett has offered an alternative account to the anthropomorphism hypothesis. His "preparedness" hypothesis posits that children are prepared conceptually at very early ages to think about God's *unique*, not human, qualities. When preschoolers begin to understand basic properties of the mind (e.g., perspective taking), they attribute those skills differently (nonanthropomorphically) to God than to humans. Barrett and Richert (2003) speculate that even though cultural contributions are necessary to help create God concepts, children may need "little direct training or tuition to acquire fairly rich theological concepts" (p. 310).

God concepts have been examined in children of different religions. For example, Pitts (1976) sampled 6- to 10-year-old children from Jewish, Lutheran, Mennonite, Methodist, Mormon, Roman Catholic, and Unitarian families. Pitts used multiple measures: children's drawings of God, interviews with children, and questionnaires for parents. Drawings were analyzed for different themes, including the degree to which children anthropomorphized God. This "A-score," as Pitts called it, varied widely across groups. God was anthropomorphized most by Mormon, Mennonite, and Lutheran children (all very similar in their scores), followed closely by Roman Catholic and Methodist children (who were identical in score). Jewish children drew the least personified pictures of God, and Unitarian children had A-scores between Jewish children and the other groups. The highest ratio of religious-to-nonreligious symbolism appeared in Roman Catholic children's art, the lowest in Unitarian children's; Jewish children's drawings were abstract and nonrepresentational. Thus, children's religious backgrounds clearly influence their God concepts.

In another study, Heller (1986) found that Hindu children, more than Jewish, Baptist, or Roman Catholic children, described a multifaceted God that feels close and like a person in some ways yet is also an abstract and intangible form of energy. These Hindu beliefs reflect their doctrine about different Gods with different natures and functions. Taken together, these studies suggest that children do extend a folk psychology and theory of mind to their God images but also conceptualize God as considerably more than human. The studies also demonstrate the value of sampling children from diverse religious backgrounds.

Thinking about God Is Not Just Cognitive

The mystery of the divine seems to capture much of children's (and adults') attention. But thinking about God is not just a cognitive act; it is deeply emotional, personal, and social. Though some have argued (Harris, 2000a, p. 176) that, to children themselves, there is "nothing special" about their God questions and that they are questions like any other, the assertion here is that the child's contemplations about God can have serious personal implications—especially for children who believe in God, come from faithful families, or are immersed in a culture where "God talk" is commonplace. This personal impact of thinking about God is underscored by the fact that the spiritual entity in question is one that, in monotheistic cultures, is upheld as *the* ultimate and divine being. Thus, thinking about God connects the child to a divine transcendent as well as to a broader social community of belief. Indeed, thinking about God does not occur in a social vacuum. Parents' reports of discussions about religion show that a large proportion of children's questions and comments are about God (Boyatzis & Janicki, 2003; Lawrence, 1965). The child's interpersonal contexts—family, church, peers—help children articulate their views on the metaphysical, and these contexts are, for much of the world's children, embedded in cultures that publicly discuss or worship the divine (see, e.g., Rizzuto, 1979). Thus, thinking about God is very much a social act, as these two conversations show. The first remarks come from an 11-year-old girl thinking about the skin color of Jesus (in Coles, 1990, pp. 57–58):

> "My daddy says there weren't any cameras then, so there's no picture of Him. . . . I know that in the black churches they'll tell you Jesus is black; he's colored. Our maid told us that's how He looks in her church—the pictures of Him—so there's the difference. I asked my grandma who's right, and she said . . . 'Honey, I don't think it makes any difference up there—skin color.' "

Here is a conversation between a father and his daughter when she was 8½ (in Boyatzis, 2004):

> C: "I just thought about how people think God is perfect, but do they mean He *knows* everything is perfect."
>
> F: "Do *you* think He knows everything?"
>
> C: "I don't know. I think we might find that out when we go to heaven. But, um, I sort of think there are some things that He might not—or *She*—might not know."
>
> F: "So you think we find out when we go to heaven."
>
> C: "Yes, I think that's where you can talk to God and ask God lots of questions."
>
> F: "Is there any other way to talk to God *now*, here on earth?"
>
> C: "If you pray. But when I pray, I'm . . . ah, I just, I'm very impatient. When I can't hear God I go, I go (*in mock whiny tone*), 'Mommy, It's *not talking to me*! It's *not talking to me*!' See, cuz I just can't hear God very well."
>
> F: "When you pray, what do you expect to hear? Do you think you'll hear God?"
>
> C: "Oh, I expect to hear . . . I expect to hear . . . I expect to hear somebody going (*in deep voice*) 'OK, thank you for that prayer.' If I ask any questions, I expect to hear the answers later on, next time I pray. But unfortunately I can't really hear the voice. I don't know if God's talking to me and I *just can't hear it*, or if God's *not* talking to me."
>
> F: "I think it's hard to know what God thinks."
>
> C: (*emphatically*) "You just *don't know*."

These excerpts also convey the richness of children's thinking and feeling that can be captured by qualitative and ethnographic methods, which are discussed later.

Children's Concepts of the Soul

In contrast to children's God concepts, their thoughts about the soul have received little empirical attention. The only empirical investigations I know of that have explicitly studied children's concepts of the soul include a study of Russian children (published in Russian; Savina, 1997), a study of Chinese children (published in Hungarian; Hui & Chou, 1991), and a study of U.S. children from mainline Protestant, Roman Catholic, and Mennonite traditions (Boyatzis, 1997).

Some work (see Evans, 2000) suggests that children use creationist explanations for human but not nonhuman animals, thus giving humans "privileged" status. If humans had such privileged status in soul concepts, children may make a human (have souls)/nonhuman (don't have souls) distinction. Or, if children conceive of the soul as an élan vital in living beings, a living/nonliving distinction could emerge (i.e., plants, animals, and humans have souls/artifacts don't). In interviews with preschoolers, Boyatzis (1997) found that 20% of children attributed a soul to furniture, 40% to plants, and 45% to cats and dogs. Children's judgment of the soul-fulness of humans was higher but varied by the age group in question: 48% of children attributed a soul to "babies" (strikingly similar to plants, cats, and dogs!), 64% to "children," and 75% to "parents." Children claiming that babies have souls may relate to the finding that many preschoolers say babies can make wishes or pray (Woolley, 2000). Overall, there was some but not sharp distinction between human/nonhuman and living/nonliving, and a trend toward more "soulfulness" as humans get older. In the Boyatzis study, a different picture emerged in a small group of Mennonite children from rural Pennsylvania. In these conservative Christians who attended a Mennonite school and had limited contact with U.S. culture, a human/nonhuman distinction emerged: none of the children said furniture, plants, or animals had a soul, whereas 88% said babies and children had souls and 100% of parents did. Together, these data support the notion that children's soul concepts are influenced by their family and religious backgrounds.

Religious and Spiritual Cognition: Parent–Child Correspondence or Independence?

The family functions as "the interpreters of religious ideology" for children (Heller, 1986, p. 32) and parents' practices and beliefs provide "cognitive anchors" (Ozorak, 1989). But is there *correspondence* or *independence* between the child's and the parents' beliefs in religious, spiritual, and metaphysical matters? The traditional social-learning approach, with its implicit "tabula rasa" child, would suggest a correspondence model: children's beliefs would be strongly similar to their parents' beliefs. However, a cognitive approach, with its depiction of the child as actively constructing and assimilating his or her reality, may thus predict only a loose association, or an independence, between parent and child beliefs. These opposing hypotheses are important to test, primarily because of their relevance to the two dominant approaches in the field of RSD.

Many researchers have examined children's and parents' beliefs about mythical figures (e.g., Santa Claus). This research is relevant to children's religious beliefs and cognitions as both topics have widespread endorsement in our culture and entail a mingling of human and supernatural qualities. In some studies, parents' endorsement of mythical characters such as Santa, the Easter Bunny, and the Tooth Fairy was positively related to their children's belief in them (Prentice, Manosevitz, & Hubbs, 1978; Rosengren, Kalish, Hickling, & Gelman, 1994). However, the correspondence between parents and children was not so strong as to suggest children think what their parents want them to think. In Prentice et al. (1978), of the parents who encouraged their children to believe in the Easter Bunny, 23% of their children did *not* believe, and of the parents who discouraged their children's belief, 47% of the children *did* believe in the Easter Bunny. In interviews with fundamentalist Christian families, Clark (1995) found that many children believed that Santa was real even though their parents discouraged such belief. A study of 3- to 10-year-old Jewish children revealed the children's belief in these mythical figures was unrelated to parents' encouragement of these beliefs (Prentice & Gordon, 1986).

Intriguing work by Taylor and Carlson (2000) investigated parents' attitudes about children's fantasy play through ethnographies and interviews with subjects from Mennonite and fundamentalist Christian religions. They also reviewed research on Hindu families. Parents' religious ideologies influenced their reactions to and beliefs about children's fantasy behavior and engagement with imaginary companions. The Hindu parents often reacted positively, because their children's talking with invisible companions may be a way the children interact with a spirit from a past life. This parental interpretation reflects their religious tradition of belief in reincarnated and metaphysical entities. In contrast, Mennonite parents had strongly negative reactions to their children's imaginary companions.

A similar pattern emerges in studies on parent–child religious beliefs. Evans (2000, 2001) examined children in secular families and in fundamentalist Christian families who also attended religious schools or were home-schooled to learn whether children from these different backgrounds endorse creationist or evolutionist accounts. To some degree, family type did matter—fundamentalist Christian children overwhelmingly embraced creationist views with virtually no endorsement of evolutionist ones. However, even young children (7 to 9 years of age) from *secular* homes embraced creationist views. Not until early adolescence did youth in secular homes began to consistently share their families' evolutionist cosmologies. Evans notes that even a "saturated" belief environment, as Evans called it, with consistent beliefs between parents and between the parents and local community norms, would still be filtered through the child's intuitive belief system. These data suggest that parent–child correspondence or independence will reflect children's cognitive level and construction of knowledge around them.

In another study, Carl Johnson (2000) interviewed Roman Catholic (RC) and Unitarian Universalist (UU) 13- and 14-year-old girls. These traditions embrace different views of the supernatural. Catholicism asserts that there are many supernatural forces (God, the Holy Ghost, saints, etc.) whereas the UU tradition does not doctrinally assert a supernatural God. In their comments, RC girls believed in God, miracles, supernatural beings, and related matters. In contrast, UU girls dismissed the notion of a supernatural being and argued that, for example, the recovery of a terminally ill child was not due to a miracle but to an unknown process or the power of human willpower. Johnson noted that UU teenagers were not solely materialists and indeed speculated about spiritual forces. The key distinction was that the UU girls endorsed the power of the human will and spirit whereas RC girls embraced a divine God who permeates all of reality.

A study on religious coping demonstrates both correspondence and independence at work. Pendleton, Cavalli, Pargament, and Nasr (2002) studied children sick with cystic fibrosis on multiple measures (e.g., interviews, artwork, parent report) and found that some children used religious coping even though their families were not religious. For example, a 10-year-old boy drew a picture of God embracing him to make him feel better. When the boy's mother saw the drawing, she was taken aback by her son's religious imagery, saying, "My kids have never even been to church in their lives!" (Pendleton et al., 2002, p. 5).

Other research makes clear that children's *perceptions* of parents' religious views and behavior are more related to the children's religious development than are the parents' *actual* views and behaviors (Bao, Whitbeck, Hoyt, & Conger, 1999; Okagaki & Bevis, 1999). What parents do and believe is less important than what *children think* parents do and believe.

The studies reviewed generate several important conclusions. One is that we must study children growing up in different religions to capture the complexity and variety in children's religious cognition and ontologies. Another is that researchers must determine how children's ideas are affected by different inputs: parents, school, community, church, religious education, and so on. Together, the findings reveal ample correspondence *and* independence between parent and child beliefs. There is evidence for both. Now, one's choice to prioritize either correspondence or independence will reflect one's core presumptions about children, families, and RSD. To advance our thinking, the position here is that the independence model of parent–child belief is theoretically more illuminating and stimulating, and for this reason: it confirms children's active role in their own RSD and thus raises serious doubts about the depiction in socialization theories of the child as a passive recipient in top-down transmission of parental belief.

Better Ways to Understand Family Mechanisms of Socialization

Many parents and children talk about religious issues, confronting the unknowability and ineffability of the spiritual and metaphysical. Sometimes children have experiences or insights that parents find anomalous or "inappropriate" to either reason or faith. Researchers might study how parents react to such experiences (see Boyatzis, 2004; Harris, 2000a, 2000b; Woolley, 1997). Parental *openness* to the varieties of children's religious and mystical experience may foster the child's relational consciousness to what is beyond oneself. Indeed, parents' acceptance of children's belief in imaginary figures (Santa, etc.) may help the child develop faith in the transcendent sacred figures that are central to religious traditions (Clark, 1995).

Family processes are described elsewhere (Mahoney & Tarakeshwar, Chapter 10, this volume). While we know that in some ways children's RSD is related to their parents' religiosity, we know little about specific mechanisms at work. Parents may influence their children's RSD as they do in other realms, through verbal induction and indoctrination of beliefs, disciplinary tactics, different reinforcements, and behavioral modeling. Some scholars have extended these constructs to spiritual modeling and spiritual observational learning (Silberman, 2003; Strommen & Hardel, 2000). Adults' retrospective reports confirm that "embedded routines"—regular family rituals—were common in families of those who grew up to be religious (Wuthnow, 1999).

A common family activity is parent–child conversation about religion. Boyatzis and Janicki (2003) asked a small sample of Christian families with children ages 3 to 12 to complete a survey on parent–child communication and to keep a diary of all conversations about religious and spiritual issues. Data were collected in two time periods, about 2 months apart, to assess the frequency, structure, and content of parent–child conversations about religious topics. The results indicated that parent–child communication about religion is a *reciprocal, bilateral dynamic* with mutual influence. This characterization of family interaction contrasts sharply with the unilateral "transmission" model that has dominated socialization models for decades. Data from surveys and diaries demonstrate that in conversations about religion children are active, initiate and terminate about half of them, speak as much as parents do, and ask questions and offer their own views. Parents ask many more open-ended questions than test questions (e.g., "What do you think heaven is like?" vs. "Who built the Ark?") and did not impose their own beliefs too strongly. On a "conviction rating" 5-point scale, parents indicated in each diary the degree to which their comments reflected their actual beliefs about the topic. The average rating was only a 3.7, suggesting that parents were not strongly stating their own views. This modest conviction could mean that parents attempted to accommodate their children's views and/or that parents "watered down" their statements to help their children better understand their views. These communication styles should be analyzed in families of different religions.

Although Boyatzis and Janicki (2003) did not measure the impact of communication style on children's beliefs (and this is a crucial step in future research), a 2-year longitudinal study on adolescents' moral reasoning seems relevant. Children's moral reasoning developed most when parents asked questions about the child's opinions, discussed the child's moral reasoning, and paraphrased the child's own words (Walker & Taylor, 1991). We may expect a similar relationship between communication style and children's RSD. Another longitudinal topic is the long-term consequence of growing up with a particular kind of religious communication style in childhood. Might early family communication styles predict different forms of later religiosity?

The diary and survey data (Boyatzis & Janicki, 2003) support the notion that most families' natural conversations about religion consist of a mutual give-and-take with reciprocal influence. This is consistent with two different but compatible models of development. One model emphasizes the role of knowledgeable adults who use scaffolding and guided participation to help the child move in a zone of proximal development to higher understandings (Rogoff, 1990; Vygotsky, 1978). A second, transactional model of development posits that children and parents influence each other in recurrent reciprocal exchanges (Kuczynski, 2003).

The bidirectional and transactional models differ from the unilateral transmission model in several key ways (Kuczynski, 2003). First, unilateral transmission models assume a static asymmetry of power between parent and child; in transactional models, there is an interdependent asymmetry. In addition, instead of positing a direct cause–effect link, transactional models presume circular causality: causes and effects are recursive and indeterminate (in Yeats's apropos phrase, it is impossible to separate the dancer from the dance). Causality is not within the parent or the child per se, but within the exchange between them. Beyond individual parent–child exchanges, children's beliefs and impressions undergo many "secondary adjustments" through "third-party discussions" that are common in the "underworld of everyday family life" (Kuczynski, 2003, p. 10). Unfortunately, the study of this complicated and messy "underworld" has been ignored in research that has emphasized the priority of parents as socializing agents.

To illustrate these issues, imagine a conversation between a child, parents, and a sibling. A young girl initiates it with a question: "Dad, will God be mad that I didn't say my prayers last night?" The father says that God cares a lot about hearing from children and that she has to try to remember to pray. With a frown, the daughter brings the father's take on the issue to the mother and says, "Mom, Dad said God's really mad at me," at which point the mother notes her daughter's worry and says, "Well, I'm sure God won't be *too* mad. What do *you* think?" The child says she is pretty sure that God will forgive her but wants her to pray tonight, and the girl then presses the mother for comment, whereupon the mother says, "I'm sure you're right, honey—God forgives all of us." The girl brings her position and the mother's view back to the father, and the discussion dwindles but continues with multiple directions of information flow. That evening in the children's room, the girl deliberates with her sibling about what the mother and father said. The siblings together then add their own interpretations of the matter, including the observation that Dad usually gets more angry than Mom when the kids forget to do things. The girl who initiated the discussion now has a houseful of ideas about God's reaction to her not saying her prayers. Within all of these subsequent exchanges the girl is affecting others, and she can retain, revise, or reject her earlier position to arrive at her "final" understanding of the matter. The girl may continue to reflect privately about the issue and modify her views through her own thinking. Later that week the family may have another conversation about saying prayers, and the girl's latest iteration will again be examined and modified. And on and on.

In light of this scenario, which is probably rather common, it is surprising that scientists ever concocted the idea of a simple unidirectional transmission of religion. The plea here is that socialization researchers embrace a bidirectional, reciprocal, and transactional model as an antidote to earlier transmission models. A bidirectional model will more accurately reveal what actually occurs in families and illuminate how children influence their parents' religious growth. Sadly, psychologists know virtually nothing about child → parent influence that is an inherent aspect of transactional models. It is possible (see Boyatzis, 2004) that some families may have distinct parent-as-mentor, child-as-apprentice roles; in other families, the two may be teacher and student to the other indistinguishably. Finally, in some families children may be viewed as "spiritual savants" who inspire parents' spiritual growth. Some cultures (e.g., the Beng of West Africa or the Warlpiri of north-central Australia), attribute to children "spiritual emissary" status as having recently passed through a liminal veil from a realm of ancestral spirits to the living (see DeLoache & Gottlieb, 2000). These examples are raised to underscore the need to move beyond the ubiquitous model of parents' unilateral transmission to passive children.

FUTURE DIRECTIONS IN THE STUDY
OF RELIGIOUS AND SPIRITUAL DEVELOPMENT

In their recent review, Emmons and Paloutzian (2003, p. 395) argued that any "single disciplinary approach is incapable of yielding comprehensive knowledge of phenomena as complex and multifaceted as spirituality." The remedy, they suggest, is a "multilevel interdisciplinary paradigm" that calls for data at multiple levels of analysis within multiple subdisciplines of psychology, and even beyond psychology. In addition to the call for a more sophisticated analysis of family processes, I suggest new directions for the field.

Future Direction 1: Refinements in Research Design and Methodology

Researchers have long called for more rigorous and longitudinal designs to explore the trajectories of RSD over time (see Boyatzis & Newman, 2004; Hood & Belzen, Chapter 4, this volume, on methodology). At the least, researchers could employ between-group comparisons and pretest–posttest studies. For example, Thananart, Tori, and Emavardhana (2000) used a pretest–posttest design with adolescents in Thailand who completed a 6-week Buddhist monastic training program. These youth were compared to a matched control group of adolescents on a variety of religiosity and outcome measures. Data were also collected from parents of the youth in both groups. Stonehouse (2001) conducted a between-group posttest study at a Christian church with children enrolled in a popular religious education curriculum called Godly Play (Berryman, 1991). These children were compared to control children from the same church not in Godly Play classes; both groups were similar on religious and family measures and all children came from highly religious families. Children drew pictures of religious figures and biblical events and discussed their art with an interviewer, discussed Bible stories, and completed a semistructured interview about their religious experiences and sense of God. A content analysis of the children's art and comments revealed that Godly Play children scored higher than control children on most variables, including meaningful insights, curiosity about religion (e.g., utterances such as "I wonder about . . . "), and expression of pleasure while discussing God. As in these two studies, future research should strive for multiple measures of different groups of subjects on different variables at different points in time.

Need for Multiple Measures

Multiple measures reveal different insights into the same topic. For example, Barrett and Keil (1996) found that subjects' God concepts were somewhat different if the measure was a Likert scale of God attributes or a response to a vignette about God. Boyatzis and Janicki (2003) found that a quantitative survey and a qualitative diary measure yielded slightly different pictures of parent–child communication about religion. Across two data collection periods, the survey showed strong stability but the diary lower stability. Surveys might tap parents' *global* schemas about family communication whereas the diaries capture *actual* conversations (that may reveal more variability over time). The important point is not that the different measures fail to converge on a single conclusion but that different measures yield different impressions of the same phenomenon. The use of multiple measures of any single variable will thus provide a more comprehensive picture of the behavior.

Interviews

Interview measures are common with children. Researchers might assess children's expressive vocabulary to test its correlation with the sophistication of children's descriptions of spiritual phenomena. Researchers could also consider demand characteristics of rapport (on this matter, see Coles, 1990; Heller, 1986, Chap. 2). When discussing God with an unfamiliar adult, children may reveal less detail and depth than with a parent, a teacher from church, or researchers who spend extensive time with them and treat them as conversation partners rather than interview subjects (see Coles, 1990; Hay & Nye, 1998).

Drawing Tasks

Children's drawings of God and heaven are commonly used windows into children's feelings and thoughts, but researchers often see through the glass dimly. First, asking a child to draw God increases the odds for an anthropomorphized deity (Barrett, 1998; Hyde, 1990). Second, the analysis of drawings must proceed carefully. As Hood (2003) argued, if a child draws God with large hands, the drawing *may* reflect an anthropomorphized

God—but the large hands may instead serve to express the child's belief that God has a unique power to create. One child drew diamonds on the roads of heaven; this may not be the child's actual image of heaven but could be her symbolic way to express that it is a beautiful place. Third, researchers ought not to presume that drawings capture a child's image of God in a way that is either veridical or static. Art is a process as well as a product, and the act of drawing may give rise to new insights in children (see Gunther-Heimbrock, 1999). Finally, task characteristics may affect drawings; when asked to draw God first and a person second, children's drawings of God seemed more abstract and the person pictures included more religious imagery (Pitts, 1976).

Future Direction 2: Virtue Development

The study of virtue is "making a comeback in psychology" (Emmons & Paloutzian, 2003, p. 386). The ascendance of positive psychology has given character traits such as forgiveness and gratitude new empirical attention. There is a rich history of developmental research on prosocial behavior, altruism, empathy, and even donating behavior (see Eisenberg & Fabes, 1998). Although virtues and their manifestations are explicitly encouraged in major religions, psychologists have operationalized these qualities through a secular, not a religious, lens.

Wise people have long debated the origins of virtue (e.g., see Plato's dialogue *The Meno*). What is the developmental trajectory of gratitude, forgiveness, and humility? When do such qualities first appear? What would constitute valid, age-appropriate measures of virtues? Parents and communities probably use different socialization and induction mechanisms to cultivate these behaviors in children, and we need to learn how religion has a hand in these processes. For example, Jewish and Christian traditions espouse different doctrines about forgiveness. Do these doctrinal differences show up in children's understanding and acts of forgiveness? If so, at what age, and to what personal and social benefits?

Within the family, are children more prosocial—or in religious terms, more kind, merciful, and charitable—if their parents frame and motivate behavior within religious language and imperatives? That is, it would be worthwhile to learn how children's levels of kindness, empathy, and charity are related to their parents' secular endorsements of such actions (say, "Be nice") versus religious motivations (say, "Love your neighbor as yourself" or "God tells us to feed the hungry and clothe the naked"). What parenting styles are associated with children's virtues? Do families possess a measurable "climate" of forgiveness or gratitude or humility that affects the child's capacity to enact such traits? In Heller's (1986) study, Roman Catholic children discussed forgiveness more than did Jewish, Baptist, and Hindu children; Heller suggested that forgiveness is central in Catholic doctrine and the Catholic family milieu. Recent data indicate links between parents' and children's forgiveness. Elementary-school children's understanding of forgiveness in an interview measure was positively predicted by mothers' forgiveness but negatively by fathers' forgiveness (Denham, Neal, & Bassett, 2004; Getman, Bassett, & Denham, 2004). Another study from the Denham team (Wyatt, Bassett, & Denham, 2004) found that children's scores on an interview measure they designed, the Child Forgiveness Inventory, were related positively to existential orientation scores in their mothers but negatively to such scores in their fathers. Future research on various aspects of parents' religiosity—worship attendance, praying, theological conservatism vs. liberalism, and so on—will reveal which predict virtues in children. Clearly, the family is a rich locus of study for the complex cultivation of virtues.

Children's virtues may be linked to peer relations. A recent study (Pickering & Wilson, 2004) found that the more first-graders are viewed as forgiving, the more popular and less aggressive their peers rated them and the more their teachers described them as having fewer social problems and as sharing with and helping others more. These two research groups—Denham and colleagues at George Mason University, and Wilson and Pickering at Seattle Pacific University—are conducting crucial work on the development and consequences of forgiveness in children, and other scholars should emulate their use of multiple measures and multiple groups of informants in the study of other virtues in childhood.

Future Direction 3: Religious Experience and Religion/Spirituality in Children's Lives

The field of RSD is quiet, too quiet, on children's religious and spiritual *experience*. Others have noted this: "That there is a paucity of rigorous developmentally focused studies of religious experience and mysticism is almost an understatement" (Spilka & McIntosh, 1997, p. 233). Emmons and Paloutzian (2003) charged that "experience is the most ignored dimension of spirituality" (p. 386). I submit this is not just a case of "yet another neglected topic" but is in fact a serious problem, and here's why: the core of spirituality is a sense of self-transcendence and the core of religion is seeking or being in relationship with the sacred. Thus, the crux of spirituality and religion is *experience*, as we were taught long ago (James, 1902/1982).

Do children experience and feel God? Carl Johnson (2000) suggested that in their frequent "why" questions, "young children are already oriented to the existence of 'something more' beyond the given world" (p. 208). Almost half a sample of Finnish children claimed to feel God's nearness "very often" (Tamminen, 1991). In Hardy's database of adults' retrospective accounts of such experiences, 15% occurred in childhood (Robinson, 1983). Retrospective studies have converged on several themes (Farmer, 1992; Robinson, 1983): One, children's experiences were often charged with joy, wonder, awe, and a sense of connectedness to something greater than the self. Two, many adults could recall their childhood experiences decades later and were still affected by them (e.g., an enhanced compassion or sensitivity).

Qualitative and ethnographic work provide ample instances of children's religious experiences, from hearing God's voice (Coles, 1990) to reacting to their First Communion (Bales, 2000) to seeing apparitions of the Virgin Mary (Anderson, 1998). Hay and Nye (1998) share a 6-year-old's description of his experience: " . . . in the night and I saw this bishopy kind of alien. I said, 'Who are you?' And he said, 'I am the Holy Spirit.' I did think he was the Holy Spirit" (p. 102). How do scholars of RSD understand children's visions of the Virgin Mary or this boy's report of a "bishopy kind of alien"?

On an emotional and experiential level, children may grasp the inherent relationality at the core of spirituality, even if this sense or awareness surpasses their ability to verbalize such a consciousness. It is a challenge to find theoretical and methodological means to understand the phenomenological reality and significance *to the child* of the religious or spiritual experience. Some experiences (for children and adults) may be amenable to linguistic expression; some will surpass linguistic capabilities. In either case, verbal measures create the risk of studying not children's experience but the language they use to describe it (see Boyatzis, 2001).

For insight into the interplay between language and experience, a most valuable work is Robert Coles's (1990) *The Spiritual Life of Children*. Coles depicts children's spiritual struggle and search for transcendent meaning by sharing many rich excerpts from interviews with school-age children from different religious backgrounds and cultures. The children's remarks are always informative and often profound. Coles's method is rather straightforward: he talks with children—at length, on many occasions, in various locations comfortable to the children. He also asks children to draw pictures and tell him about them. This time-consuming, personal approach may not work for all researchers, but his qualitative and ethnographic method demonstrates, among other things, a way to cultivate an authenticity and rapport that may be crucial to reveal the deeper functions of religion in children's lives.

Another benefit of a qualitative approach is its illumination of individual differences. Consider the idea that children have their own "spiritual signatures," a personalized expression of their experience of relational consciousness (Hay & Nye, 1998). Also, given the intangibility of transcendent entities, it is not surprising that skepticism is a personal quality that varies between children (Harris, 2000b). And in personality psychology, the trait of "spiritual transcendence" has begun receiving attention (Emmons & Paloutzian, 2003). How do these constructs of spiritual signature, skepticism, and spiritual transcendence manifest themselves in children's lives? How would we measure them? Beyond these questions, we should also address religious experience within the context of organized religion.

Some religions are sacramental and all have rituals. Public rituals and sacraments are essential mechanisms within organized religion to provide children the transcendent experiences that are at the core of religion and spirituality: connectedness to the sacred transcendent, and connectedness to people and community around the child. Important sacraments for children in many traditions include baptism, first communion, confirmation, confession, bar or bat mitzvah, and so on. Psychologists might want to learn how children understand and experience them. Organized religions prioritize these events, but do *children* feel transformed by them? Qualitative and ethnographic work is needed. How large is the discrepancy between formal doctrine and catechesis in organized religions and what children actually believe and understand? An interesting ethnographic study (Bales, 2000) on Catholics' first communion revealed that, in contrast to clergy and parental perceptions about this paramount rite, many children receiving their first communion focused not on sacred but more mundane matters—such as the taste and feel of the communion wafer and wine.

We must learn more of how children experience and understand the tenets of many organized religions: grace and redemption, sin and salvation, the distinction between faith and good works, reincarnation, the Trinity, the power of divine figures to heal and punish, and so on. Questions abound: How do Jewish children make sense of the mourning ritual of sitting shiva? What do Roman Catholic children feel and think when they are praying to a saint or statue of the Virgin Mary? How do Hindu youth make sense of their polytheistic tradition (especially if they live in a monotheistic culture)? How are Muslim children transformed by the hajj to Mecca? These are important theological matters. Psychologists who take the bold step into studying them would begin to inquire about what world religions actually care deeply about.

Future Direction 4: Cognition Is Not Everything

The paradigm of cognitive developmentalism has dominated the study of children's RSD (e.g., Hyde, 1990; Spilka, Hood, Hunsberger, & Gorsuch, 2003), with a focus on cognitive processes within different stages. Young children have traditionally been defined by their cognitive limitations, a presumption that has engendered problems for scholars trying to understand young children's spiritual experience or insight. The "obsession with stages" has serious consequences, among them impeding our understanding of the gradualness and the "complexity and uniqueness of individual religious development" (Spilka et al., 2003, p. 85).

Recently, psychologists of religion have called for the field to "escape from the confines of the Piagetian approach . . . which has become stale" (Spilka et al., 2003, pp. 104–105). It is necessary to emphasize to nondevelopmentalists that cognitive-developmentalists have indeed moved beyond Piaget. As one scholar put it, "this battle has since been won" (Johnson, 1997, p. 1024). Nevertheless, despite such advances, for many developmentalists it remains difficult to conceptualize RSD in anything other than a cognitive framework. Developmentalists are here urged to consider what RSD would look like through *non*-cognitive-developmental lenses.

Religious and Spiritual Development in Context

Fortunately, cognitive-developmentalists have called recently for more attention to culture and religion (e.g., Boyer & Walker, 2000; Taylor & Carlson, 2000; Woolley, 2000). Certainly religions themselves emphasize that religious and spiritual growth comes through *being in community* with others. Such growth is "not intelligible apart from the communal context and faith tradition in which people are formed" (Johnson, 1989, p. 19). However, developmental theories were surely not conceived with religions in mind (Estep, 2002). But RSD is, on one level, social and collective. As Scarlett and Perriello (1991) asserted in their analysis of prayer concepts, "mature prayer develops out of years of social interaction allowing individuals to understand what it means to be a self in intimate dialogue with another" (p. 67).

A sociocultural Vygtoskyan (1978) approach would foster a contextualized view of RSD (Estep, 2002), emphasizing its interpersonal processes of scaffolding and guided participation by adults that help children progress to higher levels (Rogoff, 1990). Through such lenses, we would consider how religious knowledge and behavior is *inter*personal before *intra*personal for the child. In stark contrast to a Piagetian cognitive-developmentalism and its offspring, this theory would require us to recognize the sociocultural embeddedness of religious and spiritual growth and to study interpersonal and cultural mediators that develop a relational consciousness. A social ecology model (Bronfenbrenner, 1979) would conceptualize RSD as occurring within and between multiple contexts. This model would assess different microsystems that have immediate and proximal impact (e.g., family, church, peer group, school) and the interactions (or mesosystems) between them. A recent study on adolescents illustrates the value of studying RSD in such a model. U.S. youth who live in high-poverty areas are more likely to stay on track academically if they are also high in church attendance, whereas those youth in the same high-poverty areas who are low in church attendance are likely to fall behind academically (Regnerus & Elder, 2003). Surrounding the many micro- and mesosystems are the macrosystem of cultural ideologies, so a contextualized approach must incorporate macrolevel culture.

Consider the Fulani, a nomadic people in Western Africa (M. Johnson, 2000). Due to their belief that many spirits exist in their midst, Fulani parents must protect their babies from evil spirits who may capture their babies' souls. To make their babies unattractive to these spirits, parents give their babies unappealing names, openly insult them, and even roll their babies in cow dung. When we study other cultures, we recognize—sometimes with a shock—that children are immersed in social communities with pervasive religious beliefs, sometimes subtle and sometimes conspicuous, which permeate children's experience in profound ways.

CONCLUSION: GOING BEYOND OURSELVES

The time has come for researchers to "diversify their efforts" (Spilka et al., 2003, p. 104) and transcend our own boundaries to explore other fields for new and diverse insights, paradigms, and methods. These fields could include theological accounts of development (Cavalletti, 1983; Loder, 1998; Westerhoff, 2000), the views of children within different religious traditions (Bunge, 2001), faith development theories (Fowler, 1981), childhood autobiographies (Angelou, 1969), and philosophers' views of childhood (Matthews, 1980). Recognizing the inherent limitations of narrow theoretical vantages, Reich (1993) has suggested that a more comprehensive theory would address internal and external influences, children's psychical and meaning-making efforts, social contexts, emotions, and universal versus individual qualities. Much work is required to build such rich and integrative theories, but let us begin. The point is not that any one approach will serve as the ideal paradigm for RSD but that psychologists can widen their apertures on the phenomena we study. Intellectual boldness on our part will entail moving toward a multilevel and multidisciplinary paradigm. The complexity and importance of children's religious and spiritual development warrant such a comprehensive and eclectic epistemological approach.

REFERENCES

Anderson, E. (1998). Changing devotional paradigms and their impact upon nineteenth-century Marian apparitions: The case of La Salette. *Union Seminary Quarterly Review, 52,* 85–122.

Angelou, M. (1969). *I know why the caged bird sings.* New York: Bantam.

Bales, S. R. (2000, November). *The sensual and the local: An ethnographic study of children's interpretations of First Communion.* Paper presented at the annual meeting of the American Academy of Religion/Society of Biblical Literature, Nashville, TN.

Bao, W-N., L., Whitbeck, D. H., Hoyt, D., & Conger, R. C. (1999). Perceived parental acceptance as a moderator of religious transmission among adolescent boys and girls. *Journal of Marriage and the Family, 61,* 362–374.

Barrett, J. L. (1998). Cognitive constraints on Hindu concepts of the divine. *Journal for the Scientific Study of Religion, 37,* 608–619.

Barrett, J. L., & Keil, F. C. (1996). Anthropomorphism and God concepts: Conceptualizing a nonnatural entity. *Cognitive Psychology, 31,* 219–247.

Barrett, J. L., & Richert, R. A. (2003). Anthropomorphism or preparedness?: Exploring children's God concepts. *Review of Religious Research, 44,* 300–312.

Benson, P. L. (2004). Emerging themes in research on adolescent spiritual and religious development. *Applied Developmental Science, 8,* 47–50.

Benson, P. L., Roehlkepartain, E. C., & Rude, S. P. (2003). Spiritual development in childhood and adolescence: Toward a field of inquiry. *Applied Developmental Science, 7,* 205–213.

Berryman, J. (1991). *Godly Play: A way of religious education.* San Francisco: Harper.

Boyatzis, C. J. (1997, April). *Body and soul: Children's understanding of a physical-spiritual distinc-*

tion. Poster presented to the biennial meeting of the Society for Research in Child Development, Washington, DC.

Boyatzis, C. J. (2001). A critique of models of religious experience. *The International Journal for the Psychology of Religion, 11*, 247–258.

Boyatzis, C. J. (2003a). Religious and spiritual development: An introduction. *Review of Religious Research, 44*, 213–219.

Boyatzis, C. J. (Ed.). (2003b). Religious and spiritual development [Special issue]. *Review of Religious Research, 44*(3).

Boyatzis, C. J. (2004). The co-construction of spiritual meaning in parent–child communication. In D. Ratcliff (Ed.), *Children's spirituality: Christian perspectives, research, and applications* (pp. 182–200). Eugene, OR: Cascade Books.

Boyatzis, C. J., & Janicki, D. (2003). Parent–child communication about religion: Survey and diary data on unilateral transmission and bi-directional reciprocity styles. *Review of Religious Research, 44*, 252–270.

Boyatzis, C. J., & Newman, B. T. (2004). How shall we study children's spirituality? In D. Ratcliff (Ed.), *Children's spirituality: Christian perspectives, research, and practices* (pp. 166–181). Eugene, OR: Cascade Books.

Boyer, P. (1994). *The naturalness of religious ideas: A cognitive theory of religion*. Berkeley: University of California Press.

Boyer, P., & Walker, S. (2000). Intuitive ontology and cultural input in the acquisition of religious concepts. In K. S. Rosengren, C. N. Johnson, & P. L. Harris (Eds.), *Imagining the impossible: Magical, scientific, and religious thinking in children* (pp. 130–156). Cambridge, UK: Cambridge University Press.

Bronfenbrenner, U. (1979). *The ecology of human development*. Cambridge, MA: Harvard University Press.

Bunge, M. J. (Ed.). (2001). *The child in Christian thought*. Grand Rapids, MI: Eerdmans.

Carey, S. (1985). *Conceptual change in childhood*. Cambridge, MA: MIT Press.

Cavalletti, S. (1983). *The religious potential of the child*. New York: Paulist Press.

Clark, C. D. (1995). *Flights of fancy, leaps of faith: Children's myths in contemporary America*. Chicago: University of Chicago Press.

Coles, R. (1990). *The spiritual life of children*. Boston: Houghton Mifflin.

DeLoache, J., & Gottlieb, A. (Eds.). (2000). *A world of babies: Imagined childcare guides for seven societies*. Cambridge, UK: Cambridge University Press.

Denham, S. A., Neal, K., & Bassett, H. H. (2004, April). "You hurt my feelings pretty bad": Parents' and children's emotions as contributors to the development of forgiveness. In S. Denham (Chair), *Children's forgiving in behavior, cognition, and affect*. Symposium conducted at the biennial meeting of the Conference on Human Development, Washington, DC.

Dowling, E., & Scarlett, W. G. (Eds.). (in press). *Encyclopedia of spiritual development in childhood and adolescence*. Thousand Oaks, CA: Sage.

Eisenberg, N., & Fabes, R. A. (1998). Prosocial development. In W. Damon (Series Ed.), N. Eisenberg (Vol. Ed.), *Handbook of child psychology* (5th ed.): *Vol. 3. Social, emotional, and personality development* (pp. 701–778). New York: Wiley.

Elkind, D. (1961). The child's conception of his religious denomination: I. The Jewish child. *Journal of Genetic Psychology, 99*, 209–225.

Elkind, D. (1963). The child's conception of his religious denomination: III. The Protestant child. *Journal of Genetic Psychology, 103*, 291–304.

Elkind, D. (1970). The origins of religion in the child. *Review of Religious Research, 12*, 35–42.

Emmons, R. A., & Paloutzian, R. F. (2003). The psychology of religion. *Annual Review of Psychology, 54*, 377–402.

Estep, J. R., Jr. (2002). Spiritual formation as social: Toward a Vygotskyan developmental perspective. *Religious Education, 97*, 141–164.

Evans, E. M. (2000). Beyond Scopes: Why creationism is here to stay. In K. S. Rosengren, C. N. Johnson, & P. L. Harris (Eds.), *Imagining the impossible: Magical, scientific, and religious thinking in children* (pp. 305–333). New York: Cambridge University Press.

Evans, E. M. (2001). Cognitive and contextual factors in the emergence of diverse belief systems: Creation versus evolution. *Cognitive Psychology, 42,* 217–266.

Farmer, L. J. (1992). Religious experience in childhood: A study of adult perspectives on early spiritual awareness. *Religious Education, 87,* 259–268.

Fowler, J. (1981). *Stages of faith: The psychology of human development and the quest for meaning.* New York: HarperCollins.

Gallup, G., & Bezilla, R. (1992). *The religious life of young Americans: A compendium of surveys on the spiritual beliefs and practices of teenagers and young adults.* Princeton, NJ: G. H. Gallup International Institute.

Getman, M., Bassett, H. H., & Denham, S. A. (2004, April). Marital conflict and child forgiveness: How marital conflict may affect the forgiveness strategies of children. In S. Denham (Chair), *Children's forgiving in behavior, cognition, and affect.* Symposium conducted at the biennial meeting of the Conference on Human Development, Washington, DC.

Goldman, R. G. (1964). *Religious thinking from childhood to adolescence.* London: Routledge & Kegan Paul.

Gunther-Heimbrock, H. (1999). Images and pictures of God: The development of creative seeing. *International Journal of Children's Spirituality, 4,* 51–60.

Harms, E. (1944). The development of religious experience in children. *American Journal of Sociology, 50,* 112–122.

Harris, P. L. (2000a). On not falling down to earth: Children's metaphysical questions. In K. S. Rosengren, C. N. Johnson, & P. L. Harris (Eds.), *Imagining the impossible: Magical, scientific, and religious thinking in children* (pp. 157–178). Cambridge, UK: Cambridge University Press.

Harris, P. L. (2000b). *The work of the imagination.* Malden, MA: Blackwell.

Hay, D., & Nye, R. (1998). *The spirit in the child.* London: Fount.

Heller, D. (1986). *The children's God.* Chicago: University of Chicago Press.

Hood, D. K. (2003, June). *Six children seeking God: Exploring childhood spiritual development in context.* Paper presented at the meeting of the Children's Spirituality Conference on Christian Perspectives, River Forest, IL.

Hui, C. H., & Chou, K. L. (1991). Halalfogalom es kulturalis orientacio [Cultural orientation and the concept of death]. *Magyar Pszichologiai Szemle, 47,* 381–392.

Hyde, K. E. (1990). *Religion in childhood and adolescence.* Birmingham, AL: Religious Education Press.

James, W. (1982). *The varieties of religious experience.* New York: Penguin Books. (Original work published 1902)

Johnson, C. N. (1997). Crazy children, fantastical theories, and the many uses of metaphysics. *Child Development, 68,* 1024–1026.

Johnson, C. N. (2000). Putting different things together: The development of metaphysical thinking. In K. S. Rosengren, C. N. Johnson, & P. L. Harris (Eds.), *Imagining the impossible: Magical, scientific, and religious thinking in children* (pp. 179–211). Cambridge, UK: Cambridge University Press.

Johnson, M. C. (2000). The view from the Wuro: A guide to child rearing for Fulani parents. In J. DeLoache & A. Gottlieb (Eds.), *A world of babies: Imagined childcare guides for seven societies* (pp. 171–198). Cambridge, UK: Cambridge University Press.

Johnson, S. (1989). *Christian spiritual formation.* Nashville, TN: Abingdon.

King, P. E., & Boyatzis, C. J. (2004). Exploring adolescent religious and spiritual development: Current and future theoretical and empirical perspectives. *Applied Developmental Science, 8,* 2–6.

Kuczynski, L. (2003). Beyond bidirectionality: Bilateral conceptual frameworks for understanding dynamics in parent–child relations. In L. Kuczynski (Ed.), *Handbook of dynamics in parent–child relations* (pp. 3–24). Thousand Oaks, CA: Sage.

Lawrence, P. J. (1965). Children's thinking about religion: A study of concrete operational thinking. *Religious Education, 60,* 111–116.

Lerner, R. M., Dowling, E. M., & Anderson, P. M. (2003). Positive youth development: Thriving as the basis of personhood and civil society. *Applied Developmental Science, 7,* 171–179.

Loder, J. E. (1998). *The logic of the spirit: Human development in theological perspective.* San Francisco: Jossey-Bass.

Long, D., Elkind, D., & Spilka, B. (1967). The child's conception of prayer. *Journal for the Scientific Study of Religion, 6,* 101–109.

Mahoney, A., Pargament, K. I., Murray-Swank, A., & Murray-Swank, N. (2003). Religion and the sanctification of family relationships. *Review of Religious Research, 44,* 220–236.

Mahoney, A., Pargament, K. I., Swank, A., & Tarakeshwar, N. (2001). Religion in the home in the 1980s and 90s: A meta-analytic review and conceptual analysis of religion. *Journal of Family Psychology, 15,* 559–596.

Matthews, G. (1980). *Philosophy and the young child.* Cambridge, MA: Harvard University Press.

Okagaki, L., & Bevis, C. (1999). Transmission of religious values: Relations between parents and daughters' beliefs. *Journal of Genetic Psychology, 160,* 303–318.

Ozorak, E. W. (1989). Social and cognitive influences on the development of religious beliefs and commitment in adolescence. *Journal for the Scientific Study of Religion, 28,* 448–463.

Pargament, K. I. (1999). The psychology of religion *and* spirituality?: Yes and no. *The International Journal for the Psychology of Religion, 9,* 3–16.

Pendleton, S. M., Cavalli, K. S., Pargament, K. I., & Nasr, S. Z. (2002). Religious/spiritual coping in childhood cystic fibrosis: A qualitative study. *Pediatrics, 109.* Retrieved June 25, 2003, from www.pediatrics.org/cgi/content/full/109/1/e8.

Pickering, S. R., & Wilson, B. J. (2004, April). Forgiveness in first grade children: Links with social preference, aggression, social problems, and reciprocal friendships. In S. Denham (Chair), *Children's forgiving in behavior, cognition, and affect.* Symposium conducted at the biennial meeting of the Conference on Human Development, Washington, DC.

Pitts, V. P. (1976). Drawing the invisible: Children's conceptualization of God. *Character Potential, 8,* 12–24.

Prentice, N. M., & Gordon, D. (1986). Santa Claus and the Tooth Fairy for the Jewish child and parent. *Journal of Genetic Psychology, 148,* 139–151.

Prentice, N. M., Manosevitz, M., & Hubbs, L. (1978). Imaginary figures of early childhood: Santa Claus, Easter Bunny, and the Tooth Fairy. *American Journal of Orthopsychiatry, 48,* 618–628.

Regnerus, M. D., & Elder, G. H., Jr. (2003). Staying on track in school: Religious influences in high- and low-risk settings. *Journal for the Scientific Study of Religion, 42,* 633–649.

Reich, K. H. (1993). Cognitive-developmental approaches to religiousness: Which version for which purpose? *The International Journal for the Psychology of Religion, 3,* 145–171.

Reimer, K. S., & Furrow, J. L. (2001). A qualitative exploration of relational consciousness in Christian children. *International Journal of Children's Spirituality, 6,* 7–23.

Rizzuto, A-M. (1979). *The birth of the living God: A psychoanalytic study.* Chicago: University of Chicago Press.

Robinson, E. (1983). *The original vision: A study of the religious experience of childhood.* New York: Seabury Press.

Roehlkepartain, E. C., King, P. E., Wagener, L. M., & Benson, P. L. (Eds.). (2005). *Handbook of religious and spiritual development in childhood and adolescence.* Thousand Oaks, CA: Sage.

Rogoff, B. (1990). *Apprenticeship in thinking.* New York: Oxford University Press.

Rosengren, K. S., Johnson, C. N., & Harris, P. L. (Eds.). (2000). *Imagining the impossible: Magical, scientific, and religious thinking in children.* Cambridge, UK: Cambridge University Press.

Rosengren, K. S., Kalish, C. W., Hickling, A. K., & Gelman, S. A. (1994). Exploring the relation between preschool children's magical beliefs and causal thinking. *British Journal of Developmental Psychology, 12,* 69–82.

Savina, E. A. (1995). The peculiarities of 5- to -10-year-old children's views on a soul. *Voprosy Psychologii, 3*, 21–27.

Scarlett, W. G., & Perriello, L. (1991). The development of prayer in adolescence. In F. Oser & W. G. Scarlett (Eds.), *New directions for child development: No. 52. Religious development in childhood and adolescence* (pp. 63–76). San Francisco: Jossey-Bass.

Silberman, I. (2003). Spiritual modeling: The teaching of meaning systems. *The International Journal for the Psychology of Religion, 13*(3), 175–195.

Spilka, B., Hood, R. W., Jr., Hunsberger, B., & Gorsuch, R. (2003). *The psychology of religion: An empirical approach* (3rd ed.). New York: Guilford Press.

Spilka, B., & McIntosh, D. N. (Eds.). (1997). *The psychology of religion.* Boulder, CO: Westview Press.

Stonehouse, C. (2001) Knowing God in childhood: A study of Godly Play and the spirituality of children. *Christian Education Journal, 5*(2), 27–45.

Strommen, M. P., & Hardel, R. A. (2000). *Passing on the faith: A radical new model for youth and family ministry.* Winona, MN: Saint Mary's Press.

Subbotsky, E. (1993). *Foundations of the mind: Children's understanding of reality.* Cambridge, MA: Harvard University Press.

Tamminen, K. (1991). *Religious development in childhood and youth.* Helsinki, Finland: Suomalainen Tiedeakatemia.

Tamminen, K., Vianello, R., Jaspard, J.-M., & Ratcliff, D. (1988). The religious concepts of preschoolers. In D. Ratcliff (Ed.), *Handbook of preschool religious education* (pp. 59–81). Birmingham, AL: Religious Education Press.

Taylor, M., & Carlson, S. (2000). The influence of religious beliefs on parental attitudes about children's fantasy behavior. In K. S. Rosengren, C. N. Johnson, & P. L. Harris (Eds.), *Imagining the impossible: Magical, scientific, and religious thinking in children* (pp. 247–268). Cambridge, UK: Cambridge University Press.

Thananart, M., Tori, C. D., & Emavardhana, T. (2000). A longitudinal study of psychosocial changes among Thai adolescents participating in a Buddhist ordination program for novices. *Adolescence, 35*, 285–293.

Vergote, A., & Tamayo, A. (1981). *The parental figures and the representation of God: A psychological and cross-cultural study.* New York: Mouton.

Vygotsky, L. S. (1978). *Mind in society.* Cambridge, MA: Harvard University Press.

Walker, L. J., & Taylor, J. H. (1991). Family interaction and the development of moral reasoning. *Child Development, 62*, 264–283.

Westerhoff, J. W., III. (2000). *Will our children have faith?* (Rev. ed.). Toronto: Anglican Book Centre.

Woolley, J. D. (1997). Thinking about fantasy: Are children fundamentally different thinkers and believers from adults? *Child Development, 68*, 991–1011.

Woolley, J. D. (2000). The development of beliefs about direct mental–physical causality in imagination, magic, and religion. In K. S. Rosengren, C. N. Johnson, & P. L. Harris (Eds.), *Imagining the impossible: Magical, scientific, and religious thinking in children* (pp. 99–129). Cambridge, UK: Cambridge University Press.

Wuthnow, R. (1999). *Growing up religious: Christians and Jews and their journeys of faith.* Boston: Beacon Press.

Wyatt, T. M., Bassett, H. H., & Denham, S. A. (2004, April). Parental religiosity and its influence on the emergence of forgiveness in childhood. In S. Denham (Chair), *Children's forgiving in behavior, cognition, and affect.* Symposium conducted at the biennial meeting of the Conference on Human Development, Washington, DC.

8

Religious Development from Adolescence to Middle Adulthood

MICHAEL R. LEVENSON
CAROLYN M. ALDWIN
MICHELLE D'MELLO

There is little doubt that religion and spirituality play an important role in development across the lifespan. However, more is known about the importance of religion for adaptation in later life than in early life (see McFadden, Chapter 9, this volume). While there has been some research on religious development in children, these topics have received far less attention than they deserve (see Boyatzis, Chapter 7, this volume). Even less work, however, has been conducted on religion and development in early adulthood (specifically its role in the transition from adolescence to young adulthood). Adolescence is a period of neurological, cognitive, and emotional maturation, and, according to Erikson (1950), is the primary stage for the developmental challenge of identity formation. It is surprising that more attention has not been paid to the development of a religious identity in young adulthood.

Nonetheless, the period of transition from adolescence to young adulthood is regarded as especially significant in all cultures. In traditional cultures, this is often accompanied by rites of passage, which are usually embedded in the culture's religion (van Gennep, 1960). In modern cultures, analogous traditions are more likely to be secular (e.g., graduation from high school or college—or even graduate school), but many of the other traditional role markers of adulthood are often accompanied by religious rituals, such as getting married in a church or the baptism of infants.

Young adulthood may be especially salient for the transmission of religious values and mores, as those in their 20s are often involved in the raising of children. The correlation between parents' and children's religious beliefs typically ranges from .4 to .6, and parental influence has a much stronger effect on religious behaviors than on political or other social behaviors (Beit-Hallahmi & Argyle, 1997).

Yet in postmodern cultures such as those of North America and Western Europe, many traditions, including religious ones, are no longer passed largely unaltered from one generation to the next. Some observers have concluded that religion itself is diminishing in influence with each successive generation, which is less religious than the last. However, observation of campus life at U.S. universities leaves little doubt that there has been a resurgence of interest in religion among students (Cherry, DeBerg, & Porterfield, 2001).

The purpose of this chapter is to review the admittedly rather sparse literature on religious development between adolescence and midlife. We attempt to bring some coherence to a seriously fragmented field, and point out particularly noteworthy lacunae in the literature. If adolescence is a window on the future of religious commitment, it is well to begin by looking at the religiousness of adolescents in the present day.

RELIGIOUS INVOLVEMENT AT DIFFERENT STAGES OF THE LIFESPAN

Religiousness in Adolescence

The renewed interest in the exploration of religion in general (Beit-Hallami & Argyle, 1997; Gorsuch, 1988; Paloutzian, 1996) has included some attention to the religious lives of adolescents (Donelson, 1999; Elkind, 1971). Donelson (1999) collated the number of articles devoted to this subject in the prominent journals of adolescence. She notes that from 1995 to 1999, 11 articles on religious topics were published in the *Journal of Youth and Adolescence*, six in *Adolescence*, three in *Genetic Psychology*, one in the *Journal of Research on Adolescence*, and none in the *Journal of Early Adolescence*. Although Donelson interprets these numbers optimistically by noting that the field of adolescence has given considerably more room to religious issues relative to psychology in general, in the absolute, this speaks more to the growing pains of the psychology of religion as a whole. However, in 1999, an entire issue of the *Journal of Adolescence* was devoted to religious development during adolescence, with contributions on a variety of topics, including a historical overview, and articles on prayer and personal development. Nevertheless, knowledge about religion among U.S. adolescents remains quite limited.

Benson and his colleagues (Benson, Donahue, & Erickson, 1989; Benson, Williams, & Johnson, 1987) summarized Gallup poll data, which found that a large majority of 13- to 15-year olds found religion to be important, believed in God, and reported that they were church members. Nearly all (87%) reported that they prayed at least sometimes. However, Benson et al.'s (1989) review found that age was inversely related to religiousness among 10- to 18-year-olds. They concluded that religiousness was quite important to adolescents, although there was a slight decline with age.

In a more recent study, Smith, Denton, Faris, and Regnerus (2002) conducted a secondary data analysis of three data sets: the National Longitudinal Survey of Adolescent Health (Add Health), Monitoring the Future (MTF), and the Survey of Parents and Youth (SPY). Among the things we do know is that 85% of the surveyed 13- to 18-year-olds in the Add Health survey reported religious affiliation of some kind, compared to only 13% who claimed no religious affiliation. Affiliations were predominantly Protestant (44%), with Baptists accounting for 23%. The largest percentage for an individual denomination was Catholic (24%). The other sects, such as Judaism, Buddhism, and Islam, each represented no more than 1% of the sample.

Smith et al.'s (2002) secondary analysis of the MTF data set indicated that there has been a slight shift in religious orientation over a 20-year period between 1976 and 1996. There was been a slight decline in high-school youth claiming religious affiliation and a concomitant 5% increase in those claiming no religious affiliation. Most of this decline was for Lutheran youth (by 10%), with Catholic youth showing a small decrease and Jewish groups enjoying a slight increase.

Survey data attest not only to the salience of formal affiliation in the lives of U.S. youth, but to actual behaviors like frequency of prayer, worship attendance, and youth group participation. The Add Health data show that 80% of U.S. teenagers pray, with 40% praying daily, 22% praying at least once a week, and 9% praying once a month. More than half of the 20% who were categorized as never praying were actually nonaffiliated youth who were never asked the frequency of prayer question. Youth in relatively conservative religions, such as Latter-Day Saints and Pentecostal, prayed more frequently (more than 50% prayed daily) than some other groups such as Catholics, Methodists, and Lutherans.

Regarding the level of involvement in institutional religious activities, almost 40% of eighth to 12th graders in the Add Health Survey attend weekly services. Only 15% report never attending a religious institution. Similar to the statistics on prayer frequency, more conservative groups such as Jehovah's Witness, Holiness, and Pentecostal denominations reported more frequent church attendance (over 60% attend weekly). The MTF data show a slight dip of 8% in weekly church attendance among 12th graders over 2 decades.

Data from the MTF survey show that more than half of the adolescents reported some form of youth group participation, with about 25% having been involved for the 4 years they were in high school. Almost 70% of high-school students affiliated with the Latter-Day Saints attend youth groups. However, analyses of the Add Health data showed that, overall, conservative subgroups with high proportions of African Americans have the highest youth group membership, followed by Protestant religious denominations. Parental religious identity also influenced participation in religious youth groups, such that fundamentalist Protestant and traditional Catholic children in the SPY survey were more likely to be in youth groups. As we shall see, this may have important implications for religious socialization.

Using both the Add Health data and the MTF data, Smith et al. (2002) showed that U.S. adolescent females were more likely than adolescent males to report having a religious affiliation and to be involved in religious activities like attending church. Regarding race differences, African American youth report the highest rates of church attendance across all categories of attendance frequencies. They were also more likely to be Baptist (48%), with more Hispanic youth following Catholicism (56%). The two leading religious denominations for European Americans included Catholicism (23%) and Baptist (20%).

The above data underscore the importance of religion in the lives of modern day U.S. adolescents. Almost 60% of 12th graders surveyed reported that religion was an important part of their lives, emphasizing the need for both comprehensive national-level surveys and representative empirical studies dedicated to understanding religious development in adolescence. Note, however, that Markstrom (1999), in her review of demographic information on religiousness in adolescents, concluded that most have some form of belief, but participate only sporadically. Further, only a small minority really enjoyed their religious participation and thought it would be a major factor in their lives.

Religiousness in Young Adulthood and Midlife

If religion is thriving rather than disappearing, how is religion situated in the lives of postmodern people? Our complex lives are filled with difficult choices, competing demands on time, multiple commitments, relentless busyness, and cosmopolitan cultures that include multiple religious faiths. Coming to adulthood and negotiating the adult world of work, intimacy, childrearing, and social integration is very different today than in earlier times. What implications does all this have for the function of religion in developing into adulthood?

Religion is unique among human institutions in that religions offer explanations of meaning in our lives. Striving to understand the meaning of life reflects *ultimate concern* (Emmons, 1999). An ultimate concern engages all domains of human psychology, including emotion, cognition, and motivation. Research into how people become religious must employ multiple theoretical and methodological approaches that include both socialization and developmental perspectives.

According to Spilka, Hood, Hunsberger, and Gorsuch (2003), demographic data on religiousness and religious activities comparing cohorts are highly inconsistent across studies, with various studies showing increasing religiousness with age, no age differences, and decreasing religiousness. For example, they pulled together data from the General Social Survey from 1999, part of which we graphed here. As shown in Figure 8.1, there appears to be a nonlinear relationship between age and religiosity, such that individuals in their 30s report the highest level of religiousness on all of the items, with the exception of self-ratings of either very or extremely religious, which appear to peak in the 40s. Contrary to the general perception that religiousness increases with age (or that older cohorts are more religious), individuals in their 20s were nearly always higher on these items than were those in later adulthood.

In contrast, unpublished national survey data from a conservative think tank, www.barna.org/FlexPage.aspx?Page=Topic&TopicID=22, found markedly lower religious participation among young adults. They compared four cohorts: "Busters" (born be-

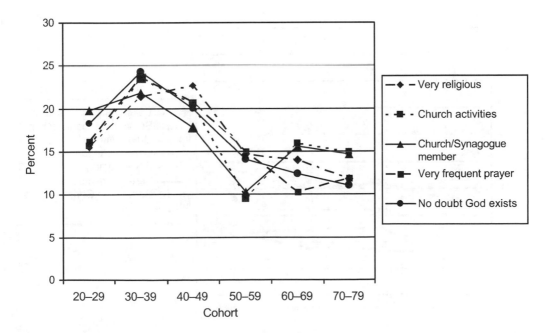

FIGURE 8.1. Cohort differences in religiousness.

tween 1965 and 1983), "Boomers" (born between 1946 and 1964), "Builders" (born between 1927 and 1945) and "Seniors" (born in 1926 and earlier). They found that the "Busters" were half as likely as any other cohort to volunteer time at their church. Only 35% attended church on a given Sunday (as compared to 50% of the "Builders"), and they were least likely to pray to God (76% as compared to 87% of the "Builders"). Although they were lowest in weekly prayer, still 76% prayed weekly. Further, the "Busters" were highest in religious seeking, arguing that young adulthood is a time of religious identity formation. Interestingly, self-ascription as a born-again Christian was highest in the "Boomer" sample (see Figure 8.2). As can be seen, different trends appear across age groups, depending upon the question. Thus, we believe that some of the contradiction in the literature is due to the form of questions asked, including the presence or absence of extreme categories.

An alternative explanation is that there is a growing split in U.S. culture between the highly religious and the highly secular. For example, the UCLA Higher Education Research Institute Annual Survey of American Freshmen (www.gseis.ucla.edu/heri/heri.html) found that, over the past 20 years, freshmen have increasingly reported no religious preference, rising from 8 to 16%. Interestingly, their fathers and mothers over the same period of time have also increased their reporting of no religious preference, although not nearly as dramatically. The same survey also asked the freshmen whether or not they were born-again Christians. The responses were remarkably uniform across 16 years, with approximately 25% reporting that they were born-again Christians. Unfortunately, the survey stopped asking this question after 2001.

One could argue from these data that understanding the formation of religious identity in young adulthood would be a highly salient area of research, given the relatively high levels of religiousness in early adulthood and the fact that at least some measures

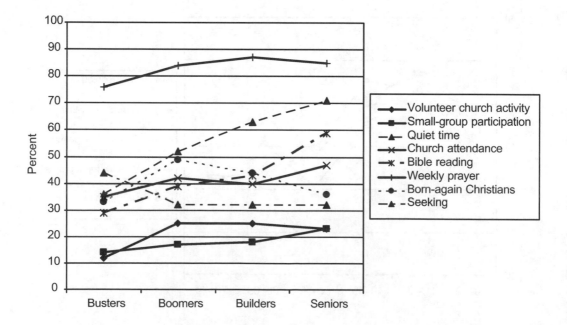

FIGURE 8.2. Religious activities by cohort.

appear to increase into the 30s and even 40s. Further, there appear to be different trajectories of religiousness, which are not captured adequately by simple cross-sectional comparisons or even aggregate longitudinal data. An interesting pattern was discovered by O'Connor, Hoge, and Alexander (2002). Their sample of Baptist, Catholic, and Methodist respondents was surveyed in 1976 and followed up 22 years later, when most of the respondents were 38 years old. Seventy-nine percent of the sample reported having lapsed in their religious involvement during that interval, but more than half of them had resumed religious activity before the second survey)although women were more likely to resume than men).

THE DEVELOPMENT OF RELIGIOUS BELIEFS AND PRACTICES IN ADULTHOOD

In the psychological literature, there are two basic models of the development of religious beliefs and practices: socialization theories and cognitive theories. Under the first heading, we discuss general issues in the socialization of religious beliefs, attitudes, and practices, as well as the special instance of conversion (more common in adolescence and young adulthood), and a more recent theory, spiritual modeling (Oman & Thoresen, 2003). We also propose some alternative perspectives that we feel merit serious attention.

Socialization Theories

Socialization can be considered from the standpoint of its influences on the individual's religiousness. It can also be viewed as a contributor to adaptation and adjustment to social roles and norms, including its potential protective role against antisocial behavior and risky health behavior.

There is no doubt that the influence of one's parents, as well as of one's peers, is important in the acquisition and maintenance of religious beliefs and behavior. Traditionally, religious forms were passed down, virtually unaltered, from one generation to the next. However automatic this transmission may have been among our ancestors, some scholars, especially around the time of the Vietnam War, detected a breakdown of generational continuity (Friedenburg, 1969), including a discontinuity of religious beliefs (Thomas, 1974). Subsequent studies could be interpreted as either supporting or contradicting this interpretation, depending on how one chooses to interpret moderate correlation coefficients (Hunsberger, 1985). It appears that the degree of closeness of parents and children in general may govern the influence of parents on adolescent children in the religious domain. Moreover, parent–child closeness varies considerably across families (Myers, 1996; Wilson & Sherkat, 1994).

In a U.S. sample, Ozorak (1989) found that cohesiveness of families was more associated with stability of religious participation than with the stability of beliefs in adolescence. Francis and Gibson (1993) obtained similar findings in a large sample of Scottish adolescents. Beliefs become more divergent as U.S. adolescents approach adulthood. This is consistent with the findings of Arnett (2001) concerning the criteria for adult status among U.S. teens and young and midlife adults. One of the most heavily endorsed criteria for all age groups was to "decide on personal beliefs and values independently of parents or other influences" (Arnett, 2001, p. 137). While this may seem an impossible exercise, it is nevertheless true that some young adults choose religious beliefs and practices at considerable variance with those of their parents. This topic is discussed in more depth later in this chapter. For the present, religious choice increasingly competes for variance with religious socialization in explaining relationships between parental influence and adult religiousness—at least in North America. This may be becoming increasingly the case in other cultures as well, with interesting implications for the study of radically politicized religious beliefs.

Evidence points toward a greater influence of mothers on adolescents' religiousness (Hertel & Donahue, 1995). This would not be surprising on the assumption of a parental division of labor in modern and postmodern households, with the primary breadwinner (still usually the father) away from home during most waking hours. Even when mothers also work, they take on most of the parenting role (Cowan & Cowan, 2000). It would be interesting to conduct studies in more agrarian societies in which both parents are available to the children during the day. Fathers who occupy the primary caregiving role may also be more influential in the religious socialization of their children.

It is certainly true that socialization remains an important source of religiousness. However, Spilka and his colleagues (2003) appear to grant little credence to the notion of an increase in religious decision making. Granted the influence of socialization from a kind of "black box" analysis, we remain in the dark about the process by which it occurs. Indeed, the importance of socialization may have been overrated. Loveland (2003), working with the 1988 General Social Survey data set, found that childhood religious socialization had no effect on the likelihood of an individual switching to another religion in adulthood, while education and marriage outside of one's religion were strong predictors of switching. On the other hand, being raised Catholic, Latter-Day Saints, Jehovah's Witness, Unitarian Universalist, or Christian Scientist was strongly protective against switching. Interestingly, having made a formal choice to join a religion while growing up was also fairly strongly negatively related to switching. This is consistent with the position taken by Arnett's respondents that making choices about important beliefs and values is vital in defining the transition to adulthood. Of course, it must be remembered that both Loveland's and Arnett's data are taken from U.S. samples. Apparently, Americans are socialized to make choices.

O'Connor et al. (2002) found that none of their multiple indices of religious socialization by parents, when the participants were 16, were significant predictors of religious participation at age 38. Besides lapsing itself, the best predictors were religious denomination, with Baptists more likely than Methodists or Catholics to be religiously involved in adulthood, and youth religious group participation. Moreover, Baptists were more likely than the other two denominations to have a personal religious practice (prayer or Bible reading) as adults.

Spiritual Models

Oman and Thoresen (2003) introduced a long overdue focus on spiritual models as sources of spiritual development. Based on the importance of observational learning in all human activities (Bandura, 1986), it is reasonable to think that this applies to religious activity and spiritual practice. All spiritual traditions emphasize the importance of teachers of spiritual practice who not only know how to instruct verbally, but who exemplify the practices and their results. Oman and Thoresen go further and propose that the exemplary behavior of spiritual models can serve as interventions to promote better mental and physical health. They are actually proposing that spiritual development, facilitated by models, can be an important source of positive human development, beyond mere religious socialization, a position long espoused by spiritual traditions themselves. Interestingly, the most influential examples of the power of spiritual models has appeared in the political sphere in which such noteworthy exemplars as Gandhi and Martin Luther King, Jr., have had wide-ranging influence well beyond their specific religious traditions.

Having recognized the importance of spiritual models, it is important to recognize that such models may work against human development and in favor of narrow, intolerant, divisive, and inhumane attitudes and behavior. In responding to a similar point made by Silberman (2003), Oman and Thoresen assert that research on spiritual modeling no more needs to clearly define the meaning of positive and negative modeling "any more than child psychology needs to define very clearly what is meant by good and bad parenting" (Oman & Thoresen, 2003, p. 200). It most certainly is incumbent on child psychology to address good and bad parenting. The recent examples of destructive spiritual modeling by religious teachers who encourage political violence, as well as the plethora of examples of "spiritual teachers" evidently largely motivated by greed and narcissism, sometimes with the involvement of obvious mental illness (as with Jim Jones and David Koresh) strongly suggest that reliance on spiritual models should be accompanied by reliance on critical thinking. Reliance on spiritual models holds much promise and, at the same time, is fraught with perils as a pathway for development in young adulthood.

Conversion

Conversion is a phenomenon of adolescence through midlife. Paloutzian (1996) makes the interesting observation that what is generally called "religious conversion" is a form of religious socialization. Conversion might be considered a more or less quick form of socialization, although some conversions arise from a conscious search for meaning. This process can result in a relatively gradual conversion that is not sudden but is also not a process spanning the two decades of "growing up" usually regarded as the time of religious socialization. Others appear to result from repressed inner conflict that "explodes" as sudden conversion (Paloutzian, 1996).

Rambo (1993) has presented the most ambitious conceptualization of religious conversion. The centerpiece of Rambo's theory is his extension of Epstein's (1985) theory of human motivation. In addition to Epstein's four basic needs for pleasure versus pain, a system of meaning, self-esteem, and relationships, Rambo added two others, power and transcendence (see also Paloutzian, Chapter 18, this volume). He theorizes seven stages of conversion including context, crisis, quest, encounter (contact with representative of the new system), interaction (with the new system's teachers, disciples, liturgy, etc.), commitment, and consequences. Rambo unpacks these stages in considerable detail. While Rambo's conceptualization is rooted in the recognition of conscious quest as the impetus for conversion, he emphasizes that it may also occur as a quest for power.

Beckford (1983) also observed that the emphasis on religion as a source of meaning had obscured the role of religion as a source of power over success and health. In a small sample of British young adult respondents, Loewenthal and Cornwall (1993) found that causal attribution to God among religious respondents, in contrast to nonreligious respondents, was largely limited to health. There were few attributions to God for financial/occupational or relationship success. There can be no doubt that religion is involved in the perception of power over death (Beckford, 1983). This issue is certainly related to Pargament's (1992) critique of the division of religiousness to that of means versus ends central to the intrinsic/extrinsic distinction (Allport, 1966). It would be interesting to explore the power aspect of religiousness in contemporary religious adolescents and young adults.

In contrast, Conn (1986, 1987) argued that conversion can be driven by an innate need for self-transcendence that may constitute a major developmental task in adulthood, as Jung (1933) theorized. This developmental perspective has given rise to a literature on transcendent experiences in adulthood and their relationship to mental health and life satisfaction (Coward & Reed, 1996; Le & Levenson, 2005; Levenson, Jennings, Aldwin, & Shiraishi, 2005).

From a developmental perspective, it is noteworthy that conversion, especially sudden conversion, may be most likely in adolescence and young adulthood (Argyle & Beit-Hallahmi, 1975). Although there is little evidence to support this view, it makes sense in light of the developmental task of identity formation at these ages (Erikson, 1950). However, Jung (1933) recognized that the process of personal integration and finding meaning was a lifelong one, with religions serving as schools for the middle-aged, preparing them for approaching the end of life. Thus, the finding by Scroggs and Douglas (1976) that conversion often happens in early middle age is not surprising. It is also worth considering that life expectancy has increased dramatically in the past century, allowing more "room for change" in midlife. The centrality of the need for self-transcendence in Rambo's theory is consistent with Jung's (1933) characterization of development as an illumination of psychic life.

Does conversion result in personality change? Paloutzian, Richardson, and Rambo (1999), in a review of the literature on the causes and consequences of conversion, found little evidence for a change in personality traits, such as the "Big Five," but did find change in second- and third-order personality processes, such as goals, identity, and meaning, as well as positive changes in behavior and mental health. This finding held regardless of whether conversion was to a more conventional religious denomination or to a less conventional one. Their review also suggests that personality may be more likely to predict conversion than to be changed by it. Paloutzian et al. (1999) also present the available data on the incidence and prevalence of religious conversion, suggesting that the possibilities for conversion research are vast and still largely unrealized. There is a great need for longitudinal, multicohort research on the phenomenon of conversion.

Education

Education is a force for socialization in all cultures that is inescapably linked to maturation. Education is both an extension of parental socialization and a challenge to it. Obviously education's influence differs in accordance with the agendas of educational institutions, prior religious socialization of the students, their age, and their academic ability. These issues have been addressed only sketchily in the empirical literature. Kuhlen and Arnold (1944) found, in a sample of U.S. adolescents age 12–18, that the older youth were more likely than the younger to express curiosity about religious beliefs than absolute belief in them. Later studies have reached similar conclusions (Benson, Yeager, Wood, Guerra, & Manno, 1986), culminating in Tamminem's (1991) study of Finnish youth that showed an increase in agnosticism and a concomitant decrease in certainty of God's existence with increasing school grade and, of course, age. It is not unlikely that the extent to which a curriculum deemphasizes religious explanations for one's personal problems and religious solutions for them influences the observed decline in religious certainty. This obvious hypothesis has not yet, to our knowledge, been tested.

On the other hand, rigid religious beliefs may be defenses against strong doubt. Among Canadian university students, Altemeyer (1988) found that, by suggesting the possibility of religious doubt by a "hidden observer" (Hilgard, 1973), students high in right-wing authoritarianism, who also had the most fundamentalist religious beliefs, were the most likely to experience their hidden observer as doubtful of the validity of their religious beliefs. Unlike Hilgard's respondents, these students were not hypnotized, yet the study's intriguing result deserves replication.

One conclusion that can be drawn so far is that religious doubt increases with age and education, even among those with the most extreme religious convictions. Late adolescence and young adulthood may be times of religious uncertainty. Apostasy, not surprisingly, was associated with less emphasis on religion by parents but seemed to have little to do with political orientation, while small amounts of variance were accounted for by intellectual orientation and difficult relationships with parents (Hunsberger, 1980, 1983; Hunsberger & Brown, 1984). Nevertheless, the general trend is toward less religious certainty in late adolescence. It must be cautioned that these studies involve small, ethnically and religiously rather homogeneous samples.

This raises a question concerning the possibility of stages of development of religious thinking across the life course. To the extent that religious affiliation, behavior, and beliefs are based on individual choices as well as by religious socialization, we must consider religious thought in addition to religious socialization as a source of religiousness.

Stages of Religious Cognition

Fowler (1981) pioneered the contemporary study of religious cognition. Following other stage theories of development, especially that of Kohlberg (1984), Fowler's theory of stages of faith development follows the time-honored developmental tradition of positing universal, sequential stages of development. These stages are consistent with stages of cognitive development. The stages move from the "intuitive-projective" faith of small children, corresponding to Kohlberg's obedience through fear stage, through the stage of "universalizing faith," corresponding to Kohlberg's stage seven (Kohlberg & Ryncarz, 1990). Interestingly, the latter stage does appear to correspond to "unity of being" systems such as those found in Sufism (Islamic mysticism; Shah, 1964) and unitive Buddhism (Cleary, 1995). There is great appeal in the theory, but the universality of the intervening stages is problematic, suggesting, for example, that one must negotiate the stage of relativism before reaching universalizing faith. This thoroughly modern notion may not be reflected in premodern but highly sophisticated systems such as those just mentioned.

Oser (1991; cf. Oser & Gmunder, 1991) have presented another stage theory of the development of religious cognition that has a decidedly motivational aspect. The theory describes stages of religious judgment based on the "solutions" of seven simultaneous tensions with respect to the influence of the divine on human life. These are freedom versus dependence, transcendence versus immanence, hope versus despair (of the influence of the divine), the hiddenness versus the transparency of divine will, faith versus fear, the sacred versus the profane aspects of life circumstances, and the eternal versus the ephemeral import of life choices. The solutions of these dilemmas are reflected in five stages of development of religious judgment. These stages begin with religious heteronomy in which divine intervention influences produce effects, followed by a stage reflecting the ability of the individual to influence the divine (by prayers and good or bad deeds). The third stage has the divine withdraw to a place of hidden influence while the individual is, for all practical purposes, completely responsible for him- or herself. This is, essentially, the opposite of stage 1. The fourth stage reintroduces the divine as self. Religious relativism becomes acceptable. Finally, in the fifth stage, the seven dimensions are coordinated, resulting (somehow) in an experience of union with the divine.

Oser and Gmunder (1991) constructed three dilemmas to reflect the stages based on the dimensions. One such dilemma concerns a young physician who thinks of God just before his airliner crashes and, in his prayer, he promises that, should his life be spared he would spend the rest of his life serving the poor of the third world. He even promises to break off his relationship with his girlfriend should she refuse to go along with this plan. The plane crashes and the young physician miraculously survives. Subsequently, he is offered a lucrative private practice. Should he keep his promise or not?

Oser and Gmunder present the dilemma and then ask a series of questions designed to assess the stages. These questions concern whether or not one has obligations to keep the promise; whether one has obligations to God at all; the reality of God's will; and the consequences of not keeping the promise. While these questions are reasonable with respect to various perceived God–human relationships, a persistent reference to God as "other" limits the degree to which higher levels of religious cognition can be assessed, especially the experience of unity of being.

This stage theory certainly pays attention to a number of well-established attitudes toward the divine, but it is not at all clear how these attitudes constitute developmental stages. It is also unclear how the stages are related to the dilemmas presented to respondents in order to determine empirically their developmental level or how they "operationalize" the seven dimensions. Stage 5 is clearly dependent on religious/spiritual experience, often based on spiritual practice, of which no mention is made. In any case, the oldest of the respondents in the study by Oser (1991) was 25, offering no lifespan data to support a stage theory. In fact, the empirical data support the well-established increase in religious doubt in later adolescence, with stage 3 (ego autonomy with the divine having little influence) in the ascendant and stage 5 nowhere to be found. What we find most interesting about this approach is the extent to which renunciation of worldly success is presented as a terrible sacrifice. In the traditional religious developmental systems of Buddhism, contemplative Christianity, and others, renunciation is regarded as the doorway to spiritual attainment. For Oser and Gmunder, renunciation is presented as a materialist tragedy, entailing the loss of material success, "paying" (grudgingly, it would appear) for one's survival, rather than gaining liberation from worldly desires.

Reich (1991), reflecting upon the theories of Fowler (1981) and Oser and Gmunder (Oser, 1991; Oser & Gmunder, 1991), observed that these theories are consistent with an inclusive logic that allows for the incorporation of contradictory positions in a new, overarching framework. In Reich's analysis and synthesis of stage theories, cognitive religious development consists of either/or reasoning based on familiar Aristotelean logic being supplanted by complementarity reasoning. In the latter, different, seemingly contradictory explanations are increasingly understood to be provisional and perspectival.

From the standpoint of developmental theory, Reich's synthesis is consistent with Overton's (1999) critique of "split metanarratives" that arbitrarily divide phenomena into real and spurious. One great problem in the explanation of religious belief, cognition, and motivation has been the persistent reductionism of psychologists in their treatment of religion. This position is still fully present, although not persuasively defended, in the most recent edition of perhaps the most prominent text in the psychology of religion (Spilka et al., 2003). This refers to the typical unwillingness of psychologists to acknowledge that religious explanations of religion have any validity. Rather, as noted by Wulff (1997), the objective has been to replace such explanations with putatively scientific ones. An appealing feature of stage theories of religious development, at least for non-reductionists, is that they are able to take religious explanations of religious cognition seriously. They are also capable of accommodating rare forms of religious experience and thought that would be lost to an actuarial approach (see Levenson, Jennings, Le, & Aldwin, in press). Wulff (1993) criticized the universal stage model of religious development on grounds similar to those applied to other universal stage theories (Levenson & Crumpler, 1996), the most important of which is that they are not universal. On the other hand, as Levenson et al. (in press) argue, there are universalizable aspects of spiritual understanding in the wisdom traditions of the world's major religions. Specifically, these are comparable practices (e.g., meditation) that decenter consciousness from the self.

Clore and Fitzgerald (2002) have presented data based on a stage conceptualization of faith development that at least supports the existence of different forms of faith, ranging from common sense, through formal and postformal reasoning, culminating in transcendent faith. The questionnaire that they developed to assess these levels of development merits longitudinal study to examine the claim that these are true stages of development.

CONSEQUENCES OF RELIGIOUSNESS IN ADOLESCENCE AND EARLY ADULTHOOD

Religion, Ethics, and Destructive Behavior

A natural question arising from the examination of how people "get religion" concerns whether and how religion affects social and political beliefs and behavior. It is probably a mistake to seek objective relationships between religion and "morality" inasmuch as people acting on religious premises have been the most divisive precisely on the question of what constitutes morality and immorality. Cochran and Beeghley (1991) found that more conservative Protestants were five times as likely as the religiously nonaffiliated to view premarital sex as "almost always" or "always" wrong. The more liberal denominations (e.g., Jewish and Episcopalian) fell in between the nonaffiliated and the conservative. Regarding homosexuality, Jews and the nonaffiliated were the only groups in which homosexuality was considered "wrong" by less than half of the respondents. Among Baptists, 89% considered homosexuality wrong. It is also worth noting that religiousness is more strongly related to sexual restraint among women than among men (Poulson, Eppler, Satterwhite, Wuensch, & Bass, 1998; Sheeran, Spears, Abraham, & Abrams, 1996).

Keeping in mind the ambiguous status of morality, is there a way in which religiousness can be adjudged helpful or harmful in promoting any more or less objective ethical behavior? Such an effect might include the avoidance of behavior that demonstrably harms others. Results of the considerable research in this area constitute a veritable model of inconclusive findings. Clearly, most antisocial behavior, as defined above, is most prevalent in adolescents and young adults. However, economic crimes may be an exception to this rule, especially among executives who abuse their authority. In a recent meta-analysis of data spanning 30 years, Baier and Wright (2001) concluded that there was a modest protective effect of religious beliefs and participation on overtly criminal behavior. As Baier and Wright (2001) observe, however, there is no consistent definition of criminality and religiousness in the 60 investigations they examined. Spilka et al.

(2003) correctly observed that most of the studies are correlational, and therefore causal directionality cannot be inferred. As they point out, conclusive evidence awaits longitudinal research designs. We might add that a large amount of destructive behavior is not officially criminal, such as destructive corporate raiding (see Levenson, 1993).

Another issue, especially pertinent to the relationship of religiousness to development in young adulthood, that has largely escaped detection by psychologists of religion, is the putatively religious motivation of considerable destructive behavior by young adults. This phenomenon is well known to Hindus and Muslims in India, for example, but moved to center stage with the events in the United States on September 11, 2001, events entirely perpetrated by young adults (although planned by older ones), but there is a steady stream of news reports of murders and atrocities by young fundamentalists of many faiths, most strikingly the "honor killings" of women who are perceived to have violated the sexual ethics of Islam (see Silberman, Chapter 29, this volume). Fundamentalist Christians may also be more likely to perpetrate violence in the family (Mahoney, Pargament, Tarakeshwar, & Swank, 2001), although the evidence is somewhat mixed (Cunradi, Caetano, & Shafer, 2002; Mahoney & Tarakeshwar, Chapter 10, this volume).

Altemeyer (1988, 2003) began, almost alone, to investigate the phenomenon of aggressive fundamentalism (see Hunsberger & Altemeyer, Chapter 21, this volume). In 1992, Altemeyer and Hunsberger found, in a sample of parents of Canadian university students, that fundamentalists tend to be aggressively prejudiced. This finding might suggest an approach to understanding putatively religiously motivated destructive behavior that does not single out one religion for criticism, but concerns itself with the psychological patterns involved in aggressive fundamentalism regardless of specific religion. It is difficult to disentangle the various threads that are woven together in the process of socialization and enculturation. However, religion can be used as a justification for all kinds of behavior, some of it undoubtedly destructive.

Religion and Altruism

If religiousness is not conclusively protective against destructive behavior, might it promote altruistic behavior? In a review of the literature, Youniss, Mclellan, and Yates (1999) found that adolescents who professed a high level of interest in religion were much more likely than other adolescents to participate in volunteer activities. Many of these activities were conducted under explicitly religious auspices. Indeed, religiousness did not predict greater participation in nonreligious volunteering. Youniss et al.'s qualitative data showed volunteering with the needy had an impact on an adolescent's thinking concerning poverty, homelessness, and discrimination.

However, in a study of willingness to help, students who scored high on intrinsic religious orientation were less likely to help people who disclosed that they were gay, even when the help needed was not associated with their homosexuality (Batson, Floyd, Meyer, & Winner, 1999). This led the authors to conclude that "devout, intrinsic religion appeared to be associated with tribal rather than universal compassion" (Batson et al., 1999, p. 455). On the other hand, persons who scored high on the Quest Scale were prepared to help, regardless of the recipient's homosexuality, consistent with the definition of quest as an open minded, nondogmatic religious attitude. One developmental conclusion that can be drawn from these studies is that strong religious involvement does not necessarily offer a pathway to the development of impartial ethics.

The Conundrum of Religion on Campus

Observation of the social scene on university campuses over the past 30 years leaves us with the strong impression that religion has become far more important to students in the past two decades. The evidence for this is admittedly impressionistic, including increasing prevalence of signs on campus inviting participation in religious groups as well as an increased blending of the religious and the political in speechmaking by students. However, impressions can be misleading. The Higher Education Research Institute (HERI) at UCLA has conducted surveys of freshmen at colleges and universities in the United States for the past four decades. In 1966, the survey began to assess religious preference and, in 1984, self-attribution as a born-again Christian. Over almost 30 years, those expressing no religious preference have increased from 6.6% to 17.6%. Those considering themselves to be born-again Christians remained at a high but stable percentage of the sample, with percentages ranging from the mid- to high 20s. Unfortunately, the born-again item was not collected after 2001 when a quarter of the sample was positive for this attribute.

The HERI data indicate a sharp increase in interest in raising a family as well as a commensurate increase in materialistic values (wanting to be wealthy) and a decrease in "developing a meaningful philosophy of life." It would be interesting to know more about the relationship between religiousness and materialism versus meaning in this sample.

Spiritual Practices

Wink and Dillon (2002) presented a critique of Fowler's theory of stages of faith development that can actually be applied to all of the stage theories touched on here. First, according to this critique, these theories are almost entirely cognitive. They do not refer to religious or spiritual practices. That is, there is no concern with the method of contacting or evoking the sacred or with observing the experiences that arise through such methods. However, all religions contain prescriptions for such practices (see Levenson et al., in press). In a longitudinal analysis using the intergenerational study sample of the Institute of Human Development at the University of California, Berkeley, Wink and Dillon (2002) found that spiritual practices and experiences increased in later life for participants who were introspective, insightful, intellectually curious, religious, and unconventional in young and middle adulthood. Women who evidenced these qualities and who had experienced negative life events in young to middle adulthood were more spiritual in later life. This study is groundbreaking in presenting an approach that is sensitive to the effects of life events (Aldwin & Levenson, 2001) and spiritual practice on spiritual development in adulthood. It reflects the growing sophistication among psychologists of religion and students of human development concerning the role of spiritual practice in spiritual development.

Religion, Spirituality, and Adult Development

There is considerable interest in religiousness and spirituality among scholars of adult development, yet the research basis for this connection remains thin though promising.

Several broad conclusions can be drawn from the information reviewed here. First, religiousness and spirituality continue to be influential in adolescence and young adulthood. While the evidence is mixed regarding the effects of religiousness and spirituality on social behavior, there may be particular stages or levels of spiritual development that are central to the full spectrum of human development. Longitudinal studies are of the greatest importance in establishing a relationship between religiousness and spirituality, on the one hand, and higher levels of human development, on the other hand. For those moving from adolescence into and through young adulthood, the question of how religiousness and spirituality serve as developmental pathways deserves careful attention.

Spiritual Experience

One specific topic that stands out as a needed focus of future research is the relationship of religious/spiritual experience to adult development. We are in complete agreement with Boyatzis, who asserts that "the core of spirituality is a sense of self-transcendence and the core of religion is seeking or being in relationship with the sacred. Thus, the crux of spirituality and religion is *experience*" (Boyatzis, Chapter 7, this volume, p. 136). We are also in agreement with those who have pointed out the fact that this is, nevertheless, the least studied aspect of religion and spirituality (Spilka & McIntosh, 1997; Emmons & Paloutzian, 2003). Indeed, this situation perfectly reflects psychology's discomfort with its most obvious subject matter, conscious experience, in favor of the apparently comforting confines of mechanistic constructs such as behavior and cognition. The founder of U.S. psychology, William James, put experience at the center of psychology and wrote about religion in entirely experiential terms (James, 1902). Boyatzis (Chapter 7, this volume) points out the impressive amount of religious experience reported by young children. Boyatzis urges us to study the connections between religious experience and belief and the need to establish this understanding on the basis of cross-cultural research. We believe that religious/spiritual experience is central to the study of religiousness and spirituality across the lifespan.

REFERENCES

Aldwin, C. M., & Levenson, M. R. (2001). Stress, coping, and health at mid-life: A developmental perspective. In M. E. Lachman (Ed.), *The handbook of midlife development* (pp. 188–214). New York: Wiley.

Allport, G. (1966). The religious context of prejudice. *Journal for the Scientific Study of Religion, 5*, 447–457.

Altemeyer, B. (1988). *Enemies of freedom: Understanding right wing authoritarianism.* San Francisco: Jossey-Bass.

Altemeyer, B. (2003). Why do religious fundamentalists tend to be prejudiced? *The International Journal for the Psychology of Religion, 13*, 17–28.

Altemeyer, B., & Hunsberger, B. (1992). Authoritarianism, religious fundamentalism, quest, and prejudice. *The International Journal for the Psychology of Religion, 2*, 113–133.

Argyle, M., & Beit-Hallahmi, B. (1975). *The social psychology of religion.* London: Routledge & Kegan Paul.

Arnett, J. J. (2001). Conceptions of the transition to adulthood: Perspectives from adolescence through midlife. *Journal of Adult Development, 8*, 133–143.

Baier, C. J., & Wright, B. R. E. (2001). "If you love me, keep my commandments": A meta-analysis of the effect of religion on crime. *Journal of Research on Crime and Delinquency, 38*, 3–21.

Bandura, A. (1986). *Social foundations of thought and action: A social cognitive theory.* Englewood Cliffs, NJ: Prentice-Hall.

Batson, C. D., Floyd, R. B., Meyer, J. M., & Winner, A. L. (1999). "And who is my neighbor?": Intrinsic religion as a source of universal compassion. *Journal for the Scientific Study of Religion, 38,* 31–41.

Beckford, J. A. (1983). The restoration of "power" to the sociology of religions. *Sociological Analysis, 44,* 11–33.

Beit-Hallahmi, B., & Argyle, M. (1997). *The psychology of religious behaviour, belief, and experience.* London: Routledge.

Benson, P. L., Donahue, M. J., & Erickson, J. A. (1989). Adolescents and religion: A review of the literature from 1970–1986. *Research in the Social Scientific Study of Religion, 1,* 153–181.

Benson, P. L., Williams, D. L., & Johnson, A. L. (1987). *The quicksilver years: The hopes and fears of young adolescents.* San Francisco: Harper & Row.

Benson, P. L., Yeager, P. K., Wood, M. J., Guerra, M. J., & Manno, B. V. (1986). *Catholic high schools: Their impact on low-income students.* Washington, DC: National Catholic Education Association.

Cherry, C., DeBerg, B. A., & Porterfield, A. (2001). *Religion on campus.* Chapel Hill, NC: University of North Carolina Press.

Cleary, T. (1995). *Entry into the inconceivable: An introduction to Hua-Yen Buddhism.* Honolulu: University of Hawaii Press.

Clore, V., & Fitzgerald, J. (2002). Intentional faith: An alternative view of faith development. *Journal of Adult Development, 9,* 97–107.

Cochran, J. K., & Beeghley, L. (1991). The influence of religion on attitudes toward non-marital sexuality: A preliminary assessment of reference group theory. *Journal for the Scientific Study of Religion, 30,* 45–62.

Conn, W. (1986). Adult conversions. *Pastoral Psychology, 34,* 225–236.

Conn, W. (1987). Pastoral counseling for self-transcendence: The integration of psychology and theology. *Pastoral Psychology, 36,* 29–48.

Cowan, C. P., & Cowan, P. A. (1999). *When partners become parents: The big life change for couples.* New York: Lea.

Coward, D., & Reed, P. G. (1996). Self-transcendence: A resource for healing at the end of life. *Issues in Mental Health Nursing, 17,* 275–288.

Cunradi, C. B., Caetano, R., & Shafer, J. (2002). Religious affiliation, denominational homogamy, and intimate partner violence among U. S. couples. *Journal for the Scientific Study of Religion, 41,* 139–151.

Donelson, E. (1999). Psychology of religion and adolescence in the United States: Past to present. *Journal of Adolescence, 22,* 187–204.

Elkind, D. (1971). The origins of religion in the child. *Review of Religious Research, 12,* 35–42.

Emmons, R. A. (1999). *The psychology of ultimate concerns: Motivation and spirituality in personality.* New York: Guilford Press.

Emmons, R. A., & Paloutzian, R. F. (2003). The psychology of religion. *Annual Review of Psychology, 54,* 377–402.

Epstein, S. (1985). The implications of cognitive-experimental self-theory for research in social psychology and personality. *Journal for the Theory of Social Behavior, 15,* 283–310.

Erikson, E. H. (1950). *Childhood and society.* New York: Norton.

Fowler, J. W. (1981). *Stages of faith: The psychology of human development and the quest for meaning.* San Francisco: Harper & Row.

Francis, L. J., & Gibson, H. M. (1993). Parental influence and adolescent religiosity: A study of church attendance and attitude toward Christianity among adolescents 11–12 and 15–16 years old. *The International Journal for the Psychology of Religion, 3,* 241–253.

Friedenburg, E. (1969). Current patterns of a generation conflict. *Journal of Social Issues, 25,* 21–38.

Gorsuch, R. L. (1988). Psychology of religion. *Annual Review of Psychology, 39,* 201–221.

Hertel, B. R., & Donahue, M. J. (1995). Parental influence on God images among children: Testing Durkheim's metaphoric parallelism. *Journal for the Scientific Study of Religion, 34,* 186–199.

Hilgard, E. R. (1973). A neodissociation interpretation of pain reduction in hypnosis. *Psychological Review, 80*, 396–411.

Hunsberger, B. (1980). A reexamination of the antecedents of apostasy. *Review of Religious Research, 21*, 158–170.

Hunsberger, B. (1983). Apostasy. *Review of Religious Research, 25*, 21–38.

Hunsberger, B. (1985). Parent–university student agreement on religious and non-religious issues. *Journal for the Scientific Study of Religion, 24*, 314–320.

Hunsberger, B., & Brown, L. B. (1984). Religious socialization, apostasy, and the impact of family background. *Journal for the Scientific Study of Religion, 23*, 239–251.

James, W. (1902). *Varieties of religious experience: A study in human nature.* London: Longmans, Green.

Jung, C. G. (1933). *Modern man in search of a soul.* San Diego: Harcourt Brace Jovanovich.

Kohlberg, L. (1984). *Psychology of moral development: The nature and validity of moral stages.* New York: Addison Wesley.

Kohlberg, L., & Ryncarz, R. A. (1990). Beyond justice reasoning: Moral development and consideration of a seventh stage. In C. N. Alexander & E. J. Langer (Eds.), *Higher stages of human development* (191–207). New York: Oxford University Press.

Kuhlen, R. G., & Arnold, M. (1944). Age differences in religious beliefs and problems during adolescence. *Journal of Genetic Psychology, 65*, 291–300.

Le, T., & Levenson, M. R. (2005). Wisdom: What's love (and culture) got to do with it? *Journal of Research in Personality, 39*(4).

Levenson, M. R. (1993). Psychopaths are not necessarily impulsive, etc.: Reply to Feelgood & Rantzen. *Theory and Psychology, 3*, 229–234.

Levenson, M. R., & Crumpler, C. A. (1996). Three models of adult psychological development. *Human Development, 39*, 135–194.

Levenson, M. R., Jennings, P. A., Aldwin, C. M., & Shiraishi, R. W. (2005). Self-transcendence: Conceptualization and measurement. *International Journal of Aging and Human Development, 60*, 127–143.

Levenson, M. R., Jennings, P. A., Le, T., & Aldwin, C. M. (2005). Contemplative psychologies as theories of self-transcendence in adulthood. In D. Wulff (Ed.), *Handbook of the psychology of religion.* Oxford: Oxford University Press.

Loewenthal, K. M., & Cornwall, N. (1993). Religiosity and perceived control of life events. *The International Journal for the Psychology of Religion, 3*, 39–45.

Loveland, M. W. T. (2003). Religions switching: Preference development, maintenance, and change. *Journal for the Scientific Study of Religions, 42*, 147–157.

Mahoney, A., Pargament, K. I., Tarakeshwar, N., & Swank, A. B. (2001). Religion in the home in the 1980s and 1990s: A meta-analytic review and conceptual analysis of links between religion, marriage, and parenting. *Journal of Family Psychology, 15*, 559–596.

Markstrom, C. A. (1999). Religions involvement in adolescent psychosocial development. *Journal of Adolescence, 22*, 205–221.

Myers, S. M. (1996). An interactive model of religiosity in inheritance: The importance of family context. *American Sociological Review, 6*, 858–866.

O'Connor, T. P., Hoge, D. R., & Alexander, E. (2002). The relative influence of youth and adult experiences on personal spirituality and church involvement. *Journal for the Scientific Study of Religious, 41*, 723–732.

Oman, D., & Thoresen, C. E. (2003). Spiritual modeling: A key to spiritual and religious growth. *The International Journal for the Psychology of Religion, 13*, 149–165.

Oser, F. (1991). The development of religious judgement. In. F. K. Oser & W. G. Scarlett (Eds.), *Religious development in childhood and adolescence* (pp. 5–25). San Francisco: Jossey-Bass.

Oser, F., & Gmunder, P. (1991). *Religious judgement: A developmental perspective.* Birmingham, AL: Religious Education Press.

Overton, W. F. (1999). Developmental psychology: Philosophy, concepts, and methodology. In W.

Damon & R. Lerner (Eds.), *Handbook of child psychology* (5th ed.): *Vol. 1. Theoretical models of human development* (pp. 107–188). New York: Wiley.

Ozorak, E. W. (1989). Social and cognitive influences on the development of religious beliefs and commitment in adolescence. *Journal for the Scientific Study of Religion, 28,* 448–463.

Paloutzian, R. F. (1996). *Invitation to the psychology of religions* (2nd ed.). Needham Heights, MA: Allyn & Bacon.

Paloutzian, R. F., Richardson, J. R., & Rambo, L. R. (1999). Religious conversion and personality change. *Journal of Personality, 67,* 1047–1079.

Pargament, K. I. (1992). Of means and ends: Religion and the search for significance. *The International Journal for the Psychology of Religion, 9,* 3–16.

Poulson, P. L., Eppler, M. A., Satterwhite, T. N., Wuensch, K. L., & Bass, L. A. (1998). Alcohol consumption, strength of religious beliefs, and risky sexual behavior in college students. *Journal of American College Health, 46,* 227–232.

Rambo, L. R. (1993). *Understanding religious conversions.* New Haven, CT: Yale University Press.

Reich, K. H. (1991). The role of complementarity reasoning in religious development. In F. K. Oser & W. G. Scarlett (Eds.), *Religions development in childhood and adolescence* (pp. 77–89). San Francisco: Jossey-Bass.

Scroggs, J. R., & Douglas, W. G. T. (1976). Issues in the psychology of religious conversion. *Journal of Religion and Health, 6,* 204–216.

Shah, I. (1964). *The Sufis.* New York: Doubleday.

Sheeran, P., Spears, R., Abraham, S. C. S., & Abrams, D. (1996). Religiosity, gender, and the double standard. *Journal of Psychology, 130,* 23–33.

Silberman, I. (2003). Spiritual role modeling: The teaching of meaning systems. *The International Journal for the Psychology of Religion, 13,* 175–195.

Smith, C., Denton, M. L., Faris, R., & Regnerus, M. (2002). Mapping American adolescent religious participation. *Journal for the Scientific Study of Religion, 41,* 597–612.

Spilka, B., & McIntosh, D. N. (Eds.). (1997). *The psychology of religion: Theoretical approaches.* Boulder, CO: Westview Press/Harper Books.

Spilka, B., Hood, R. W., Jr., Hunsberger, B., Gorsuch, R. (2003). *The psychology of religion: An empirical approach* (3rd ed.). New York: Guilford Press.

Tamminem, K. (1991). *Religious development in childhood and youth: An empirical study.* Helsinki, Finland: Suomalainen Tiedeakatemia.

Thomas, L. E. (1974). Generational discontinuity in beliefs: An exploration of the generation gap. *Journal of Social Issues, 30,* 1–22.

van Gennep, A. (1960). *The rites of passage.* Chicago: University of Chicago Press.

Wilson, J., & Sherkat, D. E. (1994). Returning to the fold. *Journal for the Scientific Study of Religion, 33,* 148–161.

Wink, P., & Dillon, M. (2002). Spiritual development across the adult life course: Findings from a longitudinal study. *Journal of Adult Development, 9,* 79–94.

Wulff, D. M. (1997). *Psychology of religion: Classic and contemporary views* (2nd ed.). New York: Wiley.

Youniss, J., Mclellan, J. A., & Yates, M. (1999). Religion, community service, and identity in American youth. *Journal of Adolescence, 22,* 243–253.

9

Points of Connection:
Gerontology and the Psychology of Religion

SUSAN H. MCFADDEN

In a footnote to the first chapter of *The Varieties of Religious Experience*, William James pronounced old age "the religious age *par excellence*" (1902/1961, pp. 28–29). When he wrote that at the beginning of the 20th century, the average life expectancy in the United States was 47 years and persons 65 and older represented about 3.1% of the U.S. population. By 2030, demographers expect that 70 million people in the United States—about 20% of the total population—will be 65 and older (Administration on Aging, 2003). This "longevity revolution" represents an unprecedented change in the age structure of human societies and has significant implications for the practice and the study of religion and of psychology. Presently, older adults' preferred approach to coping with the challenges of aging involves religion (Koenig, George, & Siegler, 1988). Compared to all other age groups, older people demonstrate the highest levels of religiosity and receive many important forms of support from religious institutions (McFadden, 1995). Both the experience of aging and the inevitability of death produce profound questions about life's meaning and purpose—questions to which the world's religions respond with affirmations of human value regardless of age or nearness to death.

Against the backdrop of the dramatic increase in the number of persons living longer, this chapter reviews studies of religion and aging conducted in the last two decades of the 20th century. The chapter opens with a consideration of time and the meaning of age and aging. It then addresses issues related to definition, measurement, theory, methods, design, and diversity in research on religion and aging. Readers should consult Chapter 2 of this *Handbook* for background on the definitional question and Chapter 3 for a more complete elaboration on measurement issues. Because other chapters review studies that included older adults in research on religion's contributions to physical health (Chapter 24), mental health (Chapter 25), and coping (Chapter 26), these topics are not addressed here. Much of this research on late life religiosity was conducted by sociologists of religion (see Moberg, 1997, for a review), who devoted little attention to the "basic psychology subdisciplines" addressed in Part III of this *Handbook*. The last section of this chapter asserts that research in these subdisciplines—especially on the cognitive psychology of aging and the psychology of late life emotion—can contribute to the psychology of religion in the 21st century, the first half of which will be dominated by the "longevity revolution." In addition, the chapter suggests that the psychology of religion can raise important questions for research on late life cognition and emotion.

TIME AND THE PSYCHOLOGY OF RELIGION AND AGING

Aging is a highly complex process unfolding in time and regulated by interrelated biological, psychological, and social systems (McFadden & Atchley, 2001). Whether viewed from the "bottom up" in light of molecular structures affected by genes, or from the "top down" in terms of the regulating function of consciousness enabled by the human nervous system, aging cannot be separated from the passage of time. Gerontologists generally agree that the amount of time a person has lived—chronological age—tells very little about functional capacity. Nearly everyone knows persons in their 70s who suffer from dementia and others who lead major organizations and run marathons.

Recognizing that there are usually significant differences between people age 60 and age 90, gerontologists sometimes refer to the young old (65–74), the middle old (75–84), and the oldest old (85 and older). However, this does not eliminate the problem that chronological age is a poor predictor of functional age. For this reason, some are starting to use the term the "third age" to refer to the time between the first retirement and the onset of disabling conditions that severely restrict activity (Weiss & Bass, 2002). Some individuals continue in the "third age" until death, maintaining high levels of physical, cognitive, and social functioning, while others slip into frailty. Thus, what seems to be a rather simple question—"How old is old?"—becomes very complex upon closer examination. Although the *psychology of aging* has been defined as the study of "regular changes in behavior after young adulthood" (Birren & Schroots, 1996, p. 8), most of the studies reviewed here focus upon persons in their late 60s and beyond.

The inescapable factor of time in the study of aging and older persons raises two additional issues: cohort effects and period effects produced by the sociohistorical circumstances that can affect researchers' questions and their data. In regard to cohort effects, it is important to recognize that persons now in their mid-70s entered adulthood when World War II ended. Jews who experienced the Holocaust are elderly and their suffering has affected their religious beliefs and worldviews, causing some to reject religious faith and others to center it in their lives (Myerhoff, 1978; Thomas, 1999). In the mid-20th century, U.S. mainline Protestantism rapidly expanded and embraced the values of science and modernism; elders socialized into adult religious life at that time rarely explored the mysteries of transcendence, so now, in old age, they may find themselves bereft of spiritual resources and religious beliefs that can provide a sense of meaning (Payne, 1984; Roof & McKinney, 1987). In the 1960s, as Catholic parents were launching their own children into adulthood, the Second Vatican Council (1962–1965) introduced profound changes in Roman Catholic religious life that some older adults celebrate and others grieve (Fahey & Lewis, 1984). Finally, after affecting numerous U.S. institutions due to its size, the baby-boom cohort entered adulthood challenging religious and political authority and producing a widespread debate about the relation between religion and spirituality (Marler & Hadaway, 2002).

Although religious meaning enables many older people to cope with suffering (Krause, 2003), it remains to be seen whether this will be true for new cohorts moving into old age. Some research indicates that a high percentage of persons in younger cohorts claim to be neither religious nor spiritual (Marler & Hadaway, 2002) and that persons who show no interest in religion in adolescence do not turn to it "by the time they have trudged well into middle age" (Altemeyer, 2004, p. 88). These examples suggest that the psychology of religion and aging must attend to the sociocultural factors that shape perspectives on religion held by persons belonging to different cohorts.

Students of religion and aging must also recognize that the historical period in which research is conducted can influence both researchers and research participants. As noted by Emmons and Paloutzian (2003), during the 1990s, the psychological study of religion rapidly acquired legitimacy through important publications and significant research support. Similarly, this chapter documents the proliferation of research on religion and aging that occurred at the end of the 20th century when federal agencies like the National Institute on Aging and private funding sources like the Fetzer Institute and the John D. Templeton Foundation began to support this research. Future historians will need to examine these and other social forces that challenged the taboo against the study of religion in both psychology and gerontology.

FACTORS AFFECTING RESEARCH ON RELIGION AND AGING

Definitions and Measures

Chapter 2 of this *Handbook* describes the debates about defining religion and spirituality that attracted so much attention in the 1990s. Gerontology was not immune to controversies over the relation between religion and spirituality, although researchers have often noted that many older people do not consider religion and spirituality to be distinct constructs. For example, Nelson-Becker's (2003) interviews with low-income, community-dwelling elders about the meanings of "religion" and "spirituality" showed that most could not define spirituality. Also, as a reminder of the importance of attending to ethnicity as well as to age in shaping understandings of these constructs, Nelson-Becker found that a group of predominantly Jewish immigrants had much more difficulty talking about religion than the African American Christians she interviewed.

Most research with older persons has focused on religiousness as expressed through organizational participation, nonorganizational activities (prayer, meditation, reading sacred texts), and subjective evaluations of religiosity. This multidimensional approach to older adults' religiosity began with research that showed that a drop in religious attendance did not predict a similar decline in nonorganizational religiosity (Ainlay & Smith, 1984; Mindel & Vaughan, 1978). Another important early study employed a multidimensional instrument to investigate religion and health in older people (Koenig, Smiley, & Gonzales, 1988). For their research on older black persons, Chatters, Levin, and Taylor (1992) developed a measure that assessed organizational and nonorganizational religiosity, as well as "subjective religiosity," which they described as the "psychological aspects of religiosity" (p. S270), including beliefs, experiences, and whether religion was central in an older person's life.

Despite these efforts to bring a multidimensional perspective on religion to studies of older adults, a report prepared in the mid-1990s for a conference on religion, health, and aging, sponsored by the National Institute on Aging (NIA) and the Fetzer Institute

(Futterman & Koenig, 1995) argued that gerontologists as a group still had "little sense of the scope and breadth of the religious domain" (p. 24) compared to sociologists and psychologists. After this conference, a working group convened and produced a publication with 13 measures of religiousness and spirituality related to physical and mental health. These included specific measures of phenomena such as meaning, values, beliefs, forgiveness, and coping, along with a multidimensional measure of religiousness and spirituality (Fetzer Institute/National Institute on Aging Working Group, 1999).

In their report on religiosity measures used by gerontologists, Futterman and Koenig (1995) noted that few researchers included items related to intrinsic, extrinsic, and quest religious orientations. Although this distinction has a long and contentious history in the psychology of religion, many gerontologists are unfamiliar with this literature. There are some exceptions, however. For example, from the beginning of his research program, Koenig has consistently employed items measuring intrinsic religiosity in his studies of religion and well-being in older people and has generally found high levels of intrinsic religiosity in older people (e.g., Koenig, Moberg, & Kvale, 1988). Differences between black elders and white elders have also been consistently identified, with the former showing higher levels of intrinsicness (Chatters et al., 1992). A study comparing Canadian Christian elders to Thai Buddhist elders found that in both groups those with a greater intrinsic religious orientation worried less (Tapanya, Nicki, & Jarusawad, 1997). Only a few researchers have examined the quest religious orientation in older adult samples. In a longitudinal study of older adults, a revised version of the Quest Scale produced two factors: a search for meaning in later life and doubt related to negative experiences with religious institutions and authorities (Futterman, Dillon, Garand, & Haugh, 1999). A subsample of widows from that longitudinal study showed higher levels of the quest orientation at the first observation, but a year later this group of elderly women showed little inclination toward questing (Thompson, Noone, & Guarino, 2003).

Recognizing that older people sometimes have different views on the meaning of terms used by researchers, the need for multidimensional measures, and the weak psychometric testing conducted on many measures, Krause (2002a) recently proposed a nine-step strategy for developing closed-end survey items for studies of religion and aging. He used focus groups, a panel of experts, individual interviews with older persons, and a nationwide random probability sample. Krause's approach is highly labor-intensive, but he presents a strong argument for the need to take this careful, multifaceted approach to the study of religion. For example, after developing a set of closed-end items, he conducted cognitive interviews with older adults, first asking for a response to each item, and then using focused probe questions to inquire about interpretations of the item. This led to the observation that a well-known question from Pargament's (1997) work on religious coping (turning to God for strength and guidance) was confusing because older people viewed "strength" and "guidance" as two different reasons for turning to God.

One of the great gaps in the development of multidimensional measures of religiosity lies in the lack of knowledge about how to assess religiosity in persons with dementia. A *PsycInfo* search on "dementia" and "religiosity" yielded only one study that included persons with dementia, but only nine out of 109 participants had dementia and most of them could not complete the 88-item questionnaires by themselves (Koenig, Moberg, & Kvale, 1988). Currently, about 10% of persons over 65 and 50% of persons over 85 have Alzheimer's disease, the most common cause of dementia in older people (Alzheimer's Association, 2003). Given the high degree of religiousness observed in elders who do not suffer dementia, one might assume many persons with dementia once led active and meaningful religious lives. Observations by chaplains, social workers, and others who work with institutionalized persons with dementia reveal that many participate in religious activities, often showing startling lucidity as they recite texts, sing hymns, and participate in rituals (Shamy, 2003).

Researchers rarely attempt to interview people with dementia to learn about their hopes, sources of meaning, and perceived quality of life. If we are indeed entering an era when the personhood of people with dementia will be honored (Kitwood, 1998), then researchers are going to need to devise ways of assessing their religious and spiritual needs and whether they are being met. Paper-and-pencil surveys will probably yield little usable data, so other methods will have to be devised. In addition to interviews, careful behavioral observations can be conducted. An example was a study of a group of persons living in a small dementia care unit that noted behaviors reflecting aspects of Emmons's (1999) construct of "spiritual intelligence" (McFadden, Ingram, & Baldauf, 2000).

Theories and Research Methods

Considerable gerontological research has been designed and conducted with little explicit reference to the metatheoretical perspectives and theoretical frameworks that guided the development of hypotheses, selection of participants, measures and research design, and interpretations of findings. One of the "founding fathers" of geropsychology, James Birren, has often described studies of aging as "data-rich and theory-poor" (1988, p. 155). Two books devoted to correcting this situation have made important contributions (Bengston & Schaie, 1999; Birren & Bengston, 1988), but neither contains any reference to research on the psychology of religion, nor does a collection of theoretical essays on the psychology of religion contain any specific reference to the study of aging and older adults except for one table addressing religious development from birth through old age (Reich, 1997).

One notable exception to the "theory-poor" condition in studies of religion and aging is found in the work of Neal Krause and his colleagues. In research on aging, religious doubt, and well-being, they tested Festinger's theory of cognitive dissonance (doubt as detrimental) and Piaget's theory of disequilibrium in cognitive development (doubt as beneficial) (Krause, Ingersoll-Dayton, Ellison, & Wulff, 1999). Identity theory predicted that older adults would experience more deleterious effects of religious doubt due to their loss of multiple role identifications. In contrast, Erikson's work on the late life struggle between integrity and despair suggested that doubt would be less problematic for older people because they are actively engaged in a life review process to formulate an integrated perspective on the life span. The research that tested these four theories showed that religious doubt was related to a reduction in psychological well-being and older people experienced less vulnerability to the effects of religious doubt than younger people. Other examples of Krause's care in establishing the theoretical basis of his research include a study on forgiveness and older adults' well-being (Krause & Ellison, 2003) and an examination of the relation between church-based social support and older adults' health (Krause, 2002b).

In addition to his insistence on clearly delineating the theoretical underpinnings of his research, Krause's work is notable also because of his use of large, national probability samples as well as small focus groups and interviews with older persons (Krause, 2002a; Krause, Chatters, Meltzer, & Morgan, 2000). Interest in qualitative gerontology as a complement to quantitative methods is growing as researchers broaden their epistemological perspectives, pay attention to outliers instead of focusing only on central tendency, and recognize the active, interrelated subjectivity of researchers and research participants (Reinharz & Rowles, 1988; Rowles & Schoenberg, 2001). Susan Eisenhandler (2003), a longtime proponent of qualitative gerontology, has identified two dimensions of older adults' religious faith: *reflexive faith* based on "religious folkways" that guide behaviors without a person's conscious investment in their meaning, and *reflective faith* that involves wrestling with what is believed, why religion is important, and the way faith shapes responses to the challenges of late life. Another example of a qualitative approach is Ramsey and Blieszner's (1999) investigation of spiritual resiliency in older women. Their interviews and focus groups uncovered the significance of the communal component of religious life, emotions shared in religious settings, and the religious roots of interpersonal relationships. Ramsey and Blieszner's work not only employed qualitative methodology, but it was also guided by feminist theorizing about human relationships and the social construction of meaning. Their work exemplifies the postmodern feminist perspective on gerontology that has the potential to produce new ways of theorizing about and investigating late life religiousness and spirituality (Ray & McFadden, 2001).

Longitudinal Research

Gerontologists agree that longitudinal research offers the best way of understanding the factors that shape late life religiosity and its effects on variables like well-being. Most longitudinal research takes two forms: follow-ups of populations originally examined in cross-sectional studies and secondary analysis of archived longitudinal data sets (Schaie & Hofer, 2001). An example of the former approach comes from Idler and Kasl's studies of the relation between religion and health. Cross-sectional and longitudinal analyses showed a greater effect on functional ability from religious attendance than from subjective religious involvement. Their research also showed that persons experiencing short-term reduction in function, and thus a decline in religious participation, went back to previous levels of attendance as soon as possible (Idler & Kasl, 1997a, 1997b). Several years later, Idler, Kasl, and Hays (2001) returned to this large, religiously diverse sample of older people and studied religious practices and beliefs among persons who died within 6 or 12 months of the last interview and those who survived past 12 months. Their prospective design allowed them to conclude that only those persons in the last 6 months of life declined in their levels of religious participation; subjective religiousness showed no decline at all, and in some cases it increased.

Wink and Dillon studied spiritual development across the life course using archived data collected from two birth cohorts (1920/1921 and 1928/1929) originally involved in research conducted by the Institute for Human Development at the University of California, Berkeley. This data set, generated from interviews conducted from childhood to old age, was not originally meant to disclose insights on religion and spirituality. However, Wink and Dillon coded for spirituality by defining it as a "search for connectedness with a sacred Other" (2002, p. 84) and coded for religiosity through answers to questions about religious attendance and the centrality of religion in participants' lives. They found a significant increase in spirituality from midlife to older adulthood (late 60s and beyond), particularly among women. Other analyses of this data set have related personality characteristics of self-confidence, intellectual engagement, and dependability in youth to a continuity of religious involvement across adulthood into old age (Clausen, 1993; see also McFadden, 1999).

In recent years, there has been an important convergence of developments in statistical analyses with the availability of longitudinal data. For example, the fifth edition of the *Handbook of the Psychology of Aging* contains a chapter on structural equation modeling in longitudinal research (Rudinger & Rietz, 2001), a topic not addressed in previous editions. This statistical technique is rapidly changing the study of aging and older adults and has begun to attract attention from researchers interested in religion. A recent paper addressed how structural equation modeling and latent growth curve analysis can be applied to the study of aging persons' religiousness and spirituality (Brennan & Mroczek, 2002).

Diversity

An important contribution of the last two decades of study of older adults' religiousness and spirituality has been the attention given to gender, racial, and religious differences. The observation that men are less religious than women is, as Rodney Stark has declared, a phenomenon that "holds around the world and across the centuries" (2002, p. 495), as well as across age groups. Many researchers have noted that older African Americans are more likely to reap the protective benefits of public religious involvement and private religious practices than older whites (Krause, 2002b). In his research on older adults' views about death, Cicirelli (2002) addressed racial and gender differences, as well as the effects of class, educational level, and marital status. The persons who had the greatest confidence in the existence of a loving, forgiving God and an afterlife were African American women, all of whom were categorized as having low socioeconomic status.

Like many studies of religion and aging, Cicirelli's sample was primarily Christian. One aspect of diversity among older people needing more attention is in the area of religious diversity. Although most studies of older persons' religiousness use samples of Christians and Jews, one notable exception is the work of the late psychologist L. E. Thomas. He compared the religious worldviews and spiritual maturity of British Anglican men and Indian Hindu men (Thomas & Chambers, 1989; Thomas, 1994), concluding that the religious worldview of the Indian men provided both an individual and a cultural ground of meaning that was lacking in the British men's lives. Thomas (2001) later studied elderly Turkish Sufis in order to test Tornstam's (1994) theory of "gerotranscendence," which suggests that with aging comes increased life satisfaction due to a shift to a more cosmic, transcendent view of life compared to an earlier focus on pragmatism and materialism. Thomas concluded that Sufis high in gerotranscendence also showed high life satisfaction, but he also noted that persons can have high life satisfaction without experiencing gerotranscendence.

AT THE INTERSECTION OF THE PSYCHOLOGY OF RELIGION AND THE PSYCHOLOGY OF AGING

The call by Emmons and Paloutzian (2003) for a multilevel interdisciplinary paradigm for the psychology of religion comes at an important time for continued theoretical development and empirical investigation of religion and aging. The psychological level of analysis has been largely absent from studies of late life religiosity and spirituality primarily because sociologists have conducted most of this research. Thus, the last section of this chapter briefly suggests how knowledge accrued from studies of the psychology of aging can contribute to a psychology of religion. In addition, this section argues that researchers studying cognition and emotion in older persons need to be informed by the work of psychologists of religion.

Cognition

We now have considerable evidence regarding changes in the cognitive abilities of older adults and the person- and situation-specific factors that influence these changes (Wilson et al., 2002). However, there has been little effort to address the implications of these changes for religious life. For example, we know that older persons often experience difficulties with explicit memory for recently learned material as well as age-related declines in working memory. Whether this has any effect upon the ways elders process information in public religious activities like worship or in their private devotional lives has not been empirically investigated.

Frail persons often experience a diminution of cognitive resources, but they too can retain connection with the sacred. An example is a woman in her 90s who stated that she used to think about God, wondering if her behavior was acceptable, and musing over difficult and complex theological issues. Now, in very old age, she said, "I can't do much any more and I can't even think much, either. I forget a great deal." But she went on to state that she believed that her days spent looking out her window and *appreciating* the world were a deep expression of her faith. "Am I neglecting God because I don't think about him or talk to him any more? I don't think so. Somehow, I feel that my looking and loving is enough for God" (Thibault, 1993, p. 93). Her minimally cognitive experience of appreciation compensated for her lost ability for theological inquiry. In order to understand whether this woman's experience is normative in very elderly, frail persons with deep faith commitments, psychologists of religion need to collaborate with psychologists who study aging and cognition.

In addition to the need to study effects of normal and disease-related cognitive changes on religious beliefs and practice, researchers should pay closer attention to changes in the organization of thought that come with age. For example, Sinnott (1994) has written that spiritual development in later life should be addressed in light of theoretical developments in the area of postformal thought. Two necessary skills for this type of thinking are "cognizance of interpersonal cocreated reality . . . [and] knowledge of how to rise above a series of conflicting truths to choose among them" (p. 93). Although Sinnott suggested a number of testable hypotheses on postformal cognition and spirituality in 1994, researchers and funding sources invested most of their time and resources in studies of religion, health, and well-being.

The characteristics of postformal thought depicted by Sinnott relate to certain work on moral reasoning and decision making, another area of research that has received far too little attention from psychologists who study older persons. There is some evidence that older persons may decline in their ability to take the moral perspective of others and to think in a complex way about other persons' situations (Pratt, Diessner, Pratt, Hunsberger, & Pancer, 1996), but whether this might be affected by active engagement in religious activities is unknown. Much work is needed on the impact of religious faith on social-cognitive processes. This is a prime example of how knowledge from the psychology of religion could contribute significantly to understanding older adult functioning. Another example concerns our lack of knowledge about how religious fundamentalism affects social cognition in older persons. Pratt, Golding, and Hunter (1983) have suggested that older people show "increasing philosophical reflectiveness" (p. 286) in their moral judgments, but we do not know how they might be influenced by religious funda mentalism.

Emotion

Research by Laura Carstenen and her colleagues has shown that emotional salience does not decline with age (Carstensen & Turk-Charles, 1994), but that older adults become more selective about their social interactions as a way of regulating emotion (Carstensen, 1992). Socioemotional selectivity theory has been supported by research showing that older adults feel emotions no less keenly; however, they make decisions about the persons with whom they will interact and the situations in which they place themselves where emotions may be elicited. This could be one explanation for the findings of Idler and Kasl (1997a, 1997b) regarding the continued religious attendance even by older people with serious disabilities. Idler and Kasl suggest that positive emotions elicited in worship and the emotional support received from fellow congregants represent powerful motivators for religious attendance. Sometimes when older people are ill, the weather is bad, or transportation is unavailable, they stay home and listen to religious services on the radio or watch them on television. In other words, they are still selectively optimizing their experiences but with a form of compensation. This description reflects the metamodel of "selective optimization with compensation" developed by Baltes and Lang (1997) to describe behaviors related to older people's everyday functioning. Much more work needs to be done in order to get a richer picture of older adults' motivation, emotion, and social behavior in religious settings.

Patterns of specifically religious emotions in older persons also need to be investigated, particularly in relation to responses to stressful situations. Although Pargament and his colleagues have written several papers applying his theory of religious coping to clinical work with older adults (Devor & Pargament, 2003; Pargament, Van Haitsma, & Ensing, 1995), and have often included older people in their studies, we lack a body of research bringing what is presently known about late life emotionality together with the psychology of religious coping. Again, this is an area where the psychology of religion—especially the psychology of religious coping—could make an important contribution to gerontology.

An indication of the potential for this kind of cross-fertilization between research areas is found in a study that showed a strong relation between "hardiness" in older people and religiosity (Magai, Consedine, King, & Gillespie, 2003). *Hardiness* was defined as the ability to engage in activities of daily living; some persons display a physically robust, "intrinsic" hardiness, while others demonstrate "earned hardiness" despite their physical decline. Persons in the latter group cope adaptively with multiple health challenges and other adversities. Religious faith strongly contributed to this kind of hardiness. In addition, persons who showed high levels of negative emotion were less likely to manifest either type of hardiness. Does this mean that religious faith and participation might support positive emotions? As suggested by Idler and Kasl's work, religious participation not only can provide multiple sources of positive emotion, but the faith that motivates people to engage in this behavior also offers support for regulating and coping with negative emotions (McFadden, 2003).

Beginning in the 1980s, evidence emerged that older adults spontaneously mention religious coping far more often than other forms of coping with major life stressors

(Koenig, George, & Siegler, 1988). As McFadden and Levin (1996) noted, religious coping points older persons toward the protective haven provided by a secure relationship with the divine; likewise, those secure relationships provide the base from which elders can venture into daily life with its many challenges and threats. Kirkpatrick's (1992) theoretical and empirical contributions in showing the application of attachment theory to religion demonstrate how work in the psychology of religion can suggest new lines of research on late life religiosity. In addition, researchers need to attend to the attachment dynamics expressed by some persons with dementia whose behavior in religious settings indicates their continued ability to connect emotionally with the transcendent.

Several recent studies have shown that the social support found in faith communities significantly contributes to physical and mental health (Krause, 2002b; Nooney & Woodrum, 2002). Often these communities are viewed as familial, and in some, fellow congregants refer to one another as "sister" and "brother." Thus, in addition to an emotional attachment to the sacred, older persons may develop emotional attachments to their faith communities, attachments that provide succor in times of trouble and courage to resolve problems, grow spiritually, and experience joy in late life (McFadden & Levin, 1996). This is an area wide open to future research.

Finally, some have suggested that later adulthood may be a time when people can become more open to emotional experiences of the transcendent, even to the point of mystical experiences (Atchley, 1997), but little systematic study of this possibility has been done. This represents yet another area in which collaborations between gerontologists and psychologists of religion could be very fruitful. In addition, the emotions evoked by art, music, drama, poetry, dance, and other arts that point elders toward the sacred have not been widely studied, although recent evidence from Wuthnow's (2003) research indicates that people interested in the arts also are more likely to be interested in spiritual growth. Given the intense interest in the arts expressed by many older people, as well as the recognition by some continuing care retirement communities of the importance of providing high-quality arts experiences for residents, it would seem reasonable to expect that for some older persons the arts represent an important pathway to religious emotion and meaning.

SOME CONCLUDING THOUGHTS

The multilevel, interdisciplinary paradigm for the psychology of religion proposed by Emmons and Paloutzian (2003) has the potential to bring the psychology of religion into conversation with gerontology to form a relationship that can benefit both fields. Gerontology has embraced this paradigm since its inception in the middle of the 20th century. A few gerontologists have always shown some interest in religion (e.g., Maves, 1960), but it has only been in the last two decades that research on religion and aging has become more widely accepted in the field due to the use of multidimensional measures, national probability samples, and more sophisticated designs and analyses. Sociologists conducted most of this research, but, as this chapter has demonstrated, there is much work yet to be done by psychologists of religion. In addition, philosophers, theologians, artists, and others representing the humanities need to be brought into the conversation in order to understand more fully a time of life uniquely "colored by awareness of a powerfully ambiguous future" (Rubinstein, 2002, p. 39).

William James never explicated his reasons for calling late life the "religious age *par excellence,*" but perhaps he was thinking about the way aging illuminates existential questions about the meaning of longevity along with religious questions about ultimate meaning. Students of the human lifespan generally agree that aging produces both growth and decline of adaptive capacity (Baltes, 1987). However, individual, cultural, and cosmic meanings that might grant some coherent perspective on the melding of gain and loss in old age have been severely eroded (Cole, 1992; Moody, 1985). Thus, the contextual backdrop for the research and scholarship reviewed in this chapter has been characterized as postmodernity, a period of profound uncertainty about the value and meaning of old age (Polivka, 2000).

As the 21st century opens with anticipation of so many people living longer, the issues addressed in this *Handbook* will become increasingly important for understanding older adults' responses to late life challenges. For many, but certainly not all older people, faith communities, religious beliefs, and experiences of the sacred will contribute to life quality and meaning. As the "longevity revolution" continues through the next 50 years, psychologists will need to employ multilevel, interdisciplinary approaches in order to understand more fully the varieties and the fruits of the "search for significance" in old age and how that search is "related to the sacred" (Pargament, 1997, p. 32).

REFERENCES

Administration on Aging. (2003). *A profile of older Americans 2002.* Retrieved October 2, 2003, from www.aoa.gov/prof/Statistics/profile/2.asp.

Ainlay, S. C., & Smith, D. R. (1984). Aging and religious participation. *Journal of Gerontology, 39,* 357–363.

Altemeyer, B. (2004). The decline of organized religion in Western civilization. *The International Journal for the Psychology of Religion, 14,* 77–89.

Alzheimer's Association. (2003). *Statistics about Alzheimer's disease.* Retrieved October 2, 2003, from www.alz.org/AboutAD/Statistics.htm.

Atchley, R. C. (1997). Everyday mysticism: Spiritual development in later adulthood. *Journal of Adult Development, 4,* 123–234.

Baltes, M. M., & Lang, F. R. (1997). Everyday functioning and successful aging: The impact of resources. *Psychology and Aging, 12,* 433–443.

Baltes, P. B. (1987). Theoretical propositions of life-span developmental psychology: On the dynamics between growth and decline. *Developmental Psychology, 23,* 611–626.

Bengston, V. L., & Schaie, K. W. (Eds.). (1999). *Handbook of theories of aging.* New York: Springer.

Birren, J. E. (1988). A contribution to the theory of the psychology of aging: As a counterpart of development. In J. E. Birren & V. L. Bengston (Eds.), *Emergent theories of aging* (pp. 153–176). New York: Springer.

Birren, J. E., & Bengston, V. L. (Eds.). (1988). *Emergent theories of aging.* New York: Springer.

Birren, J. E., & Schroots, J. J. F. (1996). History, concepts, and theory in the psychology of aging. In J. E. Birren & K. W. Schaie (Eds.), *Handbook of the psychology of aging* (4th ed., pp. 3–23). San Diego: Academic Press.

Brennan, M., & Mroczek, D. K. (2002). Examining spirituality over time: Latent growth curve and individual growth curve analyses. *Journal of Religious Gerontology, 14*(1), 11–29.

Carstensen, L. L. (1992). Social and emotional patterns in adulthood: Support for socioemotional selectivity theory. *Psychology and Aging, 7,* 331–338.

Carstensen, L. L., & Turk-Charles, S. (1994). The salience of emotion across the adult life span. *Psychology and Aging, 9,* 259–264.

Chatters, L. M., Levin, J. W., & Taylor, R. J. (1992). Antecedents and dimensions of religious involvement among older black adults. *Journal of Gerontology: Social Sciences*, 47, S269–S278.

Chatters, L. M., & Taylor, R. J. (1989). Age differences in religious participation among black adults. *Journal of Gerontology: Social Sciences*, 44, S183–S189.

Cicirelli, V. G. (2002). *Older adults' views on death*. New York: Springer.

Clausen, J. (1993). *American lives: Looking back at the Great Depression*. New York: Free Press.

Cole, T. R. (1992). *The journey of life: A cultural history of aging in America*. New York: Cambridge University Press.

Devor, N. G., & Pargament, K. I. (2003). Understanding religious coping with late-life crises. In M. A. Kimble & S. H. McFadden (Eds.), *Aging, spirituality, and religion: A handbook* (Vol. 2, pp. 195–205). Minneapolis: Fortress Press.

Eisenhandler, S. A. (2003). *Keeping the faith in late life*. New York: Springer.

Emmons, R. A. (1999). *The psychology of ultimate concerns: Motivation and spirituality in personality*. New York: Guilford Press.

Emmons, R. A., & Paloutzian, R. F. (2003). The psychology of religion. *Annual Review of Psychology*, 54, 377–402.

Fahey, C. J., & Lewis, M. A. (1984). Catholics. In E. B. Palmore (Ed.), *Handbook on the aged in the United States* (pp. 145–154). Westport, CT: Greenwood Press.

Fetzer Institute/National Institute on Aging Working Group. (1999). *Multidimensional measurement of religiousness/spirituality for use in health research*. Kalamazoo, MI: Fetzer Institute.

Futterman, A., Dillon, J. J., Garand, F., & Haugh, J. (1999). Religion as a quest and the search for meaning in later life. In L. E. Thomas & S. A. Eisenhandler (Eds.), *Religion, belief, and spirituality in late life* (pp. 153–177). New York: Springer.

Futterman, A., & Koenig, H. G. (1995, March). *Measuring religiosity in later life: What gerontology can learn from the psychology and sociology of religion*. Paper presented at the National Institute on Aging/Fetzer Institute conference, "Methodological approaches to the study of religion, health, and aging," Bethesda, MD.

Idler, E. L., & Kasl, S. V. (1997a). Religion among disabled and nondisabled persons: I. Cross-sectional patterns in health practices, social activities, and well-being. *Journal of Gerontology: Social Sciences*, 52B, S294–S305.

Idler, E. L., & Kasl, S. V. (1997b). Religion among disabled and nondisabled persons: II. Attendance at religious services as a predictor of the course of disability. *Journal of Gerontology: Social Sciences*, 52B, S306–S316.

Idler, E. L., Kasl, S. V., & Hays, J. C. (2001). Patterns of religious practice and belief in the last year of life. *Journal of Gerontology: Social Sciences*, 56B, S326–S334.

James, W. (1961). *The varieties of religious experience*. New York: Collier Books. (Original work published 1902)

Kirkpatrick, L. A. (1992). An attachment-theory approach to the psychology of religion. *The International Journal for the Psychology of Religion*, 2, 3–28.

Kitwood, T. (1998). *Dementia reconsidered: The person comes first*. Philadelphia: Open University Press.

Koenig, H. G., George, L. K., & Siegler, I. C. (1988). The use of religion and other emotion-regulating coping strategies among older adults. *The Gerontologist*, 28, 303–310.

Koenig, H. G., Moberg, D. O., & Kvale, J. N. (1988). Religious activities and attitudes of older adults in a geriatric assessment clinic. *Journal of the American Geriatrics Society*, 36, 362–374.

Koenig, H. G., Smiley, M., & Gonzales, J. A. P. (1988). *Religion, health, and aging: A review and theoretical integration*. New York: Greenwood Press.

Krause, N. (2002a). A comprehensive strategy for developing closed-end survey items for use in studies of older adults. *Journal of Gerontology: Social Sciences*, 57B, S263–S274.

Krause, N. (2002b). Church-based social support and health in old age: Exploring variations by race. *Journal of Gerontology: Social Sciences*, 57B, S323–S347.

Krause, N. (2003). Religious meaning and subjective well-being in late life. *Journal of Gerontology: Social Sciences, 58B*, S160–S170.

Krause, N., Chatters, L. M., Meltzer, T., & Morgan, D. L. (2000). Using focus groups to explore the nature of prayer in late life. *Journal of Aging Studies, 14*, 191–212.

Krause, N., & Ellison, C. G. (2003). Forgiveness by God, forgiveness of others, and psychological well-being in late life. *Journal for the Scientific Study of Religion, 42*, 77–93.

Krause, N., Ingersoll-Dayton, B., Ellison, C. G., & Wulff, K. M. (1999). Aging, religious doubt, and psychological well-being. *The Gerontologist, 39*, 525–533.

Magai, C., Consedine, N. S., King, A. R., & Gillespie, M. (2003). Physical hardiness and styles of socioemotional functioning in later life. *Journal of Gerontology: Psychological Sciences, 56B*, P269–P279.

Marler, P. L., & Hadaway, C. K. (2002). "Being religious" or "being spiritual" in America: A zero-sum proposition? *Journal for the Scientific Study of Religion, 41*, 289–300.

Maves, P. B. (1960). Aging, religion, and the church. In C. Tibbitts (Ed.), *Handbook of social gerontology* (pp. 698–749). Chicago: University of Chicago Press.

McFadden, S. H. (1995). Religion and well-being in aging persons in an aging society. *Journal of Social Issues, 51*(2), 161–175.

McFadden, S. H. (1999). Religion, personality, and aging: A life span perspective. *Journal of Personality, 67*, 1081–1104.

McFadden, S. H. (2003). Older adults' emotions in religious contexts. In M. A. Kimble & S. H. McFadden (Eds.), *Aging, spirituality, and religion: A handbook* (Vol. 2, pp. 47–58). Minneapolis: Fortress Press.

McFadden, S. H., & Atchley, R. C. (Eds.). (2001). *Aging and the meaning of time: A multidisciplinary exploration.* New York: Springer.

McFadden, S. H., Ingram, M., & Baldauf, C. (2000). Actions, feelings, and values: Foundations of meaning and personhood in dementia. *Journal of Religious Gerontology, 11*(3–4), 67–86.

McFadden, S. H., & Levin, J. S. (1996). Religion, emotions, and health. In C. Magai & S. H. McFadden (Eds.), *Handbook of emotion, adult development, and aging* (pp. 349–365). San Diego: Academic Press.

Mindel, C. H., & Vaughan, C. E. (1978). A multidimensional approach to religiosity and disengagement. *Journal of Gerontology, 33*, 103–108.

Moberg, D. O. (1997). Religion and aging. In K. F. Ferraro (Ed.), *Gerontology: Perspectives and issues* (2nd ed., pp. 193–220). New York: Springer.

Moody, H. R. (1985). The meaning of life and the meaning of old age. In T. R. Cole & S. Gadow (Eds.), *What does it mean to grow old?: Reflections from the humanities* (pp. 9–40). Durham, NC: Duke University Press.

Myerhoff, B. (1978). *Number our days.* New York: Simon & Schuster.

Nelson-Becker, H. B. (2003). Practical philosophies: Interpretations of religion and spirituality by African American and European American elders. *Journal of Religious Gerontology, 14*, 85–99.

Nooney, J., & Woodrum, E. (2002). Religious coping and church-based social support as predictors of mental health outcomes: Testing a conceptual model. *Journal for the Scientific Study of Religion, 41*, 359–368.

Pargament, K. I. (1997). *The psychology of religion and coping.* New York: Guilford Press.

Pargament, K. I., Van Haitsma, K. S., & Ensing, D. (1995). Religion and coping. In M. A. Kimble, S. H. McFadden, J. W. Ellor, & J. J. Seeber (Eds.), *Aging, spirituality, and religion: A handbook* (pp. 47–67). Minneapolis: Fortress Press.

Payne, B. P. (1984). Protestants. In E. B. Palmore (Ed.), *Handbook on the aged in the United States* (pp. 181–198). Westport, CT: Greenwood Press.

Polivka, L. (2000). Postmodern aging and the loss of meaning. *Journal of Aging and Identity, 5*, 225–235.

Pratt, M. W., Diessner, R., Pratt, A., Hunsberger, B., & Pancer, S. M. (1996). Moral and social reasoning and perspective taking in later life: A longitudinal study. *Psychology and Aging, 11*, 66–73.

Pratt, M. W., Golding, G., & Hunter, W. J. (1983). Aging as ripening: Character and consistency of moral judgment in young, mature, and older adults. *Human Development, 26,* 277–288.

Ramsey, J. L., & Blieszner, R. (2000). *Spiritual resiliency in older women: Models of strength for challenges through the life span.* Thousand Oaks, CA: Sage.

Ray, R. E., & McFadden, S. H. (2001). The web and the quilt: Alternatives to the heroic journey toward spiritual development. *Journal of Adult Development, 8,* 201–211.

Reich, K. H. (1997). Integrating differing theories: The case of religious development. In B. Spilka & D. N. McIntosh (Eds.), *The psychology of religion: Theoretical approaches* (pp. 105–113). Boulder, CO: Westview Press.

Reinharz, S., & Rowles, G. D. (Eds.). (1988). *Qualitative gerontology.* New York: Springer.

Roof, W. D., & McKinney, W. (1987). *American mainline religion: Its changing shape and future.* New Brunswick, NJ: Rutgers University Press.

Rowles, G. D., & Schoenberg, N. E. (Eds.). (2001). *Qualitative gerontology: A contemporary perspective.* New York: Springer.

Rubinstein, R. L. (2002). The third age. In R. S. Weiss & S. A. Bass (Eds.), *Challenges of the third age: Meaning and purpose in later life* (pp. 29–40). New York: Oxford University Press.

Rudinger, G., & Rietz, C. (2001). Structural equation modeling in longitudinal research on aging. In J. E. Birren & K. W. Schaie (Eds.), *Handbook of the psychology of aging* (5th ed., pp. 29–52). San Diego: Academic Press.

Schaie, K. W., & Hofer, S. M. (2001). Longitudinal studies in aging research. In J. E. Birren & K. W. Schaie (Eds.), *Handbook of the psychology of aging* (5th ed., pp. 53–77). San Diego: Academic Press.

Shamy, E. (2003). *A guide to the spiritual dimension of care for people with Alzheimer's disease and related dementia: More than body, brain, and breath.* London: Jessica Kingsley.

Sinnott, J. D. (1994). Development and yearning: Cognitive aspects of spiritual development. *Journal of Adult Development, 1,* 91–99.

Stark, R. (2002). Physiology and faith: Addressing the "universal" gender difference in religious commitment. *Journal for the Scientific Study of Religion, 41,* 495–507.

Tapanya, S., Nicki, R., & Jarusawad, O. (1997). Worry and intrinsic/extrinsic religious orientation among Buddhist (Thai) and Christian (Canadian) elderly persons. *International Journal of Aging and Human Development, 44,* 73–83.

Thibault, J. M. (1993). *A deepening love affair: The gift of God in later life.* Nashville, TN: Upper Room Books.

Thomas, L. E. (1994). The way of the religious renouncer: Power through nothingness. In L. E. Thomas & S. A. Eisenhandler (Eds.), *Aging and the religious dimension* (pp. 51–64). Westport, CT: Auburn House.

Thomas, L. E. (1999). Quarreling with God: Belief and disbelief among elderly Jewish immigrants from the former USSR. In L. E. Thomas & S. A. Eisenhandler (Eds.), *Religion, belief, and spirituality in late life* (pp. 73–92). New York: Springer.

Thomas, L. E. (2001). The Job hypothesis: Gerotranscendence and life satisfaction among elderly Turkish Muslims. In S. H. McFadden & R. C. Atchley (Eds.), *Aging and the meaning of time: A multidisciplinary exploration* (pp. 207–227). New York: Springer.

Thomas, L. E., & Chambers, K. O. (1989). "Successful aging" among elderly men in England and India: A phenomenological comparison. In L. E. Thomas (Ed.), *Research on adulthood and aging: The human science approach* (pp. 183–203). Albany: State University of New York Press.

Thompson, E. H., Noone, M. E., & Guarino, A. B. (2003). Widows' spiritual journeys: Do they quest? *Journal of Religious Gerontology, 14,* 119–138.

Tornstam, L. (1994). Gero-transcendence: A theoretical and empirical exploration. In L. E. Thomas & S. A. Eisenhandler (Eds.), *Aging and the religious dimension* (pp. 203–225). Westport, CT: Auburn House.

Weiss, R. S., & Bass, S. A. (2002). *Challenges of the third age: Meaning and purpose in later life.* New York: Oxford University Press.

Wilson, R. S., Beckett, L. A., Barnes, L. L., Schneider, J. A., Bach, J., Evans, D. A., & Bennett, D. A. (2002). Individual differences in rates of change in cognitive abilities of older persons. *Psychology and Aging, 17*, 179–193.

Wink, P., & Dillon, M. (2002). Spiritual development across the adult life course: Findings from a longitudinal study. *Journal of Adult Development, 9*, 79–94.

Wuthnow, R. (2003). *All in sync: How music and art are revitalizing American religion.* Berkeley: University of California Press.

10

Religion's Role in Marriage and Parenting in Daily Life and during Family Crises

ANNETTE MAHONEY
NALINI TARAKESHWAR

In a 1995 Gallup poll of U.S. families, 65% of mothers and 57% of fathers said that religion was "extremely" or "very" important in their lives (Mahoney et al., 1999). About 90% of the U.S. population desire religious training for their children (Gallup & Castelli, 1989) and 55% of married individuals (Heaton & Pratt, 1990) attend religious services at least several times a year. Thus, a vast audience in the United States is presumably receptive to messages that can be drawn from religion about family relationships. In turn, empirical studies from past decades indicate that religion is an important factor linked to marital and parental functioning (e.g., Dollahite, Marks, & Goodman, 2004; Mahoney, Pargament, Tarakeshwar, & Swank, 2001).

Yet psychologists have produced little theory or research on the role of religion in family life. In hopes of stimulating more psychological research on religion and family relationships, we begin this chapter with a review of empirical findings on key aspects of religion and family life over the past 25 years. In this section, we discuss the role of religion in marital and parent–child subsystems in daily life as well as during various family crises. We also delineate major conceptual and methodological challenges left to be tackled in the field of religion and family life. We end the chapter by offering illustrative theoretical constructs for how religion might operate during normative family transitions and family crises.

EMPIRICAL RESEARCH ON RELIGION AND FAMILY LIFE

Family psychology encompasses the study of different family relationships during normative stages of the family life cycle and family crises. Several comprehensive reviews of research on religion and family life have recently been published (Dollahite et al., 2004; Mahoney et al., 2001; Sherkat, & Ellison, 1999). In this section, we review research on religion and daily life across the domains of marital functioning, the transition to parenthood, and the parenting of children and adolescents. We then discuss research on family crises including marital infidelity, divorce, domestic violence, child abuse, and raising a child with special needs.

To convey well-documented empirical findings in this chapter, we cite effect sizes calculated in a study by Mahoney et al. (2001) where meta-analytical techniques were used to summarize religion–family links reported at least five times across three or more studies. These quantitative studies reported bivariate associations between religious variables and marital and parental functioning and were published during the 1980s and 1990s. The majority of these studies (87%) involved national or community samples. This minimizes the concern that findings were biased by the selection of highly religious individuals from religious organizations. But, as is typical of large surveys, most of the marital (80%) and parenting (66%) studies relied only on single-item markers of religiousness, such as religious affiliation, frequency of church attendance or prayer, and overall importance of religion. Not surprisingly, the average effect sizes were therefore small in size. Nevertheless, such associations across large heterogenous samples are impressive since global items have very limited variability. For less well-established findings, we discuss studies that are especially noteworthy on conceptual or methodological grounds.

Religion and Daily Life in Families

Marital Functioning

Global Marital Satisfaction. Two pieces of evidence indicate that greater involvement in religion is tied to spouses' global satisfaction with their marriage based on a single items (e.g., "Taking all things together, how would you describe your marriage: very happy, pretty happy, not too happy") or brief questionnaires surveying a wide range of marital issues. First, more frequent church attendance covaries with greater marital satisfaction (average $r = .07$; Mahoney et al., 2001). Second, and more compelling, the personal relevance of religion relates to greater marital satisfaction with an average r of .15 (Mahoney et al., 2001). The latter variable includes single-item ratings of the importance of religion and frequency of prayer or Bible reading, as well as more complex questionnaires about personal religiousness. This suggests more in-depth indices of religiousness could better account for marital satisfaction.

Two important moderators of links between religion and marital satisfaction have been identified. First, in a methodologically rigorous longitudinal study, Sullivan (2001) found that global religiosity promoted marital satisfaction for newlyweds over time, but only for couples with husbands with relatively greater mental health. Both husbands and wives in more religious couples with a more "neurotic" (reactive, negative) husband were less satisfied. Thus, in marriages where both partners fulfill normative expectations of healthy behavior, religion may heighten marital satisfaction; but in couples with a distressed partner, greater religiousness may exacerbate marital difficulties. Second, personal religiousness is especially predictive of marital happiness for churchgoing people ($r = .27$; Mahoney et al., 2001). But contrary to the notion that greater religiousness is merely a marker of marital conventionalization, religiousness remains tied to marital satisfaction after controlling this variable (Wilson & Filsinger, 1986).

Marital Commitment. Several researchers have examined the idea that more religious people are more committed to marriage than less religious people (Mahoney et al., 2001). Efforts to assess commitment have included direct inquiry about investment in the marriage and inferring commitment from the costs of losing the marriage. Greater individual religiousness, as reflected by global items, is consistently tied to greater commitment (average effect size of $r = .19$; Mahoney et al., 2001). Furthermore, two studies have found that greater church attendance relates to marital commitment even after taking into account demographic factors and marital or family satisfaction (Larson & Goltz, 1989; Wilson & Musick, 1996). In addition, couples' religious homogamy (i.e., shared religious affiliation, church attendance, and/or beliefs) has been repeatedly tied to greater marital commitment (average $r = .097$; Mahoney et al., 2001). Sharing deeply held religious values about investing in their marriage over the long term may help couples cement a long-range "couple identity," which other research has tied to greater sacrifices and harmony within the relationship (Stanley & Markman, 1992).

Marital Verbal Conflict and Conflict-Resolution Strategies. Research indicates that religion is a topic about which couples rarely directly argue (Oggins, 2003). Also, contrary to concerns that more religious people may tolerate conflict to stay together, spouses' personal religiousness is unrelated to the frequency of marital disputes (Mahoney et al., 2001). However, the extent to which couples share religiously based views of particular topics may inhibit conflict about these issues (Mahoney, 2005). For example, greater religious similarity between spouses has been tied to fewer arguments (Curtis & Ellison, 2002) and lower divorce rates (Call & Heaton, 1997). Conversely, marked disparities in spouses' beliefs about the Bible generate more conflict about housework and money (Curtis & Ellison, 2002). Although few couples report such polarization, couples argue more often about how they spend time and about in-laws when the wife holds much more conservative biblical beliefs than her husband, and more childrearing disputes arise for couples when the husband is more conservative than his wife (Curtis & Ellison, 2002).

Religion also offers couples guidelines to resolve conflict after it erupts (Mahoney, 2005). Several studies indicate that greater religiousness is tied to more constructive conflict-resolution strategies. For instance, Brody, Stoneman, Flor, and McCrary (1994) found that greater self-rated religiousness was tied to better marital communication skills during direct observations of African American families. Mahoney et al. (1999) also found that Caucasian couples who engaged in more joint religious activities and viewed their marriage as sacred said they more often resolved conflict via collaborative discussion. Further, greater religiousness has not been linked to counterproductive problem-solving strategies, such as yelling or stonewalling (Mahoney et al., 1999). Likewise, no differences have emerged in the level of negative communication patterns in marriages of fundamentalist than nonfundamentalist Protestants (e.g., Schumm, Ja Jeong, & Silliman, 1990). In sum, evidence suggests that greater religiousness is linked to less frequent marital conflict and better communication patterns. More research is needed on how (dis)similarities in spouses' religiously based values could moderate conflict.

Transition to Parenthood

Greater church attendance has been consistently tied to higher birthrates (Krishnan, 1993). Other research suggests that the birth of a child may trigger a transformation in the spiritual orientation of parents, such that mothers in particular attend church more frequently and experience a heightened sense of the importance of God (Becker & Hofmeister, 2001). One qualitative study has also found that the birth or presence of children prompted religious introspection or involvement for some men (Palkovitz, 2002). Although such evidence implies that religion may ease the transition from childlessness to parenthood, only a few studies have directly addressed this topic.

In terms of obstetric outcomes, King and Hueston (1994) found that rates of maternal complications and neonatal intensive care were lowest for mainline Christian women, intermediate for evangelical Christians, and highest for patients with no religious preference. Even after controlling for socioeconomic confounds, mothers from mainline churches had a lower rate of complications, and mothers who reported any type of religious affiliation had infants with a lower risk of neonatal intensive care. In addition, Magana and Clark (1995) argue that religious factors partly account for the well-established but paradoxical findings on obstetric outcomes for Mexican American women. Despite their relatively low socioeconomic status, Mexican American women deliver significantly fewer low-birth-weight babies and lose fewer babies to all causes during infancy than do women of other non-Angelo ethnic groups and are on par with more socioeconomically advantaged Caucasian groups. Magana and Clark speculate that more religiously devout Mexican American women turn to feminine religious figures (e.g., the Virgin of Guadalupe) as positive role models, which facilitates pre- and postnatal health care and coping with an infant.

To our knowledge, only one longitudinal study has assessed the role of religion and marital adjustment before and after the birth of a child. Wilcox and Wolfinger (2003) found that urban mothers who attend church regularly were more likely to be married at the time of birth than those who rarely attend church, and women who had a nonmarital birth were more likely to marry within a year if they attend church frequently. These religious effects were partly mediated by the relationship-related beliefs and behaviors promoted by churches. Churchgoing mothers expressed higher levels of commitment to the institution of marriage. They were also more likely to receive higher levels of supportive behavior (e.g., affection) from the child's father and have less conflict with the father over sexual fidelity. These findings imply that religion may serve as a protective resource for marriages during the transition to parenthood.

Parenting of Children

Discipline Practices. The bulk of research on religion and parenting has focused on whether Christian conservatism is tied to attitudes about, and the use of, corporal punishment with preschoolers and schoolage children. Such hypotheses are consistent with conservative theological views about discipline practices (see Ellison, 1996, for an excellent discussion). Adults who are affiliated with conservative Christian groups or who hold literalistic beliefs about the Bible have repeatedly been found to be more likely than other people to value child obedience (average $r = .18$) and believe in corporal punishment (average $r = .21$; Mahoney et al., 2001). Most of this attitudinal research has not, however, focused on parents. Fortunately, a study by Gershoff, Miller, and Holden (1999) provides unique insight into the topic. These researchers found that conservative Protestant parents of 3-year-olds are more likely than other parents to believe that spanking is a necessary, effective way to gain immediate and long-term obedience, and less likely to believe spanking has negative consequences, such as engendering fear or resentment. When asked to respond to vignettes that portrayed their child exhibiting increasing noncompliance, conservative Protestant parents also were more likely to select spanking and less likely to select reasoning to handle defiance. Finally, they were less likely to report feeling guilty about spanking. In terms of the actual use of corporal punishment, Christian conservatism is related to parental spanking of preadolescents with an average r = .09 (Mahoney et al., 2001). This effect is about half as robust as attitudinal links found in general adult samples. Research has also failed to substantiate concerns that conservative Christian membership or beliefs increase parents' use of nonphysical, aversive punishments (e.g., time-outs, threats, yelling; Gershoff et al., 1999) or severe physical discipline (e.g., hitting with fist; Mahoney et al., 2001).

When considering these findings, it is important to realize that the degree to which parents endorse biblical literalism (e.g., "The Bible is the actual word of God and is to be taken literally, word for word") or Christian fundamentalism (e.g., "The Bible is the answer to all important human problems") is more critical in predicting disciplinary attitudes or behavior than mere membership in a conservative Christian group. The former variables mediate links between religious denomination and both corporal punishment attitudes and behavior (e.g., Ellison, Bartkowski, & Segal, 1996). Finally, an interactive effect has been found between parents' orientation toward the Bible (liberal vs. conservative) and view parenting as a sacred endeavor when predicting corporal punishment. Murray-Swank, Mahoney, and Pargament (2003) found that greater sanctification of parenting was associated with decreased use of corporal punishment for mothers of young children who had more liberal beliefs about the Bible. In contrast, among more biblically conservative mothers, sanctification of parenting was unrelated to the frequency of corporal punishment. Thus, viewing parenting as a divine endeavor is tied to lower rates of corporal punishment, but only for parents who have a more liberal Christian religious orientation. Overall, these studies highlight the need to assess directly how much parents personally integrate particular religious beliefs into their views of parenting.

Warmth and Effective Parenting of Children. Numerous studies suggest that religion may be tied to more effective parenting, parental warmth, and family cohesiveness, but the diversity of samples and methodologies precludes the quantification of summary effect sizes (Mahoney et al., 2001). Thus, we highlight here five especially sophisticated studies. First, two excellent studies examining African American families of 9- to 12-year-olds indicate that parents' self-reported religiousness (church attendance rate multiplied by self-rated importance) is tied to better observed parenting and coparenting processes. Specifically, in Brody et al.'s study (1994), mothers' religiousness was related to more skilled parenting, less coparenting conflict, and better marital quality during observed family interactions. Greater religiousness of fathers was also tied to less coparenting conflict and better marital quality. Moreover, associations between parental religiousness and parenting skills were mediated through marital quality and coparenting skills. In the second study (Brody, Stoneman, & Flor, 1996), measures of child adjustment were used. Greater maternal and paternal religiousness were directly tied to fewer child behavior problems. Moreover, parental religiousness indirectly influenced youth self-regulation by promoting family cohesiveness and lowering marital conflict.

Wilcox (1998) also found that parents' level of endorsement of theologically conservative views about the Bible was related to self-reports of more frequent hugging and praising of preschool and schoolage children after controlling for religious and demographic factors. In a follow-up study, Wilcox (2002) found that conservative parents were also less likely than their nonconservative Protestant counterparts to yell at their preschool and schoolage children. Further, Murray-Swank et al. (2003) found that greater sanctification of parenting was tied to increased positive mother–child interactions when mothers had more conservative beliefs about the Bible. But among more liberal mothers, no link was found. Thus, even as parents with more conservative Christian beliefs are more inclined to spank their children, they are also likely to be warmer toward them, especially if they view parenting to be a sacred calling.

Parenting of Adolescents

Research clearly indicates that greater parental religiousness influences adolescents' adoption of religious beliefs and practices (e.g., Sherkat, 2003). In turn, adolescents' personal religiousness has been consistently tied to lower rates of delinquency, substance use, and premarital sexuality (e.g., Donahue & Benson, 1995) as well as to higher levels of positive outcomes (e.g., Regnerus, 2003). Surprisingly few studies, however, have directly investigated parental religiousness and parent–adolescent interactions, but available findings are encouraging.

Discipline Practices. We were unable to locate published empirical studies that directly address the overlap between religion and physical discipline of adolescents. However, in national surveys that combine youth from ages 2 to 18, significant correlations have not emerged between corporal punishment and either Christian conservatism (Alwin, 1986) or the general importance of religion (Jackson et al., 1999). Thus, links between conservative Christianity and corporal punishment seem to be restricted to families of younger children. A longitudinal study by Regnerus (2003) uncovered complex dynamics that may occur when highly devout religious parents try to control teenagers. Greater global religiousness by parents and adolescents was directly tied to less frequent serious delinquency for girls, but not boys. In addition, via the degree to which parents granted freedoms to their teenagers and the extent of teenagers' happiness with the family, parent religiosity predicted less teenage delinquency. However, these indirect pathways of influence were much stronger for girls. Taken together, this suggests that high levels of parental religiousness may "backfire" for sons who resist efforts to control their behavior, while daughters may be more open to similar efforts by highly religious parents.

Warmth and Positivity. Two rigorous studies suggest that religion facilitates positive parent–adolescent relationships. In a rare longitudinal study, Pearce and Axinn (1998) found that greater maternal religiousness when an adolescent was 18 predicted more positive parent–child relationship when the youth was 23 as reported by both parties. In addition, congruence at the end of high school between mothers' and youths' religious attendance and self-ratings of religion also predicted more positive mother–child relationship satisfaction 5 years later. Likewise, using a large national sample, Gunnoe, Hetherington, and Reiss (1999) found robust direct links between parental self-reports of greater personal religiousness and observations of greater authoritative parenting during dyadic problem-solving discussions between adolescents and both parents. Moreover, indirect pathways of influence were found for parental religiousness leading to greater social responsibility by adolescents through authoritative parenting.

Parental Gender and Family Life

Fathering. Since about 1995, a rapidly growing body of research has focused on religion and fatherhood (Dollahite et al., 2004). Based on national surveys, greater church attendance has been tied to more involvement by fathers' in youth activities (Wilcox, 2002) and greater paternal supervision, father–child interaction, and affection (Bartkowski & Xu, 2000). Further, King (2003) persuasively demonstrated that global paternal religiousness is tied to greater father–child relationship quality, positive expectations for future relationship, felt obligation, and effort devoted to parenting for married and divorced fathers, after controlling for demographic, marital, and family attitudinal mediators. Further, a series of papers by Dollahite and colleagues (e.g., Dollahite, Marks, & Olson, 1998, 2002) based on interviews with religious fathers of special needs children who are affiliated with the Church of the Latter Day Saints indicate that religious faith provides a unique source of motivation and support to devote time and effort into fathering.

Mothering. As Dollahite et al. (2004) note, feminist scholars have theorized at length about complex intersections between women, religion, and families. Yet, in puzzling contrast to the rest of family psychology, mothers as a group seem to be overlooked in studies of religion and family life. Existing research on religion and motherhood predominately involve descriptive studies of African American (e.g., Brodsky, 2000) and Mexican American mothers (e.g., Garcia, Perez, & Ortiz, 2000). Findings suggest that religious faith can facilitate adaptive parenting and the personal well-being of mothers struggling with difficult circumstances (e.g., single parenthood, poverty). Given ample research that women are more likely than men to attend religious services, to pray, to feel that religion is important, and to use religious coping behaviors, and may benefit more than men from such practices (e.g., Koenig, McCullough, & Larson, 2001), more systematic research needs to occur on the intersection between mothering and religion.

Religion and Family Crises

The findings reviewed thus far indicate that religion is linked to better marital and parental functioning in families selected from the general population. Thus, under normative conditions, religion appears to benefit family relationships. This raises the question about what are the circumstances, if any, in which religion goes awry for family dynamics? Given that religious systems of meaning provide people with fundamental assumptions about appropriate, "God-given" family values and processes (Mahoney, Pargament, Murray-Swank, & Murray-Swank, 2003) events that violate these assumptions may trigger individual and relationship distress. We now discuss family crises that would seem likely to have important religion dimensions.

Divorce

Multiple studies indicate that religion is a protective factor against divorce. People who endorse a religious affiliation have a lower risk of divorce than those who indicate no affiliation (average $r = -.08$). This translates into a divorce rate of approximately 49% for affiliated versus 62% for nonaffiliated people (Mahoney et al., 2001). Likewise, more frequent church attendance is associated with lower divorce rates (average $r = -.13$). This roughly corresponds to a 44% divorce rate for frequent churchgoers compared to a 60% rate for infrequent churchgoers. Several longitudinal studies indicate that church attendance is a predictor, not merely a consequence, of divorce (Booth, Johnson, Branaman, & Sica, 1995), even after controlling for more proximal variables (e.g., alcohol or drug use, infidelity) associated with divorce (Amato & Rogers, 1997).

Given that divorce is a less normative event for more religious people, the dissolution of a marriage may be an especially potent crisis for these families. More religious adults and children may experience divorce as a spiritual failure and struggle to reconcile this event with their religious values. Empirical research apparently has not been done on the role of religion to either facilitate or undermine the postdivorce adjustment of family members or family relationships. However, adults who have divorced (Feigelman, Gormand, & Varacalli, 1992) and their children (Lawton & Bures, 2001) are more likely to repudiate religion, and would presumably have less access to the positive psychosocial resources that religion offers.

Domestic Violence

Three large-scale, sophisticated studies have found that frequent churchgoers are about half as likely as infrequent attenders to experience marital physical aggression over time (Fergusson, Horwood, Kershaw, & Shannon, 1986) and to use physical aggression against their partners (Ellison, Bartkowski, & Anderson, 1999). However, in the small percentage of couples where marked dissimilarity exists between spouses' biblical beliefs, Ellison et al. (1999) found that more conservative men married to more liberal wives were 2.5 times more likely to be aggressive than men married to women with similar biblical views. Thus, overall, religion appears to typically be a protective factor against marital violence. But questions remain about if and when perpetrators may use religion to justify aggression, and how more devout believers may react when they are victims of domestic violence. For example, Nason-Clark (1997) observes that some religious beliefs of Evangelical Christian women may increase their reluctance to leave a physically abusive husband. Clearly, more research needs to untangle how religious practices or beliefs can become intertwined with domestic violence.

Marital Infidelity

Although sexual fidelity in marriage is a hallmark value promoted by major religions, scarce research has focused on religion and sexual attitudes or behaviors within marriage, as most research deals only with premarital sex. Nevertheless, a few studies imply that sexual infidelity may be especially distressing for more religious people. For instance, greater church attendance has been linked with greater disapproval of extramarital sex in the United States, West Germany, and Poland (Scott, 1998). Cochran and Beeghley (1991) also found that the strength of U.S. adults' professed commitment to their church doctrines for affiliates of Catholic and Protestant denominations (the exception was Episcopalians) was related to stronger disapproval of extramarital sex. In terms of behavior, in a national U.S. survey, frequent churchgoers said they had engaged in extramarital sex less often than people who never attended services (Atkins, Baucom, & Jacobson, 2001). This link was especially robust for individuals within "very happy" marriages, whereas rates of extramarital sex in "pretty happy" and "not too happy" marriages were constant regardless of church attendance rates. Thus, religious values may bolster fidelity for the very happily married, but marital discontent may override religious prohibitions for others. Overall, research implies that more religious people hold higher expectations of sexual monogamy and would feel especially guilt-ridden if they engaged in sexual infidelity or devastated if their spouse had an affair, particularly if they thought their marriage was a success. Such speculations, however, have yet to be empirically confirmed.

Child Physical Abuse

In contrast to findings about corporal punishment, current research does not support the idea that greater religiousness encourages child physical abuse. In fact, a rigorous, large-scale, longitudinal study yielded opposite findings: namely, young children whose parents rarely attended church in 1975 were more than twice as likely to suffer from physical abuse during the subsequent 17 years than children whose parents attended church regularly (Brown, Cohen, Johnson, & Salzinger, 1998). The two other studies we located on this topic were only descriptive in nature. Neither found a greater incidence of child physical abuse in Latter-Day Saint (Rollins & Oheneba-Sakyi, 1990) or Quaker (Brutz & Ingoldsby, 1984) families relative to the general population. Further, links between conservative Christian variables and physical discipline appear to be limited to families with young children and commonly used acts of corporal punishment in this age group (e.g., spanking). Overall, it is unclear what specific religious beliefs buffer or exacerbate parents' use of excessive physical force with youth.

Parenting a Child with Special Needs

A sizable body of literature, primarily descriptive and qualitative in nature, has examined how families rely on religion to cope with children with a developmental disability or serious illness (Dollahite et al., 2004). Many parents spontaneously report during interviews that they use religion in a positive manner to cope with children who have special needs. One positive form of parental religious coping consists of benevolent reappraisals of a child's problems and the parent's role as a caregiver. For example, Skinner, Bailey, Correa, and Rodriguez (1999) found that 71% of Latino mothers viewed their disabled child as a gift from God who found them worthy of the responsibility of raising such a child or wanted them to grow from the experience. Another positive form of religious coping consists of religious rituals and practices, such as praying, attending religious services, or making pilgrimages to holy places on behalf of oneself or one's child (Bailey, Skinner, Rodriguez, Gut, & Correa, 1999). However, in examining religious coping among parents of children with autism, Tarakeshwar and Pargament (2001) found that mothers can also experience negative emotions, such as being abandoned by their church and by God. Notably, such feelings were predictive of greater depressive affect and anxiety. Overall, research on religious coping per se in families of special needs children has involved only mothers. However, Dollahite and colleagues have found that fathers' religious beliefs, religious practices, and religious communities facilitated meaningful father–child relationships among Latter-Day Saint families with special needs children, although there were some congregational challenges (Dollahite et al., 1998, 2002, 2004).

Child Psychopathology

Research indicates that global markers of greater parental and familial religiousness are linked to better child psychological adjustment. This includes youth exhibiting fewer externalizing and internalizing behavior problems, greater prosocial traits, lower alcohol usage, less marijuana usage, and less serious antisocial behavior (see Mahoney et al., 2001). As noted earlier, a few studies suggest that parents' religiousness promotes children's functioning by facilitating effective parenting (Brody et al., 1994; 1996; Gunnoe et al., 1999).

Given that more religious families tend to have better behaved children, it may be especially challenging for such families to deal with child psychopathology when it does occur. Consistent with this idea, Strawbridge et al., (1998) found that more involvement in religious activities exacerbated the negative impact of family dysfunction (e.g., marital or child problems) on depressive symptoms of elderly adults, whereas religiousness buffered the negative effects of more "uncontrollable" types of problems (e.g., chronic health problems, poverty). While similar research has yet to be conducted with families of clinic-referred youth, certain religious beliefs and practices could exacerbate as well as buffer the maladjustment of clinically distressed youth.

Summary of Empirical Research and Future Challenges

Overall, social science research indicates that greater religiousness is clearly tied to multiple aspects of family life. However, this body of research is best described as embryonic. Several challenges lie ahead to develop this subfield. First, current findings are overwhelmingly based on markers of religiousness that fail to delve into the multifaceted nature of religion (Mahoney et al., 2001). Religion is unique because it infuses peoples' perceptions of daily life with religious significance (Pargament & Mahoney, 2005). While religions might differ on notions of God and other supernatural constructs, religions provide family members with prescriptive guidelines about family relationships that are reinforced through religious rituals, myths, and belief systems (Mahoney, 2005). Moreover, it is important to distinguish between two types of theological messages (Mahoney, 2005). One involves constructs, such as commitment or forgiveness, that may be advocated by both religious and nonreligious worldviews. The second type of substantive message emphasized by religion involves constructs, such as the sanctification of marriage or parenting (Mahoney et al., 2003), that directly assess perceptions about the sacred realm and are specific to religious worldviews. Such explicitly religious processes do not have direct parallels within secular systems of meaning.

A second challenge for the psychology of religion is to take seriously the notion that religiously based beliefs and practices about family life could be integrated into (1) individuals' appraisals and experiences of family relationships; (2) the dynamics of dyadic family interactions; and (3) the functioning of a family system as a whole. To date, the prevailing conceptual theory and findings in the psychology of religion address individual religious functioning (e.g., private prayer; Koenig et al., 2001). However, religion also has profound implications for social relationships. For example, people may use religion as a guide for how to respond to the behavior of other family members. Family dyads may engage in spiritual activities together or pull religious figures into the relationship as a third party. Whole family systems can call on religion to reinforce values to which all family members are expected to adhere. Research on such religiously based interpersonal processes, and their effects, is scarce.

A third challenge is to address ways in which religion can help or harm family relationships. While many messages offered by mainstream religions would seem to promote desirable family dynamics, certain religious beliefs and practices may be detrimental, especially for distressed family systems. Critics' warnings about the negative effects of religion on families seem implicitly concerned with how religion may be used to justify pathological processes. However, current empirical studies focus primarily on non-distressed samples. Thus, while religion seems to facilitate family life in normative conditions, an enormous amount of work remains to untangle the pros and cons of religion in different family circumstances. Finally, when studying families, the costs and benefits of religion need to be addressed at both the individual and relationship level of system. While a particular religious belief or practice may be beneficial for a family relationship, this may sometimes come at a cost to individual well-being.

A fourth challenge is to establish causal links between religion and family life. Divorce rates or proneness represent the sole outcome that has been repeatedly linked to religiousness in longitudinal studies. Research on other constructs is mostly cross-sectional in design. Thus, even well-established findings could be interpreted as positive family dynamics causing greater religiousness, not the other way around. Reciprocal influences are, of course, also possible. In any case, longitudinal studies would help to clarify the interplay of religion and family factors over time, including the role of "third variables" as mediators or moderators. Although many large-scale sociological studies have statistically controlled for demographic covariates, more research is needed on the salience of religion in the context of other protective family factors.

A fifth challenge is to better differentiate how religion operates for subsets of the general population, including different religious communities, ethnic groups, and family systems. Nominal religious membership (e.g., Jewish, Latter-Day Saint, Catholic, various Protestant groups) reveals little about individual differences or the function of beliefs or practices within a given religious group. Overall, ample room remains for the development of in-depth assessment about religiously based beliefs about marriage or parenting for Western religious groups. Moreover, questions remain about how diverse ethnic groups integrate different religions with family life (Dollahite et al., 2004). Although some research has been conducted on religion and African American families (e.g., Brody et al., 1994, 1996), other American racial minorities including Asians and Hispanics are understudied. Further, a glaring gap concerns non-Western religions despite the fact that there are roughly 1.1 billion Muslims (Koenig et al., 2001) and 800 million Hindus worldwide (Almeida, 1996). Finally, there has been a lack of diversity in the types of families studied, with most empirical research focused on traditional, two-parent, married households. Thus, nontraditional family systems are not well represented; this includes single-parent, gay, and blended families, as well as multigenerational and grandparent-led households.

In sum, psychologists have a great deal to offer and gain by helping to discover factors that drive religion–family links. The scarcity of psychological research on religion and family life may lead psychologists to underestimate the salience of the spiritual realm, or reduce its influence to generic psychosocial mechanisms (e.g., social support) also served by nonreligious institutions and belief systems. We contend, however, that religion has important implications for family life that deserve recognition from social scientists (Mahoney et al., 2001).

EMERGING THEORETICAL CONSTRUCTS TO ADVANCE RESEARCH ON RELIGION AND FAMILY DYNAMICS

Constructive Religious Constructs and the Transition to Parenthood

Snarey and Dollahite (2001) argue that there is an "urgent need" for good middle-range theories that address the complex relationships between familial and religious processes. In this section, we offer an illustrative model of a constructive religious construct, called "sanctification," that could facilitate family adjustment during normative family life changes. Namely, the sanctification of pregnancy is proposed as a process that could aid the transition to parenthood. Sanctification refers to perceiving an aspect of life as having "divine" significance and character (Pargament & Mahoney, 2005). Sanctification can occur in two ways. Theistic sanctification refers to perceiving an aspect of life as a manifestation of God (e.g., God is present in my marriage). Nontheistic sanctification refers to imbuing an aspect of life with qualities that characterize divinity (e.g., sacred, blessed, holy). Elsewhere, various theological positions have been delineated in support of the sanctification of marriage and of parenting (Mahoney et al., 2003). In a similar manner, a pregnancy can be much more than a biological event; it can have spiritual significance. Many religions attach deep spiritual meaning to conceiving and giving birth, particularly in the context of a marriage. Pregnancy in this light becomes a blessing from God and can be described in terms of sacred adjectives, such as "miraculous" and "divine."

Initial studies on sanctification have been conducted on marriage (Mahoney et al., 1999), parenting (Murray-Swank et al., 2003), major life strivings (Mahoney, Pargament, et al., 2005), one's physical body (Mahoney, Carels, et al., 2005), the environment (Tarakeshwar, Swank, Pargament, & Mahoney, 2001), and premarital sexuality (Murray-Swank, Pargament, & Mahoney, 2005). Overall, findings on sanctification suggest that viewing an aspect of life through a sacred lens has four important implications for family and individual functioning (Mahoney et al., 2003; Pargament & Mahoney, 2005). First, people tend to make major investments in sacred matters. As applied to the transition to parenthood, parents who sanctify pregnancy would be expected to invest more time and energy into prenatal care and make greater personal sacrifices for the emerging family. Second, when people perceive aspects of their lives through a sacred lens, they enter a spiritual world, one that contains a variety of spiritual resources to draw upon to preserve and protect sanctified aspects of life. For example, the transition to parenthood places significant stress on marriages and parents themselves. Those who sanctify pregnancy would be expected to draw on spiritual resources to help them cope. Individual-level resources include prayer, benevolent spiritual appraisals of situations, a collaborative relationship with God, and spiritual support (Pargament, 1997). The couple could also tap into family-based resources, such as joint prayer and spiritual intimacy, to help protect the emerging family (Mahoney et al., 2003). Third, sanctification is likely to elicit spiritual emotions. For example, pregnancy could be seen not only as a psychological and social turning point, but also as a "signal of transcendence" (cf. Berger, 1969), a sign that mother, father, and child are part of a larger reality, a greater unfolding design in the universe. Such perceptions are both cognitive and deeply emotional in nature. Although research on sanctification has not evaluated emotional outcomes, the sanctification of pregnancy could trigger strong emotions, especially "spiritual emotions," including feelings of gratitude, awe, humility, faith, and hope about life in general and about the infant specifically.

Finally, sanctification has been linked to psychological and spiritual benefits (Mahoney et al., 2003; Pargament & Mahoney, 2005). Thus, the sanctification of pregnancy would be expected to be tied directly to positive outcomes as well as indirectly relate to benefits by way of the aforementioned processes of investment, spiritual emotions, and spiritual resources. For example, greater sanctification of pregnancy by mothers would be expected to be tied to greater satisfaction with the pregnancy, a smoother labor and delivery, less postpartum depression, and enhanced spiritual growth and well-being. Husbands would presumably also experience many of these individual benefits. The effects of sanctification should also encompass the marriage and the family as a whole. This would include better marital and parental functioning as well as stronger parent–infant bonds. The infant, in turn, should exhibit better well-being at birth and during early infancy. While speculative in nature, this model of the sanctification of pregnancy is consistent with previous findings on the sanctification of marriage (Mahoney et al., 1999) and parenting (Murray-Swank et al., 2003). More importantly, it is presented here as an illustration of one approach to examine more closely how religiously based beliefs could facilitate a normative transition in the family life cycle.

Counterproductive Religious Constructs and Divorce

We now turn to one family crisis, namely, divorce, in which religiously based beliefs and behaviors about family relationships could exacerbate individual and relationship distress.

Sacred Loss and Desecration

Given that marriage is typically sanctified (Mahoney et al., 1999), divorce often could be appraised as a "sacred loss," which is defined as the loss of an aspect of life that previously had been viewed as a manifestation of the divine and/or invested with sacred qualities (Pargament, Magyar, Benore, & Mahoney, 2005). An alternative negative religious appraisal would be to view divorce as a desecration. This refers to perceiving a sanctified aspect of life as having been knowingly violated (Pargament et al., 2005). A recent study on desecration and college students' experiences of betrayal in romantic relationship (Magyar, Pargament, & Mahoney, 2000) suggests that desecration attributions may often occur when a spouse or child feels that one of the spouses did something that violated the marriage (e.g., deception, infidelity). In an initial study of sacred loss and desecration with a community sample (Pargament et al., 2005), higher levels of both constructs were related to more intrusive thoughts for adults who rated their most negative life event in the past 2 years (8% identified divorce or separation as the event). However, only sacred loss was related to depression and only desecration was related to greater anger. Furthermore, sacred loss was linked to greater posttraumatic growth and positive spiritual change; in contrast, desecration was associated with less posttraumatic growth. These results imply that the spiritual meaning people attach to traumatic events is linked to different types of psychological distress. Thus, within the context of a divorce, people's reactions may partly depend on the spiritual meaning attached to the event.

Spiritual Guilt

In addition to appraisals of the divorce itself, people may make religious appraisals of their own role in the dissolution of a marriage. To the degree that spouses or children feel responsible for the divorce, they may experience a profound sense of spiritual failure, accompanied by a heightened sense of religious guilt (Mahoney et al., 2003). For example, divorced spouses may reason that because they had not been able to be perfectly accepting, giving, and healing to one another in their marriage, they deserve to be cut off from the presence of God (Livingston, 1985). Systematic research on parents' or children's religious guilt in connection with divorce or other family crises appears to be sparse.

Demonization

In divorce cases where one party has violated a traditional religious wedding vow (e.g., by adultery, abandonment during a serious illness), the other spouse may demonize this partner. "Demonization" refers to viewing the perceived perpetrator of a traumatic event as operating under the influence of demonic forces, either intentionally or unwittingly. An initial study of demonization focused on college students' perceptions of the terrorists involved in the September 11, 2001, attacks on the World Trade Center and found that demonization was linked to more extreme retaliation toward, and fear of, the terrorists (Mahoney et al., 2002). In some divorce situations, one partner may similarly experience more intense negative reactions if the spouse is seen as being aligned with evil demonic forces. Such perceptions could undermine a child's relationship with the other parent and set the stage for greater postdivorce conflicts.

Theistic Triangulation

Finally, theistic triangulation is a potentially powerful negative religious process that could occur between family members as they work through a divorce. Based on a Bowenian and/or structural family systems approach, clinicians have highlighted how couples may triangulate God into the marital system when conflict emerges (Butler & Harper, 1994). That is, God could be drawn into three types of counterproductive theistic triangles that block resolution of conflict between family dyads: coalition (i.e., God takes one party's side), displacement (i.e., adversity is God's fault), or substitutive (i.e., each party seeks God's support but avoids dealing directly with the conflict). In a study of theistic triangulation, Yanni (2003) found that higher rates of theistic triangulation between college students and their parents was related to more relationship conflict and distance between the parties. Divorcing couples in which one or both spouses attempt to take a "spiritually one-up" position may likewise have more conflict and difficulty establishing effective coparenting relationships postdivorce.

   In sum, in addition to typical postdivorce readjustment challenges, family members who perceive a divorce in negative spiritual terms may experience additional personal difficulties and greater interpersonal conflict between family members (e.g., heightened coparenting conflicts). Parents may engage in negative forms of religious coping that undermines their personal recovery from divorce, parenting skills, and coparenting relationship. Such problems may affect children's postdivorce adjustment. Children may also directly experience spiritual struggles and personal distress in coming to terms with the dissolution of their parents' marriage.

Religious Resources to Recover from Family Crises

Theory and prior research in the psychology of religion has identified a variety of spiritual mechanisms that families could access to recover from family difficulties. Considerable research has focused on individual-level resources, especially within the framework of religious coping as individuals cope with difficulties related to the self (e.g., Pargament, 1997). However, empirical research on how "family" members may employ religious coping strategies specifically with "family" difficulties appears limited (Mahoney et al., 2001). The following section discusses existing evidence and highlight areas for exploration along these lines.

Family-Based Religious Practices and Rituals

A recent descriptive study found that long-married, religious couples say they engage in religious practices as a couple (e.g., praying together) to resolve marital conflict (Butler, Stout, & Gardner, 2002). Though it seems unlikely that divorcing couples would pray together, some religious communities have created religious rituals to provide a concrete ceremony for families to mark the dissolution of a marriage (Paquette, n.d.). Further habitual engagement in family prayer and attendance at religious services might also offer parents a structured mechanism when a divorce does occur to communicate apologies, hopes, and shared goals to their children within a context overseen by an authority whose power supersedes even that of parents. This may help prevent resentment and hostility from escalating out of control. Controlled studies about the effectiveness and general pervasiveness of such family-based religious activities to cope with divorce, or other family crises, need to be conducted.

Theistic Mediation

In contrast to "theistic triangulation," religion also offers family members constructive strategies to resolve interpersonal conflict (Mahoney, 2005). In theistic mediation, for instance, God (or other supernatural forces) is pulled into a dyadic relationship as a third party who mediates conflict. In this case, God would be perceived as (1) being interested in maintaining a compassionate relationship with each person, (2) taking a neutral stance about each person's "side" of the story, and (3) insisting that each person take responsibility for change in the relationship. Divorcing couples who view God this way may more readily disengage from destructive communication patterns and explore options for compromise or healthy acceptance of one another. Case examples of marriage (e.g., Butler & Harper, 1994) highlight the power of these processes. A recent study indicates that college students and parents who incorporate God into their relationship as a spiritual mediator experience fewer conflicts, higher levels of relationship satisfaction, and more adaptive communication styles (Yanni, 2003).

CONCLUSIONS

In conclusion, available empirical research indicates that greater religiousness is linked to more positive marital and parental functioning. However, much work is needed to create theoretical models and appropriate measurement tools that would lead to a more fine-grained understanding of how religion functions in family systems during significant family events. As was illustrated in this chapter, the type of influence that religion has for families is likely to depend on the specific types of religiously-based beliefs and behaviors that family members use to deal with normative family transitions and crises. Psychologists are especially equipped and encouraged to pursue these questions. When found, the answers will help inform policymakers, clergy, clinicians, and the millions of families who participate in religion about the helpful and harmful roles that religion can play in family dynamics.

REFERENCES

Almeida, R. (1996). Hindu, Christian, and Muslim families. In M. McGoldrick, J. Giordano, & J. K. Pearce (Eds.), *Ethnicity and family therapy* (pp. 395–423). New York: Guilford Press.

Alwin, D. F. (1986). Religion and parental child-rearing orientations: Evidence of a Catholic–Protestant convergence. *American Journal of Sociology, 92,* 412–440.

Amato, P. R., & Rogers, S. J. (1997). A longitudinal study of marital problems and subsequent divorce. *Journal of Marriage and the Family, 59,* 612–624.

Atkins, D. C., Baucom, D. H., & Jacobson, N. S. (2001). Understanding infidelity: Correlates in a national random sample. *Journal of Family Psychology, 15,* 735–749.

Bailey, D. B., Skinner, D., Rodriguez, P., Gut, D., & Correa, V. (1999). Awareness, use, and satisfaction with services for Latino parents of young children with disabilities. *Exceptional Children, 65,* 367–381.

Bartkowski, J. P., & Xu, X. (2000). Distant patriarchs or expressive dads?: The discourse and practice of fathering in conservative Protestant families. *Sociological Quarterly, 41,* 465–485.

Becker P. E., & Hofmeister, H. (2001). Work, family, and religious involvement for men and women. *Journal for the Scientific Study of Religion, 40,* 707–722.

Berger, P. L. (1969). *A rumor of angels: Modern society and the rediscovery of the supernatural.* Garden City, NY: Doubleday.

Booth, A., Johnson, D. R., Branaman, A., & Sica, A. (1995). Belief and behavior: Does religion matter in today's marriage? *Journal of Marriage and the Family, 57,* 661–671.

Brodsky, A. E. (2000). The role of religion in the lives of resilent, urban, African American, single mothers. *Journal of Community Psychology, 28,* 199–219.

Brody, G. H., Stoneman, Z., & Flor, D. (1996). Parental religiosity, family processes, and youth competence in rural, two-parent, African-American families. *Developmental Psychology, 32,* 696–706.

Brody, G. H., Stoneman, Z., Flor, D., & McCrary, C. (1994). Religion's role in organizing family relationships: Family process in rural, two-parent, African-American families. *Journal of Marriage and the Family, 56,* 878–888.

Brown, J., Cohen, P., Johnson, J. G., & Salzinger, S. (1998). A longitudinal analysis of risk factors for child maltreatment: Findings of a 17–year prospective study of officially recorded and self-reported child abuse and neglect. *Child Abuse and Neglect, 22,* 1065–1078.

Brutz, J., & Ingoldsby, B. B. (1984). Conflict resolution in Quaker families. *Journal of Marriage and the Family, 46,* 21–26.

Butler, M. H., & Harper, J. M. (1994). The divine triangle: God in the marital system of religious couples. *Family Process, 33,* 277–286.

Butler, M. H., Stout, J. A., & Gardner, B. C. (2002). Prayer as a conflict resolution ritual: Clinical implications of religious couples' report of relationship softening, healing perspective, and change responsibility. *American Journal of Family Therapy, 30,* 19–37.

Call, V. R. A., & Heaton, T. B. (1997). Religious influence on marital stability. *Journal for the Scientific Study of Religion, 36,* 382–392.

Cochran, J. K., & Beeghley, L. (1991). The influence of religion on attitudes toward nonmarital sexuality: A preliminary assessment of reference group theory. *Journal for the Scientific Study of Religion, 30,* 45–62.

Curtis, K. T., & Ellison, C. G. (2002). Religious heterogamy and marital conflict: Findings from the National Survey of Families and Households. *Journal of Family Issues, 23,* 551–576.

Dollahite, D. C., Marks, L. D., & Goodman, M. A. (2004). Families and religious beliefs, practices, and communities: Linkages in a diverse and dynamic cultural context. In M. J. Coleman & L. H. Ganong (Eds.), *The handbook of contemporary families: Considering the past, contemplating the future* (pp. 411–431). Thousand Oaks, CA: Sage.

Dollahite, D. C., Marks, L. D., & Olson, M. M. (1998). Faithful fathering in trying times: Religious beliefs and practices of Latter Day Saint fathers of children with special needs. *Journal of Men's Studies, 7,* 71–93.

Dollahite, D. C., Marks, L. D., & Olson, M. M. (2002). Fathering, faith, and family therapy: Generative narrative therapy with religious fathers. *Journal of Family Psychotherapy, 13,* 263–294.

Donahue, M., & Benson, P. L. (1995). Religion and the well-being of adolescents. *Journal of Social Issues, 51,* 145–160.

Ellison, C. G. (1996). Conservative Protestantism and the corporal punishment of children: Clarifying the issues. *Journal for the Scientific Study of Religion, 35,* 1–16.

Ellison, C. G., Bartkowski, J. P., & Anderson K. L. (1999). Are there religious variations in domestic violence? *Journal of Family Issues, 20,* 87–113.

Ellison, C. G., Bartkowski, J. P., & Segal, M. L. (1996). Do conservative Protestants spank more often?: Further evidence from the National Survey of Families and Households. *Social Science Quarterly, 77,* 663–673.

Feigelman, W., Gormand, B. S., & Varacalli, J. A. (1992). Americans who give up religion. *Sociology and Social Research, 76,* 138–143.

Fergusson, D. M., Horwood, L. J., Kershaw, K. L., & Shannon, F. T. (1986). Factors associated with reports of wive assault in New Zealand. *Journal of Marriage and the Family, 48,* 407–412.

Foshee, V. A., & Hollinger, B. R. (1996). Maternal religiosity, adolescent social bonding, and adolescent alcohol use. *Journal of Early Adolescence, 16,* 451–468.

Gallup, G., Jr., & Castelli, J. (1989). *The people's religion: American faith in the 90s.* New York: Macmillan.

Garcia, S. B., Perez, A. M., & Ortiz, A. A. (2000). Mexican American mothers' beliefs about disabilities: Implications for early childhood intervention. *Remedial and Special Education, 21,* 90–100.

Gershoff, E. T., Miller, P. C., & Holden, G. W. (1999). Parenting influences from the pulpit: Religious affiliation as a determinant of corporal punishment. *Journal of Family Psychology, 13,* 307–320.

Gunnoe, M. L., Hetherington, E. M., & Reiss, D. (1999). Parental religiosity, parenting style, and adolescent social responsibility. *Journal of Early Adolescence, 19,* 199–225.

Heaton, T. B., & Pratt, E. L. (1990). The effects of religious homogamy on marital satisfaction and stability. *Journal of Family Issues, 11,* 191–207.

Jackson, S., Thompson, R. A., Christiansen, E. H., Colman, R. A., Wyatt, J., Buckendahl, C. W., Wilcox, B. L., & Peterson, R. (1999). Predicting abuse-prone parental attitudes and discipline practices in a nationally representative sample. *Child Abuse and Neglect, 23,* 15–29.

King, D., & Hueston, W. (1994). Religious affiliation and obstetric outcome. *Southern Medical Journal, 87,* 1125–1128.

King, V. (2003). The influence of religion on fathers' relationships with their children. *Journal of Marriage and Family, 65,* 382–395.

Koenig, H. G., McCullough, M. E., & Larson, D. B. (Eds.). (2001). *Handbook of religion and health.* New York: Oxford University Press.

Krishnan, V. (1993). Religious homogamy and voluntary childlessness in Canada. *Sociological Perspectives, 36,* 83–93.

Larson, L. E., & Goltz, J. W. (1989). Religious participation and marital commitment. *Review of Religious Research, 30,* 387–400.

Lawton, L. E., & Bures, R. (2001). Parental divorce and the "switching" of religious identity. *Journal for the Scientific Study of Religion, 40,* 99–111.

Livingston, P. H. (1985). Union and disunion. *Studies in Formative Spirituality, 6,* 241–253.

Magana, A., & Clark, N. M. (1995). Examining a paradox: Does religiosity contribute to positive birth outcomes in Mexican American populations? *Health Education Quarterly, 22,* 96–109.

Magyar, G. M., Pargament, K. I., & Mahoney, A. (2000, August). *Violating the sacred: A study of desecration among college students.* Paper presented at the meeting of the American Psychological Association, Washington, DC.

Mahoney, A. (2005). Religion and conflict in family relationships. *Journal of Social Issues, 61*(4).

Mahoney, A., Carels, R. A., Pargament, K. I., Wachholtz, A., Edwards Leeper, L. Kaplar, M., & Frutchey, R. (2005). The sanctification of the body and behavioral health patterns of college students. *The International Journal for the Psychology of Religion, 15,* 221–238.

Mahoney, A., Pargament, K. I., Ano, G., Lynn, Q., Magyar, G., McCarthy, S., Pristas, E., & Wachholtz, A. (2002). *The devil made them do it?: Demonization and the 9/11 attacks.* Paper presented at the annual meeting of the American Psychological Association, Chicago.

Mahoney, A. , Pargament, K. I., Cole, B., Jewell, T., Magyar, G. M., Tarakeshwar, N., & Murray-Swank N. (2005). A higher purpose: The sanctification of strivings. *The International Journal for the Psychology of Religion, 15,* 239–262.

Mahoney, A., Pargament, K. I., Jewell, T., Swank, A. B., Scott, E., Emery, E., & Rye, M. (1999). Marriage and the spiritual realm: The role of proximal and distal religious constructs in marital functioning. *Journal of Family Psychology, 13,* 1–18.

Mahoney, A., Pargament, K. I., Murray-Swank, A., & Murray-Swank, N. (2003). Religion and the sanctification of family relationships. *Review of Religious Research, 40,* 220–236.

Mahoney, A., Pargament, K. I., Tarakeshwar, N., & Swank, A. (2001). Religion in the home in the 1980s and 90s: A meta-analytic review and conceptual analysis of religion, marriage, and parenting. *Journal of Family Psychology, 15,* 559–596.

Murray-Swank, A., Mahoney, A., & Pargament, K. I. (2003). *Sanctification of parenting: Influences on corporal punishment and warmth by liberal and conservative Christian mothers.* Manuscript under review.

Murray-Swank, N. A., Pargament, K. I., & Mahoney, A. (2005). At the crossroads of sexuality and spirituality: The sanctification of sex by college students. *The International Journal of the Psychology of Religion, 15,* 199–220.

Nason-Clark, N. (1997). *The battered wife: How Christians confront family violence.* Louisville, KY: Westminster John Knox Press.

Oggins, J. (2003). Topics of marital disagreements among African-American and Euro-American newlyweds. *Psychological Reports, 92,* 419–425.

Palkovitz, R. (2002). *Involved fathering and men's adult development: Provisional balances.* Hillsdale, NJ: Erlbaum.

Paquette, J. M. (n.d.). *Guide to religious divorce rituals.* Retrieved May 18, 2004, from www.beliefnet.com/story/75/story_7560_1.html.

Pargament, K. I. (1997). *The psychology of religion and coping: Theory, research, practice.* New York: Guilford Press.

Pargament, K. I., Magyar, G. M., Benore, E., & Mahoney, A. (2005). Sacrilege: A study of sacred loss and desecration and their implications for health and well-being in a community sample. *Journal for the Scientific Study of Religion, 44,* 59–78.

Pargament, K. I., & Mahoney, A. (2005). Sacred matters: Sanctification as vital topic for the psychology of religion. *The International Journal for the Psychology of Religion, 15,* 179–198.

Pearce, L. D., & Axinn, W. G. (1998). The impact of family religious life on the quality of mother–child relations. *American Sociological Review, 63,* 810–828.

Regnerus, M. D. (2003). Religion and positive adolescent outcomes: A review of research and theory. *Review of Religious Research, 44,* 394–413.

Rollins, B. C., & Oheneba-Sakyi, Y. (1990). Physical violence in Utah households. *Journal of Family Violence, 5,* 301–309.

Schumm, W. R., Ja Jeong, G. A., & Silliman, B. (1990). Protestant fundamentalism and marital success revisited. *Psychological Reports, 66,* 905–906.

Scott, J. (1998). Changing attitudes to sexual morality: A cross-national comparison. *Sociology, 32,* 815–845.

Sherkat, D. E. (2003). Religious socialization: Sources of influence and influences of agency. In M. Dillon (Ed.), *Handbook of the sociology of religion* (pp. 151–163). New York: Cambridge University Press.

Sherkat, D. E., & Ellison, C. G. (1999). Recent developments and current controversies in the sociology of religion. *Annual Review of Sociology, 25,* 363–394.

Skinner, D., Bailey, D. B., Correa, V., & Rodriguez, P. (1999). Narrating self and disability: Latino mothers' construction of identities vis-à-vis their child with special needs. *Exceptional Children, 65,* 481–495.

Snarey, J. R., & Dollahite, D. C. (2001). Varieties of religion–family linkages. *Journal of Family Psychology, 15,* 646–651.

Stanley, S. M., & Markman, H. J. (1992). Assessing commitment in personal relationships. *Journal of Marriage and the Family, 54,* 595–608.

Strawbridge, W. J., Shema, S. J., Cohen, R. D., Roberts, R. E., & Kaplan, G. A. (1998). Religiosity buffers effects of some stressors on depression but exacerbates others. *Journal of Gerontology, 53B,* S118–S126.

Sullivan, K. T. (2001). Understanding the relationship between religiosity and marriage: An investigation of the immediate and longitudinal effect of religiosity on newlywed couples. *Journal of Family Psychology, 15,* 610–626.

Tarakeshwar, N., & Pargament, K. I. (2001). Use of religious coping in families of children with autism. *Focus on Autism and Other Developmental Disabilities, 16*(4), 247–260.

Tarakeshwar, N., Swank, A. B., Pargament, K. I., & Mahoney, A. (2001). Theological conservatism and the sanctification of nature: A study of opposing religious correlates of environmentalism. *Review of Religious Research, 42,* 387–404.

Wilcox, W. B. (1998). Conservative Protestant childrearing: Authoritarian or authoritative? *American Sociological Review, 63,* 796–809.

Wilcox, W. B. (2002). Religion, convention, and parental involvement. *Journal of Marriage and Family, 64,* 780–792.

Wilcox, W. B., & Wolfinger, N. H. (2003). *Then comes marriage?: Religion and marriage in urban America.* Manuscript under review.

Wilson, M. R., & Filsinger, E. E. (1986). Religiosity and marital adjustment: Multidimensional interrelationships. *Journal of Marriage and the Family, 48,* 147–151.

Wilson, J. & Musick, M. (1996). Religion and marital dependency. *Journal for the Scientific Study of Religion, 35,* 30–40.

Yanni, G. (2003). *Religious and secular dyadic variables and their relation to parent–child relationships and college students' psychological adjustment.* Unpublished dissertation, Bowling Green State University, Bowling Green, OH.

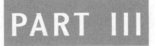

PART III

RELIGION AND BASIC PSYCHOLOGY SUBDISCIPLINES

11

The Neuropsychology of Religious and Spiritual Experience

ANDREW B. NEWBERG
STEPHANIE K. NEWBERG

Religious and spiritual experiences such as meditation, prayer, and ritual have been described in the biomedical, psychological, anthropological, and religious literature. Specific descriptions and religious texts can date back several thousand years. More recently, there has been a growth in the number of studies that have examined the neurophysiological and physiological correlates of such experiences. From an evolutionary perspective, it is likely that such experiences became possible with the development of various structures in the brain of early primates and eventually of *Homo sapiens*. The concatenation of "religiogenic" brain mechanisms in *Homo sapiens* appears to be accompanied historically by an explosion of religious traditions that have continued to permeate human societies since prehistoric times. In light of this evolutionary pattern, neurobiological and neuropsychological correlates of religious and spiritual experiences have begun to be identified. Furthermore, by considering other relevant studies in neurobiology, a more complex model of neurophysiological events during religious and spiritual experiences can be developed. More specifically, brain function can be considered in relation to its interconnection with other body physiology that can be mediated by the autonomic nervous system as well as by the neuroendocrine system. A consideration of this relation between cognitive processes in the brain and the autonomic nervous system may yield a more complete understanding of a variety of spiritual experiences ranging from "awe" to intense mystical states. Thus, from the current literature, a foundation for the development of a neuropsychological model can be considered in order to guide future studies in the neurobiology of religious and spiritual experiences. The use of state-of-the-art brain imaging techniques that can now measure various neurotransmitter systems, as well as other physiological measures, can be applied to investigate brain function during experiences such as meditation, prayer, and ritual experiences.

This chapter considers the neuropsychology of religious and spiritual experience.

This includes a brief review of the phenomenological aspects of such experiences, as well as a synthesis of existing data toward the development of a comprehensive model that can provide a foundation for future analyses into the biological roots of these experiences and the relationship between these experiences and psychological well-being.

BRAIN EVOLUTION AND SPIRITUAL EXPERIENCE

Evolution has led to the development of the complex neuronal connections that exist within the brain's cerebral hemispheres. The higher centers in the brain are also connected to the more primitive structures, such as the limbic system. For the most part, the brain evolved its complexity to provide human beings with improved abilities to delineate order in the external environment and to solve cognitive problems necessary for survival. In addition to purely cognitive aspects, the evolution of the brain led to human socialization. This ability to form family units, communities, and societies had a tremendous evolutionary advantage. The question is, then, How did these evolutionary changes in the brain lead to the development of spiritual experience, religion, and ritual?

The brain can be divided functionally into several primary cognitive functions (d'Aquili, 1978, 1983, 1986). We have previously referred to these functions as cognitive operators. The term "cognitive operator" simply refers to the neurophysiological mechanisms that underlie certain broad categories of cognitive function. Thus, these operators do not exist in the literal sense, but can be useful when considering overall brain function. The notion of cognitive operators is similar to that of the more commonly used concept of cognitive modules. However, we have proposed that cognitive operators refer to more general functions of the brain. The cognitive operators include abstraction of generals from particulars, the perception of causality in external reality, the perception of spatial or temporal sequences in external reality, and the ordering of elements of reality into causal chains. This latter function is what may give rise to explanatory models of the external world, whether scientific or mythical. Space does not permit us to describe here in detail the neurophysiological substrates and neuroanatomical networks of all these operators. However, several operators may be useful to consider when describing the neuropsychology of religious and spiritual experiences.

The *causal operator* accounts for the causal sequencing of elements of reality as abstracted from sense perceptions (d'Aquili, 1978). This causal operator derives its function from the inferior parietal lobule in the left hemisphere, the anterior convexity of the frontal lobes, primarily in the left hemisphere, and their reciprocal neural interconnections (Luria, 1966; Pribram, 1973). The causal operator is likely of critical importance in the development of religious and spiritual concepts and experiences (d'Aquili, 1978). This operator organizes any given strip of reality into what is subjectively perceived as causal sequences back to the initial terminus of that strip. In view of the apparently universal human trait of positing causes for any given strip of reality, it has been postulated that if the initial terminus is not given by sense data, the causal operator generates automatically an initial terminus (d'Aquili & Newberg, 1993). Western science refuses to postulate an initial terminus or first cause for any strip of reality unless it is observed or can be immediately inferred from observation. Under "everyday life" (nonscientific) conditions, the causal operator simply generates an initial terminus or first cause for a strip of reality. We have proposed that when no observational or "scientific" causal explanation is forthcoming for a strip of reality, gods, powers, spirits, or some other causative construct is automatically generated by the causal operator (d'Aquili & Newberg, 1997). If this is the case, the causal operator would likely operate spontaneously on reality, positing an initial causal terminus when none is given.

If it is true that the causal operator necessarily analyzes reality, then human beings have no choice but to construct myths filled with personalized power sources to explain their world. The myths may be social in nature or they may be individual in terms of dreams, daydreams, or other fantasy aspects of the individual person. Nevertheless, as long as human beings are aware of the contingency of their existence in the face of what often appears to be a capricious universe, they must construct myths to orient themselves within that universe. Thus, they construct gods, spirits, demons, or other personalized power sources with whom they can deal contractually in order to gain control over a capricious environment.

A second operator that we have suggested that has particular significance regarding spiritual experience is the *holistic operator*. The proposed holistic operator permits reality to be viewed as a whole or as a gestalt, as well as the abstraction from particulars or individuals into a larger contextual framework. The holistic operator likely resides in the parietal lobe in the right (or nondominant) hemisphere, more specifically in the posterior superior parietal lobule and adjacent areas that have been found to be involved in generating gestalt understanding about both sensory input and various abstract concepts (Bogen, 1969; Gazzaniga & Hillyard, 1971; Nebes & Sperry, 1971; Sperry, Gazzaniga, & Bogen, 1969). It is also interesting to note that this area sits opposite the area in the left hemisphere that provides the neuroanatomical substrate for logical–grammatical operations. Thus, the right parietal lobe is involved in a holistic approach to things and the left parietal lobe is involved in more reductionist processes. We will consider below how these various structures and associated structures might be involved more specifically in religious and spiritual experiences.

METHODS OF ATTAINING SPIRITUAL EXPERIENCES

In considering a neuropsychological model of religious and spiritual experiences, it is important to describe how such experiences are attained. We have previously suggested that there are two general categories of methods for attaining such experiences: group ritual and individual contemplation, such as prayer or meditation. A phenomenological analysis reveals that the two types of practices are similar in kind, if not in intensity, along two dimensions: (1) intermittent emotional discharges involving the subjective sensation of awe, peace, tranquillity, or ecstasy; and (2) varying degrees of unitary experience correlating with the emotional discharges just mentioned (d'Aquili & Newberg, 1993). These unitary experiences consist of a decreased sense or awareness of the boundaries between the self and the external world (d'Aquili, 1986; d'Aquili & Newberg, 1993; Smart, 1958, 1967, 1969; Stace, 1961). The latter dimension can also lead to a sense of oneness between other perceived individuals, thereby generating a sense of community. At the extreme, unitary experiences can eventually lead to the abolition of all boundaries of discrete being, thus generating a state of undifferentiated oneness or what we have called Absolute Unitary Being (AUB; d'Aquili & Newberg, 1999).

It should be noted that the experiences of group ritual and individual meditation have a certain degree of overlap such that each may play a role in the other. In fact, it may be that human ceremonial ritual actually provides the "average" person access to mystical experience ("average" in distinction to those regularly practicing intense contemplation, such as highly religious monks). This by no means implies that the mystic or contemplative is impervious to the effects of ceremonial ritual. Precisely because of the intense unitary experiences arising from meditation, mystics might actually be more affected by ceremonial ritual than the average person, although this has not been demonstrated yet. It might be concluded that ceremonial ritual, at its most effective, is an incredibly powerful technology, whether for good or ill. Further, because of its essentially communal aspects, it tends to have immeasurably greater social significance than meditation or contemplation. Although meditation and contemplation may produce more intense and more extended unitary states compared to the relatively brief flashes generated by group ritual, the former are almost always solitary experiences.

With regard to human ceremonial ritual, it appears to be a morally neutral technology in the sense that it might be utilized toward both positive and destructive goals. Therefore, depending on the myth in which it is imbedded and which it expresses, ritual can either promote or minimize the structural aspects of a society and promote or minimize overall aggressive behavior. Utilizing Turner's (1969) concept of *communitas* as the powerful unitary social experience usually arising out of ceremonial ritual, we can state that if a myth achieves its incarnation in a ritual that defines the unitary experience as applying only to the group or tribe, then the result is only the *communitas tribus*. It is certainly true that aggression within the group has been minimized or eliminated by the unifying experience generated by the ritual. However, this may only serve to emphasize the special cohesiveness of the group vis-à-vis the contradistinction with other groups. The result may be an increase in intergroup aggression even though intragroup aggression is diminished. The myth and its embodying ritual may, of course, apply to all members of a religion, a nation-state, an ideology, all of humanity, and all of reality. Obviously, as one increases the scope of what is included in the unitary experience, the amount of overall aggressive behavior decreases. If indeed a ceremonial ritual were giving flesh to a myth of the unity of all being, then one would presumably experience brief senses of *communitas omnium*. Such a myth-ritual experience approaches meditative states such as Bucke's (1961) cosmic consciousness or even AUB. However, such a grand scope is, unfortunately, unusual for group ritual in human ethnographic experiences.

A NEUROPHYSIOLOGICAL MODEL
OF RELIGIOUS AND SPIRITUAL EXPERIENCES

The model described below is an elaboration upon a previously described model that now incorporates recent neuroimaging, neurochemical, hormonal, and physiological studies (Newberg & Iversen, 2003). The purpose of this model is to provide a foundation from which many different types of religious experiences and practices can be considered and compared. As shown in Figure 11.1, the model begins with the prefrontal cortex and suggests a number of complex interactions with the thalamus, posterior superior parietal lobe, limbic system, and autonomic nervous system. Furthermore, a number of both excitatory and inhibitory neurotransmitters can now be proposed to play a role in such practices and experiences. Dopamine, serotonin, acetylcholine, and several other molecules may be associated with various phenomenological aspects of such experiences, and these are also considered in this model. It would be anticipated that depending upon the specific practice, ritual, tradition, and individual involved, the specific mechanisms might

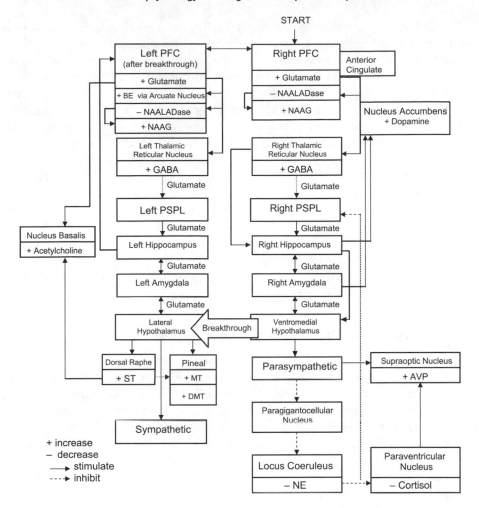

FIGURE 11.1. Schematic overview of the neurophysiological model proposed to be associated with meditative states. The circuits generally apply to both hemispheres; however, much of the initial activity is on the right.

be somewhat different. However, focusing on the phenomenology of such experiences, this model provides information regarding the diversity of experiences, whether sensory, cognitive, and affective, that can be associated with religious and spiritual experiences. The model was initially developed utilizing information from studies primarily on meditative practices due to the relatively large amount of data available. However, this model can likely be applied to many different types of practices and experiences.

Activation of the Prefrontal and Cingulate Cortex

Most meditative, prayer, or other contemplative practices require some degree of sustained attention. This can be directed to a visualized object, a mantra, prayer, or some other spiritual focus. Brain imaging studies suggest that willful acts and tasks that require sustained attention are initiated via activity in the prefrontal cortex (PFC), particularly in the right hemisphere (Frith, Friston, Liddle, & Frackowiak, 1991; Ingvar, 1994; Pardo,

Fox, & Raichle, 1991; Posner & Petersen, 1990). The cingulate gyrus has also been shown to be involved in focusing attention, probably in conjunction with the PFC (Vogt, Finch, & Olson, 1992). Thus, since spiritual practices require an intense focus of attention, it seems appropriate that a model for meditation begin with activation of the PFC (particularly the right hemisphere) as well as the cingulate gyrus. This notion is supported by the increased activity observed in these regions on several of the brain imaging studies of volitional types of meditation including that from our laboratory in which eight Tibetan Buddhist meditators were studied at baseline and during meditation (Newberg et al., 2001). Quantitative analysis demonstrated increased activity in the PFC bilaterally (though greater on the right hemisphere) and the cingulate gyrus during meditation. Therefore, meditation appears to start by activating the prefrontal and cingulate cortex associated with the will or intent to clear the mind of thoughts or to focus on an object. One positron-emission tomography (PET) study of a guided type of meditation did not demonstrate increased prefrontal activity; however, a recent study showed decreased frontal activity during externally guided word generation compared to internal or volitional word generation (Crosson et al., 2001). Thus, prefrontal and cingulate activation may be associated with the volitional aspects of meditation.

Thalamic Activation as Part of an Attentional Network

The thalamus is a major relay in the brain that connects other structures as well as communicates "higher order" processing to the areas of the brain that subserve emotion and ultimately regulate various physiological processes. Several animal studies have shown that the PFC, when activated, innervates the reticular nucleus of the thalamus (Cornwall & Phillipson, 1988), particularly as part of a more global attentional network (Portas et al., 1998). Such activation may be accomplished by the PFC's production and distribution of the excitatory neurotransmitter glutamate, which the PFC neurons use to communicate among themselves and to innervate other brain structures (Cheramy, Romo, & Glowinski, 1987). The thalamus itself governs the flow of sensory information to cortical processing areas via its interactions with the lateral geniculate and lateral posterior nuclei and also likely uses the glutamate system in order to activate neurons in other structures (Armony & LeDoux, 2000). It is known that the lateral geniculate nucleus receives raw visual data from the optic tract and routes it to the striate cortex for processing. The lateral posterior nucleus of the thalamus provides the posterior superior parietal lobule (PSPL) with the sensory information it needs to determine the body's spatial orientation (Bucci, Conley, & Gallagher, 1999).

When excited, the reticular nucleus secretes the inhibitory neurotransmitter gamma-aminobutyric acid (GABA) onto the lateral posterior and geniculate nuclei, cutting off input to the PSPL and visual centers in proportion to the reticular activation (Destexhe, Contreras, & Steriade, 1998). During meditation, because of the increased activity in the PFC, particularly on the right, there should theoretically be a concomitant increase in the activity in the reticular nucleus of the thalamus. While brain imaging studies of meditation have not had the resolution to distinguish the reticular nuclei, our recent single photon emission computed tomography (SPECT) study did demonstrate a general increase in thalamic activity that was proportional to the activity levels in the PFC. This is consistent with, but does not confirm, the specific interaction between the PFC and reticular nuclei. If the activation of the right PFC causes increased activity in the reticular nucleus during meditation, the result may be decreased sensory input entering into the PSPL. Several studies have demonstrated an increase in serum GABA during meditation, possibly reflecting increased central GABA activity (Elias, Guich, & Wilson, 2000). This functional deafferentation related to increased GABA would mean that fewer distracting outside stimuli would arrive at the visual cortex and PSPL, enhancing the sense of focus during the meditative practice.

It should also be noted that the dopaminergic system, via the basal ganglia, is believed to participate in regulating the glutamatergic system and the interactions between the prefrontal cortex and subcortical structures. A recent PET study measured the dopaminergic tone during Yoga Nidra meditation and demonstrated a significant increase in dopamine levels during the meditation practice (Kjaer et al., 2002). Kjaer and colleagues hypothesized that this increase may be associated with the gating of cortical–subcortical interactions that leads to an overall decrease in readiness for action that is associated with this particular type of meditation. Future studies will be necessary to elaborate on the role of dopamine during meditative practices as well as the interactions between dopamine and other neurotransmitter systems.

PSPL Deafferentation

Studies have indicated that the PSPL is involved in the analysis and integration of higher order visual, auditory, and somaesthetic information (Adair, Gilmore, Fennell, Gold, & Heilman, 1995; see also Joseph, 1990). As suggested earlier, this structure likely plays an important role in both holistic and reductionistic cognitive processes. It is also involved in a complex attentional network that includes the PFC and thalamus (Fernandez-Duque & Posner, 2001). Through the reception of auditory and visual input from the thalamus, the PSPL is able to help generate a three-dimensional image of the body in space, provide a sense of spatial coordinates in which the body is oriented, help distinguish between objects, and exert influences in regard to objects that may be directly grasped and manipulated (Mountcastle, Motter, & Anderson, 1980; Lynch, 1980). These functions of the PSPL might be critical for distinguishing between the self and the external world. It should be noted that a recent study has suggested that the superior temporal lobe may play a more important role in body spatial representation, although this has not been confirmed by other reports (Karnath, Ferber, & Himmelbach, 2001). However, it remains to be seen what is the actual relationship between the parietal and temporal lobes in terms of spatial representation.

Regardless, deafferentation of these orienting areas of the brain, we propose, is an important concept in the physiology of meditation. If, for example, deafferentation of the PSPL by the reticular nucleus's GABAergic effects occurs, the person may begin to lose his or her usual ability to spatially define the self. Such a notion is supported by clinical findings in patients with Balint's syndrome, in which parietal lobe damage results in marked difficulty orienting themselves in three-dimensional space. The effects of meditation are likely to be more selective and do not destroy the sense of self, but do alter the perception of it. Deafferentation of the PSPL has also been supported by two imaging studies demonstrating decreased activity in this region during intense meditation (Newberg et al., 2001; Herzog et al., 1990–1991). Further, our SPECT study showed a correlation between increasing activity in the thalamus and decreasing activity in the PSPL. The implication is that the more individuals increased the activity in their PFC, the more they deafferented the PSPL. Hence, one might suggest that the deeper and more intense the focus, the more likely one might ultimately attain unitary states.

Hippocampal and Amygdalar Activation during Spiritual Practices

In addition to the complex cortical–thalamic activity, meditative and spiritual practices might also be expected to alter activity in the limbic system, especially since stimulation of limbic structures is associated with experiences similar to those described during these practices (Fish, Gloor, Quesney, & Olivier, 1993; Saver & Rabin, 1997). The hippocampus acts to modulate and moderate cortical arousal and responsiveness, via rich and extensive interconnections with the prefrontal cortex, other neocortical areas, the amygdala, and the hypothalamus (Joseph, 1990). Hippocampal stimulation has been shown to diminish cortical responsiveness and arousal; however, if cortical arousal is initially at a low level, then hippocampal stimulation tends to augment cortical activity (Redding, 1967). The ability of the hippocampus to stimulate or inhibit neuronal activity in other structures likely relies upon the glutamate and GABA systems, respectively (Armony & LeDoux, 2000). In our neuropsychological model of meditation, we have suggested that during meditation, there is partial deafferentation of the right PSPL. This deafferentation could further result in stimulation of the right hippocampus because of the inverse modulation of the hippocampus in relation to cortical activity. If, in addition, there is simultaneous direct stimulation of the right hippocampus via the thalamus (as part of the known attentional network) and mediated by glutamate, then we suggest that a powerful recruitment of stimulation of the right hippocampus occurs. Right hippocampal activity may ultimately enhance the stimulatory function of the PFC on the thalamus via the nucleus accumbens, which is capable of gating the neural input from the PFC to the thalamus via the neuromodulatory effects of dopamine (Newman & Grace, 1999).

The hippocampus greatly influences the amygdala, such that they complement and interact in the generation of attention, emotion, and certain types of imagery (Joseph, 1990). It seems that much of the prefrontal modulation of emotion is via the hippocampus and its connections with the amygdala (Poletti & Sujatanond, 1980). Because of this reciprocal interaction between the amygdala and the hippocampus, we have suggested that activation of the right hippocampus during meditation likely stimulates the right lateral amygdala as well. The results of the functional magnetic resonance imaging (fMRI) study by Lazar and colleagues (2000) support the notion of increased activity in the regions of the amygdala and hippocampus during meditation.

Hypothalamic and Autonomic Nervous System Changes

It is known that the hypothalamus is extensively interconnected with the limbic system. Stimulation of the right lateral amygdala has been shown to result in stimulation of the ventromedial portion of the hypothalamus with a subsequent stimulation of the peripheral parasympathetic system (Davis, 1992). Increased parasympathetic activity should be associated with the subjective sensation first of relaxation, and eventually, of a more profound quiescence. Activation of the parasympathetic system would also cause a reduction in heart rate and respiratory rate. All of these physiological responses have been observed during meditation (Jevning, Wallace, & Beidebach, 1992).

Typically, when breathing and heart rate slow down, the paragigantocellular nucleus of the medulla ceases to innervate the locus coeruleus (LC) of the pons. The LC produces and distributes norepinephrine (NE) (Foote, 1987), a neuromodulator that increases the susceptibility of brain regions to sensory input by amplifying strong stimuli, while simultaneously gating out weaker activations and cellular "noise" that fall below the activation threshold (Waterhouse, Moises, & Woodward, 1998). Decreased stimulation of the LC results in a decrease in the level of NE (Van Bockstaele & Aston-Jones, 1995). The breakdown products of catecholamines such as NE and epinephrine have generally been found to be reduced in the urine and plasma during meditation (Walton, Pugh, Gelderloos, & Macrae, 1995), which may simply reflect the systemic change in autonomic balance. However, it is not inconsistent with a cerebral decrease in NE levels as well. During a meditative practice, our model suggests that reduced firing of the paragigantocellular nucleus cuts back its innervation of the locus ceruleus, which in turn is known to supply the PSPL and the lateral posterior nucleus with NE (Foote, 1987). Thus, a reduction in NE would decrease the impact of sensory input on the PSPL, contributing to its deafferentation.

The locus coeruleus would also deliver less NE to the hypothalamic paraventricular nucleus. The paraventricular nucleus of the hypothalamus typically secretes corticotropin-releasing hormone (CRH) in response to innervation by NE from the locus coeruleus (Ziegler, Cass, & Herman, 1999). This CRH stimulates the anterior pituitary to release adrenocorticotropic hormone (ACTH) (Livesey, Evans, Mulligan, & Donald, 2000). ACTH, in turn, stimulates the adrenal cortex to produce cortisol, one of the body's stress hormones (Davies, Keyon, & Fraser, 1985). Decreasing NE from the locus ceruleus during meditation would likely decrease the production of CRH by the paraventricular nucleus and ultimately decrease cortisol levels. Most studies have found that urine and plasma cortisol levels are decreased during meditation (Jevning, Wilson, & Davidson, 1978; Sudsuang, Chentanez, & Veluvan, 1991), supporting the notion that there is an overall decrease in cortisol secretion. This also has implications for the relationship between meditative practices and decreased stress since cortisol is frequently considered to be a primary "stress hormone."

The drop in blood pressure associated with parasympathetic activity during meditation practices might be expected to relax the arterial baroreceptors, leading the caudal ventral medulla to decrease its GABAergic inhibition of the supraoptic nucleus of the hypothalamus. In certain circumstances, this lack of inhibition can provoke the supraoptic nucleus to release the vasoconstrictor arginine vasopressin (AVP), thereby tightening the arteries and returning blood pressure to normal (Renaud, 1996). AVP has also been shown to contribute to the general maintenance of positive affect (Pietrowsky, Braun, Fehm, Pauschinger, & Born, 1991), decrease self-perceived fatigue and arousal, and significantly improve the consolidation of new memories and learning (Weingartner et al., 1981). In fact, plasma AVP has been shown to increase dramatically during meditation (O'Halloran et al., 1985). The increase in AVP might therefore result in a decreased subjective feeling of fatigue and an increased sense of arousal. It could also help to enhance the meditator's memory of the experience, perhaps explaining the subjective phenomenon that meditative and spiritual experiences are remembered and described in very vivid terms.

PFC Effects on Other Neurochemical Systems

As a spiritual practice continues, there should be continued activity in the PFC associated with the persistent will to focus attention. In general, as PFC activity increases, it produces ever-increasing levels of free synaptic glutamate in the brain. Increased glutamate can stimulate the hypothalamic arcuate nucleus to release beta-endorphin (BE) (Kiss, Kocsis, Csaki, Gorcs, & Halasz, 1997). BE is an opioid produced primarily by the arcuate nucleus of the medial hypothalamus and distributed to the brain's subcortical areas (Yadid, Zangen, Herzberg, Nakash, & Sagen, 2000). BE is known to depress respiration, reduce fear, reduce pain, and produce sensations of joy and euphoria (Janal, Colt, Clark, & Glusman, 1984). That such effects have been described during meditation may implicate some degree of BE release related to the increased PFC activity. Meditation has been found to disrupt diurnal rhythms of BE and ACTH, while not affecting diurnal cortisol rhythms (Infante et al., 1998). However, it is likely that BE is not the sole mediator in such experiences during meditation because simply taking morphine-related substances does not produce equivalent spiritual experiences. Furthermore, one very limited study demonstrated that blocking the opiate receptors with naloxone did not affect the experience or electroencephalogram (EEG) associated with meditation (Sim & Tsoi, 1992).

Glutamate activates N-methyl-D-aspartate receptors (NMDAr), but excess glutamate can kill these neurons through excitotoxic processes (Albin & Greenamyre, 1992). We propose that if glutamate levels approach excitotoxic concentrations during intense states of meditation, the brain might limit its production of N-acetylated alpha-linked acidic dipeptidase, which converts the endogenous NMDAr antagonist N-acetylaspartylglutamate (NAAG) into glutamate (Thomas, Vornov, Olkowski, Merion, & Slusher, 2000). The resultant increase in NAAG would protect cells from excitotoxic damage. There is an important side effect, however, since the NMDAr inhibitor NAAG is functionally analogous to the disassociative hallucinogens ketamine, phencyclidine, and nitrous oxide (Jevtovic-Todorovic, Wozniak, Benshoff, & Olney, 2001). These NMDAr antagonists produce a variety of states that may be characterized as either schizophrenomimetic or mystical, such as out-of-body and near-death experiences (Vollenweider et al., 1997).

Autonomic Nervous System Activity

In the early 1970s, Gellhorn and Kiely developed a model of the physiological processes involved in meditation based almost exclusively on autonomic nervous system (ANS) activity, which, while somewhat limited, indicated the importance of the ANS during such experiences (Gellhorn & Kiely, 1972). These authors suggested that intense stimulation of either the sympathetic or the parasympathetic system, if continued, could ultimately result in simultaneous discharge of both systems (what might be considered a "breakthrough" of the other system). Several studies have demonstrated predominant parasympathetic activity during meditation associated with decreased heart rate and blood pressure, decreased respiratory rate, and decreased oxygen metabolism (Travis, 2001). However, a recent study of two separate meditative techniques suggested a mutual activation of parasympathetic and sympathetic systems by demonstrating an increase in the variability of heart rate during meditation (Peng et al., 1999). The increased variation in heart rate was hypothesized to reflect activation of both arms of the ANS. This notion also fits the characteristic description of meditative states as involving a sense of overwhelming calmness as well as significant alertness. Also, the notion of mutual activation of both arms of the ANS is consistent with recent developments in the study of autonomic interactions (Hugdahl, 1996).

Serotonergic Activity

Activation of the ANS can result in intense stimulation of structures in the lateral hypothalamus and median forebrain bundle that are known to produce both ecstatic and blissful feelings when directly stimulated (Olds & Forbes, 1981). Stimulation of the lateral hypothalamus can also result in changes in serotonergic activity. In fact, several studies have shown that after meditation, the breakdown products of serotonin (ST) in urine are significantly increased, suggesting an overall elevation in ST during meditation (Walton et al., 1995). Serotonin is a neuromodulator that densely supplies the visual centers of the temporal lobe, where it strongly influences the flow of visual associations generated by this area (Joseph, 1990). The cells of the dorsal raphe produce and distribute ST when stimulated by the lateral hypothalamus (Aghajanian, Sprouse, & Rasmussen, 1987) and also when activated by the prefrontal cortex (Juckel, Mendlin, & Jacobs, 1999). Moderately increased levels of ST appear to correlate with positive affect, while low ST often signifies depression (Van Praag & De Haan, 1980). This relationship has clearly been demonstrated with regard to the effects of the selective serotonin reuptake inhibitor medications that are widely used for the treatment of depression. It should also be noted that several clinical studies have found that meditative and related spiritual practices can lower rates of depression or relapse into depression. The relationship between spiritual practices and decreased depression supports a serotonin role in spiritual practices.

When cortical ST receptors (especially in the temporal lobes) are activated, however, the stimulation can result in a hallucinogenic effect. Tryptamine psychedelics such as psylocybin and LSD seem to take advantage of this mechanism to produce their extraordinary visual associations (Aghajanian & Marek, 1999). The mechanism by which this appears to occur is that ST inhibits the lateral geniculate nucleus, greatly reducing the amount of visual information that can pass through (Funke & Eysel, 1995; Yoshida, Sasa, & Takaori, 1984). If combined with reticular nucleus inhibition of the lateral geniculate, ST may increase the fluidity of temporal visual associations in the absence of sensory input, possibly resulting in the internally generated imagery that has been described during certain meditative states.

Increased ST levels can affect several other neurochemical systems. An increase in serotonin has a modulatory effect on dopamine, suggesting a link between the serotonergic and dopaminergic systems that may enhance feelings of euphoria (Vollenweider, Vontobel, Hell, & Leenders, 1999), which is frequently described during meditative states. ST, in conjunction with the increased glutamate, has been shown to stimulate the nucleus basalis to release acetylcholine, which has important modulatory influences throughout the cortex (Manfridi, Brambilla, & Mancia, 1999). Increased acetylcholine in the frontal lobes has been shown to augment the attentional system and in the parietal lobes to enhance orienting without altering sensory input. While no studies have evaluated the role of acetylcholine in meditation, it appears that this neurotransmitter may enhance the attentional component as well as the orienting response in the face of progressive deafferentation of sensory input into the parietal lobes during meditation. Increased ST combined with lateral hypothalamic innervation of the pineal gland may lead the latter to increase production of the neurohormone melatonin (MT) from the conversion of ST (Moller, 1992). Melatonin has been shown to depress the central nervous system and reduce pain sensitivity (Shaji & Kulkarni, 1998). During meditation, blood plasma MT has been found to increase sharply (Tooley, Armstrong, Norman, & Sali, 2000), which may contribute to the meditator's feelings of calmness and decreased awareness of pain (Dollins et al., 1993). Under circumstances of heightened activation, pineal enzymes can also endogenously synthesize the powerful hallucinogen 5-methoxy-dimethyltryptamine (DMT) (Monti & Christian, 1981). Several studies have linked DMT to a variety of mystical states, including out-of-body experiences, distortion of time and space, and interaction with supernatural entities (Strassman & Clifford, 1994; Strassman, Clifford, Qualls, & Berg, 1996). Hyperstimulation of the pineal at this step, then, could also lead to DMT production that can be associated with the wide variety of mystical-type experiences associated with that hallucinogen.

CONCLUSION: SPIRITUAL EXPERIENCE IN PSYCHOLOGICAL PRACTICE

While other chapters in this book address the diverse relationship between spirituality and psychology, the review presented here raises several important points regarding the nature of this association. Western society has historically emphasized the importance of causality, technological advances, and empiricism. It is from these values that Western medicine, psychiatry, and psychology have developed. We propose that regardless of the connotation of the concept of spirituality in Western society, mystical and meditative experiences are natural and probably measurable processes that are and can be experienced by a diversity of people of different races, religions, and cultures. Those having spiritual experiences can have a variety of neuropsychological constitutions. In addition, it is important for clinicians to be sensitive and knowledgeable regarding spiritual and philosophical beliefs (Worthington, McCullough, & Sandage, 1996). Professionals need to be capable of distinguishing normal, healthy spiritual growth from psychopathology. We hope that some of the neurophysiological analysis described above might allow for a distinction between "normal" spiritual experiences and pathological states. In fact, such a nomenclature may be valuable for future psychological analysis of religious experiences. However, the fact that spiritual experiences have an effect on autonomic function as well as other cortically mediated cognitive and emotional processes suggests that such experiences not only affect the human psyche, but also can be carefully crafted to assist in the therapy of various disorders. It has already been shown that prayer and meditation can improve both physical and psychological parameters (Carson, 1993; Kabat-Zinn, Lipworth, & Burney, 1985; Kaplan, Goldenberg, & Galvin-Nadeu, 1993; Worthington et al., 1996). The more the underlying neurophysiological correlates of spiritual experiences are understood, the more such experiences can be analyzed and utilized in clinical practice. Therefore, spiritual experience can be very useful in clinical psychological and psychiatric practice. Furthermore, clinicians themselves can be instrumental in helping their patients toward personal and spiritual growth by discussing various meditative and/or spiritual practices and encouraging patients to approach these practices in an unambiguous manner. According to Rowan (1983), a humanistic psychologist, it is the self that is the missing link between the psychological and the spiritual. Therefore, it seems natural that spiritual experiences, such as those encountered in meditation and prayer, could become an adjunct to Western therapeutic practices and that developing oneself spiritually can become an important part of psychosocial as well as neuropsychological development.

ACKNOWLEDGMENT

We would like to thank Thomas G. Fikes for his helpful comments on this chapter.

REFERENCES

Adair, K. C., Gilmore, R. L., Fennell, E. B., Gold, M., & Heilman, K. M. (1995). Anosognosia during intracarotid barbiturate anaesthesia: Unawareness or amnesia for weakness. *Neurology, 45,* 241–243.

Aghajanian, G. K., & Marek, G. J. (1999). Serotonin and hallucinogens. *Neuropsychopharmacology, 21,* 16S–23S.

Aghajanian, G., Sprouse, J., & Rasmussen, K. (1987). Physiology of the midbrain serotonin system. In H. Meltzer (Ed.), *Psychopharmacology: The third generation of progress* (pp. 141–149). New York: Raven Press.

Albin, R., & Greenamyre, J. (1992). Alternative excitotoxic hypotheses. *Neurology, 42,* 733–738.

Armony, J. L., & LeDoux, J. E. (2000). How danger is encoded: Toward a systems, cellular, and computational understanding of cognitive-emotional interactions in fear. In M. S. Gazzaniga (Ed.), *The new cognitive neurosciences* (pp. 1073–1074). Cambridge, MA: MIT Press.

Bogen, J. E. (1969). The other side of the brain: II. An appositional mind. *Bulletin of Los Angeles Neurological Society, 34,* 135–162.

Bucci, D. J., Conley, M., & Gallagher, M. (1999). Thalamic and basal forebrain cholinergic connections of the rat posterior parietal cortex. *Neuroreport, 10,* 941–945.

Bucke, R. M. (1961). *Cosmic consciousness.* Secaucus, NJ: Citadel Press.

Burton, H., & Jones, E. G. (1976). The posterior thalamic region and its cortical projections in new world and old world monkeys. *Journal of Comparative Neurology, 168,* 249–302.

Carson, V. B. (1993). Prayer, meditation, exercise, special diets: Behaviors of the hardy person with HIV/AIDS. *Journal of the Association of Nurses in AIDS Care, 4,* 18–28.

Cheramy, A., Romo, R., & Glowinski, J. (1987). Role of corticostriatal glutamatergic neurons in the presynaptic control of dopamine release. In M. Sandler, C. Feuerstein, & B. Scatton (Eds.), *Neurotransmitter interactions in the basal ganglia.* New York: Raven Press.

Cornwall, J., & Phillipson, O. T. (1988). Mediodorsal and reticular thalamic nuclei receive collateral axons from prefrontal cortex and laterodorsal tegmental nucleus in the rat. *Neuroscience Letter, 88,* 121–126.

Crosson, B., Sadek, J. R., Maron, L., Gokcay, D., Mohr, C. M., Auerbach, E. J., Freeman, A. J., Leonard, C. M., & Briggs, R. W. (2001). Relative shift in activity from medial to lateral frontal cortex during internally versus externally guided word generation. *Journal of Cognitive Neuroscience, 13,* 272–283.

d'Aquili, E. G. (1978). The neurobiological bases of myth and concepts of deity. *Zygon, 13,* 257–275.

d'Aquili, E. G. (1983). The myth–ritual complex: A biogenetic structural analysis. *Zygon, 18,* 247–269.

d'Aquili, E. G. (1986). Myth, ritual, and the archetypal hypothesis: Does the dance generate the word? *Zygon, 21,* 141–160.

d'Aquili, E. G., & Newberg, A. B. (1993). Religious and mystical states: A neuropsychological substrate. *Zygon, 28,* 177–200.

d'Aquili, E. G., & Newberg, A. B. (1999). *The mystical mind: Probing the biology of religious experience.* Minneapolis, MN: Fortress Press.

Davies, E., Keyon, C. J., & Fraser, R. (1985). The role of calcium ions in the mechanism of ACTH stimulation of cortisol synthesis. *Steroids, 45,* 551–560.

Davis, M. (1992). The role of the amygdala in fear and anxiety. *Annual Review of Neuroscience, 15,* 353–375.

Destexhe, A., Contreras, D., & Steriade, M. (1998). Mechanisms underlying the synchronizing action of corticothalamic feedback through inhibition of thalamic relay cells. *Journal of Neurophysiology*, 79, 999–1016.

Dollins, A. B., Lynch, H. J., Wurtman, R. J., Deng, M. H., Kischka, K. U., Gleason, R. E., & Lieberman, H. R. (1993). Effect of pharmacological daytime doses of melatonin on human mood and performance. *Psychopharmacology*, 112, 490–496.

Elias, A. N., Guich, S., & Wilson, A. F. (2000). Ketosis with enhanced GABAergic tone promotes physiological changes in transcendental meditation. *Medical Hypotheses*, 54, 660–662.

Fernandez-Duque, D., & Posner, M. I. (2001). Brain imaging of attentional networks in normal and pathological states. *Journal of Clinical Experimental Neuropsychology*, 23, 74–93.

Fish, D. R., Gloor, P., Quesney, F. L., & Olivier, A. (1993). Clinical responses to electrical brain stimulation of the temporal and frontal lobes in patients with epilepsy. *Brain*, 116, 397–414.

Foote, S. (1987). Extrathalamic modulation of cortical function. *Annual Review of Neuroscience*, 10, 67–95.

Frith, C. D., Friston, K., Liddle, P. F., & Frackowiak, R. S. (1991). Willed action and the prefrontal cortex in man: A study with PET. *Proceedings of the Royal Society of London*, 244, 241–246.

Funke, K., & Eysel, U. T. (1995). Possible enhancement of GABAergic inputs to cat dorsal lateral geniculate relay cells by serotonin. *Neuroreport*, 6, 474–476.

Gazzaniga, M. S., & Hillyard, S. A. (1971). Language and speech capacity of the right hemisphere. *Neuropsychologia*, 9, 273–280.

Gellhorn, E., & Kiely, W. F. (1972). Mystical states of consciousness: Neurophysiological and clinical aspects. *Journal of Nervous and Mental Disease*, 154, 399–405.

Herzog, H., Lele, V. R., Kuwert, T., Langen, K.-J., Kops, E. R., & Feinendegen, L. E. (1990–1991). Changed pattern of regional glucose metabolism during yoga meditative relaxation. *Neuropsychobiology*, 23, 182–187.

Hugdahl, K. (1996). Cognitive influences on human autonomic nervous system function. *Current Opinion in Neurobiology*, 6, 252–258.

Infante, J. R., Peran, F., Martinez, M., Roldan, A., Poyatos, R., Ruiz, C., Samaniego, F., & Garrido, F. (1998). ACTH and beta-endorphin in transcendental meditation. *Physiology and Behavior*, 64, 311–315.

Ingvar, D. H. (1994). The will of the brain: Cerebral correlates of willful acts. *Journal of Theoretical Biology*, 171, 7–12.

Janal, M., Colt, E., Clark, W., & Glusman, M. (1984). Pain sensitivity, mood and plasma endocrine levels in man following long-distance running: Effects of naxalone. *Pain*, 19, 13–25.

Jevning, R., Wallace, R. K., & Beidebach, M. (1992). The physiology of meditation: A review. A wakeful hypometabolic integrated response. *Neuroscience Biobehavioral Review*, 16, 415–424.

Jevning, R., Wilson, A. F., & Davidson, J. M. (1978). Adrenocortical activity during meditation. *Hormones and Behavior*, 10, 54–60.

Jevtovic-Todorovic, V., Wozniak, D. F., Benshoff, N. D., & Olney, J. W. (2001). A comparative evaluation of the neurotoxic properties of ketamine and nitrous oxide. *Brain Research*, 895, 264–267.

Joseph, R. (1990). *Neuropsychology, neuropsychiatry, and behavioral neurology*. New York: Plenum Press.

Juckel, G. J., Mendlin, A., & Jacobs, B. L. (1999). Electrical stimulation of rat medial prefrontal cortex enhances forebrain serotonin output: Implications for electroconvulsive therapy and transcranial magnetic stimulation in depression. *Neuropsychopharmacology*, 21, 391–398.

Kabat-Zinn, J., Lipworth, L., & Burney, R. (1985). The clinical use of mindfulness meditation for the self-regulation of chronic pain. *Journal of Behavioral Medicine*, 8, 163–190.

Kaplan, K. H., Goldenberg, D. L., & Galvin-Nadeu, M. (1993). The impact of a meditation-based stress reduction program on fibromyalgia. *General Hospital Psychiatry*, 15, 284–289.

Karnath, H. O., Ferber, S., & Himmelbach, M. (2001). Spatial awareness is a function of the temporal not the posterior parietal lobe. *Nature*, 411, 950–953.

Kiss, J., Kocsis, K., Csaki, A., Gorcs, T. J., & Halasz, B. (1997). Metabotropic glutamate receptor in

GHRH and beta-endorphin neurons of the hypothalamic arcuate nucleus. *Neuroreport, 8,* 3703–3707.

Kjaer, T. W., Bertelsen, C., Piccini, P., Brooks, D., Alving, J., & Lou, H. C. (2002). Increased dopamine tone during meditation-induced change of consciousness. *Cognitive Brain Research, 13*(2), 255–259.

Lazar, S. W., Bush, G., Gollub, R. L., Fricchione, G. L., Khalsa, G., & Benson, H. (2000). Functional brain mapping of the relaxation response and meditation. *Neuroreport, 11,* 1581–1585.

Livesey, J. H., Evans, M. J., Mulligan, R., & Donald, R. A. (2000). Interactions of CRH, AVP and cortisol in the secretion of ACTH from perifused equine anterior pituitary cells: "Permissive" roles for cortisol and CRH. *Endocrinology Research, 26,* 445–463.

Luria, A. R. (1966). *Higher cortical functions in man.* New York: Basic Books.

Lynch, J. C. (1980). The functional organization of posterior parietal association cortex. *Behavioral Brain Sciences, 3,* 485–499.

Manfridi, A., Brambilla, D., & Mancia, M. (1999). Stimulation of NMDA and AMPA receptors in the rat nucleus basalis of Meynert affects sleep. *American Journal of Physiology, 277,* R1488–R1492.

Moller, M. (1992). Fine structure of pinealopetal innervation of the mammalian pineal gland. *Microscope Research Technology, 21,* 188–204.

Monti, J. A., & Christian, S.T. N.-N. (1981). Dimethyltryptamine: An endogenous hallucinogen. *International Review of Neurobiology, 22,* 83–110.

Mountcastle, V. B. (1976). The world around us: Neural command functions for selective attention. *Neurosciences Research Progress Bulletin, 14,* 1–47.

Mountcastle, V. B., Motter, B. C., & Andersen, R. A. (1980). Some further observations on the functional properties of neurons in the parietal lobe of the waking monkey. *Brain Behavioral Sciences, 3,* 520–529.

Nebes, R. D., & Sperry, R. W. (1971). Hemispheric disconnection syndrome with cerebral birth injury in the dominant arm area. *Neuropsychologia, 9,* 249–259.

Newberg, A. B., Alavi, A., Baime, M., Pourdehnad, M., Santanna, J., & d'Aquili, E. G. (2001). The measurement of regional cerebral blood flow during the complex cognitive task of meditation: A preliminary SPECT study. *Psychiatry Research: Neuroimaging, 106,* 113–122.

Newberg, A. B., & d'Aquili, E. G. (1994). The near death experience as archetype: A model for "prepared" neurocognitive processes. *Anthropology of Consciousness, 5,* 1–15.

Newberg, A. B., & Iversen, J. (2003). The neural basis of the complex mental task of meditation: Neurotransmitter and neurochemical considerations. *Medical Hypotheses, 61,* 282–291.

Newman, J., & Grace, A. A. (1999). Binding across time: The selective gating of frontal and hippocampal systems modulating working memory and attentional states. *Consciousness and Cognition, 8,* 196–212.

O'Halloran, J. P., Jevning, R., Wilson, A. F., Skowsky, R., Walsh, R. N., & Alexander, C. (1985). Hormonal control in a state of decreased activation: Potentiation of arginine vasopressin secretion. *Physiology and Behavior, 35,* 591–595.

Olds, M. E., & Forbes, J. L. (1981). The central basis of motivation: Intracranial self-stimulation studies. *Annual Review of Psychology, 32,* 523–574.

Pardo, J. V., Fox, P. T., & Raichle, M. E. (1991). Localization of a human system for sustained attention by positron emission tomography. *Nature, 349,* 61–64.

Peng, C. K., Mietus, J. E., Liu, Y., Khalsa, G., Douglas, P. S., Benson, H., & Goldberger, A. L. (1999). Exaggerated heart rate oscillations during two meditation techniques. *International Journal of Cardiology, 70,* 101–107.

Pietrowsky, R., Braun, D., Fehm, H. L., Pauschinger, P., & Born, J. (1991). Vasopressin and oxytocin do not influence early sensory processing but affect mood and activation in man. *Peptides, 12,* 1385–1391.

Poletti, C. E., & Sujatanond, M. (1980). Evidence for a second hippocampal efferent pathway to hypothalamus and basal forebrain comparable to fornix system: A unit study in the monkey. *Journal of Neurophysiology, 44,* 514–531.

Portas, C. M., Rees, G., Howseman, A. M., Josephs, O., Turner, R., & Frith, C. D. (1998). A specific role for the thalamus in mediating the interaction attention and arousal in humans. *Journal of Neuroscience, 18*, 8979–8989.

Posner, M. I., & Petersen, S. E. (1990). The attention system of the human brain. *Annual Review of Neuroscience, 13*, 25–42.

Pribram, K. H. (1973). The primate frontal cortex: Executive of the brain. In K. H. Pribram & A. R. Luria (Eds.), *Psychophysiology of the frontal lobes*. New York: Academic Press.

Redding, F. K. (1967). Modification of sensory cortical evoked potentials by hippocampal stimulation. *Electroencephalography and Clinical Neurophysiology, 22*, 74–83.

Renaud, L. P. (1996). CNS pathways mediating cardiovascular regulation of vasopressin. *Clinical and Experimental Pharmacology and Physiology, 23*, 157–160.

Rowan, J. (1983). The real self and mystical experiences. *Journal of Humanistic Psychology, 23*(2), 9–27.

Saver, J. L., & Rabin, J. (1997). The neural substrates of religious experience. *Journal of Neuropsychiatry and Clinical Neuroscience, 9*, 498–510.

Shaji, A. V., & Kulkarni, S. K. (1998). Central nervous system depressant activities of melatonin in rats and mice. *Indian Journal of Experimental Biology, 36*, 257–263.

Sim, M. K., & Tsoi, W. F. (1992). The effects of centrally acting drugs on the EEG correlates of meditation. *Biofeedback Self Regulation, 17*, 215–220.

Smart, N. (1958). *Reasons and faiths: An investigation of religious discourse, Christian and non-Christian*. London: Routledge & Kegan Paul.

Smart, N. (1967). History of mysticism. In P. Edwards (Ed.), *Encyclopedia of philosophy*. London: Macmillan.

Smart, N. (1969). *The religious experience of mankind*. London: Macmillan.

Sperry, R. W., Gazzaniga, M. S., & Bogen, J. E. (1969). Interhemispheric relationships: The neocortical commisures; syndromes of hemisphere disconnection. In P. J. Vinken & C. W. Bruyn (Eds.), *Handbook of clinical neurology, Vol. 4*. Amsterdam: North Holland.

Stace, W. T. (1961). *Mysticism and philosophy*. London: Macmillan.

Strassman, R. J., & Clifford, R. (1994). Dose–response study of N,N-Dimethyltrypamine in humans: I. Neuroendocrine, autonomic, and cardiovascular effects. *Archives of General Psychiatry, 51*, 85–97.

Strassman, R. J., Clifford, R., Qualls, R., & Berg, L. (1996). Differential tolerance to biological and subjective effects of four closely spaced doses of N,N-Dimethyltrypamine in humans. *Biological Psychiatry, 39*, 784–795.

Sudsuang, R., Chentanez, V., & Veluvan, K. (1991). Effects of Buddhist meditation on serum cortisol and total protein levels, blood pressure, pulse rate, lung volume and reaction time. *Physiology and Behavior, 50*, 543–548.

Thomas, A. G., Vornov, J. J., Olkowski, J. L., Merion, A. T., & Slusher, B. S. (2000). N-Acetylated alpha-linked acidic dipeptidase converts N-acetylaspartylglutamate from a neuroprotectant to a neurotoxin. *Journal of Pharmacology and Experimental Therapies, 295*, 16–22.

Tooley, G. A., Armstrong, S. M., Norman, T. R., & Sali, A. (2000). Acute increases in night-time plasma melatonin levels following a period of meditation. *Biological Psychology, 53*, 69–78.

Travis, F. (2001). Autonomic and EEG patterns distinguish transcending from other experiences during transcendental meditation practice. *International Journal of Psychophysiology, 42*, 1–9.

Turner, V. (1969). *The ritual process: Structure and anti-structure*. Ithaca, NY: Cornell University Press.

Van Bockstaele, E. J., & Aston-Jones, G. (1995). Integration in the ventral medulla and coordination of sympathetic, pain and arousal functions. *Clinical and Experimental Hypertension, 17*, 153–165.

Van Praag, H., & De Haan, S. (1980). Depression vulnerability and 5–Hydroxytryptophan prophylaxis. *Psychiatry Research, 3*, 75–83.

Vogt, B. A., Finch, D. M., & Olson, C. R. (1992). Functional heterogeneity in cingulate cortex: The anterior executive and posterior evaluative regions. *Cerebral Cortex, 2*, 435–443.

Vollenweider, F. X., Leenders, K. L., Scharfetter, C., Antonini, A., Maguire, P., Missimer, J., & Angst, J. (1999). Metabolic hyperfrontality and psychopathology in the ketamine model of psychosis using positron emission tomography (PET) and [18F]fluorodeoxyglucose (FDG). *European Neuropsychopharmacology, 7,* 9–24.

Vollenweider, F. X., Vontobel, P., Hell, D., & Leenders, K. L. (1999). 5-HT modulation of dopamine release in basal ganglia in psilocybin-induced psychosis in man—a PET study with [11C]raclopride. *Neuropsychopharmacology, 20,* 424–433.

Walton, K. G., Pugh, N. D., Gelderloos, P., & Macrae, P. (1995). Stress reduction and preventing hypertension: Preliminary support for a psychoneuroendocrine mechanism. *Journal of Alternative Complementary Medicine, 1,* 263–283.

Waterhouse, B. D., Moises, H. C., & Woodward, D. J. (1998). Phasic activation of the locus coeruleus enhances responses of primary sensory cortical neurons to peripheral receptive field stimulation. *Brain Research, 790,* 33–44.

Weingartner, H., Gold, P., Ballenger, J. C., Smallberg, S. A., Summers, R., Rubinow, D. R., Post, R. M., & Goodwin, F. K. (1981). Effects of vasopressin on human memory functions. *Science, 211,* 601–603.

Worthington, E. L., McCullough, M. E., & Sandage, S. J. (1996). Empirical research on religion and psychotherapeutic processes and outcomes: A 10-year review and research prospectus. *Psychological Bulletin, 119,* 448–487.

Yadid, G., Zangen, A., Herzberg, U., Nakash, R., & Sagen, J. (2000). Alterations in endogenous brain beta-endorphin release by adrenal medullary transplants in the spinal cord. *Neuropsychopharmacology, 23,* 709–716.

Yoshida, M., Sasa, M., & Takaori, S. (1984). Serotonin-mediated inhibition from dorsal raphe neurons nucleus of neurons in dorsal lateral geniculate and thalamic reticular nuclei. *Brain Resolution, 290,* 95–105.

Ziegler, D. R., Cass, W. A., & Herman, J. P. (1999). Excitatory influence of the locus coeruleus in hypothalamic–pituitary–adrenocortical axis responses to stress. *Journal of Neuroendocrinology, 11,* 361–369.

12

Cognitive Approaches to Religion

ELIZABETH WEISS OZORAK

In the lead essay for the 2001 issue of the *Annual Review of Psychology*, Albert Bandura noted that a paradigm shift has occurred in the field in the past few decades. Psychology no longer views human behavior only as a set of predetermined responses to environment, or as the output of a complexly programmed computer; instead, people are recognized as agents capable of performing intentional acts with a view toward achieving goals that are congruent with a particular set of beliefs. In this view, belief systems are pivotal, as they provide people with a working model of the world that helps them make behavioral choices. Under this paradigm, research on all aspects of cognition has flourished and a number of intriguing theoretical frameworks have been advanced.

As Andresen (2001) notes, this productive climate offers great opportunities to develop cognitive approaches to the study of religion. In spite of these opportunities, cognitive-psychological research on religion remains—with a few exceptions—sporadic and incompletely connected: it is indicative that of the 10 contributors to the Andresen volume, just one is a psychologist (Barrett) and just one is a psychiatrist (McNamara). The fields of anthropology and comparative religion are heavily represented in current cognitive research, with important contributions from sociology, philosophy, and cognitive neuroscience. The good news for psychologists of religion who feel they may be toiling in obscurity (Pargament, 2002) is that there are some exciting opportunities for collegiality beyond our own backyard.

This chapter illuminates some of the connections between existing lines of work and suggest ways in which researchers might capitalize, within and across disciplinary lines, on the field's developments to date. In the first sections, I introduce current cognitive models and briefly describe research on religion that has looked at some aspect of that model. The following sections describe the main directions cognitive research on religion has taken in the last several years and questions that remain open in each. The concluding section reviews some of the cutting-edge issues in cognitive research and suggests ways in which these might be applied to research on religion, to the benefit of both.

INFORMATION PROCESSING

The Modal Model

Textbooks of cognitive psychology almost always include a discussion of the so-called modal model of cognition, initially described by Atkinson and Shiffrin (1971). In this model, environmental input enters the sensory registers and from there is encoded into short-term, or working, memory. Some of this material makes it into long-term memory, where it is organized according to existing knowledge structures, such as categories, schemas, and scripts in a richly interconnected network. Although there have been some recent criticisms of this model (Nairne, 2002), it undergirds most cognitively oriented work over the past 30 years and today.

At each stage of encoding, the information becomes less precisely like the original input and relies more heavily on meaning provided by reference to preexisting knowledge and beliefs. For example, a colleague's friendly greeting goes into the sensory registers as a fairly accurate visual image and auditory trace, but the words and expression become fuzzy in working memory as part of my attention is occupied with choosing an appropriate response. The resulting long-term memory is gist only, and if I greet this colleague regularly, eventually my long-term memories of these occasions will mush together into one collective generic account.

As the disparity between original information and encoded information increases, the effects of prior knowledge and beliefs are more clearly observed. Memories of conversations, to use the preceding example, owe much to our cultural scripts as well as to our impressions of the conversational partner. Over time, the dialogue we recall bears more resemblance to the roles we imagine for ourselves and our conversational partner than to the original utterances. In addition, our schemas about the relationship between the two of us (i.e., relational schemas) and the kinds of conversations we habitually have will strongly influence the conversations we recall (Baldwin, 1992). What we experience and what we know—or think we know—is always framed by what we experienced before and believed already. Through these framing effects, both our personal histories and our group identities (culture, ethnicity, faith community, gender, etc.) have substantial impact on what we perceive and remember.

Applications to Religion Research

A number of theorists maintain that religious cognition is produced by exactly the same processes as other kinds of cognition. Contributors to the Andresen (2001) volume largely support this perspective (notably Barrett, Guthrie, Lawson, and McCauley), as does Boyer (e.g., 2001), whose work informs many of the chapters in the book. Boyer maintains that the human mind has evolved with certain adaptive predispositions and restrictions, and that religious forms invariably reflect those characteristics, just like other cognitions and cultural practices. This produces a limited set of recurring concepts across religious and cultural groups. Concepts of agency, social exchange, moral sense and misfortune, Boyer (2003) argues, show distinct family resemblances even across cultures that superficially seem very different, and religious versions of these are similar to nonreligious versions (e.g., many religions involve one or more omniscient beings, but this is similar to the ways in which a close relative or friend might be able to guess a person's intent without hearing it articulated).

In addition to their focus on innate cognitive mechanisms, these theorists seem to concur at least implicitly that normal cognitive processes are sufficient to explain religious belief and experience. Guthrie (2001) focuses largely on perception and interpretation; McCauley (2001) and Whitehouse (2002) emphasize the role of memory in determining religious practice and experience; Barrett (2002) and Lawson (2001) concentrate on knowledge structures. A parallel analysis from a behaviorist perspective, relational frame theory (Barnes-Holmes, Hayes, & Gregg, 2001), takes a similar view, although the vocabulary used is more behavioral in flavor.

A few theorists (e.g., Oser & Gmeunder, 1991; Sinnott, 2000) assert that religious cognition is indeed distinctive, raising the possibility of a sacred agency being partially responsible for the patterns of religious cognition that are observed. Most cognitive research neither affirms nor denies such a possibility, but it remains a contentious implicit question. I return to the question of "true or not" later in the chapter because it continues to affect the development of the field.

Perception

As Hill (1997) notes, association to cognitive networks can occur in automatic processing, such as pattern recognition, as well as in controlled processing, such as reasoning. Religion, which often involves strongly ingrained knowledge representations and habits of thought, probably relates to effects in every aspect of information processing in those to whom it is deeply important. Recent evidence supports the priming effect of religious terms (Wenger, 2004), as well as perceptual differences related to religious style (Ash, Crist, Salisbury, & Dewell, 1996). Possibly people with different perceptual styles are drawn to different manifestations of religious faith; longitudinal data from the teen years into adulthood would help to establish which comes first. Watts and Williams (1988) suggest that divergences in perception, both between religious and nonreligious individuals and among those of different faiths, are partly a matter of selective attention, which in turn would limit what is available to memory.

Memory

I have described at length elsewhere a general model of how memory might shape and be shaped by religious experience (Ozorak, 1997). Briefly, since memory content is extensively structured by preexisting patterns, both culturally given and personally salient, our experiences tend to confirm our expectations, religious and otherwise. To give one example, Szuchewicz (1994) has documented how a prayer group's selective attention to contributions that related to the day's Scripture reading produced a shared impression that the Holy Spirit "always" guided the group in terms of a specific theme. A combination of priming by the Scripture itself, the group's reinterpretation of contributions to make them match in some way, and a failure to rehearse contributions that could not be made to fit accounted for the consequent strength of this impression, which was then overtly confirmed by the leader at each session.

McCauley and Lawson (McCauley, 2001; McCauley & Lawson, 2002) point out that memory is essential for ongoing transmission of religious practice, particularly in preliterate cultures. They postulate—and support with anecdotal evidence from various cultures—a predictable underlying grammar of ritual due to the specific functions and limitations of human memory. For example, rituals believed to involve the direct intervention of a superhuman agent rely on high sensory and emotional stimulation rather than rehearsal to be memorable. By contrast, the ritual frequency hypothesis (Whitehouse, 2002) maintains that it is frequency of performance (rehearsal) alone that dictates the need for sensory and emotional extremes.

Clarification and elaboration of these hypotheses might benefit from systematic study of individuals with imperfect or incomplete memory of various important rituals. For example, anecdotal evidence from pastors and lay ministers who visit elderly shut-ins (e.g., Cartwright, 1995, personal communication) suggests that certain rituals become deeply ingrained and the ability to access them persists even in the face of massive general memory deterioration. A cognitive analysis might show which prayers and practices are recalled verbatim, and perhaps discern some patterns: frequency of rehearsal, early age of encoding, emotional valence, overall significance to the religious group, and McCauley's (2001) dimension of proximity to a supernatural agent are all candidates for producing resilience in recall.

Knowledge Structures and Framing

Religion has been described as a schema (McIntosh, 1995) or perhaps a cluster of schemas (Ozorak, 1997) that are used to organize new information and to guide decision making, even outside an explicitly religious context (of course, for some religious adherents, there is no such thing as an aspect of life outside the religious context). The framing of choices and interpretation of outcomes has substantial long-term effects for motivation and persistence (Bandura, 2001). Religious frames may not be rational (Chaves & Montgomery, 1996), but that does not mean they are not adaptive. As Cantor (2002) points out, people may use irrational beliefs to keep themselves motivated and actually spur better performance. Religious or other supernatural causal attributions may be used in this way (Deconchy, Hurteau, Quelen, & Ragot, 1997). In addition, definitions of success and failure in religious systems may be different from success and failure according to the cultural status quo (Patzer & Helm, 2001). Certainly, many religions and some nonreligious philosophies help believers to distance themselves from past failures and approach the future with a positive outlook (Barnes-Holmes et al., 2001).

Judgment, Decision Making, and Problem Solving

Retrieval from memory is easier than reasoning, so people tend to stick with earlier solutions, whether or not they still work. When there is no earlier solution, people rely on schemas, scripts, and causal theories to shape courses of action rather than bottom-up problem solving. Subjective utility theory—the notion that people choose on the basis of what they want tempered by what they expect—is the dominant model of decision making (Hastie, 2001). However, what utility theory fails to supply is information about how people arrive at what they want (past history and cultural scripts largely determine what they expect).

Religious values provide one impetus toward choice, either through assent to the religious organization's position (applying a past solution) or through weighing that position against other values (Dillon, 1999). However, research on religion and decision making has focused mainly on choices involving contraception (Iyer, 2002) and sexual abstinence (Paul, Fitzjohn, Eberhart-Phillips, Herbison, & Dickson, 2000) or explicitly religious choices (e.g., Chaves & Montgomery, 1996). For those with highly elaborated religious schemas, many choices likely reflect religious values. Exploring these would address decision theory's need for more information about how values and goals contribute to perceptions of utility (Hastie, 2001).

Religion-based problem-solving research has focused mainly on coping (see Parga-ment, Ano, & Wachholz, Chapter 26, this volume). This research often has a strong cog-nitive component insofar as it focuses on appraisal. Maltby and Day (2003) found that positive religious coping is associated with tendencies to appraise problems as challenges rather than as threats or losses. Reich (2002) suggests that problem solving involves a comparison of appraisals such that "rivaling descriptions" are coordinated and set in a larger context (p. 15). If Reich is correct, some of the inconsistencies Maltby and Day (2003) found in appraisal effects may be due to participants' attempts to reconcile com-peting appraisals. It would be interesting to extend the study of religious appraisal effects beyond crisis situations.

Insight and Intuition (Implicit Knowing)

If there is a unique form of religious cognition, Watts and Williams (1988) argue, it is in the form of insight and intuitive knowing. Miller and C'De Baca (2001) suggest that in-sight is "more than cognitive" (p. 38), involving the opportunity for self-transformation through recognition of an "authentic truth" (p. 40) that demands a new way of acting. They point out that not all insight is religious in nature; and of course, all religiously in-clined people may not be equally open to intuitive knowing. Psychiatrists in a Canadian sample claimed that therapy is more likely than religion to yield transformational insights (Baetz, Larson, Marcoux, Jokic, & Bowen, 2002); by contrast, Miller and C'De Baca (2001) lamented that transformational insight seemed to occur almost everywhere but in therapy.

Obviously, the jury is more than out on religious insight—it has barely convened. However, good studies of insight in problem solving exist, and two plausible theories are currently being tested. MacGregor, Ormerod, and Chronicle (2001) suggest that people look for insight only after it becomes apparent that the current approach cannot lead to a solution (progress-monitoring theory). Knoblich, Ohlsson, and Raney (2001) propose that people often need to revisit their initial construal of the problem in order to attain in-sight (representational change theory).

Although the theories differ on some points, they concur that self-imposed con-straints on the definition of the problem or the strategies considered for solving it are fre-quently the cause of mental impasse, and that insight occurs when these restraints are re-moved or tempered. Religion, because of its strong affective components, might provoke such impasses as well as resolve them. However, both models have been tested only on well-defined problems like dot connection or matchstick arithmetic problems, and need to be explored in ill-defined problem situations (i.e., when the rules, the criteria for suc-cess, and/or the problem itself remain unclear; most significant real-world problems fall into this category). It would be worth examining people's reported experiences of apply-ing their faith to problem solving to see whether the patterns of thought predicted by ei-ther theory occur, and, if so, what factors seem to make one or the other prevail—for ex-ample, quest orientation, rigidity of belief system, or group norms for doubt and disagreement.

Counterintuitive Ideas

A shared quality of religious belief systems is that they deal with mysterious or counterintuitive phenomena—events or entities that cannot be fully accounted for by mundane explanations. Contrary to the commonsense notion that religion is used to provide explanations for such phenomena, Boyer (2003) argues that religious belief systems generate mysteries, much like other supernatural thinking (such as magic, folk legends, and dreams). Certainly, in many societies, religious explanations often run counter to the kinds of explanations found in other domains, creating tension for believers rather than resolving it (Evans, 2001). Boyer and Ramble (2001) have shown that information with counterintuitive features is more easily remembered and has greater impact over time than similar information with no intuitive violations. On the other hand, supernatural agents and events typically rely on schemas that largely conform to normal schemas; in other words, there is an optimal level of bizarreness (Boyer, 2003). For example, ghosts and spirits violate our understanding of physics but not our understanding of psychology: they go through walls, but have human-like passions and, if they talk, converse in recognizable patterns. In a less common pattern of intuitive violation, zombies conform to the normal physical properties of bodies, but are psychologically peculiar.

Sinnott (2000) argues, in contrast, that the ability to assimilate counterintuitive religious ideas is a consequence of what she calls *postformal cognition*, a mature ability to hold apparently contradictory logics in dialogue with one another. This capacity develops through experience and makes possible a unified sense of reality, much like Reich's relational and contextual reasoning (Reich, 2002). The problem with both this line of thought and Boyer's is that cognitive capacities may explain what it is possible for us to believe, but they do not tell us why particular beliefs emerge from the set of possible beliefs. In addition, paradoxical beliefs do not seem to be limited to people with mature cognitive abilities.

SOCIAL COGNITION

Schemas and Scripts

Social cognition is thought involving social interaction and ourselves as social beings. Like other forms of cognition, it relies heavily on schemas and scripts. Since religion is an important part of many people's self-concept and provides numerous contexts for interaction, it is sure to play a role in social perception, social memory, and relational reasoning. It is worth asking how religion figures into people's schemas and scripts and how it affects social-cognitive processes that have been widely studied, since religion sometimes engages people in scripts that diverge abruptly from the cultural norm (e.g., Ingram, 1989). In addition, the variations induced by social group memberships such as race, class, gender, and the like need to be addressed.

Basic Dimensions of Religious Schemas

Twenty years ago, Moehle (1983) analyzed an extensive set of reported religious experiences in an attempt to identify the salient dimensions along which they varied. The three dimensions that emerged were level of personal control, spiritual–temporal, and social–individual. Schemas involving personal control are obviously central to coping with crisis (e.g., McIntosh, 1995; see Park, Chapter 16, this volume), but pertain to many other aspects of cognition as well. Given the vast amount of work on locus of control in the past two decades, Moehle's dimensions deserve to be revisited (see Haidt & Rodin, 1999, who argue that control and efficacy are natural bridges to a wide variety of topics in- and outside of psychology). One natural connection might be with prayer, which also has been analyzed for categorical differences (Ladd & Spilka, 2002). Ladd and Spilka's *inward*, *outward*, and *upward* distinction appears to relate to Mochle's social–individual dimension, while intercession and petition, and possibly other categories of prayer, seem based in locus-of-control appraisals. Likewise, the patterns of perceived ritual efficacy found by Barrett (2002) suggest specific scripts about control by a god with extraordinary powers versus by others. Such scripts undoubtedly reflect both cultural and religious variations in locus of control as well as possibly universal ways of constructing causal equations (Boyer, 2003).

Attributions of Causality

Perceptions of control and efficacy are part of the general grammar of causal attribution. An attribution theory for religious applications has been mapped (Spilka, Shaver, & Kirkpatrick, 1985) and tested in a number of ways. There is evidence that religious attributions are favored for events with far-reaching consequences, especially positive ones (Lupfer, Tolliver, & Jackson, 1996). Both religious orientation (Hovemyr, 1998) and religious conservatism (Kunst, Bjorck, & Tan, 2000) affect the way in which individuals make attributions. When religious attributions are made, individuals often perceive divine or supernatural causes working indirectly (e.g., through other people) rather than through direct action (Weeks & Lupfer, 2000). It would be useful to analyze religious attributions with respect to violations of intuition, to see whether these attributions differ from mundane explanations as Boyer (2001) would predict.

Relational Schemas

As previously discussed, relational schemas predict and shape interactions with others (Baldwin, 1992). These schemas seem to fit with utility theory in that they involve a combination of expectancies and values, although they also involve strongly associated scripts or predictable sequences of behavior. Baldwin and his colleagues have demonstrated in several studies that these schemas prime self-evaluations, interpretations of ambiguous behavior, and personal goals for the interaction (see Baldwin & Baccus, 2003, for an overview).

For religious believers in some traditions, including Christianity, Judaism, and Islam, the faith tradition suggests certain kinds of relational schemas that do or should operate between the individual and God and between the individual and the community. Hill and Hall (2002) examine several classic theories of relationship, such as attachment theory and object relations theory, for patterns that might characterize relational schemas between Christians and the God they worship. Ozorak (2003b) found that volunteer service activated religious relational schemas for college students who described themselves as religious.

Judgment and Framing

Schemas affect judgment in part by the way in which they frame the options. A number of researchers have looked at the role of religious contexts and beliefs in framing judgments, with mixed results. Cohen and Rozin (2001), for example, found that Jews and Christians reached different conclusions about the moral wrongness of thinking about a sinful action, although participants of both faiths tended to agree about the wrongness of related actions. Cobb, Ong, and Tate (2001), in contrast, found no religious differences in judgments of wrongdoing, and in fact concluded that religious reasoning was similar to nonreligious moral reasoning; however, they asked only about wrong actions, not about wrong thoughts. Turiel and Neff (2000) are probably right to insist that culture, religion, gender, and social position interact in complex ways to produce moral judgments, and that individuals' choices may distinguish between the morally best choice and the pragmatically best choice given the social context.

The way in which information about religion itself is introduced in studies seems to exert some influence on judgment. Peeters and Hendrickx (2002) demonstrated that judgments of hypothetical people followed two patterns, a Self–Other narrative response that generated a single representation with affective connotations and a Third Person response that compiled information in a more science-like fashion. Judgments of the person's religious attitudes, like judgments of personality, triggered the Self–Other response, while information about the person's doctrine generated the Third Person response.

Cognitive Dissonance

Just as religion may be said to create as many counterintuitive notions as it explains, it causes as much cognitive dissonance as it resolves (Exline, 2002). Given the recent national focus on issues surrounding homosexuality, both inside and outside of mainline churches, it is unsurprising that identifying oneself as a homosexual Christian often creates cognitive dissonance internally and externally (Mahaffy, 1996). Homosexual Christians whose own beliefs were at odds with one another had more difficulty resolving the dissonance than those who attributed the dissonance they felt to external causes such as other people's prejudices. When the church is actually supportive, dissonance is minimized (Rodriguez & Ouellette, 2000).

In the case of conflicting beliefs that pit two culturally supported identities against one another, such as creationism, which pits fundamentalist Christianity against the scientific establishment, believers who cannot withdraw comfortably from either one may simply opt to live with both in tension (Evans, 2001). Deconchy et al. (1997) found that religion-like "fantastic" explanations seemed to buffer problem solvers from learned helplessness, but their participants were not put in the position of having to defend these explanations in social contexts.

Social Perception

Social Identity

The cognitive dissonance we feel when some aspect of a strongly held belief or cherished behavior runs counter to a prevailing social norm reveals the presence of a complex self-schema that incorporates elements of our various social identities as well as a sense of continuity based on prior experiences. Culturally weighted categories such as race or ethnicity, gender, sexual orientation, or social class may entail constraints that shape the individual's construction of identity and so take on a personal meaning over time (Frable, 1997). Level of commitment to a particular reference group affects how much an individual will be influenced by the norms of that group. Those whose religion is highly salient to them show different patterns of values than those without a strong religious identity

(Lau, 1989) and adhere more to religious group norms of behavior and cognition (Wimberly, 1989).

Dufour (2000) proposes that we construct our identities as we mature, in part by sifting through the cognitive and behavioral components provided by our various reference groups, including the faith community for those who are raised with one. Where the components seem to conflict, they are "tried on" in turn to see how the individual might reconcile them, perhaps through a process of reinterpretation. In some cases, where practice has been suppressed among a persecuted religious minority, this sifting reaches back across generations to preserve something that is newly valued (Jacobs, 2000).

Many Americans describe their acquisition of religious beliefs as a logical process (Kenworthy, 2003), perhaps because this fits the preferred cultural script for attitude formation. However, relationships appear to be central to the development of religious identity (Ganzevoort, 1998a; Jacobs, 2000), especially close family relationships (Ozorak, 1989). Social comparisons with peers from the same faith group can cause polarization of belief and entrench oneself more firmly in a religious identity. Perhaps both peer and family influences are based partly in spiritual modeling, as described by Oman and Thoresen (2003). Porpora (1996) found that religiously oriented people are more likely to have personal heroes whom they try to emulate, perhaps in part because they feel themselves at odds with the dominant culture.

Self-Perception

A religious identity can have strong effects on self-perception. For African Americans, religion seems to buffer self-esteem (Ellison, 1993); the reverse can be true for gay and lesbian Christians who feel rejected by their church (Mahaffy, 1996). Among samples of university students, intrinsic religiosity has predicted a tendency to see oneself as more virtuous than others (Rowatt, Ottenbreit, Neesselroade, & Cunningham, 2002), especially in the face of negative feedback (Burris & Jackson, 2000). In fairness, others may be equally likely to resort to religious stereotypes: a huge archival study found that religious people are generally perceived as nicer (Brennan & London, 2001).

Judgments of Others

Religious people's judgments of others are not always nice (see Donahue & Nielsen, Chapter 15, this volume, for a fuller treatment of religion and prejudice). However, it appears that the mixed relationship between religion (or at least Christianity) and prejudice is the result of separable factors, including right-wing authoritarianism and Christian orthodoxy (Laythe, Finkel, Bringle, & Kirkpatrick, 2002). Begue (2001) has also demonstrated a "black sheep" internal prejudice effect among Catholics with respect to other Catholics who practice or favor abortion.

Simple framing effects such as the *halo effect*—the tendency toward evaluative consistency, positive or negative—account for some bias in perceptions of others. We tend to like those who are like us and project additional good traits onto those already identified with; the reverse is true for those unlike us or identified with a bad trait. Beyond these, Hewstone, Rubin, and Willis (2002) have described several theoretical models of biases in social perception that help to explain how religion might affect the perception of others. Optimal distinctiveness theory posits that we need to see ourselves as both assimilated and different, leading us to compare and contrast ourselves with others so as to bolster both perceptions. This is related to the self-esteem bias, which encourages us to see ourselves as first among equals in general. Subjective uncertainty theory and terror management theory both suppose that we forge identity with groups having clear norms in order to build our confidence, but believe ourselves to be superior examples of those norms so as to allay anxiety. These theories fit the data on self-perception discussed earlier, and they clearly apply to religion.

Group Identity Effects

A recent review article on identity discussed the roles of gender, ethnicity or race, sexual orientation, and class in shaping social schemas (Frable, 1997). The omission of religion was odd in light of the article's focus on Latino Americans, whose Catholicism was likely an important part of their identity. Even in the so-called melting pot of the United States, cultural groups like the Amish are identified primarily by religion, although they also use a unique German dialect (Hostetler, 1993). To complicate matters, these group identities interact in multifarious ways, as is obvious from a brief mental review of the churches (let alone the temples, mosques, etc.) in any city familiar to the reader. These group identities must be kept in view when studying religion, even though most studies cannot include them all as variables.

Gender is probably the group variable most widely included in studies of religion, since it is easy to identify participants, or ask them to self-identify, as male or female. Women have different religious experiences and roles from men even in relatively egalitarian U.S. churches and synagogues. Women also think about religion differently than men do (Neitz, 1995; Ozorak, 1996), affecting the religiously based choices they make (Ozorak, 2003a).

Culture is trickier to include because there are so axes of difference: important divergences can emerge between even apparently similar Western countries (Dillon, 1996; Jablonski, Grzymala Moszczynska, & van der Lans, 1994). The best solution is probably to encourage research with a wide variety of ethnic, religious, and cultural groups so as to avoid reaching erroneous conclusions about what is universal (Boyer, 2003).

LANGUAGE

Social Responses to Language

Language is a social medium; language choices on all levels can have tremendous significance for speaker and audience alike (Edwards, 1985). Ethnic and religious minorities have strong responses to the use of the home language rather than the majority tongue (Edwards, 1985; Hostetler, 1993). It is no surprise that Hebrew has powerful meaning even for Jews who do not speak it or that Catholics are still divided over whether the Mass should be said in Latin. Changing from traditional masculine language for God and for humanity to more inclusive terminology remains a sticking point in many U.S. churches, although clergy who use inclusive language are not necessarily disparaged (Greene & Rubin, 1991). Given the concern among the faithful about these social aspects of religious language and the well-demonstrated psychological effects of language use (Romaine, 2000), this area of research deserves much more attention.

Discourse and Narrative

Religions, Niebuhr (1941) has argued, survive on their stories. What has proved especially vexatious to Jews and Christians is that they share key elements of their central stories, and yet the same story seems to have different meanings for the two faiths (Goldberg, 1991). There is some evidence that even within faith groups the same narratives are understood in slightly different ways, with important implications (Dillon, 1999). Widely publicized Scripture-based disagreements over issues like the ordaining of women and the status of homosexual members dominate U.S. Christianity. Discourse analysis, with its attention to levels of language, illuminates such debates and misunderstandings.

Discourse analysis distinguishes between the surface code (what is actually said, verbatim), the textbase (the meaning of the words that are used), and the situational model (the view of the world on which the meanings rest). For example, the contrasts drawn by Goldberg (1991) between Jewish and Christian interpretations of the Exodus story might be explained as an identical surface code masking differences in the situational model— here, the assumptions made about the nature of God. The cultural scripts shared by American Jews and Christians may obscure the differences of underlying worldview in this context.

Christian arguments about "literal" interpretation of Scriptures—bearing in mind that most Christians cannot read the original biblical languages—are fundamentally about discourse, in particular the difficulty for modern readers to be certain about the textbase underlying some of the surface code as well as a social context that was very different our own (Borg, 2004). The interpretation issue dominates the painful deliberations about the acceptability of homosexual relationships (e.g., what exactly did the writer of Leviticus 18:22 mean by the word that has been translated, centuries later, as "abomination"?). These are psychological issues, not just linguistic ones, both because language is always collectively constructed in a particular social context and because the consequences of interpretation bear so much emotional weight.

In addition to the shared discourse that underlies religious faith, individuals construct their own religious narrative. These stories, while intensely personal, substantially reflect the social constraints provided by the faith and by the culture generally (Ganzevoort, 1998b). The process of putting oneself in the context of the wider religious narrative and of ordering one's experiences to make them coherent to oneself and others seems to be essential to religion. A religion "works" to the extent that its story plays out satisfactorily in the lives of those who believe in it (Day, 1993; Goldberg, 1991). Religious knowing that derives from experience seems able to transform lives in a way that no amount of doctrine or teaching can do (Watts & Williams, 1988). It seems fair to conclude with Day (1993) that religious narratives are always performative rather than merely descriptive.

Narrative as a Vehicle for Transformation

If religious narratives are performative, they offer consequential opportunities for transformation. Just as the individual who says "I do" in the course of a marriage ceremony emerges as, in some sense, a different person, the religious individual can be changed by the process of assenting to a new narrative. In fact, this seems to occur often in Christian conversions (Stromberg, 1993), and the conscious construction of the narrative seems to enhance the result (Liu, 1991).

Some people actively choose a new narrative or a new interpretation of an older narrative because they want to change (Miller & C'De Baca, 2001). The processing of reconfiguring a story gives power to the one who does it (Carlson & Erickson, 2000) and can offer the opportunity to build in a higher purpose or a role for God. Religious communities sometimes support their members in such reconstructive efforts (Mankowski & Thomas, 2000; Rappaport & Simkins, 1991). Mattis and Jagers (2001) found that this kind of empowerment through individual and shared narrative work is commonly used by African Americans, frequently drawing on their religious tradition.

SUGGESTIONS FOR FUTURE RESEARCH

The Truth Question

The question of whether religion is "true" or not has haunted the psychology of religion for decades (Pargament, 2002). Some cognitive theorists argue for a clearer focus on mechanisms, so as to avoid any suspicion of "defensive motives" (e.g., Belzen, 1999, p. 236) or a "metaphysical agenda" (McCallister, 1995, p. 314). Others have insisted that the "truth question" must remain open (e.g., Argyle, 2002; Ozorak, 1997), in part because psychological inquiries are about the human end of the equation, not about what, if anything, is on the other end of our perceptions. Most psychologists of religion have chosen to ignore this elephant in the living room. However, many good researchers are probably dissuaded from studying religion at all because they don't want to share space with an elephant, real or not.

Public discussion of religion is now mainstream, but as the gaps described in this chapter show, research needs to catch up with that shift. If psychology were to adopt the multilevel interdisciplinary paradigm proposed by Emmons and Paloutzian (2003), which welcomes data from many levels of analysis without devaluing either the other levels or religious phenomena themselves, the field would be well on its way. What follows are some specific suggestions for implementing such a paradigm.

Measures and Method

Grant (2001) has suggested that the study of religion would be greatly helped by the adoption of more sophisticated methods from other areas of his discipline (sociology). Expanding his point to include psychology, two areas of fruitful inquiry emerge.

Narrative Analysis

Many studies of religion, including a substantial percentage of those cited here, use some form of narrative data (see Hood & Belzen, Chapter 4, this volume). However, as Grant (2001) points out, most of these do not make use of the sophisticated methods now available for analyzing discourse, including optimal matching strategies modeled after DNA research and semantic network analysis borrowed from cognitive anthropology. Psychology itself has taken a renewed interest in narrative research (see, e.g., McAdams, Josselson, & Lieblich, 2001). With the groundswell of interest in related disciplines, the time seems ripe to try some of these more positivistic approaches along with the qualitative approaches already in use. In addition, narrative data seem particularly appropriate for the longitudinal studies that are needed to confirm direction of effects.

Implicit Measures

Implicit measures of cognitive function are at the cutting edge of the field (Fazio & Olson, 2003). Association tests with selective priming are often used in research on attitudes to avoid alerting participants to the focus of the research. To my knowledge, this kind of test has not been used on religion, but it could be. In addition, a wide variety of linguistic measures has been developed, such as counts of specific word types and changes in the structure of explanations (Pennebaker, Mehl, & Niederhoffer, 2003). Strong emotional states have been shown to generate predictable patterns of change in language. These would be appropriate for the study of religion, and would fit well with a narrative research agenda.

Applications

A popular proverb says "Well begun is half done." What follows are three areas of research that are already "well begun." In each case there is substantial public interest and a burgeoning record of research that includes religion in some way. What is needed, in each case, is more work on the cognitive aspects of the connection to religion.

Health

Ten years after physician Larry Dossey published his first book on the power of prayer in healing (Dossey, 1993), the topic made it to the front cover of *Newsweek*: "God & Health: Is religion good medicine? Why science is starting to believe" (Kalb, 2003). At the same time, linkages between religion and health were already being explored in mainstream psychological journals (e.g., George, Ellison, & Larson, 2002; Powell, Shahabi, & Thoresen, 2003; see Oman & Thoreson, Chapter 24, this volume). In this case, a cognitive model of these linkages has been suggested (Dull & Skokan, 1995), but it has yet to be taken up by other researchers. Systematic tests of the model's propositions and perhaps some theoretical tinkering are in order.

Psychological Well-Being

Subjective well-being is emphasized in U.S. culture and has begun to receive attention from psychologists. A plethora of research confirms connections between religion and well-being (e.g., Fabricatore, Handal, Rubio, & Gilner, 2004; Taylor, 2001; see Miller & Kelley, Chapter 25, this volume), although such connections are far from absolute or automatic (Exline, 2002; see Exline & Rose, Chapter 17, this volume). Clinical literature—much of it involving narrative—suggests that religion can be used to reinvent the self in ways that improve subjective quality of life (Carlson & Erickson, 2000; Magee, 2001). Such research would benefit from a cognitive model and some experimental tests of the model using the kinds of linguistic techniques already described.

Politics

In post-9/11 America, religion and politics have become habitual strange bedfellows. Researchers had already begun exploring the relationship of religion to political action or inaction in particular groups, including African Americans (e.g., Lee, 2003) and Christian fundamentalists (e.g., Hood & Smith, 2002), along with a few general studies (e.g., Djupe & Grant, 2001). However, the political events of the past few years seem to have lent the topic a new urgency, both in the United States and elsewhere (e.g., Brewer, Kersh, & Petersen, 2003; Duriez, Luyten, Snauwaert, & Hutsebaut, 2002; Gopin, 2002). Researchers are beginning to ask whether religions affect the nature and extent of political participation in the same way as membership in other social groups or there is something special about the role of religious imperatives in political activity; and not only that, but whether religion can be used to encourage peace as well as war and violence (see Silberman, Chapter 29, this volume).

Cognitive psychology is just one component of the theoretical approaches needed here. Religion needs to be factored into broader cognitive theories of political participation (e.g., Lavine, 2002), and social cognitive mechanisms need to be identified more clearly in studies of war and peacemaking (e.g., Gopin, 2002); interestingly, a recent Associated Press (2003) story described a social-cognitive approach to rehabilitating Al-Qaeda recruits that is apparently proving somewhat successful.

CONCLUSION

As Bandura (2001) observes, fortuitous events shape fate, but people can "make chance happen" by the actions they take and by putting themselves in the way of particular experiences (p. 12). Thus, just as environments shape people, people shape environments—particularly social ones—and they do so, most frequently, on the basis of their beliefs. Religions are an important core of highly primed beliefs for many people. Cognitive research that fails to take this into account will inevitably fall short of what it might discover. The literature shows that religious beliefs and associations impact information processing from its initial stages through all kinds of complex reasoning, especially in social contexts.

Bandura (2001) notes that the dawn of the 21st century finds the Western world in a period of social fragmentation. The complex problems we face require collective action, and yet for a variety of reasons, mental as well as environmental, we have a strikingly low sense of collective efficacy. It could be argued that religions, with their counterintuitive notions of efficacy, extensive effects on information processing, and extended social connections, provide one of the few remaining sources of collective efficacy—a capacity that, as history shows, can be used for good or ill. Understanding the ways in which religious cognition shapes human action is overdue to become a top priority for psychological research.

REFERENCES

Andresen, J. (2001). Introduction: Towards a cognitive science of religion. In J. Andresen (Ed.), *Religion in mind: Cognitive perspectives on religious belief, ritual, and experience* (pp. 1–44). New York: Cambridge University Press.

Argyle, M. (2002). State of the art: Religion. *Psychologist, 15,* 22–26.

Ash, C. A., Crist, C. L., Salisbury, D., & Dewell, M. (1996). Unilateral and bilateral brain hemispheric advantage on visual matching tasks and their relationship to styles of religiosity. *Journal of Psychology and Theology, 24,* 133–154.

Associated Press. (2003). Saudi interrogators use new technique. abcnews.go.com/wire/World/ap20031201_126.html.

Atkinson, R. C., & Shiffrin, R. M. (1971). The control of short term memory. *Scientific American*, *225*, 82–90.

Baetz, M., Larson, D. B., Marcoux, G., Jokic, R., & Bowen, R. (2002). Religious psychiatry: The Canadian experience. *Journal of Nervous and Mental Disease*, *190*, 557–558.

Baldwin, M. W. (1992). Relational schemas and the processing of social information. *Psychological Bulletin*, *112*, 461–484.

Baldwin, M. W., & Baccus, J. R. (2003). An expectancy-value approach to self-esteem. In S.J. Spencer & S. Fein (Eds.), *The Ontario Symposium: Vol. 9. Motivated social perception* (pp. 171–194). Mahwah, NJ: Erlbaum.

Bandura, A. (2001). Social cognitive theory: An agentic perspective. *Annual Review of Psychology*, *52*, 1–26.

Barnes-Holmes, D., Hayes, S. C., & Gregg, J. (2001). Religion, spirituality, and transcendence. In S. C. Hayes, D. Barnes-Holmes, & B. Roche (Eds.), *Relational frame theory: A post-Skinnerian account of human language and cognition* (pp. 239–251). New York: Kluwer/Plenum.

Barrett, J. L. (2002). Smart gods, dumb gods, and the role of social cognition in structuring ritual intuitions. *Journal of Cognition and Culture*, *2*, 183–193.

Begue, L. (2001). Social judgment of abortion: A black sheep effect in a Catholic sheepfold. *Journal of Social Psychology*, *141*, 640–649.

Belzen, J. A. (1999). The cultural psychological approach to religion: Contemporary debates on the object of the discipline. *Theory and Psychology*, *9*, 229–255.

Borg, M. (2004). *The heart of Christianity: Rediscovering a life of faith*. San Francisco: HarperCollins.

Boyer, P. (2001). *Religion explained*. New York: Basic Books.

Boyer, P. (2003). Religious thought and behaviour as by-products of brain function. *Trends in Cognitive Sciences*, *7*, 119–124.

Boyer, P., & Ramble, C. (2001). Cognitive templates for religious concepts: Cross cultural evidence for recall of counter intuitive representations. *Cognitive Science*, *25*, 536–584.

Brennan, K. M., & London, A. S. (2001). Are religious people nice people?: Religiosity, race, interview dynamics, and perceived cooperativeness. *Sociological Inquiry*, *71*, 129–144.

Brewer, M. D., Kersh, R., & Petersen, E. (2003). Assessing conventional wisdom about religion and politics: A preliminary view from the pews. *Journal for the Scientific Study of Religion*, *42*, 125–136.

Burris, C. T., & Jackson, L. M. (2000). Social identity and the true believer: Responses to threatened self stereotypes among the intrinsically religious. *British Journal of Social Psychology*, *39*, 257–278.

Cantor, N. (2002). Constructive cognition, personal goals, and the social embedding of personality. In L. G. Aspinwall & U. M. Staudinger (Eds.), *A psychology of human strengths* (pp. 49–60). Washington, DC: American Psychological Association.

Carlson, T. D., & Erickson, M. J. (2000). Re-authoring spiritual narratives: God in persons' relational identity stories. *Journal of Systematic Therapies*, *19*, 65–83.

Chaves, M., & Montgomery, J. D. (1996). Rationality and the framing of religious choices. *Journal for the Scientific Study of Religion*, *35*, 128–144.

Cobb, N. J., Ong, A. D., & Tate, J. (2001). Reason based evaluations of wrongdoing in religious and moral narratives. *The International Journal for the Psychology of Religion*, *11*, 259–276.

Cohen, A. B., & Rozin, P. (2001). Religion and the morality of mentality. *Journal of Personality and Social Psychology*, *81*, 697–710.

Day, J. M. (1993). Speaking of belief: Language, performance, and narrative in the psychology of religion. *The International Journal for the Psychology of Religion*, *3*, 213–229.

Deconchy, J. P., Hurteau, C., Quelen, F., & Ragot, I. (1997). The psychology of religion and cognitive models (the "learned helplessness" case). *The International Journal for the Psychology of Religion*, *7*, 263–268.

Dillon, M. (1996). Cultural differences in the abortion discourse of the Catholic Church: Evidence from four countries. *Sociology of Religion, 57,* 25–36.

Dillon, M. (1999). The Catholic Church and possible "organizational selves": The implications for institutional change. *Journal for the Scientific Study of Religion, 38,* 386–397.

Djupe, P. A., & Grant, J. T. (2001). Religious institutions and political participation in America. *Journal for the Scientific Study of Religion, 40,* 303–314.

Dossey, L. (1993). *Healing words: The power of prayer and the practice of medicine.* San Francisco: HarperCollins.

Dufour, L. R. (2000). Sifting through tradition: The creation of Jewish feminist identities. *Journal for the Scientific Study of Religion, 39,* 90–106.

Dull, V. T., & Skokan, L. A. (1995). A cognitive model of religion's influence on health. *Journal of Social Issues, 51,* 49–64.

Duriez, B., Luyten, P., Snauwaert, B., & Hutsebaut, D. (2002). The importance of religiosity and values in predicting political attitudes: Evidence for the continuing importance of religiosity in Flanders (Belgium). *Mental Health, Religion and Culture, 5,* 35–54.

Edwards, J. (1985). *Language, society and identity.* New York: Blackwell.

Ellison, C. G. (1993). Religious involvement and self perception among Black Americans. *Social Forces, 71,* 1027–1055.

Emmons, R. A., & Paloutzian, R. F. (2003). The psychology of religion. *Annual Review of Psychology, 54,* 377–402.

Evans, E. M. (2001). Beyond Scopes: Why creationism is here to stay. In K. S. Rosengren, C. N. Johnson, & P. L. Harris (Eds.), *Imagining the impossible: Magical, scientific, and religious thinking in children* (pp. 305–333). New York: Cambridge University Press.

Exline, J. J. (2002). Stumbling blocks on the religious road: Fractured relationships, nagging vices, and the inner struggle to believe. *Psychological Inquiry, 13,* 182–189.

Fabricatore, A. N., Handal, P. J., Rubio, D. M., & Gilner, F. H. (2004). Stress, religion, and mental health: Religious coping in mediating and moderating roles. *The International Journal for the Psychology of Religion, 14,* 91–108.

Fazio, R. H., & Olson, M. A. (2003). Implicit measures in social cognition research: Their meaning and use. *Annual Review of Psychology, 54,* 297–327.

Frable, D. E. S. (1997). Gender, racial, ethnic, sexual, and class identities. *Annual Review of Psychology, 48,* 139–162.

Ganzevoort, R. R. (1998a). Religious coping reconsidered, part one: An integrated approach. *Journal of Psychology and Theology, 26,* 260–275.

Ganzevoort, R. R. (1998b). Religious coping reconsidered, part two: A narrative reformulation. *Journal of Psychology and Theology, 26,* 276–286.

George, L. K., Ellison, C. G., & Larson, D. B. (2002). Explaining the relationships between religious involvement and health. *Psychological Inquiry, 13,* 190–200.

Goldberg, M. (1991). *Jews and Christians: Getting our stories straight.* Philadephia: Trinity Press International.

Gopin, M. (2002). *Holy war, holy peace: How religion can bring peace to the Middle East.* New York: Oxford University Press.

Grant, D. S., II. (2001). Symbols, stories, and practices: New empirical directions in the study of religious meaning. *Sociological Quarterly, 42,* 233–251.

Greene, K., & Rubin, D. L. (1991). Effects of gender inclusive/exclusive language in religious discourse. *Journal of Language and Social Psychology, 10,* 81–98.

Guthrie, S. (2001). Why gods?: A cognitive theory. In J. Andresen (Ed.), *Religion in mind: Cognitive perspectives on religious belief, ritual, and experience* (pp. 94–111). New York: Cambridge University Press.

Haidt, J., & Rodin, J. (1999). Control and efficacy as interdisciplinary bridges. *Review of General Psychology, 3,* 317–337.

Hastie, R. (2001). Problems for judgment and decision making. *Annual Review of Psychology, 52,* 653–683.

Hewstone, M., Rubin, M., & Willis, H. (2002). Intergroup bias. *Annual Review of Psychology, 53,* 575–604.

Hill, P. C. (1997). Toward an attitude process model of religious experience. In B. Spilka & D. N. McIntosh (Eds.), *The psychology of religion: Theoretical approaches* (pp. 184–193). Boulder, CO: Westview Press.

Hill, P. C., & Hall, T. W. (2002). Relational schemas in processing one's image of God and self. *Journal of Psychology and Christianity, 21,* 365–373.

Hood, M. V., III, & Smith, M. C. (2002). On the prospect of linking religious-right identification with political behavior: Panacea or snipe hunt? *Journal for the Scientific Study of Religion, 41,* 697–710.

Hostetler, J. A. (1993). *Amish society* (4th ed.). Baltimore: Johns Hopkins University Press.

Hovemyr, M. (1998). The attribution of success and failure as related to different patterns of religious orientation. *The International Journal for the Psychology of Religion, 8,* 107–124.

Ingram, L. C. (1989). Evangelism as frame intrusion: Observations on witnessing in public places. *Journal for the Scientific Study of Religion, 28,* 17–26.

Iyer, S. (2002). Religion and the decision to use contraception in India. *Journal for the Scientific Study of Religion, 41,* 711–722.

Jablonski, P., Grzymala Moszczynska, H., & Van der Lans, J. (1994). Interpretation of religious language among Poles and the Dutch: Cognitive competence or cultural construction? *Polish Psychological Bulletin, 25,* 283–302.

Jacobs, J. L. (2000). The spiritual self-in-relation: Empathy and the construction of spirituality among modern descendants of the Spanish crypto-Jews. *Journal for the Scientific Study of Religion, 39,* 53–63.

Kalb, C. (2003, November 10). Faith and healing. *Newsweek,* pp. 44–56.

Kenworthy, J. B. (2003). Explaining the belief in God for self, in group, and out group targets. *Journal for the Scientific Study of Religion, 42,* 137–146.

Knoblich, G., Ohlsson, S., & Raney, G. E. (2001). An eye-movement study of insight problem solving. *Memory and Cognition, 29,* 1000–1009.

Kunst, J. L., Bjorck, J. P., & Tan, S.-Y. (2000). Causal attributions for uncontrollable negative events. *Journal of Psychology and Christianity, 19,* 47–60.

Ladd, K. L., & Spilka, B. (2002). Inward, outward, and upward: Cognitive aspects of prayer. *Journal for the Scientific Study of Religion, 41,* 475–484.

Lau, S. (1989). Religious schema and values. *The International Journal of Psychology, 24,* 137–156.

Lavine, H. (2002). On-line versus memory-based process models of political evaluation. In K. R. Monroe (Ed.), *Political psychology* (pp. 225–247). Mahwah, NJ: Erlbaum.

Lawson, E. T. (2001). Psychological perspectives on agency. In J. Andresen (Ed.), *Religion in mind: Cognitive perspectives on religious belief, ritual, and experience* (pp. 141–172). New York: Cambridge University Press.

Laythe, B., Finkel, D. G., Bringle, R. G., & Kirkpatrick, L. A. (2002). Religious fundamentalism as a predictor of prejudice: A two-component model. *Journal for the Scientific Study of Religion, 41,* 623–635.

Lee, S. (2003). The church of faith and freedom: African-American Baptists and social action. *Journal for the Scientific Study of Religion, 42,* 31–41.

Liu, C. (1991). Becoming a Christian consciously versus nonconsciously. *Journal of Psychology and Theology, 19,* 364–375.

Lupfer, M. B., Tolliver, D., & Jackson, M. (1996). Explaining life-altering occurrences: A test of the "God-of-the-gaps" hypothesis. *Journal for the Scientific Study of Religion, 35,* 379–391.

MacGregor, J. N., Ormerod, T. C., & Chronicle, E. P. (2001). Information processing and insight: A process model of performance on the nine-dot and related problems. *Journal of Experimental Psychology: Learning, Memory and Cognition, 27,* 176–201.

Magee, J. (2001). Mysticism and reframing memories in life review groups. *Journal of Religious Gerontology, 13,* 65–73.

Mahaffy, K. A. (1996). Cognitive dissonance and its resolution: A study of lesbian Christians. *Journal for the Scientific Study of Religion, 35,* 392–402.

Maltby, J., & Day, L. (2003). Religious orientation, religious coping and appraisals of stress: Assessing primary appraisal factors in the relationship between religiosity and psychological well being. *Personality and Individual Differences, 34,* 1209–1224.

Mankowski, E. S., & Thomas, E. (2000). The relationship between personal and collective identity: A narrative analysis of a campus ministry community. *Journal of Community Psychology, 28,* 517–528.

Mattis, J. S., & Jagers, R. J. (2001). A relational framework for the study of religiosity and spirituality in the lives of African Americans. *Journal of Community Psychology, 29,* 519–539.

McAdams, D. P., Josselson, R., & Lieblich, A. (2001). The narrative study of lives: Introduction to the series. In D. P. McAdams, R. Josselson, & A. Lieblich (Eds.), *Turns in the road: Narrative studies of lives in transition* (pp. 3–34). Washington, DC: American Psychological Association.

McCallister, B. J. (1995). Cognitive theory and religious experience. In R. W. Hood, Jr. (Ed.), *Handbook of religious experience* (pp. 312–352). Birmingham, AL: Religious Education Press.

McCauley, R. N. (2001). Ritual, memory, and emotion: Comparing two cognitive hypotheses. In J. Andresen (Ed.), *Religion in mind: Cognitive perspectives on religious belief, ritual, and experience* (pp. 115–140). New York: Cambridge University Press.

McCauley, R. N., & Lawson, E. T. (2002). *Bringing ritual to mind: Psychological foundations of cultural forms.* New York: Cambridge University Press.

McIntosh, D. N. (1995). Religion as schema, with implications for the relation between religion and coping. *The International Journal for the Psychology of Religion, 5,* 1–16.

Miller, W. R., & C'De Baca, J. (2001). *Quantum change: When epiphanies and sudden insights transform ordinary lives.* New York: Guilford Press.

Moehle, D. (1983). Cognitive dimensions of religious experiences. *Journal of Experimental Social Psychology, 19,* 122–145.

Nairne, J. S. (2001). Remembering over the short-term: The case against the standard model. *Annual Review of Psychology, 52,* 53–81.

Neitz, M. J. (1995). Feminist theory and religious experience. In R. W. Hood, Jr. (Ed.), *Handbook of religious experience* (pp. 520–534). Birmingham, AL: Religious Education Press.

Niebuhr, H. R. (1941). The story of our life. In *The meaning of revelation* (pp. 43–81). New York: Macmillan.

Oman, D., & Thoresen, C. E. (2003). Spiritual modeling: A key to spiritual and religious growth? *The International Journal for the Psychology of Religion, 13,* 149–165.

Oser, F. K., & Gmuender, P. (1991). *Religious judgement: A developmental perspective.* Birmingham, AL: Religious Education Press.

Ozorak, E. W. (1989). Social and cognitive influences on the development of religious beliefs and commitment in adolescence. *Journal for the Scientific Study of Religion, 28,* 448–463.

Ozorak, E. W. (1996). The power, but not the glory: How women empower themselves through religion. *Journal for the Scientific Study of Religion, 35,* 17–29.

Ozorak, E. W. (1997). In the eye of the beholder: A social cognitive model of religious belief. In B. Spilka & D. N. McIntosh (Eds.), *The psychology of religion: Theoretical approaches* (pp. 194–203). Boulder, CO: Westview Press.

Ozorak, E. W. (2003a). Culture, gender, faith: The social construction of the person–God relationship. *The International Journal for the Psychology of Religion, 13,* 249–257.

Ozorak, E. W. (2003b). Love of God and neighbor: Religion and volunteer service among college students. *Review of Religious Research, 44,* 285–299.

Pargament, K. I. (2002). Is religion nothing but . . . ?: Explaining religion vs. explaining religion away. *Psychological Inquiry, 13,* 239–244.

Patzer, N. L., & Helm, H. W., Jr. (2001). Categories of success endorsed among religiously identified Seventh Day Adventist students. *Psychological Reports, 88,* 1121–1128.

Paul, C., Fitzjohn, J., Eberhart-Phillips, J., Herbison, P., & Dickson, N. (2000). Sexual abstinence at age 21 in New Zealand: The importance of religion. *Social Science and Medicine, 51,* 1–10.

Peeters, G., & Hendrickx, A. (2002). The similarity between the perception and interpretation of information in a profane and a religious context. *The International Journal for the Psychology of Religion, 12,* 41–52.

Pennebaker, J. W., Mehl, M. R., & Niederhoffer, K. G. (2003). Psychological aspects of natural language use: Our words, our selves. *Annual Review of Psychology, 54,* 547–577.

Porpora, D. V. (1996). Personal heroes, religion, and transcendental metanarratives. *Sociological Forum, 11,* 209–229.

Powell, L. H., Shahabi, L., & Thoresen, C. E. (2003). Religion and spirituality: Linkages to physical health. *American Psychologist, 58,* 36–52.

Rappaport, J., & Simkins, R. (1991). Healing and empowering through community narrative. *Prevention in Human Services, 10,* 29–50.

Reich, K. H. (2002). *Developing the horizons of the mind: Relational and contextual reasoning and the resolution of cognitive conflict.* New York: Cambridge University Press.

Rodriguez, E. M., & Ouellette, S. C. (2000). Gay and lesbian Christians: Homosexual and religious identity integration in the members and participants of a gay positive church. *Journal for the Scientific Study of Religion, 39,* 333–347.

Romaine, S. (2000). *Language in society.* New York: Oxford University Press.

Rowatt, W. C., Ottenbreit, A., Nesselroade, K. P., Jr., & Cunningham, P. A. (2002). On being holier than thou or humbler than thee: A social psychological perspective on religiousness and humility. *Journal for the Scientific Study of Religion, 41,* 227–237.

Sinnott, J. (2000). Cognitive aspects of unitative states: Spiritual self realization, intimacy, and knowing the unknowable. In M. E. Miller & A. N. West (Eds.), *Spirituality, ethics, and relationship in adulthood: Clinical and theoretical explorations* (pp. 177–198). Madison, CT: Psychosocial Press.

Spilka, B., Shaver, P. R., & Kirkpatrick, L. (1985). A general attribution theory for the psychology of religion. *Journal for the Scientific Study of Religion, 24,* 1–20.

Stromberg, P. G. (1993). *Language and self-transformation: A study of the Christian conversion narrative.* New York: Cambridge University Press.

Szuchewycz, B. (1994). Evidentiality in ritual discourse: The social construction of religious meaning. *Language in Society, 23,* 389–410.

Taylor, N. M. (2001). Utilizing religious schemas to cope with mental illness. *Journal of Religion and Health, 40,* 383–388.

Turiel, E., & Neff, K. (2000). Religion, culture, and beliefs about reality in moral reasoning. In K. S. Rosengren, C. N. Johnson, & P. L. Harris (Eds.), *Imagining the impossible: Magical, scientific, and religious thinking in children* (pp. 269–304). New York: Cambridge University Press.

Watts, F., & Williams, M. (1988). *The psychology of religious knowing.* New York: Cambridge University Press.

Weeks, M., & Lupfer, M. B. (2000). Religious attributions and proximity of influence: An investigation of direct interventions and distal explanations. *Journal for the Scientific Study of Religion, 39,* 348–362.

Wenger, J. L. (2004). The automatic activation of religious concepts: Implications for religious orientations. *The International Journal for the Psychology of Religion, 14,* 109–123.

Whitehouse, H. (2002). Religious reflexivity and transmissive frequency. *Social Anthropology, 10,* 91–103.

Wimberley, D. W. (1989). Religion and role identity: A structural symbolic interactionist conceptualization of religiosity. *Sociological Quarterly, 30,* 125–142.

13

Emotion and Religion

ROBERT A. EMMONS

Given the rapid growth in the psychology of religion (Emmons & Paloutzian, 2003) and the psychology of emotion (Lewis & Haviland-Jones, 2000) in recent years, one would expect to see considerable scholarship directed toward the interface of these two fields. While a literature search using the PsychINFO database for the period 1988–2002 returned 2,875 citations for the term *religion* and 5,116 for the term *emotion*, a scant five citations include both terms! The range of emotional phenomena is vast, and I cannot attempt to do justice to this vastness within a single chapter. Because of the recent emergence of the scientific study of positive emotions, I will emphasize the role of religion in the generation and regulation of emotional experience, focusing primarily on positive emotional experience. The study of positive emotions is a major trend in contemporary affective science (Fredrickson, 2001), and I wish to highlight the many ways in which the psychology of religion can contribute to a growing understanding of positive emotions and the functions of positive emotions in people's lives. Considerable other literature, including various chapters within this volume, also touch upon emotion-related phenomena. For example, Miller (1999), Propst (1988), Richards and Bergin (1997) and Shafranske (1996, and Chapter 27, this volume) all deal extensively with religious psychotherapy and maladaptive emotions.

This chapter has several purposes: to present a brief historical overview on the study of emotion and religion; to review recent research on emotions typically considered to be religious; to document the various ways in which religion might modulate emotional experience; and to consider various functions that religious emotions might serve. My overriding concern is to sketch the newest lines of research that are emerging now that show promise of contributing significantly to the psychology of religion and to the psychology of emotion during the next several years. I begin first by describing what I mean by emotion.

WHAT IS EMOTION?: LEVELS OF EMOTIONAL EXPERIENCE

Any discussion of religion and emotion presupposes an understanding of what emotion is. The field of affective science has been moving toward standardized terminology that provides researchers and clinicians with a common frame of reference. Thus before beginning my presentation of the literature on religion and emotion, it might be helpful to familiarize the reader with what is meant by the concept of emotion, and how an emotion differs from other related affective phenomena. In doing so I will borrow from the recent conceptual analysis of Rosenberg (1998). Rosenberg proposed that the common forms of affective experience could be structured into three hierarchical levels of analysis: affective traits, moods, and emotions.

Rosenberg (1998) placed affective traits at the top of the hierarchy of affective phenomena. She defined *affective traits* as stable predispositions toward certain types of emotional responding that set the threshold for the occurrence of particular emotional states. For example, hostility is thought to lower one's threshold for experiencing anger, or happiness could be thought of as lowering one's threshold for experiencing pleasant affect. Affective traits are relatively stable components of personality that are consistently expressed over time and across situations. Some of the research that I review in this chapter will be focused on this level of the affective hierarchy.

In contrast to affective traits, *emotions* are "acute, intense, and typically brief psychophysiological changes that result from a response to a meaningful situation in one's environment" (Rosenberg, 1988, p. 250). Emotions are a subset of a larger class of affective phenomena (Fredrickson, 2001). They are discrete states that involve the appraisal of the personal meaning of a circumstance in a person's environment. Both the type of emotion experienced and its intensity depend on cognitive interpretation or appraisal of the situation. Such appraisal involves not only assessing the nature of the external situation or event that might cause the emotional response, but also the responses of other people exposed to that same situation or event. Emotions typically motivate a particular course of action; each discrete emotion triggers a particular action tendency (Fredrickson, 2001). A major division between types of emotions are affect program theories and propositional attitude theories (Griffiths, 1997; Roberts, 2003). Affect programs pertain to the basic, universal emotions such as anger, disgust, joy, sadness, and fear, while the latter category contain a wider range of cognitively complex emotions including guilt, shame, pride, and gratitude. Basic emotions are universal and innate. There exists for each a recognizable facial expression and a distinct physiological patterning. The higher cognitively complex emotions depend heavily on cognitive appraisals and are assumed to exhibit greater cultural variation. Religion, at least when it comes to the generation of emotion, appears to have more do with the latter than with the former.

Rosenberg considered *moods*, which wax and wane, fluctuating throughout or across days, as subordinate to affective traits, but as superordinate to discrete emotion episodes. Moods are subtle and less accessible to conscious awareness than are emotions (i.e., one is less likely to be aware of anger as a mood than as an emotion). Despite their subtlety relative to emotions, however, moods are important because they are expected to have broad, pervasive effects on consciousness that emotions simply cannot because of their relatively short duration (Rosenberg, 1998). Because the majority of research on religion and affect has been at the level of affective traits of discrete emotions, I will have comparatively little to say about religion and mood.

CONCEPTUALIZING LINKS BETWEEN RELIGION AND EMOTION

The connection between religion and emotion is a long and intimate one. For one, religion has always been a source of profound emotional experience. Commenting on this historical association, Pruyser (1967) writes that "there is something about emotion that has always had a great appeal to the religionist" (p. 142). Religion likely influences both the generation of emotion and the regulation of emotional responses. I discuss religion and the generation of specific, discrete emotions below. Links between religion and emotion can also be seen in religious attitudes toward emotional experience and expression. Watts (1996) distinguishes between two main notions about the role of emotions in religious life. The charismatic movement stresses the cultivation of intense positive emotions and their importance in religious experience and collective religious rituals (see also McCauley, 2001), whereas the contemplative tradition stresses a calming of the passions and the development of emotional quietude. In addition to these two approaches to regulating emotions, there is the ascetic view (Allen, 1997) that links religion with greater awareness of emotion (possible emotional intelligence, to use a contemporary term) and the creative expression of emotion.

Silberman (2003) suggests three ways in which religious and spiritual meaning systems influence emotion. First, religion prescribes appropriate and inappropriate emotions and their level of intensity. For example, within Judaism, people are encouraged to love God with all of their hearts (Deuteronomy 6:5) and to serve God with joy (Deuteronomy 28:47). Second, beliefs about the nature and attributes of God may give rise to specific emotions as well as influence overall emotional well-being. For example, a belief about a loving personal God may have a positive effect on emotional well-being, while a belief about a punitive vengeful God may have the opposite effect. Third, religion offers the opportunity to experience a uniquely powerful emotional experience of closeness to the sacred (Otto, 1917/1958).

Concerning the intensity issue, Ben-Ze'ev (2002) hypothesizes that religion influences the intensity of emotion in three ways. First, religious belief systems influence the meaningfulness attached to events. To the degree to which people perceive a divine influence on daily events, these events will be perceived as more meaningful and hence capable of generating stronger emotions than ordinary events. Second, according to Ben Ze'ev, religious and nonreligious persons differ in their perceptions regarding issues of deservingness for life events. Because of the belief that events signify God's intention and will, religious individuals are more likely to be accepting of life events than nonreligious individuals, and deservingness is typically associated with less intense emotional reactions. Third is the issue of controllability. Religious persons, according to Ben Ze'ev, typically believe that God directs and controls everyday events. Personal controllability is positively associated with emotional intensity; thus, all things being equal, the emotional intensity of religious individuals would be lower than that of nonreligious individuals. These are intriguing hypotheses that need to be empirically tested.

RELIGION AND THE GENERATION OF EMOTION

The role of emotion in religion is central in several prominent accounts of religious experience. Jonathan Edwards described the function of religious emotions in his theological classic *A Treatise Concerning Religious Affections* (1746/1959). Edwards was so struck by the evidentiary force of emotion that he made it a cornerstone of his theology, as exemplified in this quote: "The Holy Scriptures do everywhere place religion very much in the affections; such as fear, hope, love, hatred, desire, joy, sorrow, gratitude, compassion, and zeal" (p. 96). These affections were divided into two groups according to whether they were characterized by approval (gratitude, love, joy) or disapproval (hatred, fear, sorrow). Thus an important appraisal dimension for Edwards was approval/liking versus disapproval/rejection (Pruyser, 1967). Rather than belief, which was seen as intellectual and heartless by Edwards, these affections were to be taken as the signs of genuine spiritual experience. A review of his contributions (Hutch, 1978) suggests considerable benefits can be gained from a reading of Edwards's insights into the nature of religious emotions.

Schleiermacher's (1799) notable treatise on religion also placed emotion at the center of conscious religious experience. Feeling was central. Reverence, humbleness, gratefulness, compassion, remorse, and zeal were described as essential elements of religious experience by Schleiermacher. In agreement with Edwards, Schleiermacher viewed intellectual beliefs as overly rational and lacking in spontaneity; the heart of religion was seen as the heart, not the head (Pruyser, 1967, p. 140).

Arnold (1960), in her book *Emotion and Personality*, was quite possibly the first psychology of emotion theorist to write extensively about positive human emotions. In the chapter on positive emotions, she included a section on religious emotions in which she noted that in addition to the prototypical religious emotions of reverence and awe that Otto (1917/1958) and others had identified, several other emotions can be experienced toward God (which was her criteria for a religious emotion). In particular, love, joy, and happiness are "reactions to overwhelming abundance, an infinity, of the good and the beautiful" (1960, p. 328) and contain "a hint of eternity" (p. 160). Clearly, these emotions are imbued with a spiritual significance for Arnold. They serve the function of motivating people toward states of perfection, toward total fulfillment. Her phenomenological analysis of happiness as a religious feeling and its differentiation from joy, serenity, and contentment was an early important contribution to understanding differences between discrete positive emotions.

What Makes Emotions Sacred?

What does it mean to say that certain emotions or emotional experiences are sacred? We can identify several characteristics of sacred emotions. First, sacred emotions are those emotions that are more likely to occur in religious (e.g., churches, synagogues, mosques) *settings* than in nonreligious settings. However, this does not mean that sacred emotions cannot be experienced in nonreligious settings. Second, sacred emotions are those that are more likely to be elicited through spiritual or religious activities or *practices* (e.g., worship, prayer, meditation) than by nonreligious activities. However, this does not mean they cannot be activated through nonreligious channels as well. Third, sacred emotions are more likely to be experienced by *people* who self-identify as religious or spiritual (or both) than be people who do not think of themselves as either religious or spiritual. However, sacred emotions can be felt (on occasion) by people who do not think of themselves as religious or spiritual. Fourth, sacred emotions are those emotions that religious and spiritual *systems* around the world have traditionally sought to cultivate in their adherents. Fifth, and last, sacred emotions are those emotions experienced when individuals imbue seemingly secular aspects of their lives (e.g., family, career, events) with a spiritual significance (Mahoney et al., 1999).

The search for the sacred is the defining feature of religion (Hill et al., 2000). The term "sacred" refers to a divine being, divine object, ultimate reality, or Ultimate Truth as perceived by the individual (Hill et al., 2000, p. 68). Pargament (1999) has argued that conceiving of spirituality in terms of an ability to imbue everyday experience, goals, roles, and responsibilities with sacredness opens new avenues for empirical exploration. Furthermore, perceiving aspects of life as sacred is likely to elicit spiritual emotions. Spiritual emotions such as gratitude, awe and reverence, love and hope are likely to be generated when people perceive sacredness in various aspects of their lives. Mahoney et al. (1999) found that when marital partners viewed their relationship as imbued with divine qualities, they reported greater levels of marital satisfaction, more constructive problem-solving behaviors, decreased marital conflict, and greater commitment to the relationship, compared to couples who did not see their marriage in a sacred light. Similarly, Tarakeshwar, Swank, Pargament, and Mahoney (2001) found that a strong belief that nature is sacred was associated with greater pro-environmental beliefs and a greater willingness to protect the environment. A plausible hypothesis to be tested in future research is whether sanctification of the environment leads to experiencing more frequent and more intense sacred emotions such as awe and wonder in nature.

Specific Sacred Emotions

Gratitude

Gratitude has been defined as "the willingness to recognize the unearned increments of value in one's experience" (Bertocci & Millard, 1963, p. 389), and as "an estimate of gain coupled with the judgment that someone else is responsible for that gain" (Solomon, 1977, p. 316). At its core, gratitude is an emotional response to a gift. It is the appreciation felt after one has been the beneficiary of an altruistic act. Some of the most profound reported experiences of gratitude can be religiously based or associated with reverent wonder toward an acknowledgment of the universe (Goodenough, 1998), including the perception that life itself is a gift. In the great monotheistic religions of the world, the concept of gratitude permeates texts, prayers, and teachings. Worship with gratitude to God for his many gifts and mercies are common themes, and believers are urged to develop this quality. A religious framework thus provides the backdrop for experiences and expressions of gratitude.

McCullough and colleagues (McCullough, Kilpatrick, Emmons, & Larson, 2001) recently reviewed the classical moral writings on gratitude and synthesized them with contemporary empirical findings. They suggested that the positive emotion of gratitude has three moral functions: it serves as a moral barometer (an affective readout that is sensitive to a particular type of change in one's social relationships, the provision of a benefit by another moral agent who enhances one's well-being), a moral motivator (prompting grateful people to behave prosocially themselves), and a moral reinforcer (that increases the likelihood of future benevolent actions). McCullough, Emmons, and Tsang (2002) found that measures of gratitude as a disposition were positively correlated with nearly all of the measures of spirituality and religiousness, including spiritual transcendence, self-transcendence, and the single-item religious variables. The grateful disposition was also related to measures of spiritual and religious tendencies. Although these correlations were not large (i.e., few of them exceeded $r = .30$), they suggest that spiritually or religiously inclined people have a stronger disposition to experience gratitude than do their less spiritual/religious counterparts. Thus, spiritual and religious inclinations may facilitate gratitude, but it is also conceivable that gratitude facilitates the development of religious and spiritual interests (Allport, Gillespie, & Young, 1948) or that the association of gratitude and spirituality/religiousness is caused by extraneous variables yet to be identified. The fact that the correlations of gratitude with these affective, prosocial, and spiritual variables were obtained using both self-reports and peer reports of the grateful disposition suggests that these associations are substantive and not simply the product of monomethod biases in measurement. This study may be also be useful for explaining why religiously involved people are at a lower risk for depressive symptoms or other mental health difficulties.

McCullough et al. (2002) also found that people who reported high levels of spirituality reported more gratitude in their daily moods, as did people higher in religious interest, general religiousness, and intrinsic religious orientation. Interestingly, however, the extrinsic, utilitarian religious orientation and quest-seeking religious orientation were not significantly correlated with the amount of gratitude in daily mood. These findings suggest that people high in conventional forms of religiousness, especially people for whom religion is a fundamental organizing principle (i.e., people high in intrinsic religiousness) and people who report high levels of spiritual transcendence, experience more gratitude in their daily moods than do their less religious/spiritual counterparts. Watkins, Woodward, Stone, and Kolts (2003) found that trait gratitude correlated positively with intrinsic religiousness and negatively with extrinsic religiousness. The authors suggest that the presence of gratitude may be a *positive* affective hallmark of religiously and spiritually engaged people, just as an absence of depressive symptoms is a *negative* affective hallmark of spiritually and religiously engaged people. They likely see benefits as gifts from God, "as the first cause of all benefits" (Watkins et al., 2003, p. 437).

Awe and Reverence

Few would disagree that the emotions of awe and reverence are central to religious experience. Awe was the cornerstone of Otto's (1917/1958) classic analysis of religious experience. The essence of religious worship, for Otto, was the overpowering feeling of majesty and mystery in the presence of the holy that is at the same time fascinating and dreadful. This juxtaposition of fear and fascination is a hallmark of religious awe (Wettstein, 1997).

Several philosophers of emotion have offered conceptual analyses of awe in which they define awe and distinguish it from reverence and related states. Roberts (2003) describes awe as a *sensitivity to greatness*, accompanied by a sense of being overwhelmed by the object of greatness and reverence as "an acknowledging subjective response to something excellent in a personal (moral or spiritual) way, but qualitatively above oneself" (p. 268). The major distinction between awe and reverence, for Roberts, is that awe could equally be experienced in response to something perceived as vastly evil as to something vastly good, but reverence is typically reserved for those things or persons esteemed worthy of it, in a positive or a moral sense. Similarly, Woodruff (2001) states that "reverence is the well-developed capacity to have the feelings off awe, respect and shame when these are the right feelings to have" (p. 8). Solomon (2002) argues that awe is passive whereas reverence is active: to be awestruck implies paralysis, while reverence leads to active engagement and responsibility toward that which a person reveres.

In contrast to these substantial theological and philosophical writings, little research in the psychology of religion has focused on either awe or reverence as a religious emotion. Many psychologists mention awe in their studies of religious experiences, but few have attempted to study it systematically. Maslow (1964) included the experience of awe under the broad umbrella of "peak experiences" (1964, p. 65), an umbrella that included "practically everything that, for example, Rudolf Otto defines as characteristic of religious experience" (1964, p. 54). Several other studies have included awe under the slightly less broad category of mystical experiences, but since awe is not the purpose of these studies, their research and conclusions are difficult to utilize with respect to awe. For example, though Hardy (1979) lists awe, reverence, and wonder as a category of religious experience recorded in his database, his examples merely include a description of the "it" of a particular mystical experience or mention awe as an after-effect of the experience. Interestingly, Hardy (1979) found that awe was not a particularly frequently reported experience: awe, reverence, and wonder occurred in 7% of reported religious experiences that he collected, compared to 21% for joy and happiness and 25% for peace and security. Likewise, when Hood (1975) included awe as an item on his mysticism scale he was not interested in the experience of awe per se, but in the mystical experience that might (or might not) produce awe.

Keltner and Haidt (2003) have recently offered a prototypical approach to awe that represents an important new contribution. According to their definition, an awe experience includes both a *perceived vastness* (whether of power or magnitude) and a *need for accommodation*, which is an "inability to assimilate an experience into current mental structures" (p. 304). Variation in the valence of an awe experience is due to whether the stimulus is appraised in terms of beauty, exceptional ability, virtue, perceived threat, or supernatural origin. In contrast, those experiences that do not include both perceived vastness and need for accommodation are not occurrences of awe, but are simply members of the awe family. For example, surprise involves accommodation without vastness. Feelings of deference involve vastness without accommodation. Unfortunately, there is very little empirical research on awe, and until this changes anything we say about awe as a religious emotion must be restricted to what can be gleaned from sacred writings.

As the study of awe is still in its early stages, future research should begin with the prototype approach to awe offered by Keltner and Haidt (2003) and the definition of reverence offered by philosophers and theologians (Roberts, 2003; Woodruff, 2001) and develop tests to measure individual differences in these experiences. Once a reliable measure of awe and reverence exists, individual differences in these experiences can be explored, as well as their relation to religion and spirituality, their developmental antecedents, and their relationship to emotional and physical well-being.

Wonder

Wonder is another emotion that has received scant empirical attention by psychologists but has a significant spiritual thrust. Bulkeley (2002) defined *wonder* as "the emotion excited by an encounter with something novel and unexpected, something that strikes a person as intensely powerful, real, true, and/or beautiful" (p. 6). Brand (2001) provided a phenomenological account of wonder-joy: profound and deeply moving experiences of positive emotions where there is a co-occurrence of feelings of wonder, joy, gratitude, awe, yearning, poignancy, intensity, love, and compassion. They are an opening up of the heart to the persons or profound circumstances being witnessed and are triggered by a variety of circumstances. Experiences of wonder are a significant feature of many of the world's religious, spiritual, and philosophical traditions (Bulkeley, 2002). Bulkeley proposes that the experience of wonder involves a twofold process: (1) a sudden decentering of the self when faced with something novel and unexpectedly powerful, followed by (2) an ultimate recentering of the self in response to new knowledge and understanding. It is evident that the wonder that Bulkeley describes and the sense of awe described by Haidt and Keltner have much in common; it will be up to future research to establish the unique properties of these overlapping states.

Hope

Hope is a theological virtue, one of the "Big Three," along with faith and charity. In Christian theology, hope is looking forward to the eternal world where the kingdom of God will be ushered in: "Let us hold unswervingly to the hope we profess, for he who promised is faithful" (Hebrews 10:23, *New International Version Bible* [NIV]). In its religious context, hope provides respite during trials, brings perseverance during challenges, and provides assurance of eternal joy.

Hope research has burgeoned over the past decade, with studies indicating hope's numerous positive effects on mental and physical health (see Snyder, Sigmon, & Feldman, 2002, for a review). In this light, whenever religion fosters or hinders hope, one would expect significant positive or negative effects on the whole person. In current research, the construct of hope is often couched in terms of goals, with hope requiring the thought of a goal, perceived pathways to those goals (pathway thoughts), and motivation (agency thoughts) to follow through to the goal. Snyder and colleagues (2002) use this understanding of hope to explain the link previously found between religion or religious involvement and health or well-being: Religions provide adherents with goals, paths to those goals, and incentives to reach those goals, either for good or for ill.

Sethi and Seligman (1993) found that among nine Jewish, Christian, and Muslim groups, the more fundamentalist the group was, the more hopeful and optimistic were the sermons, the liturgy, and the average participant's outlook. This finding of greater hope in persons in fundamentalist faiths is an intriguing one, given that fundamentalism is often associated with a more constricted and less spontaneous approach to life (Altemeyer and Hunsberger, Chapter 21, this volume). Could it be that persons in conservative faiths tend to present overly positive images of themselves and thus deny negative emotions? Bullard and Park (1998) tested the hypothesis that fundamentalism (measured in terms of adherence to Protestant orthodoxy) is related to the overt expression of emotions. They used a frequently employed measure of emotional expressiveness that classifies respondents into high-anxious, low-anxious, repressor, or defensively high-anxious categories. Fundamentalism was associated with anxiety such that the low fundamentalism group was more likely to be highly anxious; no significant patterns were found between the other three expressive styles and fundamentalism. Thus, the finding of greater positive emotions in fundamentalist faiths is not due to the nonexpression or repression of negative affect. This study is the only one that has examined whether adherence to religious doctrine is associated with styles of emotional expression.

RELIGION AND THE REGULATION OF EMOTION

"Emotion regulation" refers to the processes by which individuals influence which emotions they have, the intensity of these emotions, and how these emotions are expressed

(Gross, 1999). The regulatory process may be conscious or unconscious, intentional or unintentional. Emotions, both positive and negative, can be transformed or regulated by intentionally engaging in spiritual practices. Religions' teachings and texts contain information concerning how emotions should be handled. The importance of emotion regulation in everyday life provides a legitimate rationale for examining the role of religion in this process. Emotional regulation techniques that have their rationales in religious traditions can modulate everyday emotional experience (Schimmel, 1997; Watts, 1996), providing spiritual rationales and methods for handling problematic emotions such as anger, guilt, and depression. Watts and Williams (1988, Chap. 6) draw parallels between religious and clinical approaches to emotional control and cite meditational training as an activity with origins in both Western and Eastern contemplative religions. Positive emotional benefits have been reported for Zen meditation (Gillani & Smith, 2001) and for the cultivation of transpersonal states long associated with spiritual and religious traditions (McCraty, Barrios-Choplin, Rozman, Atkinson, & Watkins, 1998). Baer (2003) reviewed the literature on mindfulness-meditation interventions and found that these interventions appear to alleviate a variety of negative emotional states (primarily anxiety and depression) and may be efficacious in cultivating positive states such as compassion.

Thayer, Newman, and McClain (1994) examined the success of several behavioral and cognitive strategies for regulating unpleasant moods and raising energy levels. One category of strategies was labeled as religious/spiritual, though there was no information provided as to what these specific religious and spiritual strategies actually were. As mood management techniques, these were found to more common in older participants than in younger ones and were particularly effective for reducing nervousness, tension, and anxiety. Although spiritual and religious activity was not among the most common behaviors used to reduce tension and anxiety, it was rated as most successful. In a factor analysis, religious and spiritual techniques loaded on a pleasant distraction factor; this factor was found to be the most effective strategy for mood change. So, although low in absolute frequency (study participants were doctoral-level psychotherapists), religious practices were rated as the single best method of regulating unpleasant moods.

Forgiveness

Forgiveness is a religiously based technique that has been shown to be powerful in regulating negative emotions. Pargament (1997) suggests that forgiveness is religious in that (1) religion lends a spiritual significance to the act of forgiving, and (2) religion offers role models and concrete methods to facilitate forgiveness. Forgiveness as a contemporary psychological or social science construct has also generated popular and clinical interest as well as empirical investigation (for reviews, see McCullough, Pargament, & Thoresen, 2000; Witvliet, Ludwig, & Bauer, 2002; Witvliet, Ludwig, & Vander Laan, 2001). The scientific literature on forgiveness is growing rapidly across a number of areas of psychology, including the social–clinical interface (McCullough, 2001), though clinical applications of forgiveness probably still bear little connection to empirical research.

There have been a handful of studies that have been explicitly designed to examine the impact of forgiveness on the remediation of negative emotions. Witvliet and her colleagues (Witvliet, Ludwig, & Bauer, 2002; Witvliet, Ludwig, & Vander Laan, 2001) examined subjective emotions and emotional physiology during forgiving and unforgiving imagery. In their initial study, Witvliet et al. (2001) found that when participants visualized forgiving responses toward people who had offended them, they experienced significantly less anger, sadness, and overall negative arousal compared to when they rehearsed the offense or maintained a grudge. Paralleling the self-reports were greater sympathetic nervous system arousal (skin conductance and blood pressure increases) and facial tension during unforgiving imagery. A follow-up study examined the emotions of transgressors (Witvliet et al., 2002). When transgressors imagined seeking forgiveness from their victims, the transgressors reported lower levels of sadness, anger, and guilt and higher levels of hope and gratitude *if* they imagined the victim genuinely forgiving the transgressor. Imagining reconciliation rather than forgiveness led to a similar reduction in negative (anger, sadness, guilt) emotions and increase in positive (gratitude, hope, empathy) emotions.

Forgiveness interventions have also been shown to be successful in alleviating depression, anxiety, and grief in postabortion men (Coyle & Enright, 1997) and depression and anxiety in incest survivors (Freedman & Enright, 1996). In the latter study, the intervention group also showed significant gains in overall levels of hopefulness, suggesting, as did the work of Witvliet and colleagues, that forgiveness is involved in facilitating positive emotions as well as reducing negative emotions. The ability of forgiveness interventions to increase certain positive emotions is one of the more surprising findings in the research literature on forgiveness to date.

In one of the few cultural studies on forgiveness, Huang and Enright (2000) examined forgiveness and anger in a Taiwanese sample. Adults recalled an incident of deep interpersonal hurt, and their affective state was recorded both during and after recall. The researchers found that when participants granted forgiveness unconditionally out of a sense of compassion, self-reported levels of anger were lower than when they forgave out of a sense of duty or obligation. Thus, the effectiveness *of* forgiveness to reduce negative emotions is contingent upon the motivation *for* forgiveness.

Mindfulness

A number of philosophical, psychological, and spiritual traditions, both in the East and in the West, highlight mindfulness's importance, but are there really adaptational and mental health benefits to being more conscious of what's happening in the here-and-now? *Mindfulness*, an enhanced attention to and awareness of the present, is currently the subject of innumerable books, seminars, and workshops designed to facilitate this quality of consciousness as a means to helping people live more authentic and happier lives. But very little research has examined its direct role in psychological health and well-being.

Brown and Ryan (2003) developed a self-report instrument, called the Mindful Attention Awareness Scale (MAAS), to measure mindfulness, and administered it to subjects ranging from college students to working adults to Zen meditators to cancer patients. In mindfulness, which Brown and Ryan (2003) showed is a unique quality of consciousness, two experiences work in tandem: attending to present, ongoing events and experiences while allowing new events and experiences to come into awareness. In their research, Brown and colleagues have found that more mindful individuals, as measured by the MAAS, have a greater self-regulatory capacity and higher levels of well-being.

Regarding self-regulation, Brown and Ryan (2003, Study 3) showed that those who are more mindful are more attuned to their emotions, as reflected in a higher concordance between their explicit, or self-attributed, emotional states and implicit, or nonconscious, emotions. Because implicit measures are not susceptible to conscious control and manipulation, this suggests that more mindful individuals are more attuned to their implicit emotions and reflect that knowledge in their explicit, affective self-descriptions. This is consistent with theory positing that present-centered awareness and attention facilitates self-knowledge, a crucial element of integrated functioning.

A number of studies have shown that mindfulness has direct relations to well-being outcomes, as well. For example, Brown and Ryan (2003, Study 1) report that similar to other personal qualities, mindfulness can be cultivated and enhanced, or neglected and allowed to diminish. Brown and Ryan (2003, Study 2) showed that people who actively cultivated a heightened attention to and awareness of what's taking place in the present moment through meditative practices had higher levels of mindfulness. And in a clinical study with early-stage cancer patients who received training in mindfulness as the central element of an 8-week stress reduction program (Brown & Ryan, 2003, Study 5), those individuals who showed greater increases in mindfulness, as assessed by the MAAS, showed greater declines in mood disturbance and stress.

RELIGION AND EMOTION: REMAINING ISSUES

Functions of Religious Emotions

Current models of emotions typically aim to describe the form and function of emotions in general. Despite this aim, many models are formulated around prototypic and negative emotions like fear and anger. For instance, key to many theorists' models of emotions is the idea that emotions are, by definition, associated with specific action tendencies. What functions do religious emotions serve? Noting that traditional models based on specific action tendencies did not do justice to positive emotions, Fredrickson (2001) developed an alternative model for the positive emotions that better captures their unique effects. She called this the broaden-and-build theory of positive emotions (Fredrickson, 2001) because positive emotions appear to *broaden* people's momentary thought–action repertoires and *build* their enduring personal resources. Whereas the narrowed mind-sets of negative emotions carry direct and immediate adaptive benefits in situations that threaten survival, the broadened mind-sets of positive emotions, which occur when people feel safe and satiated, are beneficial in other ways. Specifically, these broadened mind-sets carry indirect and long-term adaptive benefits because broadening *builds* enduring personal resources (Fredrickson, 2001).

Fredrickson (2001) analyzed the functions of several distinct positive emotions. Joy, for instance, creates the urge to play, push the limits, and be creative, urges evident not only in social and physical behavior, but also in intellectual and artistic behavior. Interest, a phenomenologically distinct positive emotion, creates the urge to explore, take in new information and experiences, and expand the self in the process. Contentment, a third distinct positive emotion, creates the urge to savor current life circumstances, and integrate these circumstances into new views of self and of the world. And gratitude, a fourth distinct positive emotion, creates the urge to creatively repay kindness. These various thought–action tendencies—to play, to explore, to savor and integrate, and to repay kindness—each represent ways that positive emotions broaden habitual modes of thinking or acting. In general terms, then, positive emotions appear to enlarge the cognitive context, an effect recently linked to increases in brain dopamine levels (Ashby, Isen, & Turken, 1999).

Finding positive meaning is perhaps the most reliable path to cultivating positive emotions (Fredrickson, 2001). To the extent that religions offer their believers worldviews that help them to find positive meaning in both ordinary daily events (e.g., appreciating nature) and major life challenges (e.g., finding benefit in a cancer diagnosis), they also cultivate positive emotions such as joy, serenity, awe, gratitude, and hope. According to the broaden-and-build theory, these positive emotions should, in turn, broaden people's mind-sets, making them more creative and integrative in their thinking, and build and replenish critical personal and social resources, such as resilience, optimism, and social support. These resources, a wide range of studies have shown, enhance health and well-being.

In future research, it will be important to conceptually and empirically distinguish secular positive emotions (i.e., positive emotions felt outside religious or sacred contexts) from one or more categories of religious or sacred positive emotions, which might include positive emotions felt in religious services, toward God or a higher power, toward other believers, or otherwise connected to that which believers imbue with a sense of the sacred. Religious practices may be distinctly human ways of initiating upward spirals that enhance spiritual growth as well as health and well-being.

Are Religious Emotions Unique?

A perennial issue in the psychology of religion pertains to the uniqueness of emotions that are labeled as religious. Are these a separate class of emotions or simply ordinary emotions felt in religious contexts or elicited through religious rituals such as prayer and worship? Consider this statement from William James (1902/1958):

> In the psychologies and in the philosophies of religion, we find the authors attempting to specify just what entity it is. One man allies it to the feeling of dependence; one makes it a derivative from fear; others connect it with the sexual life; others still identify it with the feeling of the infinite; and so on. Such different ways of conceiving it ought of themselves to arouse doubt as to whether it possibly can be one specific thing; and the moment we are willing to treat the term "religious sentiment" as a collective name for the many sentiments which religious objects may arouse in alternation, we see that it probably contains nothing whatever of a psychologically specific nature. There is religious fear, religious love, religious awe, religious joy, and so forth. But religious love is only man's natural emotion of love directed to a religious object; religious fear is only the ordinary fear of commerce, so to speak, the common quaking of the human breast, in so far as the notion of divine retribution may arouse it; religious awe is the same organic thrill which we feel in a forest at twilight, or in a mountain gorge; only this time it comes over us at the thought of our supernatural relations; and similarly of all the various sentiments which may be called into play in the lives of religious persons. As concrete states of mind, made up of a feeling plus a specific sort of object, religious emotions of course are psychic entities distinguishable from other concrete emotions; but there is no ground for assuming a simple abstract "religious emotion" to exist as a distinct elementary mental affection by itself, present in every religious experience without exception. As there thus seems to be no one elementary religious emotion, but only a common storehouse of emotions upon which religious objects may draw, so there might conceivably also prove to be no one specific and essential kind of religious object, and no one specific and essential kind of religious act. (pp. 39–40)

For James, what makes religious emotion *religious* are ordinary felt emotions under circumstances that make it apparent to the person that God or a higher power is involved.

Emotion and Spiritual Transformation

A major research area in the psychology of religion has always been conversion or transformation (Paloutzian, this volume, Chapter 18; Paloutzian, Richardson, & Rambo, 1999). Many theories of the processes underlying spiritual transformations have been offered, but virtually all converge on the importance of the affective basis of spiritual transformation (Hill, 2002; Oatley & Djikic, 2002). In these perspectives, emotions are seen as agents of transformation in the spiritual self. While the emphasis is generally placed on the role of negative emotions in triggering spiritual changes, positive emotions may play an important role as well. For example, Allport, Gillespie, and Young (1948) found that gratitude was the fourth most cited reason among youth for turning to religion, and the role of gratitude and goodness (as well as awe and wonder) in G. K. Chesterton's (1936) adult conversion to Catholicism is legendary.

Ullman's (1989) study is frequently cited as supporting the hypothesis that conversion is more based in emotion than it is on an intellectual search process. In examining conversion among four different faith groups, Ullman found that the converts reported a greater degree of emotional distress in childhood than did nonconverts, and were more likely to say that emotional stress was a more important factor in their conversion than was a cognitive quest.

The research that exists is suggestive of links between emotion and transformation, but much more needs to be done. There is a great need for longitudinal studies of emotion in which emotions are both motivators and consequences of transformation. Future research should also focus more on positive emotions, both as motivators of change and potential consequences of change. The measurement of positive emotions has improved considerably in recent years and researchers have established and well-validated measures to draw upon and incorporate into their research designs.

RELIGIOUS EMOTIONS IN EMOTION HISTORY: TWO ILLUSTRATIONS

A vastly different approach to emotion and religion can be found in the field of *emotions history* (Stearns & Lewis, 1998). Emotions history examines the experience and expression of emotions among U.S. subcultures during specific historical contexts, and seeks to discern the dominant affective climate that prevailed in these groups during these periods. The formal study of history of emotions is a relatively new discipline, but two recent studies warrant mentioning here as illustrations of how religious emotions are influenced by historical context.

Working under the assumption that Judaism requires emotional involvement and emotional transactions with God, Mayer (1994) engaged in a lexigraphic study of emotion trends in biblical texts. He classified nine emotion terms (happiness, anger, fear, sadness, love, hate, contempt, guilt, and envy) in the books of the Hebrew Bible and examined changes in the frequency of occurrence over the 12-century period during which, according to general scholarly agreement, the books were written. The primary purpose of the study was to see whether emotion changed over time. As the centuries progressed, Mayer found a systematic increase in references to happiness; no other emotions were shown to systematically increase or decrease over this time period. Although he considers a number of alternative hypotheses and is cognizant of the perils and limitations of a psychohistorical analysis, Mayer suggests that this finding can be taken as evidence of the positive psychological benefits of a highly religious culture, and advocates a historical analysis of emotion and religion for understanding factors that influence emotion in the present.

A second study sought to describe the predominant emotions expressed by U.S. Pentecostal women in the first half of the 20th century (Griffith, 1998). This qualitative study of a variety of texts focused on the pious emotions of southern, rural, and poor female members of the Pentecostal Church. One of the primary hallmarks of the Pentecostal faith is the natural and authentic expression of emotion. Indeed, the Pentecostal movement has traditionally sought to provoke and sustain strong emotions in believers. Griffith's examination of narratives of conversion, reports of healing experiences, and responses to prayers revealed a high occurrence of emotions pertaining to praise, gratitude, love, joy, and exuberant happiness. Griffith hypothesized a dual role for these emotions: (1) they defined an ethic of separation, setting apart believers from nonbelievers and from members of other Christian sects, thus enhancing commitment to the ingroup; and (2) they were essential elements in constructing a testimony for communicating one's faith to others and for providing assurance and certainty of one's own faith. This study, along with Mayer's (1994), are examples of how historical and theological contexts shape emotion and provide important clues about the function of religious emotions in everyday life.

FUTURE DIRECTIONS AND CONCLUSION

There are two trends that are likely to have significant impact on emotion research within the psychology of religion in the near future.

First, further progress in religion and emotion is likely to be spurred on by the current vigorous activity in the field of religion and health (see Oman & Thoresen, Chapter 24, and Miller & Kelley, Chapter 25, this volume). Researchers are examining mechanisms that explain the effects of religious practices on health. It follows from the broaden-and-build theory (Fredrickson, 2001) that sacred positive emotions can serve as resources that a person can draw upon in times of need, including coping with stress and dealing with and recovering from physical illness. It is also plausible, for example, that the biology of emotions and related states activated during religious worship (praise, reverence, awe, gratitude, love, hope) could have neuroendocrine or immunological consequences, thus potentially accounting for the salubrious effects of religious practices on health outcomes. Any examination of the neurobiology of these states will have to rely upon the phenomenological properties of worship as well, thus producing new insights at this level of analysis.

Second, the growing cognitive science of religion field (Andresen, 2001; Pyysiäinen & Anttonen, 2002) is likely to open new vistas for understanding the functions of emotion in religious contexts and in religious cognition. The role of emotions in the adoption and transmission of religious beliefs currently plays a prominent role in several cognitive theories of religion (Andresen, 2001), particularly in accounting for the provocativeness of religious rituals (McCauley, 2001). Much of this work focuses on religion as counterintuitiveness (Boyer, 2001) and emotional responses to counterintuitive representations. Research has shown that counterintuitive representations are more effectively recalled than ordinary or even unusual representations (Boyer, 2001), which may be due to their ability to arouse strong emotions. Emotion is also assumed to play a pivotal role in resolving doubts concerning religious representations (beliefs) and in enhancing commitment to the object of those representations. Franks (2003), cites the example of positive emotions in response to perceived answers to prayer as serving to reduce doubts about the benevolence of God. Connecting the act of prayer to the experience of positive emotion provides at least a temporary resolution in the mind of the believer who may have doubted God's benevolence. Given the pervasiveness of religious doubts (Clark, 1958; Hunsberger, Pratt, & Pancer, 2002), an incorporation of the role of emotion might contribute to understanding both the development and the resolution of questions and doubts concerning religious doctrines.

In each of these two cases, it is clear that progress will require collaboration between psychologists who specialize in religion and experts in evolutionary biology, neuroscience, philosophy, anthropology, and cognitive science, so that developments in the psychology of religion take into account and build upon advances in these related scientific disciplines. It will also be necessary to take an approach of downward causation, in which individual beliefs and socioreligious contexts regulate biological systems of the body. Successful researchers who contribute to the next generation of knowledge at the interface of religion and emotion will thus likely need to be schooled not just in the sciences but in theology as well.

ACKNOWLEDGMENT

Preparation of this chapter was supported by a grant from the John Templeton Foundation.

REFERENCES

Allen, D. (1997). Ascetic theology and psychology. In R. C. Roberts & M. R. Talbot (Eds.), *Limning the psyche: Explorations in Christian psychology* (pp. 297–316). Grand Rapids, MI: Eerdmans.

Allport, G. W., Gillespie, J. M., & Young, J. (1948). The religion of the post-war college student. *Journal of Psychology, 25*, 3–33.

Andresen, J. (Ed.). (2001). *Religion in mind: Cognitive perspectives on religious belief, ritual, and experience.* Cambridge, UK: Cambridge University Press.

Arnold, M. B. (1960). *Emotion and personality.* New York: Columbia University Press.

Ashby, F. G., Isen, A. M., & Turken, A. U. (1999). A neuropsychological theory of positive affect and its influence on cognition. *Psychological Review, 106*, 529–550.

Baer, R. A. (2003). Mindfulness training as a clinical intervention: A conceptual and empirical review. *Clinical Psychology: Science and Practice, 10*, 125–143.

Ben Ze'ev, A. (2002). *The subtlety of the emotions.* New York: Cambridge University Press.

Bertocci, P. A., & Millard, R. M. (1963). *Personality and the good.* Philadelphia: Mckay.

Boyer, P. (2001). *Religion explained.* New York: Basic Books.

Brand, W. (2001). Experiencing tears of wonder-joy: Seeing with the heart's eye. *Journal of Transpersonal Psychology, 33*, 9–111.

Brown, K. W., & Ryan, R. M. (2003). The benefits of being present: Mindfulness and its role in psychological well-being. *Journal of Personality and Social Psychology, 84*, 822–848.

Bulkeley, K. (2002, November). *The evolution of wonder: Religious and neuroscientific perspectives.* Paper presented at the annual meeting of the American Academy of Religion, Toronto, Canada.

Bullard, P. L., & Park, C. L. (2001). Emotional expressive style as a mediator between religion and health. *International Journal of Rehabilitation and Health, 4*, 201–214.

Chesterton, G. K. (1936). *The autobiography of G. K. Chesterton.* New York: Sheed & Wood.

Clark, W. H. (1958). *The psychology of religion.* New York: Harper & Row.

Coyle, C. T., & Enright, R. D. (1997). Forgiveness intervention with post-abortion men. *Journal of Consulting and Clinical Psychology, 65,* 1042–1046.

Edwards, J. (1959). *Religious affections.* In J. E. Smith (Ed.), *The works of Jonathan Edwards* (Vol. 2). New Haven, CT: Yale University Press. (Original work published 1746)

Emmons, R. A., & Paloutzian, R. F. (2003). The psychology of religion. *Annual Review of Psychology, 54,* 377–402.

Franks, B. (2003). The nature of unnaturalness in religious representations: Negation and concept combination. *Journal of Cognition and Culture, 3,* 41–68.

Fredrickson, B. L. (2001). The role of positive emotions in positive psychology: The broaden-and-build theory of positive emotions. *American Psychologist, 56,* 218–226.

Fredrickson, B. L. (2002). How does religion benefit health and well-being?: Are positive emotions active ingredients? *Psychological Inquiry, 13,* 209–213.

Freedman, S. R., & Enright, R. D. (1996). Forgiveness as an intervention goal with incest survivors. *Journal of Consulting and Clinical Psychology, 64,* 983–992.

Gillani, N. B., & Smith, J. C. (2001). Zen meditation and ABC relaxation theory: An exploration of relaxation states, beliefs, dispositions, and motivations. *Journal of Clinical Psychology, 57,* 839–846.

Goodenough, U. (1998). *The sacred depths of nature.* New York: Oxford University Press.

Griffith, R. M. (1998). "Joy unspeakable and full of glory": The vocabulary of pious emotion in the narratives of American Pentecostal women, 1910–1945. In P. N. Stearns & J. Lewis (Eds.), *An emotional history of the United States* (pp. 218–240). New York: New York University Press.

Griffiths, P. E. (1997). *What emotions really are.* Chicago: University of Chicago Press.

Gross, J. J. (1999). Emotion regulation: Past, present, future. *Cognition and Emotion, 13,* 551–573.

Hardy, A. (1979). *The spiritual nature of man: A study of contemporary religious experience.* Oxford, UK: Clarendon Press.

Hill, P. C. (2002). Spiritual transformation: Forming the habitual center of personal energy. *Research in the Social Scientific Study of Religion, 13,* 87–108.

Hill, P. C., Pargament, K. I., Wood, R. W., Jr., McCullough, M. E., Swyers, J. P., Larson, D. B., & Zinnbauer, B. J. (2000). Conceptualizing religion and spirituality: Points of commonality, points of departure. *Journal for the Theory of Social Behavior, 30,* 51–77.

Hood, R., Jr. (1975). The construction and preliminary validation of a measure of mystical experience. *Journal for the Scientific Study of Religion, 14,* 29–41.

Huang, S. T., & Enright, R. D. (2000). Forgiveness and anger-related emotions in Taiwan: Implications for therapy. *Psychotherapy, 37,* 71–79.

Hunsberger, B., Pratt, M., & Prancer, M. P. (2002). A longitudinal study of religious doubts in high school and beyond: Relationships, stability, and searching for answers. *Journal for the Scientific Study of Religion, 41,* 255–266.

Hutch, R. A. (1978). Jonathan Edwards' analysis of religious experience. *Journal of Psychology and Theology, 6,* 123–131.

James, W. (1958). *The varieties of religious experience.* New York: Longmans. (Original work published 1902)

Keltner, D., & Haidt, J. (2003). Approaching awe: A moral, spiritual, and aesthetic emotion. *Cognition and Emotion, 17,* 297–314.

Lewis, M., & Haviland-Jones, J. M. (Eds.). (2000). *Handbook of emotions* (2nd ed.). New York: Guilford Press.

Mahoney, A., Pargament, K. I., Jewell, T., Swank, A. B., Scott, E., Emery, E., & Rye, M. (1999). Marriage and the spiritual realm: The role of proximal and distal religious constructs in marital functioning. *Journal of Family Psychology, 13,* 321–338.

Maslow, A. (1964). *Religions, values, and peak experiences.* New York: Penguin Books.

Mayer, J. D. (1994). Emotion over time within a religious culture: A lexical analysis of the Old Testament. *Journal of Psychohistory, 22,* 235–248.

McCauley, R. N. (2001). Ritual, memory, and emotion: Comparing two cognitive hypotheses. In J. Andresen (Ed.), *Religion in mind: Cognitive perspectives on religious belief, ritual, and experience* (pp. 115–140). New York: Cambridge University Press.

McCraty, R., Barrios-Choplin, B., Rozman, D., Atkinson, M., & Watkins, A. (1998). The impact of a new emotional self-management program on stress, emotions, heart rate variability, DHEA and cortisol. *Integrative Physiological and Behavioral Science, 33*, 151–170.

McCullough, M. E. (2001). Forgiveness: Who does it and how do they do it? *Current Directions in Psychological Science, 10*, 194–197.

McCullough, M. E., Emmons, R. A., & Tsang, J. (2002). The grateful disposition: A conceptual and empirical topography. *Journal of Personality and Social Psychology, 82*, 112–127.

McCullough, M. E., Kilpatrick, S. D., Emmons, R. A., & Larson, D. B. (2001). Is gratitude a moral affect? *Psychological Bulletin, 127*, 249–266.

McCullough, M. E., Pargament, K. I., & Thoresen, C. E. (Eds.). (2000). *Forgiveness: Theory, practice and research*. New York: Guilford Press.

Miller, W. R. (Ed.). (1999). *Integrating spirituality into treatment: Resources for practitioners*. Washington, DC: American Psychological Association.

Oatley, K., & Djikic, M. (2002). Emotions and transformations. *Journal of Consciousness Studies, 9*, 97–116.

Otto, R. (1958). *The idea of the holy* (J.W. Harvey, Trans.). London: Oxford University Press. (Original work published 1917)

Paloutzian, R. F., Richardson, J. T., & Rambo, L. R. (1999). Religious conversion and personality change. *Journal of Personality, 67*, 1047–1080.

Pargament, K. I. (1997). *The psychology of religion and coping*. New York: Guilford Press.

Pargament, K. I. (1999). The psychology of religion *and* spirituality?: Yes and no. *The International Journal for the Psychology of Religion, 9*, 3–16.

Park, Y. O., & Enright, R. D. (1997). The development of forgiveness in the context of adolescent friendship conflict in Korea. *Journal of Adolescence, 20*, 393–402.

Propst, L. R. (1988). *Psychotherapy in a religious framework: Spirituality in the emotional healing process*. New York: Human Sciences Press.

Pruyser, P. W. (1967). *A dynamic psychology of religion*. New York: Harper & Row.

Pyysiäinen, I., & Anttonen, V. (Eds.). *Current approaches in the cognitive science of religion*. New York: Continuum.

Richards, P. S., & Bergin, A. E. (1997). *A spiritual strategy for counseling and psychotherapy*. Washington, DC: American Psychological Association.

Roberts, R. C. (2003). *Emotions: An essay in aid of moral psychology*. New York: Cambridge University Press.

Rosenberg, E. L. (1998). Levels of analysis and the organization of affect. *Review of General Psychology, 2*, 247–270.

Schimmel, S. (1997). *The seven deadly sins*. New York: Oxford University Press.

Schleiermacher, F. (1799). *On religion: Speeches to its cultured despisers*. London: Kegan Paul, Trench, Tribner.

Sethi, S., & Seligman, M. E. P. (1993). Optimism and fundamentalism. *Psychological Science, 4*, 256–259.

Shafranske, E. P. (Ed.). (1996). *Religion and the clinical practice of psychology*. Washington, DC: American Psychological Association.

Silberman, I. (2003). Spiritual role modeling: The teaching of meaning systems. *The International Journal for the Psychology of Religion, 13*, 175–195.

Snyder, C. R., Sigmon, D. R., & Feldman, D. B. (2002). Hope for the sacred and vice versa: Positive goal-directed thinking and religion. *Psychological Inquiry, 13*(3), 234–238.

Solomon, R. C. (1977). *The passions*. Garden City, NY: Anchor Books.

Solomon, R. C. (2002). *Spirituality for the skeptic: The thoughtful love of life*. New York: Oxford University Press.

Stearns, P. N., & Lewis, J. (Eds.). (1998). *An emotional history of the United States*. New York: New York University Press.

Tarakeshwar, N., Swank, A. B., Pargament, K. I., & Mahoney, A. (2001). Theological conservatism and the sanctification of nature: A study of opposing religious correlates of environmentalism. *Review of Religious Research, 42*, 387–404.

Thayer, R. E., Newman, J. R., & McClain, T. M. (1994). Self-regulation of mood: Strategies for changing a bad mood, raising energy, and reducing tension. *Journal of Personality and Social Psychology, 67*, 910–925.

Ullman, C. (1989). *The transformed self: The psychology of religious conversion*. New York: Plenum Press.

Watkins, P. C., Woodward, K., Stone, T., & Kolts, R. L. (2003). Gratitude and happiness: Development of a measure of gratitude and relationships with subjective well-being. *Social Behavior and Personality, 31*(5), 431–452.

Watts, F. N. (1996). Psychological and religious perspectives on emotion. *The International Journal for the Psychology of Religion, 6*, 71–87.

Watts, F. N., & Williams, M. (1988). *The psychology of religious knowing*. Cambridge, UK: Cambridge University Press.

Wettstein, H. (1997). Awe and the religious life. *Juadaism: A Quarterly Journal of Jewish Life and Thought, 46*, 387–407.

Witvliet, C. V., Ludwig, T. E., & Bauer, D. J. (2002). Please forgive me: Transgressors' emotions and physiology during imagery of seeking forgiveness and victim responses. *Journal of Psychology and Christianity, 21*, 219–233.

Witvliet, C. V., Ludwig, T. E., & Vander Laan, K. L. (2001). Granting forgiveness or harboring grudges: Implications for emotion, physiology, and health. *Psychological Science, 12*, 117–123.

Woodruff, P. (2001). *Reverence: Renewing a forgotten virtue*. New York: Oxford University Press.

14

The Role of Personality in Understanding Religious and Spiritual Constructs

RALPH L. PIEDMONT

Spirituality and religiosity are the key concepts in the psychology of religion. In their recent review of the field, Emmons and Paloutzian (2003) noted the upsurge in interest in these constructs over the past 15 years by both applied and basic researchers. However, despite such common usage, these terms have no universally accepted definitions. Any review of the literature will reveal a large number of disparate definitions (McGinn [1993] identified 35 different definitions for spirituality). But however one defines these constructs, they are essentially individual differences dimensions: some individuals are high on these qualities, others are low, and most fall somewhere in the middle. As such, the need exists to understand, both conceptually and empirically, what variability on these dimensions indicates about people. One way of doing this is to link numinous (i.e., spiritual or mystical) constructs with established models of personality. Such theories have the value of conceptualizing spiritual and religious variables within broader motivational contexts. The purpose of this chapter is to examine several different models of personality and how they have been used to expand our understandings of spiritual constructs. These models were selected because of their demonstrated value to the field; their strengths and weaknesses will be summarized. This discussion is followed by a presentation of the five key empirical issues research needs to address in order to move the field forward.

Across the many different definitions for spirituality and religiosity (see Zinnbauer & Pargament, Chapter 2, this volume, for a review), research has shown that spiritual constructs represent genetically based cognitive and affective qualities that have behavioral implications across the lifespan (Hill et al., 2000; also see Boyatzis, Chapter 7; Levenson & Aldwin, Chapter 8; and McFadden, Chapter 9, this volume). As such, numinous constructs reflect many of the same qualities of traditional personality variables, such as being intrinsic to the person, motivational in nature, providing stability in functioning over time, and providing consistency in behavior across situations (Piedmont,

1999). Such overlap in form and function makes it only logical for one to view spiritual and religious constructs within the interpretive umbrella of broader models of personality. This provides three important benefits to those working in this area . First, personality theories provide measurement models for developing religious and spiritual scales. Such quantification allows for a psychometric understanding of what the scale represents as well as an opportunity to integrate findings within a cohesive conceptual model. This enables researchers in the psychology of religion to link their numinous constructs to mainstream theoretical models in the social sciences, thereby enhancing the relevance of their work. Second, it provides an interpretive context for understanding the broader conceptual dimensions of the variable. Personality theories provide insights into the development and expression of spiritual motivations and religious sentiments over time, their adaptive significance to the individual, and how they "fit" into the broader psychic system we call "the person." Finally, to the extent that religious and spiritual variables are independent of traditional personality theories, then the development of these constructs can be used to expand the predictive relevance of these theories.

The following section reviews five different personality models frequently used for evaluating spiritual and religious constructs. Two of these models (object relations and attachment style) are considered *theories of the midrange.* The term "theories of the midrange" refers to personality models that focus on specific, circumscribed psychological phenomena. Rather than providing a broad view of personality, theories of the midrange instead focus on salient subsystems and articulate in detail how they operate and impact functioning. Usually, such theories evolve from broad models and are presented as developments or refinements to them. The final three models (Eysenck's biological typology, Cloninger's biosocial model, and the Five-Factor Model of personality) represent *broad-band* approaches to understanding personality. Broad-band theories aim to provide comprehensive, multidimensional descriptions of personality and the processes that underlie their development and expression. Broad-band personality models are a useful point of entry for establishing an interdisciplinary dialogue between religious researchers and their colleagues in the broader social sciences.

PERSONOLOGICAL APPROACHES TO UNDERSTANDING NUMINOUS CONSTRUCTS

Object Relations

Object relations theory developed from Freud's earlier work with psychoanalysis centering on those psychic processes by which individuals "introject" environmental objects (e.g., parents) into their psychic world, and the role these objects play in how the individual comes to perceive the environment (see Kernberg, 1966, for a more detailed overview). Introjection, a more primitive form of identification, represents a process by which the person creates internal representations of significant others. These internal objects have specific affective tones and textures associated with them that will govern how the person will react not only to that object, but also to others who are similarly conceived (e.g., God). Another important aspect of object relations concerns how the individual manages these internal objects, which is developmentally linked. For example, young children will tend to view objects with specific emotions (e.g., mother is all good; father is bad). There is an "all or none" quality here; an object is either good or bad. As the person matures, he or she is able to make finer emotional discriminations regarding objects and is able to tolerate more sophisticated, and sometimes conflicting, emotions. For example, the internal father object may be seen as being both fearsome and protective simultaneously. In short, the developed psychic world contains emotionally textured objects that represent both positive and negative elements.

Object relations theory is naturally conducive to understanding both spiritual and religious motivations because at the center of each is a search for some relationship to the transcendent. To the extent that this relationship is internalized by the individual, object relations theory will be able to offer explanations for how this relationship evolves and resonates within the person. The groundwork for making this linkage with numinous constructs was laid in the pioneering work of Rizzuto (1979). For Rizzuto, the centerpiece of attention is the person's relationship to God. The person develops images of God out of his or her interactions with early caregivers. The dynamic interplay between parent and child creates the template for the child's introjection of numerous objects, including one for God. The God image is a transitional object in that it is a psychic symbol that the person can draw upon to navigate problems at a particular stage of development. As the person moves on to a higher level of development, the need for this object disappears. However, Rizzuto notes that the God image, although a transitional object, is special in that it it that makes an ongoing contribution to the quality of an individual's life. According to Rizzuto, God is always "a transitional object at the service of gaining leverage with oneself, with others, and with life itself. This is so, not because God is God, but because, like the teddy bear, he has obtained a good half of his stuffing from the primary objects the child has 'found' in his life. The other half of God's stuffing comes from the child's capacity to 'create' a God according to his needs" (p. 179).

Strengths and Weaknesses

The practical value of Rizzuto's work is that she is able to integrate an individual's relationship to the numinous within the context of a widely accepted and clinically applied theoretical framework of personality. Further, she does so in a more positive manner than Freud originally treated the subject (e.g., Freud, 1913/1950, 1927/1961). Her formulations provide a very nuanced sense of the intrapsychic forces that may create a positive or negative sense of religiosity. The clarity of her formulations about the interpersonal origins of the God image provide a platform for research in this area. In fact, numerous efforts have been made to quantitatively explore these relationships. Lawrence (1997) developed the God Image Inventory (GII) in an effort to capture those unconscious dynamics that form the God image. Others have attempted to link an individual's object relations development to God image and spiritual maturity (Brokaw & Edwards, 1994; Hall, Brokaw, Edwards, & Pike, 1998), and their results have shown some support for these formulations.

However, not all work has been supportive of the basic assumptions (e.g., Piedmont, Ciarrocchi, & Williams, 2002; Spilka, Addison, & Rosensohn, 1975). Perhaps the greatest weakness of research in this area has been its almost singular reliance on self-report measures. Psychoanalysis is a theory of the unconscious mind, and researchers in this area from its beginnings have made it quite clear that objective measures cannot access this dimension of the individual (see McClelland, 1980, for a review of the issues). When projective measures are used (e.g., Brokaw & Edwards, 1994), the results are not as supportive as with the self-report measures. Thus, the major weakness of this approach is that it relies on aspects of the personality that are difficult to measure. Additionally, there is much controversy surrounding the psychometrics of projective tests which further confounds progress in this area (e.g., Lilienfeld, Wood, & Barb, 2000). Future research will need to find measurement models that are sensitive to unconscious dynamics, yet possess acceptable levels of validity and reliability. One potential methodology may be the act-frequency approach developed by Buss and Craik (1983). This behavior-sampling methodology is based on self-reports and seems ideally suited for capturing patterns in behavior that would be linked to unconscious motives. Piedmont (1989) showed that an act-frequency measure of achievement motivation was significantly correlated to *both* projective *and* objective measures of the construct. There is no doubt that researchers in this area need to move toward more rigorous methodologies that include representative large samples and measures with stronger psychometric qualities.

Attachment Style

A related approach to understanding how personality plays a role in spiritual and religious development is attachment style (AS). Like object relations, AS sees the quality of an individual's early relationships with caregivers as forming the templates for later relationships, including those with the numinous. However, this approach is less directly tied to psychoanalytic theory and therefore employs a measurement model more conducive to quantitative research (Brennan, Clark, & Shaver, 1998). Further, attachment theory provides a sociobiological perspective that examines the evolutionary significance of these different attachment styles. These species-typical behaviors represent solutions to problems in adaptation. Thus, attachment theory provides a new level of analysis to interpersonal relationships that objects relations does not offer.

The AS approach developed from research examining toddler reactions to strangers and caregivers (e.g., Ainsworth, Blehar, Waters, & Wall, 1978). Bowlby (1973) proposed that the patterns and qualities of these early relationships with caregivers have important implications for how adults come to organize their thoughts, feelings, and behaviors in other close relationships. Further, the quality of these formative relationships also have implications for self-image and personality style. Three attachment styles have been identified: the *secure style* is defined by confidence in the availability of attachment figures during times of need; the *avoidant style* is characterized by insecurity and lack of trust in the ability of others to care for one's needs, such that the individual remains aloof interpersonally; and the *anxious-ambivalent style* is dominated by a view of others as being reluctant to get close to oneself—here there is a strong desire for closeness but a high fear of rejection. According to Bowlby, these attachment styles have been developed to promote a closeness between a child and his or her primary caregiver. In situations of stress and danger, these attachment systems are activated and the infant engages in behaviors that are aimed at bringing the caregiver into closer proximity with the child. Hazan and Shaver (1987) extended these concepts to include how adults form romantic relationships. Classifying their sample into the three attachment styles, they noted that the three groups evidenced significant differences on a variety of measures querying about their close relationships and childhood history.

Kirkpatrick (1998) has extended this line of work to include an individual's relationship to, and image of, God. He showed that at any given moment, an individual's relationship with God corresponds with his or her attachment style (e.g., secure individuals see God as comforting and secure, avoidant individuals with their fears of intimacy similarly avoid relationships with God). However, over time, attachment styles were shown to predict some changes in an individual's relationship with God. Specifically, anxious–insecure types were the most likely to find a new relationship with God that was more emotionally stable and secure. Thus attachment style operated in a compensatory manner over time. Those with the most fragile styles actively sought a closer relationship with a deity rather than evidencing their more customary pattern of interpersonal detachment.

Strengths and Weaknesses

Like object relations, AS focuses on primary interpersonal relationships as the beginning block for understanding how individuals orient themselves to others in adulthood. AS provides another facet of interpretation to this process by including an evolutionary perspective on these processes. Finding a species-wide survival value to these processes opens the door for understanding spiritual and religious constructs as basic qualities of human existence. These qualities are present because they solve adaptational problems. Further, the AS approach involves a more quantitative method for measuring constructs. Unfortunately, measurement is one of the area's greatest weaknesses (Garabino, 1998). As Bartholomew and Shaver (1998) have pointed out, there are a plethora of instruments available, some measuring the tripartite breakdown of styles noted above, while others attempt to measure a four-way typology of styles, and they may not all be assessing the same constructs.

Conceptually, the findings regarding linkages between AS and images of God are not always consistent, which may be due to the different measures of attachment that are employed. Whether AS links to images of God in a compensatory (i.e., insecure people seeking a secure relationship with God) or corresponding (i.e., insecure people feeling insecure with God) manner has yet to be determined, although the correspondence perspective seems more evident (e.g., Granqvist, 1998; Piedmont et al., 2002). As such, it is not easy to summarize the pattern of findings in this area. The sometimes bewildering array of findings makes new investigations difficult to fit into any nomological net.

Overall Comments Regarding Theories of the Midrange

It is interesting to note that the two "theories of the midrange" aimed at understanding how individuals come to orient themselves with the transcendent are founded on our interpersonal nature. These two approaches outline how our styles of relating to self and others are correlated and argue that these patterns are replicated to some degree when we turn toward the numinous. However, the relative specificity of these models is also their greatest weakness. By focusing on select aspects of functioning, they miss other contributing factors. Perhaps the inconsistencies in the findings from these two areas is evidence that limited theories of personality are insufficient for capturing the manifold factors involved in our spiritual and religious quests. Broader, more inclusive models of human personality are needed to provide the necessary perspective. The next section will examine three broad-range models of personality.

Eysenck's Biological Typology

Eysenck was interested in developing a model of personality that was rooted in the central nervous system and thus would provide a genotypic explanation for behavioral variability (Eysenck, 1967). He began with the two major personality dimensions of *neuroticism*, the tendency to experience negative affect, and *extraversion*, the tendency to experience positive affect. Taking a rigorous experimental approach, Eysenck was able to identify brain mechanisms that covaried with these observed dispositions. Ultimately, Eysenck identified two neurological structures that were responsible for these personality styles: the *ascending reticular activation system* (ARAS), a brain region located in the lower brain stem that regulates levels of physiological arousal, and the *visceral brain activation* (VBA), a set of brain structures including the limbic system and hypothalamus that regulates affect. Levels of extraversion were moderated by the level of ARAS activation, with extraverts having intrinsically lower levels of arousal and introverts having higher levels. Individuals high on neuroticism exhibited more activity in the VBA than those lower on the construct. Thus, personality was rooted in the basic capacity of the brain to regulate levels of arousal and inhibition.

Later, Eysenck included the dimension of *psychoticism*, another neurologically based dimension that is genetically based. Individuals high on this dimension care very little for the company of others and show overt hostility. Such individuals display a more antagonistic, manipulative orientation toward others. Although a high score on psychoticism does not mean that an individual is psychotic in a diagnostic sense, there is a degree of peculiarity surrounding the person. Finally, all three of these dimensions were considered to be mutually independent.

This three-dimensional biological model has generated much research interest, especially among those in the psychology of religion. The personality scale developed to capture these personality characteristics (the Eysenck Personality Questionnaire) has been used to identify personality types of ministers (Jones & Francis, 1992) and personal factors contributing to dissatisfaction in ministry (Francis & Rodger, 1994), as well as how personality factors contribute to spiritual involvement and happiness (Francis & Katz, 2003; Maltby & Day, 2001). Lewis and Maltby (1995) demonstrated that a more compassionate and caring attitude toward others (i.e., low psychoticism) was linked to greater levels of religiosity (which was defined as attitudes toward prayer, the Bible, and God). Eysenck's own prolific work with this typology has generated an extensive amount of interpretive depth to these three dimensions. As a result, research using this instrument carries with it implications for clinical and nonclinical functioning as well as an insight into underlying neurological mechanisms that may be motivating behavior.

Strengths and Weaknesses

Eysenck's pioneering work has shaped much of the neurobiological research done on these traits by demonstrating that there exist neurological substrates that control arousal levels and behavioral dispositions. Clearly, there is a biological basis to personality and Eysenck was one of the first to explore this uncharted territory. His work asserts that personality constructs are real entities in the sense that there are physical systems and processes that underlie them.

This work is being extended to research on religious and spiritual constructs as well. Newberg (see Newberg & Newberg, Chapter 11, this volume) and his colleagues applied this approach to understanding the neural mechanisms underlying spiritual activities. This work provides an interesting examination of brain activity via PET (positron-emission tomography) scans and EEGs (electroencephalograms) and demonstrates that individuals involved in prayer/meditation show significant changes in brain activity. Newberg also includes hypotheses as to the evolutionary basis to these mechanisms, asking the question, "Did we evolve directly to possess a spiritual disposition, or was spirituality a by-product of some other evolutionary process?" This type of work represents the frontier for researchers in the psychology of religion and holds great promise for (1) documenting the neurophysiological basis of numinous constructs, and therefore demonstrating that they represent "real" entities; (2) outlining the basic adaptive pressures that lead to the development of spiritual and religious strivings, thus providing a broader historical context for understanding how and why these qualities were acquired; and (3) providing new insights into the possibility of enhancing spiritual strivings through chemical and experiential interventions.

There are limitations to Eysenck's model that need to be appreciated. First, as a descriptive typology of personality dimensions, three factors may not be enough for the model to be comprehensive. The current dominant model of personality traits is the Five-Factor Model of personality (FFM; Digman, 1990). Although the FFM is discussed in more detail below, Costa and McCrae (1995) examined how Eysenck's model mapped onto these five dimensions and concluded that Eysenck's model may not provide an exhaustive listing of all aspects of personality. Another drawback to this approach is that Eysenck never considered spirituality and religiosity in his work. Because he never provided any potential explanations for these phenomena, researchers need to piece together such explanations ad hoc. Finally, although originally Eysenck's work was groundbreaking, science's understanding of brain functioning in terms of both structure and physiology has greatly improved. Eysenck's original neurological formulations were straightforward and relevant, but advances in brain chemistry and anatomy have greatly enhanced our understanding of how the brain influences behavior, especially the role played by neurotransmitters (see Zuckerman, 2003, for a review). Thus, there are limitations to this theory's ability to explain certain brain–behavior links (see Cloninger, 1988). Newer theories have been proposed that do capitalize on this more advanced knowledge base and seem to offer greater promise for understanding and predicting behavior. The biosocial theory developed by Cloninger (1987) is one such model.

Cloninger's Unified Biosocial Theory

In an effort to integrate information from diverse sources (e.g., twin and family studies, neuropharmacological and neurobehavioral studies, psychometric studies of personality, and studies of longitudinal development), Cloninger sought to provide a model of personality that was both complete personologically and anchored in specific neuropharmacological mechanisms. The result (Cloninger, 1987) was a personality model that linked brain systems (behavioral activation, behavioral inhibition, and behavior maintenance) with specific neurotransmitters (dopamine, serotonin, and norepinepherine, respectively) with particular personality temperaments (novelty seeking, harm avoidance, and reward dependence, respectively). The model has since been modified (Cloninger, Svrakic, & Przybeck, 1993) to include another dimension of temperament (persistence) and three additional *character* dimensions (character is defined in terms of insight learning and the capacity to reorganize one's self-concept) labeled self-directedness, cooperativeness, and self-transcendence. It is hypothesized that character develops out of the genetically based temperaments, which then structures how the individual perceives various stimuli, which in turn influences how an individual will consistently respond to the stimuli. Both temperament and character mutually influence one another and motivate behavior.

Research has shown value to these constructs for understanding both nonclinical and disordered personality functioning (Duijsens, Spinhoven, Goekoop, Spermon, & Eurelings-Bontekoe, 2000; Svrakic, Whitehead, Przybeck, & Cloninger, 1993). The genetic and biological foundations of these constructs provide a rich interpretive frame-work for conceptualizing those physical mechanisms that are guiding behavior in differ-ent situations and clinical contexts (Cloninger, 1998). Of particular interest is that this revision of the model explicitly included a dimension of spirituality, self-transcendence, which is defined as reflecting a "concept of self as an integral part of the universe and its source: from this self concept are derived feelings of mystical participation, religious faith, and unconditional equanimity and patience" (Cloninger, Przybeck, Svrakic, & Wetzel, 1994, p. 16). The self-transcendence character dimension breaks down into three subscales: self-forgetfulness, transpersonal identification, and spiritual acceptance. Given the origins of this scale, the inclusion of a measure of spirituality is an indication that it represents a genetically inherited quality that has associated neurophysiological sequella. Spirituality is clearly seen as being an inherent physical property of the individual.

MacDonald and Holland (2002) examined the psychometric properties of the self-transcendence dimension in a large sample of undergraduates. They found the self-transcendence scales to have adequate reliability and validity, and to represent a quality of the person that was independent of the four temperaments. However, problems were noted with the factor structure of this dimension, with fewer factors emerging than speci-fied by the model. This may be a consequence of using a student sample. Ball, Tennen, and Kranzler (1999) found strong support for the self-transcendence scales in both com-munity and inpatient substance abuse samples. Thus, there seems to be evidence support-ing self-transcendence as a psychometrically robust, factorially cohesive dimension.

Strengths and Weaknesses

Cloninger's model picks up where Eysenck left off and provides a sophisticated integra-tion of neurobiological functioning with personality styles and temperament. The dimen-sions he has identified have been documented to be genetically heritable qualities that emerge in specific biological processes and seem to covary with specific behaviors. That an index of spirituality has been included in this roster provides strong evidence of the value of numinous constructs: They are not solipsistic aspects of the individual. Rather, spiritual behaviors emerge from biologically developed mechanisms that have evolved to facilitate adaptation. These behaviors can be reliably measured and linked to a variety of salient psychosocial outcomes. The work of both Cloninger and Eysenck provides a new way of looking at spirituality in ways that involve concrete physical mechanisms and interprets these processes within an evolutionary perspective. Future research in the psy-chology of religion should see this as the new frontier for exploration. Biological models would involve the development and usage of new types of numinous variables, dimen-sions not based on simple self-report questionnaires. It would also help to move the level of discussion in the field away from denomination-specific issues to the identification of salient, universal human qualities.

For those working in this area, there are issues that need to be considered. First, the biosocial model should be seen as a "work in progress." Since its introduction in 1987, the model has gone through several revisions and modifications. Many of the problems noted in earlier models were due to the volatility of the factor structures: there have been continuous problems in replication and generalizability. The Temperament Character In-ventory, the latest operationalization of the model, suffers from similar problems (see Ball et al., 1999; MacDonald & Holland, 2002). Caution needs to be exercised in using this scale. Further, Herbst, Zonderman, McCrae, and Costa (2000) tested Cloninger's hypothesis that these temperaments are genetically based and found no such connections in a large community sample. Thus, more data are needed to firmly establish the genetic basis of these qualities. Another problem concerns the uniqueness of the spirituality dimension vis-à-vis the personality dimensions of the FFM. As can be seen in Table 14.1, the Temperament Character Inventory (TCI) dimensions correlate highly with the five personality dimensions, especially Neuroticism and Extraversion. The question arises as to whether this aspect of spirituality merely reflects qualities of personality already contained in the FFM. Finally, another problem with the TCI centers on the fact that all the items on the self-transcendence scale are positively worded, which sets up a potential acquiescence bias. McCrae, Herbst, and Costa (2001) demonstrated that when acquiescence is controlled for in the TCI, its factor structure changes, in that self-transcendence no longer forms its own dimension, and instead becomes a marker for Openness.

It is interesting to note that many numinous measures do not control for acquiescence. This is more the case for measures of spirituality than of religiosity, and for newer versus older measures. This may be the result of the difficulty in writing negatively reflected items, or it may be due to an unwillingness to conceive of spirituality as having any negative components. Whatever the case, acquiescence is a real response confound that needs to be addressed. Failing to do so may compromise our ability to reliably assess the uniquely numinous aspects of the individual. This is perhaps the most important issue to be addressed by research in this field: to determine whether numinous constructs tell us something about people not already described by current personality measures. In order to accomplish this task, one would need to have a comprehensive set of constructs that can be measured in a psychometrically sound manner. The FFM claims to be such a personality model.

Five-Factor Model of Personality

Over the past 30 years, researchers have converged on the existence of five orthogonal trait dimensions that constitute an adequate taxonomy of personality characteristics (Digman, 1990). These dimensions are known as the FFM and are labeled: (1) *neuroticism*, the tendency to experience negative emotions such as anxiety, depression, and hostility; (2) *extraversion*, the quantity and intensity of one's interpersonal interactions; (3) *openness*, the proactive seeking and appreciation of new experiences; (4) *agreeableness*, the quality of one's interpersonal interactions along a continuum from compassion to antagonism; and (5) *conscientiousness*, the persistence, organization, and motivation exhibited in goal-directed behaviors (Costa & McCrae, 1992). Research has found strong cross-observer, cross-instrument convergence indicating that these dimensions are not a product of any self-distortion or rater bias (e.g., Piedmont, 1994). These dimensions also were found to be extremely stable over the adult lifespan; 25-year stability coefficients indicate that 80% of the variance in these traits is unchanging, and 60% is estimated to remain constant over a 50-year adult lifespan (Costa & McCrae, 1994). Finally, these dimensions have a strong genetic basis (Heath, Neale, Kessler, Eaves, & Kendler, 1992), indicating that they are not mere summary descriptions of behavior, but are genotypic tendencies of individuals to think, act, and feel in consistent ways. The value of this model is twofold. Empirically this model is well defined and robust, emerging even cross-culturally (McCrae & Costa, 1997). Conceptually, these domains are well validated and provide

TABLE 14.1. Correlations between Various Spiritual and Religiosity Indices and the Domains of the Five-Factor Model of Personality.

	N	E	O	A	C
Spiritual Experience Inventory[a]					
Spiritual Support	−.09	.10	−.07	.25**	.10
Spiritual Openness	−.08	.11*	.46***	.08	.04
Religious Problem Solving[b]					
Collaborative	−.27**	.30**	.08	.20*	.33**
Self-Directing	.23**	−.18*	−.01	−.12	−.15
Deferring	−.20*	.22**	−.33**	.00	.19*
Intrinsic/Extrinsic Religiosity[c]					
Intrinsic	.00	−.04	−.09*	.09*	.11*
Extrinsic	.11*	−.04	−.07	−.07	−.09
Religious Well-Being Scale[c]					
Existential	−.51***	.34***	−.05	.20***	.39***
Religious	−.04	.05	−.11*	.11**	.13**
Hood Mysticism Scale[c]					
Factor 1	.02	.08	.23***	−.04	.02
Factor 2	−.04	.13**	.20***	.01	.09*
Spiritual Transcendence Scale[d]					
Universality	.01	.10	.20***	.21***	.10
Prayer Fulfillment	.05	.06	.09	.12*	.13*
Connectedness	−.02	.17**	.17**	.25***	.08
Faith Maturity Scale[e]					
Horizontal	−.01	.07**	.04	.14***	.12***
Vertical	−.01	.07**	.20***	.24***	.11***
Religiosity Items: Frequency[d]					
Read Bible	−.05	.00	.07	.19***	.11*
Read Religious Literature	−.13*	.09	.04	.21***	.13*
Prayer	.09	.05	.01	.23***	.13*
Attend Services	.02	.11*	−.11*	.21***	.12*
Temperament Character Inventory[f]					
Novelty Seeking	.20***	.36***	.35***	−.15**	−.48***
Harm Avoidance	.71***	−.54***	−.10*	−.08*	−.09*
Reward Dependence	.10*	.36***	.25***	.42***	.02
Persistence	.09*	.20***	−.04	.07	.62***
Self-Directed	−.69***	.27***	.05	.33***	.46***
Cooperative	−.21***	.21***	.23***	.66***	.17**
Self-Transcendent	.40***	.26***	.08*	.08*	−.03

Note. N, Neuroticism; E, Extraversion; O, Openness; A, Agreeableness; C, Conscientiousness.
[a] Csarny, Piedmont, Sneck, and Cheston (2000).
[b] Rodgerson and Piedmont (1998).
[c] Piedmont (1999).
[d] Piedmont (2001).
[e] Piedmont and Nelson (2001).
[f] Cloninger, Przybeck, Svrakic, and Wetzel (1994).
* $p < .05$; ** $p < .01$; *** $p < .001$; two-tailed.

clear definitions of very circumscribed constructs. Therefore, the FFM can serve as a useful reference point for developing and evaluating religious variables.

Saroglou (2002) conducted a meta-analysis of the relations between the FFM and measures of religiosity, spiritual maturity, religious fundamentalism, and extrinsic religion. He noted that religiosity (i.e., involvement in religious activities such as prayer) was related to the dimensions of Agreeableness and Conscientiousness. Spiritual maturity was related to all five personality dimensions, while extrinsic religion was related to high Neuroticism. Religious fundamentalism was related to all dimensions except Conscientiousness. In order to give more texture to these findings, Table 14.1 presents correlations between a number of different measures of spirituality and religiosity with the FFM personality domains gleaned from a variety of studies. These results parallel those of Saroglou, but also yield other insights. First, these numinous constructs do evidence numerous correlations with the FFM domains, and some are quite high (e.g., Existential Well-Being Scale; Spiritual Openness; the character scales of the TCI). The pattern of the relations with the FFM can provide insights into the personological qualities represented in these scales. For example, the Religious Problem Solving Scales all correlate with Neuroticism and Extraversion, underscoring their relatedness to coping abilities and levels of well-being. Note that the Existential Well-Being Scale also shares many of these same properties because it has a similar pattern of correlates with the FFM. However, the Religious Well-Being Scale does not relate to those personality dimensions that underlie well-being, and instead relates to low Openness and to high Agreeableness and Conscientiousness. This reflects more of a moralistically based altruistic orientation (i.e., helping others by calling them to walk the right path). Thus, these two scales capture very different aspects of the individual and would be predictive of very different types of outcomes.

Overall, though, correlations with the FFM show that the spirituality scales seem to correlate with the Openness and Agreeableness domains (e.g., the Spiritual Transcendence Scales), while religious behaviors appear to relate more to Agreeableness and Conscientiousness (e.g., the religiosity items). This supports the view that spirituality and religiosity share something in common (e.g., Hill & Pargament, 2003), a compassionate attitude toward others. They differ in that spirituality involves a seeking, curious attitude toward the transcendent, while religiosity involves more of the dutiful, procedural aspects of faith involvement. Patterns of relationships with the FFM can help develop the construct validity of numinous constructs as well as provide insights into the types of outcomes these constructs will predict. The FFM can also be helpful for identifying areas of personological redundancy among measures. Just because two scales have similar names *does not mean* that they assess similar constructs. For example, the Spiritual Support and Spiritual Openness scales capture independent aspects of personality even though both are considered elements of a common dimension, that is, spiritual experience.

One final note. It should be pointed out that although religious constructs share something in common with the FFM, these numinous variables are not redundant with the model. Clearly, there are significant amounts of unique, reliable variance in all these scales, which suggests that numinous constructs contain information about individuals *not represented* in traditional personality models. Numinous constructs may constitute a sixth dimension of personality (Piedmont, 2001). Ultimately, it is what religious and spiritual constructs do not have in common with the FFM that is of most importance to the field. It supports the contention that for any model of human functioning to be comprehensive, it will need to include measures of the numinous. This issue is discussed in more detail in the next section.

Strengths and Weaknesses

The obvious strength of the FFM is that it is an empirically robust, comprehensive taxonomy of traditionally defined personality constructs. The dimensions of the FFM can be accurately measured by psychometrically sound instruments (e.g., the Revised NEO Personality Inventory; Costa & McCrae, 1992), and the constructs have been empirically validated as being powerful predictors of a wide array of psychologically salient outcomes. Unlike the other models discussed in this chapter, measurement is the premier strength of this model. Conceptually, the FFM can be very useful for understanding numinous scales and can play an active role in helping to create useful nomological nets for our measures (Gorsuch, 1984). It can also serve as an empirical point of departure for the development of new measures of spirituality and religiosity that are nonredundant with these dimensions (e.g., the Spiritual Transcendence Scale; Piedmont, 2001).

The most salient weakness of the FFM is that there is little conceptual development of these factors. The FFM was empirically derived from an analysis of trait language, and as such there is little information concerning the etiology and development of these constructs. Although they are genetically heritable, exactly how these dimensions are developed and the forces that impact their expression over time are sorely lacking (see Costa & McCrae, 1998). Other criticisms center on whether these factor analytically derived dimensions are really the best interpretation of the extant data, and that other possible structural models involving more factors are equally possible (e.g., Block, 1995).

Overall Comments Regarding Broad-Band Theories

The three broad-band models contrast sharply with the earlier theories in terms of their scope of explanation, highly developed measurement models, and emphasis on biological/genetic mechanisms. Nonetheless, they do complement the theories of the midrange by providing a broader context for elaborating the value of the specific dynamics they describe. It is interesting to note how the two biological models seamlessly integrate spiritual phenomena, either indirectly, as in Eysenck's model, or directly, as in Cloninger's model. These theories underscore the assertion that numinous strivings are grounded in identifiable physical mechanisms and systems. That these systems developed over time to meet challenges in human adaptation highlights the value that religious and spiritual qualities provide for humans and the quality of the lives they build. Yet, if spiritual variables do in fact have a direct causal impact on such outcomes as coping ability, well-being, disease resistance, and mental health, then the extent to which these numinous systems can be manipulated creates the possibility for a new class of interventions that are biologically based, spiritually focused, and targeted toward the amelioration of a variety of psychological problems (Richards, 2002).

In the meantime, the trait-based approach represented by the FFM offers a more immediate avenue for understanding numinous constructs. Although more work needs to be done in developing the "theoretical depth" of the model, its empirically robust dimensions can be used in a variety of ways to support progress in the psychology of religion. Piedmont (1999) identified four ways the FFM could be useful: (1) as a method for describing the motivations of individuals who seek spiritual/religious goals; (2) as a method for describing the perceived motivational characteristics of religious figures; (3) as a method for developing the construct validity of numinous constructs; and (4) as an empirical reference point for the development of new religious and spiritual scales that more clearly capture motivations that are nonoverlapping with these five dimensions.

The existence of a trait taxonomy highlights the need for psychology of religion researchers to undertake similar taxonomic work with numinous constructs. Such an effort would help clarify how and to what degree spiritual and religious constructs are blends of these established traits and to what extent they represent something new and distinct. The data presented in Table 14.1 highlight this issue. Do the correlations between the FFM and the religious constructs suggest that being spiritual involves an open receptivity to and curiosity about the transcendent, a compassionate orientation toward others, and a sense of personal self-discipline and dutifulness in carrying out obligations? Are these essential elements to spirituality? Or are the personality dimensions merely lenses through which spiritual strivings become focused? Are there spiritually open people as well as spiritually closed people? Certainly, it is easy to see that spiritually mature individuals can be compassionate and tender, but cannot an individual with a more hard-nosed, self-reliant, "tough love" attitude be spiritually mature as well?

These are important questions that speak to the heart of how we define and understand numinous constructs. There are numerous definitions of spirituality and religiosity (e.g., McGinn, 1993), but it is unlikely that all of them are correct. There needs to be some boundaries around our variables that define what they are and what they are not. We need to develop some consensus as to what types of personological material represent spiritual and religious qualities. Contemporary personality theories offer a way to accomplish this essential descriptive task. The theories summarized here provide both a broad conceptual framework (and language) for discussing numinous variables and empirical technologies for quantifying these constructs in ways that would promote dialogue with other disciplines. Ultimately, if spirituality is indeed an additional dimension of personality, then this line of work may lead to the identification of a whole new class of potential clinical interventions (Murray-Swank, 2003). In the meantime, there are still numerous empirical issues that need to be addressed. The following section outlines five important issues that should form a core agenda for guiding future research in the field.

FIVE KEY EMPIRICAL ISSUES FOR FUTURE RESEARCH

Issue 1: Understanding the Personological Content of Religious and Spiritual Scales

The FFM has something to contribute to our understanding of religious and spiritual constructs. Although itself not based on numinous constructs, it does provide a useful starting point for evaluating the personological aspects of religious and spiritual constructs. To the extent that religious constructs do have any overlap with these personality dimensions, the FFM can be useful in outlining the motivational, attitudinal, and behavioral correlates of these scales. For example, as shown in Table 14.1, measures of spirituality overlapped with the domains of high Openness and high Agreeableness. Thus, these measures should uniformly reflect individuals who see the best in human nature, and are confident that education, innovation, and cooperation can better society. Correlations with the domains of the FFM can also lead to a set of personological expectations that can be used to establish the construct validity of a scale.

Relatedly, correlations with the FFM also provide a way for linking religious constructs to each other. Scales with similar relationships to the FFM domains would share much in common personologically, while different patterns of correlates would indicate that two scales share little in common. Ozer and Riese (1994) likened the correlation of a scale with the FFM to the establishment of latitude and longitude for a given location on Earth. As they noted, "[those] who continue to employ their preferred measure without locating it within the FFM can only be likened to geographers who issue reports of new lands but refuse to locate them on a map for others to find" (Ozer & Riese, 1994, p. 361). The taxonomic nature of the FFM provides an ideal medium for managing information about religious and spiritual scales that will enable researchers to efficiently identify areas of content redundancy among measures as well as to discover gaps in the construct validity of these instruments.

Issue 2: Establishing the Incremental Validity of Religious and Spiritual Scales

A burgeoning literature links spiritual and religious constructs to a number of mental and physical health outcomes (see Koenig, McCullough, & Larson, 2000). On its face, this literature shows the facilitative effect that religion and spirituality have on physical and mental health. Individuals with high levels of these constructs frequently are seen as experiencing less physical illness (or recovering quicker from disease) than those who score lower on these dimensions. Pargament and colleagues have shown how religious coping adds significantly to individuals' attempts to manage personal stress, burnout, and mortality (see Pargament, Ano, & Wachholtz, Chapter 26, this volume).

However, these findings do not go unchallenged. Criticisms of these findings have emerged on the basis of numerous methodological and statistical shortcomings (e.g., Sloan, Bagiella, & Powell, 2001). One issue centers on the lack of evidence documenting the predictive power of religious and spiritual variables over and above other established constructs, like social support. This failure to demonstrate incremental predictive validity for spiritual and religious constructs raises important concerns about their construct validity (see Joiner, Perez, & Walker, 2002). The question arises, "To what degree are spiritual constructs merely the 'religification' of already existing personality constructs?"

To be valuable, religious and spiritual constructs need to demonstrate that they possess predictive power over and above established personality constructs, like those represented in the FFM. For example, consider the Spiritual Well-Being Scale. What does it tell us about individuals that a more secular-oriented well-being scale does not? As shown in Table 14.1, some aspects of this construct (e.g., existential) have a high overlap with those aspects of personality that have been shown to be very predictive of well-being. What is the value added by including the "spiritual?" The incremental validity paradigm provides a methodology for addressing this issue. It enables researchers to identify those individual difference qualities unique to religious and spiritual constructs that are predictive of salient psychosocial (e.g., well-being, social styles, sexual attitudes) and health outcomes (e.g., recovery rates from illness, coping ability, physical adaptation).

Incremental validity analyses need to become a routine part of all validation research using numinous constructs. Whether employing hierarchical multiple regression analysis, structural equation modeling, or other mediational analyses, it is imperative that the unique, substantive value of religious and spiritual constructs be documented. Evidence of incremental validity will help to stop interpretations of religious constructs as being "nothing more than . . . " (see Pargament, 2002). Fortunately, a developing literature shows numinous constructs to represent aspects of the individual not contained by traditional personality dimensions (e.g., MacDonald, 2000; Piedmont, 2001; Saucier & Goldberg, 1998).

Issue 3: Structural Nature of Religious and Spiritual Constructs

Scott (cited in Hill et al., 2000) identified 31 different definitions of religiousness and 40 of spirituality. It is ironic that despite such a broad research interest in the numinous, little attention has been devoted to understanding these constructs empirically. Such broad conceptual diversity undermines efforts at summarizing the current research literature and preempts the field from integrating religious and spiritual constructs with mainstream theoretical models. The lack of conceptual clarity generates serious empirical issues that, if not resolved, threaten to strangle future progress for the field.

There are two issues that need to be addressed. The first concerns whether the constructs of religiosity and spirituality are multifaceted or multidimensional. A multidimensional scale is one that contains several independent dimensions. Scores on one of these dimensions do not correlate with scores on any other, and information contained across these dimensions are nonredundant. A multifaceted scale, on the other hand, is one that contains multiple dimensions that are all correlated to some degree. This overlap exists because the dimensions are all emerging from a common latent construct. Multidimensional scales provide breadth of coverage, while multifaceted scales provide greater fidelity of assessment for a single domain. Numinous constructs are frequently conceived of as being multidimensional in nature (e.g., Hill et al., 2000), although little data exists to support this contention. There is a surprising lack of comprehensive factor analytic studies in which multiple measures of spirituality and religiosity are analyzed jointly with personality marker scales.

MacDonald (2000) did factor-analyze 11 spirituality measures and found five spiritual dimensions that were independent of personality. However, he included measures not traditionally thought of as numinous (e.g., Paranormal Beliefs Scale; Self-Expansiveness Level) and, in a joint factor analysis with the NEO PI-R (a measure of the FFM), did not indicate how these dimensions cross-loaded with these personality factors. Piedmont, Ciarrocchi, Dy-Liacco, Mapa, and Williams (2003) report on a joint factor analysis of markers of the FFM and the Brief Multidimensional Measure of Religiousness/Spirituality (MMRS; Fetzer Institute/National Institute on Aging Working Group, 1999). The MMRS explicitly conceptualizes religiousness and spirituality as multidimensional constructs and provides items across 12 separate domains. The resulting factor analysis indicated that religiousness and spirituality each formed separate, highly correlated factors that were both independent of personality. These results suggest that these dimensions are multifaceted. Certainly, much more effort needs to be invested into this type of basic structural analysis. The key to this type of analysis is the inclusion of FFM marker scales. Jointly factor-analyzing personality and numinous constructs allows for a determination of which aspects of spirituality are related to personality and which are not. Simply factor-analyzing a set of spirituality measures is insufficient for advancing the field.

The second issue is to examine the extent of overlap between religiosity and spirituality. Conceptually, the two are believed to share many common features (Hill et al., 2000). Individuals perceive the two in very similar ways (see Zinnbauer & Pargament, Chapter, 2 this volume, for a review). The data in Table 14.1 show that spirituality and religiosity share a common personological connection on Agreeableness; Piedmont et al. (2003) found a correlation of .45 between these two dimensions in their factor analysis of the MMRS. Structural equation modeling can be useful for helping to understand the underlying level of overlap between these two variables. Given that overlap does exist, it is necessary to determine whether these two factors should be considered a single overall dimension. If not, then evidence of their discriminant validity needs to be presented in order to justify their separate usage. Why does one need to use both variables if only one (or some composite of the two) would work just as well, if not better? Thus, the incremental validity of these constructs relative to each other also needs to be established. It must be shown that each of these constructs contains sufficient unique, reliable variance to warrant separate interpretations.

Issue 4: The Causal Relationships between the Numinous and the Psychological

A conceptual question that has *not yet been asked* about these two constructs concerns the causal relationships between them and other psychological constructs. Are spirituality and religiosity better conceived of as predictors of psychological maturity, or are they merely by-products of an individual's psychological system? This is an important question that speaks to the ultimate value of these constructs. Does a person's orientation to the numinous develop out of his or her sense of personhood? If so, then it is one's level of psychological adjustment that forms the experiences of the numinous. Thus, unhappy people will tend to have unhappy relationships with the transcendent. Like any other behavior, relationships with some ultimate reality are reflections of more basic psychological dynamics. From this perspective, numinous constructs are merely the reflection of already established psychological constructs (e.g., Joiner et al., 2002), or are just a conduit or method by which individuals are able to activate other psychological mechanisms that are adaptive (e.g., Fredrickson, 2002).

However, if spirituality and religiosity are "inputs" into our psychological system, then they become important conduits through which growth and maturity can be focused. In this scenario, the quality of a person's relationship to the transcendent has important implications for his or her own psychological sense of stability. Therefore, disturbances in an individual's relationship to the transcendent would have serious repercussions for the rest of his or her mental world. Demonstrating that numinous constructs serve as causal inputs into our psychic systems would have far-reaching implications for how the social sciences conceptualize individuals. As separate qualities of the individual not contained in current personality models, numinous constructs would provide new insights into who people are and the goals they are pursuing. If religious and spiritual constructs play a significant role in driving adaptation and growth, then this creates the possibility for a whole new class of potential therapeutic strategies based on these types of dynamics (e.g., Murray-Swank, 2003; Piedmont, 2004). At a minimum, it would demand that any model of human behavior must include numinous constructs if that model were to be comprehensive.

Issue 5: Spirituality and Religiosity as Human Universals

Moberg (2002) has noted that the bulk of research in this area has been done in a predominantly Christian context (see also Gorsuch, 1984). To varying degrees, measures reflect specific aspects of spiritual and religious experiences unique to Christians (e.g., personal commitment to Jesus Christ), and thus exclude other groups from being included in the research process. Piedmont and Leach (2002) identified two possible reasons for this: (1) most researchers in the area are Christians themselves and many are often associated with Christian-based universities; and (2) Christian samples are the easiest to obtain because they are the largest faith bloc in this country. The end result, though, is a lack of theological pluralism that will ultimately undermine the field's ability to develop comprehensive models of spiritual development and experience that have broad relevance and ecological validity.

There is a need to examine these constructs across different religious faiths and to plumb their spiritual orientations. Two approaches would need to be taken: an *emic approach*, where researchers examine specific faith traditions and determine those unique features that define and describe their spirituality; and an *etic approach*, where spiritual concepts developed from one cultural context are applied to another to determine the degree to which a common set of constructs are useful for understanding all traditions. Both approaches have their strengths and limitations. Together, though, they would enable researchers to identify those broad dynamics that may be underlying all spiritual quests while also appreciating how culture, context, and faith tradition combine to focus how these broad dynamics are shaped into specific religious and spiritual orientations.

Fortunately, techniques and methodologies have been developed for conducting this type of research and these approaches can be readily generalized to spiritual and religious constructs (e.g., Berry, Poortinga, & Pandey, 1997). By assuming an inclusive religious and cultural perspective, researchers will begin to develop a body of data that will illustrate the importance of numinous constructs by virtue of their universal presence and importance.

CONCLUSIONS

This is certainly an exciting time for the psychology of religion. As this volume testifies, never have there been more resources available from which to draw for those in this area. Never has there been this level of interest in spiritual and religious phenomena from both the general public and from professionals in all disciplines, such as medicine, business, anthropology, and the arts. This interest in, and receptivity to, the numinous provides a rare opportunity for this field to make a significant and durable contribution to human knowledge.

At the heart of this interest is a growing recognition that spirituality represents not only a core element of who we are as people, but that spirituality is a *uniquely human* quality. Only our species evidences any concern for, sensitivity to, or celebration of the numinous. There are no animal models for spirituality. Every human culture across history has reserved a significant place for religious and spiritual endeavors. Religion has helped define how we think of ourselves and the world in which we live. It has influenced our law, philosophy, politics, government, education, and morality. Spirituality and religion are ways in which humans strive to create a fundamental sense of personal meaning. There is no doubt that spirituality is an important and universal element of who we are. But more than that, when we examine the numinous, we are taking an intimate look at our humanity and what it is that makes our species unique.

ACKNOWLEDGMENT

I would like to thank Rose Piedmont and Ruth Dennison-Tedesco for their efforts at proofreading and copyediting earlier versions of this chapter.

REFERENCES

Ainsworth, M. D. S., Blehar, M. C., Waters, E., & Wall, S. (1978). *Patterns of attachment: A psychological study of the Strange Situation*. Hillsdale, NJ: Erlbaum.

Ball, S. A., Tennen, H., & Kranzler, H. R. (1999). Factor replicability and validity of the Temperament and Character Inventory in substance-dependent patients. *Psychological Assessment, 11*, 514–524.

Bartholomew, K., & Shaver, P. R. (1998). Methods of assessing adult attachment: Do they converge? In J. A. Simpson & W. S. Rholes (Eds.), *Attachment theory and close relationships* (pp. 25–45). New York: Guilford Press.

Berry, J. W., Poortinga, Y. H., & Pandey, J. (Eds.). (1997). *Handbook of cross-cultural psychology: Vol. 1. Theory and method* (2nd ed.). Boston: Allyn & Bacon.

Block, J. (1995). A contrarian view of the five-factor approach to personality description. *Psychological Bulletin, 117*, 187–215.

Bowlby, J. (1973). *Attachment and loss: Separation, anxiety and anger.* New York: Basic Books.

Brennan, K. A., Clark, C. L., & Shaver, P. R. (1998). Self-report measurement of adult attachment: An integrative overview. In J. A. Simpson & W. S. Rholes (Eds.), *Attachment theory and close relationships* (pp. 46–76). New York: Guilford Press.

Brokaw, B. F., & Edwards, K. J. (1994). The relationship of God image to level of object relations development. *Journal of Psychology and Theology, 22*, 352–371.

Buss, D. M., & Craik, D. H. (1983). The act-frequency approach to personality. *Psychological Review, 90*, 105–126.

Cloninger, C. R. (1987). A systematic method for clinical description and classification of personality variants. *Archives of General Psychiatry, 44*, 573–588.

Cloninger, C. R. (1988). A unified biosocial theory of personality and its role in development. *Psychiatric Development, 6*, 83–120.

Cloninger, C. R. (1998). The genetics and psychobiology of the seven-factor model of personality. In K. R. Silk (Ed.), *Biology of personality disorders* (pp. 63–92). Washington, DC: American Psychiatric Press.

Cloninger, C. R., Przybeck, T. R., Svrakic, D. M., & Wetzel, R. D. (1994). *The Temperament and Character Inventory (TCI): A guide to its development and use.* St. Louis, MO: Center for Psychobiology of Personality.

Cloninger, C. R., Svrakic, D. M., & Przybeck, T. R. (1993). A psychobiological model of temperament and character. *Archives of General Psychiatry, 50*, 975–990.

Costa, P. T., Jr., & McCrae, R. R. (1992). *The NEO PI-R professional manual.* Odessa, FL: Psychological Assessment Resources.

Costa, P. T., Jr., & McCrae, R. R. (1994). Set like plaster?: Evidence for the stability of adult personality. In T. F. Heatherton & J. L. Weinberger (Eds.), *Can personality change?* (pp. 21–40). Washington, DC: American Psychological Association.

Costa, P. T., Jr., & McCrae, R. R. (1995). Primary traits of Eysenck's P-E-N system: Three- and five-factor solutions. *Journal of Personality and Social Psychology, 69*, 308–317.

Costa, P. T., Jr., & McCrae, R. R. (1998). Trait theories of personality. In D. F. Barone, M. Hersen, & V. B. Van Hasselt (Eds.), *Advanced personality* (pp. 103–121). New York: Plenum Press.

Csarny, R. J., Piedmont, R. L., Sneck, W. J., & Cheston, S. E. (2000). An evaluation of the incremental validity of the Spiritual Experience Index—Revised. *Research in the Social Scientific Study of Religion, 11*, 117–131.

Digman, J. M. (1990). Personality structure: Emergence of the five-factor model. *Annual Review of Psychology, 41*, 417–440.

Duijsens, I. J., Spinhoven, P., Goekoop, J. G., Spermon, T., & Eurelings-Bontekoe, E. H. M. (2000). The Dutch Temperament and Character Inventory (TCI): Dimensional structure, reliability and validity in a normal and psychiatric outpatient sample. *Personality and Individual Differences, 28*, 487–499.

Emmons, R. A., & Paloutzian, R. F. (2003). The psychology of religion. *Annual Review of Psychology, 54*, 377–402.

Eysenck, H. J. (1967). *The biological basis of personality.* Springfield, IL: Thomas.

Fetzer Institute/National Institute on Aging Working Group. (1999, October). *Multidimensional measurement of religiousness/spirituality for use in health research: A report of the Fetzer/National Institute on Aging Working Group.* Kalamazoo, MI: Fetzer Institute.

Francis, L. J., & Katz, Y. J. (2003). Religiosity and happiness: A study among Israeli female undergraduates. *Research in the Social Scientific Study of Religion, 12,* 75–86.

Francis, L. J., & Rodger, R. (1994). The influence of personality on clergy role prioritization, role influences, conflict and dissatisfaction with ministry. *Personality and Individual Differences, 16,* 947–957.

Fredrickson, B. L. (2002). How does religion benefit health and well-being?: Are positive emotions active ingredients? *Psychological Inquiry, 13,* 209–213.

Freud, S. (1950). Totem and taboo. In J. Strachey (Ed. and Trans.), *The standard edition of the complete psychological works of Sigmund Freud* (Vol. 13). New York: Norton. (Original work published 1913)

Freud, S. (1961). The future of an illusion. In J. Strachey (Ed. and Trans.), *The standard edition of the complete psychological works of Sigmund Freud* (Vol. 22). New York: Norton. (Original work published 1927)

Garabino, J. J. (1998). Comparisons of the constructs and psychometric properties of selected measures of adult attachment. *Measurement and Evaluation in Counseling and Development, 31,* 28–45.

Gorsuch, R. L. (1984). Measurement: The boon and bane of investigating religion. *American Psychologist, 39,* 228–236.

Granqvist, P. (1998). Religiousness and perceived childhood attachment: On the question of compensation or correspondence. *Journal for the Scientific Study of Religion, 37,* 350–367.

Hall, T. W., Brokaw, B. F., Edwards, K. J., & Pike, P. L. (1998). An empirical exploration of psychoanalysis and religion: Spiritual maturity and object relations development. *Journal for the Scientific Study of Religion, 37,* 303–313.

Hazan, C., & Shaver, P. (1987). Romantic love conceptualized as an attachment process. *Journal of Personality and Social Psychology, 52,* 511–524.

Heath, A. C., Neale, M. C., Kessler, R. C., Eaves, L. J., & Kendler, K. S. (1992). Evidence for genetic influences on personality from self-reports and informant ratings. *Journal of Personality and Social Psychology, 63,* 85–96.

Herbst, J. H., Zonderman, A. B., McCrae, R. R., & Costa, P. T., Jr. (2000). Do the dimensions of the Temperament and Character Inventory map a simple genetic architecture?: Evidence from molecular genetics and factor analysis. *American Journal of Psychiatry, 157,* 1285–1290.

Hill, P. C., & Pargament, K. I. (2003). Advances in the conceptualization and measurement of religion and spirituality: Implications for physical and mental health research. *American Psychologist, 58,* 64–74.

Hill, P. C., Pargament, K. I., Hood, R. W., McCullough, M. E., Sawyers, J. P., Larson, D. B., & Zinnbauer, B. J. (2000). Conceptualizing religion and spirituality: Points of commonality, points of departure. *Journal for the Theory of Social Behaviour, 30,* 51–77.

Joiner, T. E., Perez, M., & Walker, R. L. (2002). Playing devil's advocate: Why not conclude that the relation of religiosity to mental health reduces to mundane mediators? *Psychological Inquiry, 13,* 214–216.

Jones, D. L., & Francis, L. J. (1992). Personality profile of Methodist ministers in England. *Psychological Reports, 70,* 538.

Kernberg, O. (1966). Structural derivatives of object relationships. *International Journal of Psycho-Analysis, 47,* 236–253.

Kirkpatrick, L. A. (1998). God as substitute attachment figure: A longitudinal study of adult attachment style and religious change in college students. *Personality and Social Psychology Bulletin, 24,* 961–973.

Koenig, H. G., McCullough, M. E., & Larson, D. B. (2000). *Handbook of religion and health.* New York: Oxford University Press.

Lawrence, R. T. (1997). Measuring the image of God: The God Image Inventory and the God Image Scale. *Journal of Psychology and Theology, 25*, 214–226.

Lewis, C. A., & Maltby, J. (1995). Religiosity and personality among U.S. adults. *Personality and Individual Differences, 18*, 293–295.

Lilienfeld, S. O., Wood, J. M., & Garb, H. N. (2000). The scientific status of projective tests. *Psychological Science in the Public Interest, 1*(2), 27–66.

MacDonald, D. A. (2000). Spirituality: Description, measurement, and relation to the five-factor model of personality. *Journal of Personality, 68*, 153–197.

MacDonald, D. A., & Holland, D. (2002). Examination of the psychometric properties of the Temperament and Character Inventory self-transcendence dimension. *Personality and Individual Differences, 32*, 1013–1027.

Maltby, J., & Day, L. (2001). Spiritual involvement and belief: The relationship between spirituality and Eysenck's personality dimensions. *Personality and Individual Differences, 30*, 187–192.

McClelland, D. C. (1980). Motive dispositions: The merits of operant and respondent measures. In L. Wheeler (Ed.), *Review of personality and social psychology* (Vol. 1, pp. 10–41). Beverly Hills, CA: Sage.

McCrae, R. R., & Costa, P. T., Jr. (1997). Personality trait structure as a human universal. *American Psychologist, 52*, 509–516.

McCrae, R. R., Herbst, J. H., & Costa, P. T., Jr. (2001). Effects of acquiescence on personality factor structures. In R. Riemann, F. M. Spinath, & F. Ostendorf (Eds.), *Personality and temperament: Genetics, evolution, and structure* (pp. 217–231). Berlin: Pabst Science.

McGinn, B. (1993). The letter and the spirit: Spirituality as an academic discipline. *Christian Spirituality Bulletin, 1*, 1–10.

Moberg, D. O. (2002). Assessing and measuring spirituality: Confronting dilemmas of universal and particular evaluative criteria. *Journal of Adult Development, 9*, 47–60.

Murray-Swank, N. (2003). *Solace for the soul: An evaluation of a psycho-spiritual intervention for female survivors of sexual abuse.* Unpublished doctoral dissertation, Bowling Green State University, Bowling Green, Ohio.

Ozer, D. J., & Riese, S. P. (1994). Personality assessment. *Annual Review of Psychology, 45*, 357–388.

Pargament, K. I. (2002). Is religion nothing but . . . ?: Explaining religion versus explaining religion away. *Psychological Inquiry, 13*, 239–244.

Piedmont, R.L. (1989). The Life Activities Achievement Scale: An act-frequency approach to the measurement of motivation. *Educational and Psychological Measurement, 49*, 863–874.

Piedmont, R. L. (1994). Validation of the NEO-PIR observer form for college students: Toward a paradigm for studying personality development. *Assessment, 1*, 259–268.

Piedmont, R. L. (1999). Strategies for using the five-factor model of personality in religious research. *Journal of Psychology and Theology, 27*, 338–350.

Piedmont, R. L. (2001). Spiritual transcendence and the scientific study of spirituality. *Journal of Rehabilitation, 67*, 4–14.

Piedmont, R. L. (2004). Spiritual transcendence as a predictor of psychosocial outcome from an outpatient substance abuse program. *Psychology of Addictive Behaviors, 18*, 213–222.

Piedmont, R. L., Ciarrocchi, J. W., Dy-Liacco, G., Mapa, A. T., & Williams, J. E. G. (2003). *An evaluation of spirituality and religiosity as empirical constructs for personality research.* Manuscript under review.

Piedmont, R. L., Ciarrocchi, J. W., & Williams, J. E. G. (2002). A components analysis of ones' image of God. *Research in the Social Scientific Study of Religion, 13*, 109–123.

Piedmont, R. L., & Leach, M. M. (2002). Cross-cultural generalizability of the Spiritual Transcendence Scale in India: Spirituality as a universal aspect of human experience. *American Behavioral Scientist, 45*, 1888–1902.

Piedmont, R. L., & Nelson, R. (2001). A psychometric evaluation of the short form of the Faith Maturity Scale. *Research in the Social Scientific Study of Religion, 12*, 165–184.

Richards, W. A. (2002). Entheogens in the study of mystical and archetypal experiences. *Research in the Social Scientific Study of Religion, 13,* 143–158.

Rizzuto, A. M. (1979). *The birth of the living god.* Chicago: University of Chicago Press.

Rodgerson, T. E., & Piedmont, R. L. (1998). Assessing the incremental validity of the Religious Problem-Solving Scale in the prediction of clergy burnout. *Journal for the Scientific Study of Religion, 37,* 517–527.

Saroglou, V. (2002). Religion and the five-factors of personality: A meta-analytic review. *Personality and Individual Differences, 32,* 15–25.

Saucier, G., & Goldberg, L. R. (1998). What is beyond the Big Five? *Journal of Personality, 66,* 495–524.

Sloan, R. P., Bagiella, R., & Powell, T. (2001). Without a prayer: Methodological problems, ethical challenges, and misrepresentation in the study of religion, spirituality, and medicine. In T. G. Plante & A. C. Sherman (Eds.), *Faith and health: Psychological perspectives* (pp. 339–354). New York: Guilford Press.

Spilka, B., Addison, J., & Rosensohn, M. (1975). Parents, self, and God: A test of competing theories of individual–religion relationships. *Review of Religious Research, 16,* 154–165.

Svrakic, D. M., Whitehead, C., Przybeck, T. R., & Cloninger, C. R. (1993). Differential diagnosis of personality disorders by the seven-factor model of temperament and character. *Archives of General Psychiatry, 50,* 991–999.

Zuckerman, M. (2003). Biological bases to personality. In T. Millon & M. J. Lerner (Eds.), *Handbook of psychology: Vol. 5. Personality and social psychology* (pp. 85–116). Hoboken, NJ: Wiley.

15

Religion, Attitudes, and Social Behavior

MICHAEL J. DONAHUE
MICHAEL E. NIELSEN

For many, this topic is central to the social-scientific study of religion. Never mind where religion came from, how it develops, or even how to measure it, does it "work" ? Are religious people "better" than others? This chapter considers findings concerning the relation between religiousness and a variety of interpersonal attitudes and behaviors: prejudice, altruism and prosocial behavior, honesty, sexuality, family relations, crime and delinquency, and politics and peace.

THE PSYCHOLOGY OF . . . WHAT?

But first we offer some thoughts about definitions. What is "religion"? While generally some variant of "the perceived relation between an individual and a powerful supernatural agent or agents" would seem to suffice, clever discussions can be constructed about exceptions to such a rule. For example, many point to Buddhism as an example of a world religion that does not have a God. "However, this argument is based on a specious account of [it];. . . . [Many contend that Buddhists] . . . don't worship the Buddha, yet [they] treat him as a supernatural agent, especially in rituals" (Slone, 2004, p. 5; see also his Chap. 6). Others inquire whether conceptual systems that supposedly serve the same functions as religion for a given individual should be considered a sort of "implicit" religion (e.g., devotion to Apple computers; Lam, 2001). But as Lupton (1986) notes, such an overbroad definition results in unacceptably fuzzy categories, and so the interested researcher would be better served by accepting the fact that many people have no religious orientation rather than by diluting the definition of religion to the point of uselessness.

In general, most measures of religiousness are quite highly intercorrelated (e.g., Bassett et al., 1991). In addition, only a small subset of measures is used with any frequency: church attendance; single-item measures of religious commitment or salience; intrinsic and extrinsic religiousness; and so on. Thus most researchers use precisely the sort of definition of what it means to be "religious" that might be obtained from the "person-in-the-street" (but see also the discussion of the concepts of "religion" and "spirituality" in Zinnbauer and Pargament, Chapter 2, this volume).

RELIGION AS SOCIAL

Why consider religion as a social phenomenon? James (1902/1985) defines religion as "the feelings, acts, and experiences of individual men in their solitude, so far as they apprehend themselves to stand in relation to whatever they may consider the divine" (p. 31). But religion can also be defined as an inherently *social* phenomenon. For example, in Islam, the *ahadeeth* (collections of the teachings of Mohammed on various specific topics, not unlike Jesus' sermons in the Christian synoptic gospels; Matthew, Mark, and Luke) are filled with assurances from the Messenger of God that good works will ensure entrance into paradise: "Charity is prescribed for each descendant of Adam every day the sun rises . . . listening to the deaf, leading the blind . . . supporting the feeble with the strength of one's arms—all of these are charity prescribed for you" (*Fiqh-us-Sunnah*, Vol. 3, no. 98).

In the Christian tradition, and most notably in the synoptic gospels, the social nature of the teachings is quite striking. In addition to the so-called Golden Rule (Matthew 7:12) and the "second greatest commandment," love of neighbor as of self (Matthew 22:39), the Lord's Prayer calls down upon believers the condition that God forgive them only to the degree that they forgive others (Matthew 6:12). Jesus promises his presence when "*two or three* have gathered" (Matthew 18:20, emphasis added); it might be argued that there is no such thing as "one Christian." Perhaps even more to the point, when Jesus speaks of how one is to be "saved," the *failure to do good* for others is itself a sufficiently grievous offense to result in eternal damnation (Lazarus and the rich man, Luke 16:19–21; the parable of the sheep and the goats, Matthew 25:31–46).

Thus, the inherently social nature of religion, and its relation to social psychology seems clear. Indeed, prominent theories in personality-social psychology have been employed in the analysis of religious behavior, including dissonance theory (Brock, 1962), attribution theory (Bulman & Wortman, 1977), and theories of altruism (Batson, Eidelman, Higley, & Russell, 2001). Therefore attention to religion as a context for social interaction would seem, if nothing else, representative of the research in the area.

DIFFERENT WAYS OF BEING RELIGIOUS: INTRINSIC, EXTRINSIC, QUEST

In light of the social nature of religion, it is perhaps not surprising that the most commonly used scales of religiousness, at least to study its relation to social phenomena, were designed by social psychologists. Since much of the research to be cited in what follows employs these measures, a brief introduction would seem appropriate.

Intrinsic and Extrinsic

According to Gordon W. Allport, in his seminal study of the roots of discrimination, *The Nature of Prejudice* (1954/1979), "The role of religion is paradoxical. It makes prejudice and it unmakes prejudice" (p. 444). This finding lead him to hypothesize that were two contrasting types of religious motivations. After a period of conceptual development using a variety of terminologies (see Donahue, 1985, for a review), he ultimately settled on the terms intrinsic (*I*) and extrinsic (*E*) religiousness. In Allport's view, "the extrinsically motivated person uses his religion whereas the intrinsically motivated lives his religion" (Allport & Ross, 1967, p. 434). A typical item from the *I* scale is: "My whole approach to life is based upon my religion"; a typical item from the *E* scale is: "What religion offers me most is comfort in times of trouble and sorrow" (Gorsuch & McPherson, 1989).

Although *I* and *E* were originally postulated as the ends of a single bipolar continuum, it was soon discovered that *I* and *E* were better conceptualized as two separate independent variables. The ensuing years saw fairly widespread use of the scales. By the end of 1982, nearly 70 articles had been published in English employing the scales (Donahue, 1985, p. 400) as well as more than 50 doctoral dissertations. A search of English-language research citations and doctoral dissertations reveals that in the 10 years between 1986 and 1995, some 200 journal articles and 160 dissertations appeared that involved the scales. And the rate has continued unabated. The period from 1996 to 2003 produced another 200 journal articles and 140 dissertations.

The scales have not been without their critics. Dittes (1971) complained that Allport ventured into the "prophetic" by attempting to determine the nature of "true" religion. In the same year, Hunt and King published a factor analysis claiming that *I* was multidimensional, and that a single *E* factor could best be measured using only six of the 11 items in the scale. In contrast, Kirkpatrick (1989) concluded just the opposite: that *I* had a unitary structure, while *E* might involve as many as three dimensions.

Kirkpatrick and Hood (1990) published an article calling for more theoretically sophisticated research than had characterized the studies that had used *I* and *E* up to that time. Connolly (1999), presenting a review of Hunt and King's (1971) and Kirkpatrick and Hood's (1990) critiques, concluded that there was little point to continued use of the scales, and that "more able psychologists of religion" would probably stop using them and "involvement in *I–E* research may well become a banner identifying second-rate psychologists of religion" (p.183). Or not. Spilka, Hood, Hunsberger, and Gorsuch (2003) cite research involving *I* and/or *E* on 69 of the 543 pages of their text.

Quest

"Quest" (*Q*) religiousness was proposed by C. Daniel Batson to address a dimension of "growth" and "seeking" that he felt had been in Allport's original conceptualization of *I*, but that was not embodied in the *I* scale (see Batson, Schoenrade, & Ventis, 1993, for an overview). He developed a scale that was intended to focus on a "growth" or "seekership" quality in religious development. The scale includes items such as "It might be said that I value my religious doubts and uncertainties."

Critics of *Q* have questioned whether it could be a measure of religion at all, since it fails to correlate with other, more established measures, and there was no clear evidence that religious groups scored higher on *Q* than less religious groups (Donahue, 1985), but Batson et al. (1993) cited evidence to the contrary. Hood and Morris (1985) took *Q* to task on the grounds that a measure that was negatively correlated with measures of doctrinal orthodoxy could not be a measure of religiousness, but Batson and Ventis (1985) begged to differ.

In view of the ongoing controversy, many researchers in the psychology of religion have opted to use all three scales, *I*, *E*, and *Q*, to examine the relation between religiousness and behavior. That body of research, along with a variety of other measures of religiousness, are examined in what follows.

PREJUDICE

Allport and Ross (1967) correlated *I* and *E* with several measures of prejudice: negative attitudes toward blacks, Jews, other non-Europeans, and mentally disturbed individuals. He also included a scale of what he referred to as "a 'jungle' philosophy of life" reflecting the belief that "it's a dog-eat-dog world." *E* was generally correlated with such measures; *I* was not. Donahue (1985) reported that later studies found essentially the same pattern of relations.

But why is *I* uncorrelated with prejudice? Why doesn't religion inhibit prejudice, as Allport's conceptual approach predicted it would? One possible reason for a lack of negative correlation is that the relation is not linear, or "straight-line." A consistent curvilinear relation between the two (prejudice is highest for those with moderate *I* scores, and lowest for those scoring high or low on *I*) would produce a nonsignificant correlation. The "positive correlation" represented by the "rising" side of the inverted-U shape would cancel out the "negative" correlation in the second half of the curve. In fact, Allport and Ross (1967) presented this possibility, and cited seven studies with a variety of religiousness measures that obtained that finding. Gorsuch and Aleshire (1974) examined 25 religion prejudice studies in which the curvilinearity hypothesis could be addressed, and concluded that "20 were consistent with the expectation that the marginal church member manifested more prejudice than either the nonactive or the most active members" (p. 285). Spilka et al. (2003) criticized this finding, however, on the grounds that many studies did not include "nonreligious" individuals.

Most recent studies have continued to find no correlations between *I* and prejudice (Bailey, 2000; Cannon, 2001; Lundblad, 2002). Beck and Miller (2000) found that those who scored high on *I* were less likely to make snap judgments about others' religious or moral orientation (*E* scores were not reported). Herek (1987) found *intrinsics* no less prejudiced against gays and lesbians than *extrinsics*, but Fulton, Gorsuch, and Maynard (1999) found that prejudice against gay men and lesbians was correlated with *I* only in the case of morally based feelings about them rather than "nonmorally" based opinions (hate the sin, love the sinner). Using a "social distance" measure, they found that attitudes of those scoring high on *I* toward gay men and lesbians were no more negative than their attitude toward others who violated their moral code—for example, liars and racists. Among Lutheran pastors, Taylor (2000) found *I* uncorrelated with either prejudice against or positive attitudes toward gay men; *E* positively correlated with attitudes toward gay men (but not lesbians); *Q* correlated with positive attitudes toward both. A high score on an index combining both a measure of belief orthodoxy and *Q* was unrelated to attitudes toward gays and lesbians.

In general, then, *I* is uncorrelated with measures of prejudice, although devoutly religious individuals prefer to "keep their distance" from people whom they consider "sinners." A religion of social convention (as measured by *E*) is more likely to be related to prejudice against members of an outgroup.

PROSOCIAL BEHAVIOR AND HELPING

Establishing a connection between religion and helping others would seem to be a "slam dunk." The record of history points to Christianity as the inventor of the nonprofit hospital and of religious orders solely dedicated to serving in them. The presence of men and women religious ministering to the victims of various pandemics throughout history is well established. Indeed, Stark (1997) contends that it was likely that Christians' response to a plague in Rome, and their decision to stay and care for the sick, rather than flee to the countryside, provided a major impetus for Christianity's early growth. More recently, it should be noted that when the Nobel Peace Prize does not go to diplomats or organizations, it frequently goes to individuals motivated by strong religious beliefs (e.g., Jimmy Carter, Carlos F. X. Belo, the 14th Dalai Lama, Elie Wiesel, Desmond Tutu, Lech Walesa, Mother Teresa).

A variety of research studies have examined the religion-and-helping correlation. Gallup Polls, for example, periodically assess the role of religion in helping. Among people Gallup surveyed in 1984, those who were highly spiritually committed were more than twice as likely to be currently working in giving service to the elderly, poor, or otherwise needy as those who were highly uncommitted. This pattern has held consistent in follow-up studies (Colasanto, 1989; Wuthnow, 1994). Other research has found that religion is more strongly associated with planned helping, as when people consider helping an AIDS program (Omoto, Snyder, & Berghuis, 1993) or other types of volunteer service organizations (Clary & Snyder, 1991, 1993). But the help religious people extend to the needy apparently has its limits, particularly when the person in need exhibits behavior that violates a religious standard (Jackson & Esses, 1997; Thurston, 2000). Here also the religious keep their distance from outgroup members. The role of "faith-based organizations" in providing services to people in need also awaits further study (Cnaan, 2002).

Contributions of people's time and money to charities represents another area that has interested researchers. Americans donate about 1% of their incomes to religious charities and about 1% to other causes (Myers, 1992). Some suggest that much religious giving essentially serves the function of "club membership fees" rather than the function of charitable acts (Argyle, 2000). Indeed, an entire literature has grown up to examine the time "spent" in religious endeavors in the context of various "rational choice" or economic theories (Iannaccone, 1997; Young, 1996).

It is true that religious people give to religious organizations to further religious ends. But this giving is not only monetary; it also includes volunteer time. This time is estimated to be equivalent, on average, to approximately 40% of the value of their monetary contributions (Hoge, Zech, McNamara, & Donahue, 1998). To the extent that religiousness serves as a unique force to inhibit a wide variety of behaviors that are considered problematic—crime, premarital pregnancy, alcoholism, substance abuse—and does so in a way that government is forbidden to do—by instilling religious faith—then, even if indirectly, such giving is no less charitable and perhaps at least as effective as donations of time, treasure, and talent to secular charities.

HONESTY

Empirical studies of lying and religion lead to two primary conclusions. The first is that there are relatively few published studies assessing the impact of religiosity on lying. For

example, a PsycINFO search for articles published during the past 20 years that link religion with either lying or deception revealed only 34 articles, the vast majority of which
deal with social desirability, psychohistory, or clinical, therapeutic concerns. The second
is that although religiosity appears to be the best predictor of attitudes about honesty
(Katz, Santman, & Lonero, 1994), religious respondents are sometimes, but not consistently, less likely to cheat or engage in deception than their nonreligious peers, despite a
nearly universal religious injunction against dishonesty (Grasmick, Bursik, & Cochran,
1991; Perrin, 2000; Smith, Wheeler, & Diener, 1975). Indeed, one study even reported
that children who attended a religious school may have cheated more frequently than
those who attended a secular school (Guttman, 1984). What little research there is finds
no consistent difference in the degree to which members of various religions (e.g., Christianity, Hinduism, Islam, and Jainism) value honesty (Kothari, 1994; Wolfe & Mourribi,
1985).

Nearly all such studies, however, have been conducted in school settings and so offer
even less empirical evidence regarding the relation between religiousness and cheating or
lying among adults than they do among students. Furthermore, from a psychological perspective, most studies of honesty have treated religion in a relatively unsophisticated way.
This fact, combined with the inconsistent results in the area, invites additional research.
For example, there is great potential for experimental studies that would enable researchers to examine the effect of religiousness conceived as a personality variable alongside
situational inducements to perform an honest or a dishonest act. Given the paucity of
experimental studies in the psychology of religion, and the core assumption that religion
affects individuals' honesty, this is an area sorely needing research attention.

SEXUALITY

If there is a single issue about which psychology and religion are perceived to be most at
odds, it must surely be the area of sexuality. Shea (1992) asserts that by a conservative
"estimate the number of castrations, whippings, incarcerations, burnings . . . and other
executions attributable directly to [Christianity's hostility to sex] to be in the millions. . . .
[And they] continue to the present time" (p. 70). Shea offers no citations to support this
assertion, simply stating it as if it was self-validating. Aside from the patent absurdity of
the statement that they "continue to the present time," even the statement that they were
once common is no longer considered tenable. Stark's (2003) review of recent historical
research, and his own archival analyses, indicate that many beliefs about such a vicious
and violent past are modern-day stereotypes, largely the result of the biases of certain
19th- and early 20th-century historians. Such presumptions likewise ignore the place of
the medical profession, as opposed to religion, in advancing sexual repression while
"Christianity gave America an ethic of sexual pleasure" (Gardella, 1985).

So if we can allow that the influence of religion on sexuality is not one of brutal repression, what does the research tell us about the relation between the two? The effect of
religiosity on sexuality has been examined in many studies, frequently with nationally
representative samples. For example, Cochran and Beeghley (1991) examined a subset of
15,000 U.S. respondents from the National Opinion Research Center (NORC) surveys
conducted between 1971 and 1989. Analyses showed a strong ($r = .51$) correlation between religious commitment and belief that extramarital sex is wrong. Conservative denominations were more likely to condemn extramarital intercourse than were mainline

denominations; Jews reported the least condemnation of extramarital sex. Within denominations, the correlation between religious commitment and condemnation of extramarital intercourse also varies in a manner roughly consistent with the degree to which the denomination is at odds with the dominant culture: stronger correlations between religious commitment and condemnation of extramarital sex were found among sects, while the weakest correlations were found for Episcopalians.

Similar patterns of correlations have been found for self-reports of engagement in premarital sex. Indeed, Benson, Donahue, and Erickson (1989) stated that major reviews that had been conducted by adolescent pregnancy researchers (e.g., Chilman, 1980; Hayes, 1987) and major nationwide interview data (Zelnik, Kantner, & Ford, 1981) indicated strong "constraining effects of religion on the likelihood of engaging in premarital intercourse" (p. 170).

Some research on this subject generates results that invite further questions. One such study surveyed over 2,700 U.S. adults and found that religious people were less likely to report having had extramarital affairs than were nonreligious people (Janus & Janus, 1993). Curiously, however, adults reporting themselves to be "religious" were less likely to have had affairs (26%) than were adults who reported themselves to be "very religious" (31%). This finding deserves some pursuit by researchers studying the connection between religious attitudes and social behavior, as a variety of social and psychological mechanisms might be at work.

The topic of sexual orientation and religion has begun to be investigated, but substantial gaps remain in our knowledge of this issue. While it is generally found that religious orthodoxy or conservatism is associated with greater prejudice toward homosexuals (Morrison & Morrison, 2002), the more interesting questions concern the psychological dynamics for this relation. One explanation for this effect is that religious groups unwittingly exacerbate a natural "us versus them" mentality that heightens prejudice toward people who are seen as threatening to the group (Altemeyer, 2003). Another promising explanation for the effect focuses on how the content of an individual's beliefs accounts for prejudice toward homosexuals (Laythe, Finkel, & Kirkpatrick, 2001). Of course, these are not necessarily incompatible hypotheses, and we look forward to research that addresses them.

Another area worthy of further examination is the types of spiritual conflicts experienced by homosexuals (Buchanan, Dzelme, Harris, & Hecker, 2001; Rodriguez & Ouellette, 2000). Data from one small-scale study suggests that spiritual conflict affects approximately two-thirds of all gays and lesbians (Schuck & Liddle, 2001), but the extent to which this problem actually occurs remains unknown because we lack reliable statistical estimates garnered from large samples. Likewise, these analyses have not adequately addressed the extent to which cognitive dissonance theory, social identity theory, or other frameworks might best account for people's experiences with sexual orientation and religion.

RELIGION-RELATED ABUSE

Is religion a risk factor for child abuse? Vivid reports in the 1980s of "satanic ritual abuse" and of ritualistic sacrifice of infants were later found to be spurious (Richardson, Best, & Bromley, 1990). Curiously, a small number of therapists reported a relatively large number of such incidents among their clients; most therapists never worked with even a single client who claimed to be a victim of satanic abuse (Bottoms, Shaver, Goodman, & Qin, 1995). More recent headlines have focused on sexual abuse of children by Catholic priests. There is no denying that terrible incidents of abuse did occur, and that there may have been cases of malfeasance by bishops to preserve the reputation of the Catholic Church. But one of the most striking findings of the National Review Board for the Protection of Children and Young People (2004) established to examine the scandal was the lack of research into relevant questions. Is the rate of abuse by Catholic priests more or less than the rate of abuse by ministers in Protestant denominations? More or less than the rates among men in similar positions of authority, such as Boy Scout leaders or teachers? Some 80% of the priests engaged in sexual contact with postpubertal boys, an act technically known as *ephebophilia*, rather than *pedophilia*. Research indicates that the clinical profiles of ephebophiles and pedophiles differ markedly, and the two terms should not be interchanged (McGlone, 2004). The commission of these crimes peaked in 1980, with a major decline since then. Is this somehow related to Catholic Church history or was there such a pattern in society at large? No one knows the answers to these questions because there is little or no relevant research.

Child physical abuse has received somewhat more research attention but remains little understood. The most consistent effect appears to be that fundamentalist religious beliefs are associated with a greater likelihood of violence among Jewish (Shor, 1998) and Christian (Ellison, Bartkowski, & Segal, 1996) families. The effects of such abuse are just now beginning to be the subject of empirical research. Compared to a group of victims whose abuse did not involve religion, victims of religion-related physical abuse showed greater levels of depression, anxiety, hostility, psychoticism, and other psychological problems years later (Bottoms, Nielsen, Murray, & Filipas, 2004). To the extent that these data are replicated in other samples, they suggest that when abuse is connected to religion negative effects are compounded. Additional research is sorely needed so that we can better understand the extent of the problem, the psychological mechanisms by which it occurs, and the possibility that child sexual abuse, religion-related medical neglect, and other forms of abuse might show similar effects. Theoretical perspectives such as attachment theory (Kirkpatrick, 1997) and the role of God in coping (Pargament, 2001) could be useful in explaining the long-term effects of religion-related abuse (Bottoms et al., 2004). In the case of attachment theory, the notion of God as an attachment figure who substitutes for weak parental attachments would suggest that the person who suffers religion-related abuse is likely to be deprived of a close attachment to God as well as to parents. Pargament's research on religious coping suggests that the victim would be deprived of the significant positive effects of using God as a resource for coping with distressful events. These theories provide readily testable hypotheses for researchers investigating religion-related child abuse, whether physical or sexual in nature.

CRIME AND PUNISHMENT

By definition, criminal acts are antisocial. Research addressing religion's role in promoting or inhibiting crime has a long history. A recent meta-analysis of the area (Baier & Wright, 2001) examined 79 effect sizes across 60 studies. They found that "the mean reported effect size was $r = -.12$, and the median was $r = -.11$ . . . none of [the correlations reported] were positive. . . . These findings show that religious behavior and beliefs exert a significant, moderate deterrent effect on individuals' criminal behavior" (p. 14).

The authors also went on to examine some related hypotheses. One is the hypothesis that the deterrent effect of religion is increased when one is immersed within a religious community; they found that the data supported this conclusion. In addition, they found that nonvictim crimes (e.g., gambling and drug use) were also more likely to be deterred by religion.

Attitudes regarding the punishment of criminals are related to religiosity. For example, 75% of Americans in general favor the death penalty, but among those who say religion is important to them the figure increases to 84% (Gallup & Lindsay, 1999). Of course, this finding speaks of religion in general, with no fine distinctions being made among denominations or specific religious beliefs. While Christian orthodoxy correlates positively with endorsement of the death penalty, we begin to see that such attitudes are malleable when we consider the case of Roman Catholics living in the United States. Recent research conducted by Bjarnasson and Welch (2004) found that church attendance by Catholics is positively correlated with endorsement of Cardinal Bernadin's (1984) statement regarding "a seamless garment" on "life issues," which denounces both capital punishment and abortion. After Bernandin's framing of the issue in this way, U. S. Catholic support for capital punishment changed markedly. Whereas Catholics were generally more likely than non-Catholics to support the death penalty during the early 1970s, this difference has declined, particularly among parishioners who were highly integrated into their parish (Bjarnasson & Welch, 2004). This pattern also is consistent with the notion that one's social identity helps guide individual attitudes.

Many different theoretical viewpoints are available for application to these issues. Whether the subject is crime, family violence, or prosocial behavior, analytic perspectives can draw from a range of theories that emphasize the "micro," such as cognitive dissonance theory, or the "macro," such as rational choice theory. Using such a multilevel approach to do this promises at least two important benefits: it can improve our understanding of social behavior and religion, and it can facilitate interdisciplinary dialogue because of the wide variety of theories available. For example, psychological (e.g., theories of attitude–behavior consistency, social identity theory) and socioeconomic (e.g., rational choice theory) approaches could be examined profitably in the context of volunteerism. Ideally, these approaches could be examined jointly in order to gain a more nuanced understanding of the way individual- and social-level influences combine to account for people's behavior.

PSYCHOLOGY OF RELIGION, POLITICS, AND PEACE

The psychological study of religion sits at a crossroads between psychology and religious studies. Social psychology is at a similar crossroads with other social sciences, and this fact presents the opportunity for cross-fertilization among these disciplines. We focus now on the relevance of the psychology of religion on two such areas of inquiry.

Religion and Politics

The political and religious spheres are often tightly intertwined. Psychological theories can be helpful in understanding such interconnections. As one example, consider the finding that in 1990, before the demise of the Soviet Union, merely 15% of Ukrainians identified themselves as Orthodox Christians. Seven years later, however, after Ukraine established its independence, 70% of Ukrainians so identified themselves (Kolodny, 1997). Such an enormous change in religious identity illustrates the powerful interconnections among religious, political, and national identities.

Political leaders also use religion in order to garner and maintain power. For example, most Middle East studies scholars agree that the House of Saud endorses Wahabbism in order to maintain its power (Esposito, 1987). Likewise, most U.S. political scientists agree that George W. Bush reaches out to Evangelical Christians because they provide him with an important base of support (Rozell, 2003). Just as religion can serve political ends, so too can politics serve an individual's religious goals. Recent survey data illustrate this point. Most Americans (79%) agree with the notion of keeping church and state separate, but conservative Protestants and Evangelicals, a significant portion of the U.S. populace, desire religion to have a greater influence on the U.S. political scene, whereas non-Evangelicals do not (Gallup & Lindsay, 1999).

Among the more informative projects in this area is the Clergy Study Project, which examined the roles of clergy in Judaism, Unitarian-Universalism, and in 16 Christian religious bodies in the 2000 national election (Smith, 2004). The majority of clergy engaged in some form of political activity, including delivering sermons on politics, organizing study groups, or performing some form of activist work on behalf of candidates. Whether they were conservative Evangelicals who view the world as being in a state of moral decline (Guth et al., 2003) or Unitarian-Universalists working toward a more liberal social–political agenda (Green, 2004), the clergy viewed their efforts as a natural part of their moral obligation to be involved in society. Thus, religious belief expresses itself as engagement with society and with political structures. This effect is moderated, however, by the degree to which an individual's religion is accepted by society. In a separate study, U. S. Hindus, Buddhists, and Muslims expressed a high degree of alienation from society and were less likely to become involved in political activity (Wuthnow & Hackett, 2004).

History abounds with examples of the religious affecting the political, and vice versa. Psychological theories regarding attitude–behavior consistency, leadership, and decision making have much to contribute to our understanding of the way in which individuals' attitudes and values shape their decisions and are quite relevant to questions concerning when and how people construe religion and politics, and how they maintain separate versus combined goals in those spheres. As we seek to understand these phenomena, however, we must extend our knowledge base to include other disciplines, either by independent study or, more preferably, by working with colleagues in other disciplines. By drawing from the expertise of colleagues in disciplines such as political science or sociology, and by integrating their broad, "macro" analyses with more "micro" psychological theories, we will add breadth and depth to our understanding of the ways in which religion and other social institutions affect people. We also can gain insight into the underlying question of religion as a means or as an end, a question that has been a prime concern at least since Allport articulated the I/E typology (Batson, Schoenrade, & Ventis, 1993).

Religion, Peace, Conflict, and War

Significant implications exist for religious attitudes and beliefs on people's views regarding war. Indeed, the U.S. Naval War College recognizes this connection, offering an elective course titled "Faith and Force: Religion, War and Peace." This is an important, yet generally neglected, area of study by psychologists of religion (but see Silberman, Chapter 29, this volume, for a discussion of religious terrorism). A good base for examining these relations is found in the work of Christie, Wagner, and Winter (2001), who distinguish between direct and structural violence. *Direct violence* entails actions that directly, immediately, and adversely affect another person's life. It is intentional, dramatic, and can kill people outright, as in cases of war or hate crimes. *Structural violence* is more indirect and chronic, and results in long-term adverse effects that decrease one's lifespan, often dramatically.

Recent history offers examples of religious bodies and individuals advocating direct violence for religious reasons (Juergensmeyer, 2003). Religious leaders also may advocate support of war, as when the Southern Baptist Convention president announced, "We will enlist prayer warriors as special forces to pray for our troops and their families" (Graham, 2003). When leaders encourage people to draw connections between the religious and the martial by using religious language to describe the righteousness of their cause or to describe the enemy as evil, however, such "tough talk" promotes authoritarianism and polarization in a conflict, working against the prospects for a peaceful end to the conflict (Pettigrew, 2003).

The relation between religion and structural violence can be more subtle than that between religion and direct violence. To the extent that societal resources are allocated inequitably, structural violence is being done (Christie et al., 2001). Religions that support such inequities would be considered as contributing to structural violence. White supremacist Christianity in the United States and extremist interpretations of Islam in Afghanistan or Saudi Arabia, among others, illustrate religion's role in maintaining structural violence.

Efforts to reduce direct violence are known as peacemaking. While such work takes different forms, its proponents advocate nonviolent means to reduce direct violence; they react to specific events; they act in a defined time at a defined place; and they tend not to disrupt the current power structure (Christie et al., 2001). Religion can play an important role in understanding the peaceful resolution of conflict. On an institutional level, religions may issue statements (*Atlanta Journal-Constitution*, 2003), hold vigils, and make other efforts to convey their message to political leaders and to the public (e.g., National Council of Churches, 2003). Although such peacemaking efforts may be associated with relatively liberal forms of religion, peacemaking is also evident in religions that are conservative, as was the case when The Church of Jesus Christ of Latter-day Saints helped to defeat the MX intercontinental ballistic missile system in the 1980s (Nielsen, 2004). Religion also can be an important element contributing to dramatic and heroic personal interventions in the midst of war (Oliner & Oliner, 1988).

Actions to address structural violence are known as peace building. Many religions encourage such efforts, which may be consistent with their stated mission in social outreach activities and represent important expressions of religious belief and attitudes. Examples of peace building at an institutional level include the many Roman Catholic pastoral letters and encyclicals written during the past century that call for the fair and equitable distribution of the world's resources, equal access to political power, social justice, and fairness (Pennock, 2000). The 2003 World Council of Churches statement advocating peace through passive resistance, education, and other means also illustrates principles of peace building. On an individual level, religious peace building is exemplified by Mohandas Gandhi, whose promotion of peace drew from his ecumenism. Gandhi's use of civil disobedience to achieve civil rights inspired Martin Luther King, A. J. Muste, and many others (Barash & Webel, 2002; Muste, 1952/2002).

For psychologists of religion, people's efforts in peacemaking and peace building represent a prime opportunity to examine important, tangible effects of religious belief. Potentially useful theoretical perspectives for such research are truly diverse, including moral judgment, social exchange theory, theories regarding norms, social influence theory, social learning theory, conflict resolution, and many others. For example, stereotyping research could examine the effect on people's beliefs of learning that Palestinian "suicide bombers" are often educated, middle-class, and without deep religious commitment (Pettigrew, 2003). Religion can play an important part in people's efforts to cope with conflict, as it did during the contentious overthrow of Philippine president Joseph Estrada in 2001 (Macapagal & Nario-Galace, 2003; for more on religious coping, see Pargament, Ano, & Wachholtz, Chapter 26, this volume). Additional research into religion's roles in fomenting and resolving conflict and war is warranted, and would be an important contribution that psychology of religion can make to psychology.

POSSIBLE THEORETICAL FRAMEWORKS

We have described a wide range of subjects that have received, and in our view should continue to receive, research attention from psychologists of religion. There are several different theoretical frameworks that may be useful in conducting this research. We discuss a few here, recognizing that this list is brief and that there are many others that would be useful. As we improve our understanding of psychology and religion by pursuing research in these areas, we also can promote the study of religious behavior and belief by other psychologists. We move from examples illustrating distinctly "psychological" issues to those that are more sociological and philosophical.

One core issue in social psychology concerns the degree to which attitudes and behavior are consistent (Bagozzi & Burnkrant, 1979; Fazio, Herr, & Olney, 1984; Fishbein & Ajzen, 1974; Kahle & Berman, 1974; Ostrom, 1969; Salancik & Conway, 1975; Wicker, 1969, 1971; Zanna, Olson, & Fazio, 1980). Some of the classic studies relevant to the psychology of religion, such as *When Prophecy Fails* (Festinger, Riecken, & Schachter, 1956), have been based on relevant theories such as cognitive dissonance theory. While there has already been interesting and insightful research using this paradigm, its value is by no means exhausted for the psychology of religion. The same is true of related questions dealing with attitude–behavior causality and attitude change. Attitude researchers have used religion as a content area in which to test out various theories and processes, but in our view this area of research is far from exhausted.

Social identity theory is adopted by many involved in peace psychology (e.g., Christie et al., 2001), and may be of value for psychologists of religion. It appears in the *I/E/Q* paradigm as a social-extrinsic religious orientation (Kirkpatrick, 1989), although most attention has focused on intrinsicness instead. Social identity theory also resonates with some recent writing in the psychology of religion, such as Buddhist psychology (de Silva, 2000). From this view, people's alienation from society, or "identity crisis," ultimately generates a pathological society. Careful examination of the ways that religion affects identity and may be used to promote positive or harmful social interactions is warranted, as the effects appear to be vitally important (Keen, 1986).

Sociology of religion has devoted a great deal of attention to the theory of secularization: that religious adherence declines as societies become more technologically advanced. Support for this theory, while not completely gone (Bruce, 2001), has declined of late, as typified by the title of Stark's (1999) article, "Secularization, R.I.P." Similarly, the active involvement of fundamentalist groups in changing societal structures (Marty & Appleby, 1993a, 1993b), argues against the Marxist "opiate of the masses" image. But whether it is religious decline, religious ferment, or religious scandal, change in the public face of religion is highly relevant to the psychology of religion in terms of people's doubts and uncertainty (see Paloutzian, Chapter 18, this volume). A social-psychological understanding of religion is incomplete without examining how such processes apply to the individual as well as to society.

Conservatism, humanism, and other value systems provide a foundation for the psychology of religion, and for religious individuals themselves (see Geyer & Baumeister, Chapter 23, this volume). Despite this fact, the relation between values, attitudes, and religion remains a subject that has received less attention by psychologists than it deserves. Indeed, a PsycINFO search combining these terms returned merely two dozen entries, few of which were recent. Conceptual analyses of the differences between values and attitudes, the translation of general values to specific attitudes, and the various expressions of values and attitudes in everyday life all warrant further research. Religion provides an excellent context for doing this.

CONCLUSIONS AND IMPLICATIONS

Religion's impact on social life is perhaps the most vigorous area of study in the psychology of religion, not only in terms of the number of studies conducted, but in terms of the range of phenomena and relevant theories. In this brief survey, we have seen that religion affects social attitudes and behavior in myriad ways. Prejudice and helping, honesty and sexuality, child abuse and other crimes, and politics and peace all are highly impacted by one's religious beliefs and behaviors. These results point to the complex nature of religion in people's lives and in society—on the one hand, religion can promote prejudice, intolerance, and war. On the other hand, it can promote understanding, tolerance, and peace. Working out the details concerning when religion does each will undoubtedly continue to occupy researchers for years to come.

Just as the social implications of religion are diverse, so too should be the methods and theoretical perspectives of the psychologists who study them. By using different methods to examine attitudes and social behavior, researchers improve our measurement of constructs and better establish validity. Social psychology and related disciplines offer numerous methods readily applicable to the topics covered in this chapter (see Hood & Belzen, Chapter 4, this volume; Reis & Judd, 2000). Likewise, researchers can draw from a wide variety of theories selected from psychology and other relevant disciplines. Because religion represents an intersection of many interests, examining its social implications necessarily requires a willingness to consider divergent theoretical and even disciplinary perspectives. Studying religion, for example, by using the I/E/Q paradigm and variations of the "lost letter" technique, while also doing content analyses of material published by various religions or denominations, will serve the psychology of religion far better than reliance on only one research method or theoretical perspective. Depending on one's focus, theories from fields as diverse as anthropology, criminology, and political science would be useful in such research, although they are rather rarely used at present. Forming partnerships with colleagues in those disciplines who share an interest in religious phenomena is a fruitful way to begin such work.

Finally, the importance of the issues examined in this chapter can be seen on at least two levels beyond the obvious goal of advancing the psychology of religion. First, addressing the social aspects of religion can also enhance our understanding of basic psychological matters, as Festinger et al. (1956) demonstrated. Perhaps more importantly, because they also deal with significant societal issues, the topics addressed in this chapter ultimately can exert a significant practical effect on people and on society. If there is a common theme to the research in this area, it must be that religion engages others, whether for better or for ill.

REFERENCES

Allport, G. W. (1979). *The nature of prejudice* (unabridged, 25th anniv. ed.). Reading, MA: Addison-Wesley. (Original work published 1954)

Allport, G. W., & Ross, M. J. (1967). Personal religious orientation and prejudice. *Journal of Personality and Social Psychology, 5,* 432–443.

Altemeyer, B. (2003). Why do religious fundamentalists tend to be prejudiced? *The International Journal for the Psychology of Religion, 13,* 17–28.

Argyle, M. (2000). *Psychology and religion: An introduction.* New York: Routledge.

Atlanta Journal-Constitution. (2003, March 22). Statements on war by religious institutions and leaders, p. B2.

Bagozzi, R., & Burnkrant, R. E. (1979). Attitude organization and the attitude–behavior relationship. *Journal of Personality and Social Psychology, 37,* 913–929.

Baier, C. J., & Wright, B. R. E. (2001). "If you love me, keep my commandments": A meta-analysis of the effect of religion on crime. *Journal of Research in Crime and Delinquency, 38,* 3–21.

Bailey, S. D. (2000). Religious orientation and the expression of racial prejudice among graduate students in the field of psychology. *Dissertation Abstracts International-B, 61,* 3048.

Barash, D. P., & Webel, C. P. (2002). *Peace and conflict studies.* Thousand Oaks, CA: Sage.

Bassett, R. L., Camplin, W., Humphrey, D., Dorr, C., Biggs, S., Distaffen, R., et al. (1991). Measuring Christian maturity: A comparison of several scales. *Journal of Psychology and Theology, 19,* 84–93.

Batson, C. D., Eidelman, S. H., Higley, S. L., & Russell, S. A. (2001). "And who is my neighbor?" II: Quest religion as a source of universal compassion. *Journal for the Scientific Study of Religion, 40,* 39–50.

Batson, C. D., Schoenrade, P., & Ventis, W. L. (1993) *Religion and the individual: A social-psychological perspective.* New York: Oxford University Press.

Batson, C. D., & Ventis, W. L. (1985). Misconception of quest: A reply to Hood and Morris. *Review of Religious Research, 26,* 398–407.

Beck, R., & Miller, C. D. (2000). Religiosity and agency and communion: The relation to religious judgmentalism. *Journal of Psychology, 134,* 315–324.

Benson, P. L., Donahue, M. J., & Erickson, J. A. (1989). Adolescence and religion: A review of the literature from 1970 to 1986. *Research in the Social Scientific Study of Religion, 1,* 151–179.

Bernadin, J. L. (1984). *The seamless garment.* Kansas City, MO: National Catholic Reporter.

Bjarnasson, T., & Welch, M. R. (2004). Father knows best: Parishes, priests and American Catholic parishioners' attitudes toward capital punishment. *Journal for the Scientific Study of Religion, 43,* 103–118.

Bottoms, B. L., Nielsen, M. E., Murray, R., & Filipas, H. (2004). Religion related child physical abuse:

Although *Dissertation Abstracts International* citations are given in the reference list, full-text versions (rather than abstracts) were consulted via ProQuest Digital Dissertations (www.lib.umi.com/dissertations/; accessed July 9, 2004).

Characteristics and psychological outcome. *Journal of Aggression, Maltreatment and Trauma, 8,* 87–114.

Bottoms, B. I.., Shaver, P. R., Goodman, G. S., & Qin, J. (1995). In the name of God: A profile of religion-related child abuse. *Journal of Social Issues, 51,* 85–111

Brock, T. C. (1962). Implications of conversion and magnitude of cognitive dissonance. *Journal for the Scientific Study of Religion, 1,* 198–203.

Bruce, S. (2001). Christianity in Britain, R.I.P. *Sociology of Religion, 62,* 191–203.

Buchanan, M., Dzelme, K., Harris, D., & Hecker, L. (2001). Challenges of being simultaneously gay or lesbian and spiritual and/or religious: A narrative perspective. *The American Journal of Family Therapy, 29,* 435–449.

Bulman, R. J., & Wortman, C. B. (1977). Attributions of blame and coping in the real world: Severe accident victims react to their lot. *Journal of Personality and Social Psychology, 35,* 351–363.

Cannon, C. E. (2001). The influence of religious orientation and white racial identity on expressions of prejudice. *Dissertation Abstracts International-B, 62,* 598.

Chilman, C. S. (1980). *Adolescent sexuality in a changing American society: Social and psychological perspectives.* Washington, DC: U.S. Department of Health, Education, and Welfare.

Christie, D. J., Wagner, R. V., & Winter, D. D. N. (2001). *Peace, conflict and violence: Peace psychology for the 21st century.* Upper Saddle River, NJ: Prentice Hall.

Clary, E. G., & Snyder, M. (1991). A functional analysis of altruism and prosocial behavior: The case of volunteerism. In M. Clark (Ed.), *Prosocial behavior* (pp. 119–148). Newbury Park, CA: Sage.

Clary, E. G., & Snyder, M. (1993). Persuasive communications strategies for recruiting volunteers. In D. R. Young, R. M. Hollister, & V. A. Hodgkinson (Eds.), *Governing, leading, and managing nonprofit organizations* (pp. 121–137). San Francisco: Jossey-Bass.

Cnaan, R. (2002). *The invisible caring hand: American congregations and the provision of welfare.* New York: New York University Press.

Cochran, J. K., & Beeghley, L. (1991). The influence of religion on attitudes toward nonmarital sexuality: A preliminary assessment of reference group theory. *Journal for the Scientific Study of Religion, 30,* 45–62.

Colasanto, D. (1989, November). Americans show commitment to helping those in need. *Gallup Report, No. 290,* 17–24.

Connolly, P. (1999). Psychological approaches. In P. Connolly (Ed.), *Approaches to the study of religion* (pp. 135–192). London: Continuum.

de Silva, P. (2000). *An introduction to Buddhist psychology* (3rd ed.). Lanham, MD: Rowman & Littlefield.

Dittes, J. E. (1971). Typing the typologies: Some parallels in the career of church-sect and extrinsic–intrinsic. *Journal for the Scientific Study of Religion, 10,* 375–383

Donahue, M. J. (1985). Intrinsic and extrinsic religiousness: Review and meta-analysis. *Journal of Personality and Social Psychology, 48,* 400–419.

Ellison, C. G., Bartkowski, J. P., & Segal, M. L. (1996). Conservative Protestantism and the parental use of corporal punishment. *Social Forces, 74,* 1003–1028.

Esposito, J. L. (1987). *Islam and politics* (4th ed.). Syracuse, NY: Syracuse University.

Fazio, R. H., Herr, P. M., & Olney, T. J. (1984). Attitude accessibility following a self-perception process. *Journal of Personality and Social Psychology, 47,* 277–286.

Festinger, L., Riecken, H. W., & Schachter, S. (1956). *When prophecy fails: A social and psychological study of a modern group that predicted the destruction of the world.* Minneapolis: University of Minnesota Press.

Fishbein, M., & Ajzen, I. (1974). Attitudes towards objects as predictors of single and multiple behavioral criteria. *Psychological Bulletin, 81,* 59–74.

Fulton, A. S., Gorsuch, R. L., & Maynard, E. A. (1999). Religious orientation, antihomosexual sentiment, and fundamentalism among Christians. *Journal for the Scientific Study of Religion, 38,* 14–22.

Gallup, G., Jr., & Lindsay, D. M. (1999). *Surveying the religious landscape: Trends in U.S. beliefs.* Harrisburg, PA: Morehouse.

Gardella, P. (1985). *Innocent ecstasy: How Christianity gave America an ethic of sexual pleasure.* New York: Oxford University Press.

Gorsuch, R. L., & Aleshire, D. (1974). Christian faith and ethnic prejudice: A review and interpretation of research. *Journal for the Scientific Study of Religion, 13,* 281–307.

Gorsuch, R. L., & McPherson, S. E. (1983). Intrinsic/extrinsic measurement: I/E-revised and single-item scales. *Journal for the Scientific Study of Religion, 28,* 348–354.

Graham, J. (2003). Comments on war in Iraq, March 20, 2003. Accessed March 29, 2003, at www.prestonwood.org/sites/document.asp?=did3100.

Grasmick, H. G., Bursik, R. J., Jr., & Cochran, J. K. (1991). "Render unto Caesar what is Caesar's": Religiosity and taxpayers' inclinations to cheat. *Sociological Quarterly, 32,* 251–266.

Green, J. C. (2004). A liberal dynamo: The political activism of the Unitarian-Universalist clergy. *Journal for the Scientific Study of Religion, 42,* 577–590.

Guth, J. L., Beail, L., Crow, G., Gaddy, B., Montreal, S., Nelsen, B., et al. (2003). The political activity of evangelical clergy in the election of 2000: A case study of five denominations. *Journal for the Scientific Study of Religion, 42,* 501–514.

Guttman, J. (1984). Cognitive morality and cheating behavior in religious and secular school children. *Journal of Educational Research, 77,* 249–254.

Hayes, C. D. (Ed.). (1987). *Risking the future: Adolescent sexuality, pregnancy, and childbearing.* Washington, DC: National Academy Press.

Herek, G. M. (1987). Religious orientation and prejudice: A comparison of racial and sexual attitudes. *Personality and Social Psychology Bulletin, 13,* 34–44.

Hoge, D. R., Zech, C. E., McNamara, P. H., & Donahue, M. J. (1998). The value of volunteers as resources for congregations. *Journal for the Scientific Study of Religion, 37,* 470–480.

Hood, R. W., Jr., & Morris, R. J. (1985). Conceptualization of quest: A critical rejoinder to Batson. *Review of Religious Research, 26,* 391–397.

Hunt, R. A., & King, M. B. (1971). The intrinsic–extrinsic concept: A review and evaluation. *Journal for the Scientific Study of Religion, 10,* 339–356.

Iannaccone, L. R. (1997). Skewness explained: A rational choice model of religious giving. *Journal for the Scientific Study of Religion, 36,* 141–157.

Jackson, L. M., & Esses, V. M. (1997). Of Scripture and ascription: The relation between religious fundamentalism and intergroup helping. *Personality and Social Psychology Bulletin, 23,* 893–906.

James, W. (1985). *The varieties of religious experiences: A study in human nature.* New York: Penguin Classics. (Original work published 1902)

Janus, S. S., & Janus, C. L. (1993). *The Janus report.* New York: Wiley.

Juergensmeyer, M. (2003). *Terror in the mind of God: The global rise of religious violence* (3rd ed.). Berkeley: University of California Press.

Kahle, L. R., & Berman, J. J. (1974). Attitudes cause behaviors: A cross-lagged panel analysis. *Journal of Personality and Social Psychology, 37,* 315–321.

Katz, R. C., Santman, J., & Lonero, P. (1994). Findings on the revised Morally Debatable Behaviors Scale. *Journal of Psychology, 128,* 15–21.

Keen, S. (1986). *Faces of the enemy: Reflections of the hostile imagination.* San Francisco: Harper & Row.

Kirkpatrick, L. A. (1989). A psychometric analysis of the Allport–Ross and Feagin measures of intrinsic–extrinsic religious orientation. *Research in the Social Scientific Study of Religion, 2,* 3–28.

Kirkpatrick, L. A., & Hood, R. W., Jr. (1990). Intrinsic–extrinsic religious orientation: The boon or bane of contemporary psychology of religion? *Journal for the Scientific Study of Religion, 29,* 442–462.

Kolodny, A. N. (1997, September). *National churches in the context of national renaissance of*

Ukraine. Paper presented at the conference Religion at the End of the Twentieth Century, Sevastopol, Ukraine.

Kothari, S. (1994). Impact of religion upon development of moral concepts. *Psycho-Lingua, 24*(2), 65–72.

Lam, P.-Y. (2001). May the force of the operating system be with you: Macintosh devotion as implicit religion. *Sociology of Religion, 62,* 243–262.

Laythe, B., Finkel, D., & Kirkpatrick, L. A. (2001). Predicting prejudice from religious fundamentalism and right-wing authoritarianism: A multiple-regression approach. *Journal for the Scientific Study of Religion, 40,* 1–10.

Lundblad, R. T. (2002). Social, religious, and personal contributors to prejudice. *Dissertation Abstracts International-B, 63,* 589.

Lupton, H. E. (1986). Use of the notion "implicit religion" in psychological study: A discussion paper. In J. A. Belzen & J. M. van der Lans (Eds.), *Current issues in the psychology of religion: Proceedings of the Third Symposium on the Psychology of Religion in Europe* (pp. 44–55). Amsterdam, The Netherlands: Rodopi.

Macapagal, M. E. J., & Nario-Galace, J. (2003). Social psychology of People Power II in the Philippines. *Peace and Conflict: Journal of Peace Psychology, 9,* 219–233.

Marty, M. E., & Appleby, R. S. (Eds.). (1993a). *Fundamentalisms and society: Reclaiming the sciences, the family, and education.* Chicago: University of Chicago Press.

Marty, M. E., & Appleby, R. S. (Eds.). (1993b). *Fundamentalisms and the state: Remaking polities, economies, and militance.* Chicago: University of Chicago Press.

McGlone, G. J. (2004). The pedophile and the pious: Towards a new understanding of sexually offending and non-offending Roman Catholic priests. *Journal of Aggression, Maltreatment and Trauma, 8,* 115–131.

Morrison, M. A., & Morrison, T. G. (2002). Development and validation of a scale measuring modern prejudice toward gay men and lesbian women. *Journal of Homosexuality, 43,* 15–27.

Muste, A. J. (2002). *Of holy disobedience.* Wallingford, PA: Pendle Hill. (Original work published 1952)

Myers, D. M. (1992). *The pursuit of happiness.* New York: Morrow.

National Council of Churches. (2003). *Taking action to avert war.* Accessed March 17, 2003, at www.ncccusa.org.

National Review Board for the Protection of Children and Young People. (2004). *A report on the crisis in the Catholic Church in the United States.* Washington, DC: United States Conference of Catholic Bishops.

Nielsen, M. E. (2004, Spring). Mormonism and psychology: A broader vision for peace. *Dialogue: A Journal of Mormon Thought, 37*(1), 109–132.

Oliner, S. P., & Oliner, P. M. (1988). *The altruistic personality: Rescuers of Jews in Nazi Europe.* New York: Free Press.

Omoto, A. M., Snyder, M., & Berghuis, J. P. (1993). The psychology of volunteerism: A conceptual analysis and a program of action research. In J. B. Pryor & G. D. Reeder (Eds.), *The social psychology of HIV infection* (pp. 333–356). Hillsdale, NJ: Erlbaum.

Ostrom, T. M. (1969). The relationship between the affective, behavioral, and cognitive components of attitude. *Journal of Experimental Social Psychology, 5,* 12–30.

Pargament, K. I. (2001). *The psychology of religious coping: Theory, research, practice.* New York: Guilford Press.

Pennock, M. (2000). *Catholic social teaching: Learning and living justice.* New York: Ave Maria Press.

Perrin, R. D. (2000). Religiosity and honesty: Continuing the search for the consequential dimension. *Review of Religious Research, 41,* 534–544.

Pettigrew, T. F. (2003). Peoples under threat: Americans, Arabs, and Israelis. *Peace and Conflict: Journal of Peace Psychology, 9,* 69–90.

Reis, H. T., & Judd, C. M. (Eds.). (2000). *Handbook of research methods in social and personality psychology.* New York: Cambridge University Press.

Richardson, J. T., Best, J., & Bromley, D. G. (Eds.). (1991). *The satanism scare.* New York: Aldine de Gruyter.

Rodriguez, E. M., & Ouellette, S. C. (2000). Gay and lesbian Christians: Homosexual and religious identity integration in the members of a gay-positive church. *Journal for the Scientific Study of Religion, 39,* 333–347.

Rozell, M. J. (2003). Evangelicals inside the beltway. *Religion in the 2004 Election* [Special supplement]. *Religion in the News, 6*(3), pp. 6, 18.

Salancik, G. R., & Conway, M. (1975). Attitude inferences from salient and relevant cognitive content about behavior. *Journal of Personality and Social Psychology, 32,* 827–840.

Schuck, K. D., & Liddle, B. J. (2001). Religious conflicts experienced by lesbian, gay, and bisexual individuals. *Journal of Gay & Lesbian Psychotherapy, 5,* 63–82.

Shea, J. D. (1992). Religion and sexual adjustment. In J. F. Schumaker (Ed.), *Religion and mental health* (pp. 70–84). New York: Oxford University Press.

Shor, R. (1998). The significance of religion in advancing a culturally sensitive approach towards child maltreatment. *Families in Society, 79,* 400–409.

Slone, D. J. (2004). *Theological incorrectness: Why religious people believe what they shouldn't.* New York: Oxford University Press.

Smith, C. (Ed.). (2004). Clergy as political activists [Special section]. *Journal for the Scientific Study of Religion, 42,* 495–604.

Smith, R. E., Wheeler, G., & Diener, E. (1975). Faith without works: Jesus people, resistance to temptation, and altruism. *Journal of Applied Social Psychology, 5,* 320–330.

Spilka, B., Hood, R. W., Jr., Hunsberger, B., & Gorsuch, R. L. (2003). *The psychology of religion: An empirical approach* (3rd ed.) New York: Guilford Press.

Stark, R. (1999). Secularization, R.I.P. *Sociology of Religion, 60,* 249–273.

Stark, R. (2003). *For the glory of God: How monotheism led to reformations, science, witch-hunts, and the end of slavery.* Princeton, NJ: Princeton University Press.

Taylor, T. S. (2000). Is God good for you, good for your neighbor?: The influence of religious orientation on demoralization and attitudes towards lesbians and gay men. *Dissertation Abstracts International-A, 60,* 4472.

Thurston, N. S. (2000). Evangelical and fundamentalist protestants. In P. S. Richards & A. E. Bergin (Eds.), *Handbook of psychotherapy and religious diversity* (pp. 131–153). Washington, DC: American Psychological Association.

Wicker, A. W. (1969). Attitudes versus actions: The relationship of verbal and overt responses to attitude objects. *Journal of Social Issues, 25,* 41–78.

Wicker, A. W. (1971). An examination of the "other variables" explanation of attitude–behavior inconsistency. *Journal of Personality and Social Psychology, 19,* 18–30.

Wolfe, G., & Mourribi, A. (1985). A comparison of the value systems of Lebanese Christian and Muslim men and women. *Journal of Social Psychology, 125,* 781–782.

Wuthnow, R. (1994). *God and mammon in America.* New York: Free Press.

Wuthnow, R., & Hackett, C. (2004). The social integration of practitioners of non-Western religions in the United States. *Journal for the Scientific Study of Religion, 42,* 651–668.

Young, L. (1996). *Rational choice theory and religion: Summary and assessment.* New York: Routledge.

Zanna, M. P., Olson, J. M., & Fazio, R. H. (1980). Attitude–behavior consistency: An individual difference perspective. *Journal of Personality and Social Psychology, 38,* 432–440.

Zelnik, M., Kantner, J., & Ford, K. (1981). *Sex and pregnancy in adolescence.* Beverly Hills, CA: Sage.

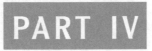

PART IV

THE CONSTRUCTION AND EXPRESSION OF RELIGION

16

Religion and Meaning

CRYSTAL L. PARK

> Religion deals with the highest levels of meaning. As a result, it can interpret each life or each event in a context that runs from the beginning of time to future eternity. Religion is thus uniquely capable of offering high-level meaning to human life. Religion may not always be the best way to make life meaningful, but it is probably the most reliable way.
>
> —BAUMEISTER (1991, p. 205)

Meaning is a central topic in psychology, or perhaps even *the* central topic (Baumeister, 1991). Meaning can be considered fundamental to understanding human nature because it has been defined both very broadly—encompassing many other psychological constructs, such as goals (e.g., Emmons, 1999), beliefs (e.g., Janoff-Bulman & Frantz, 1997; Spilka, Hood, Hunsberger, & Gorsuch, 2003), well-being and satisfaction (e.g., Debats, 2000), and life narrative (Kenyon, 2000)—and very deeply, referring to the core of human existence (e.g., Frankl, 1969). In recent years, psychologists have evinced a resurgent interest in issues of meaning (e.g., Wong & Fry, 1998).

The relationship between religion and meaning is intimate and complex. Because religion serves, for most people, as a lens through which reality is perceived and interpreted (McIntosh, 1995; see Ozorak, Chapter 12, this volume), it is closely tied to concepts of meaning. Like other systems of meaning, religion influences beliefs, goals, and emotions (Silberman, 2005). However, religion is unique in centering on what individuals hold to be sacred (Pargament, Magyar, & Murray-Swank, 2005), and this sacred content is often reflected in individuals' beliefs, goals, and emotions. It has even been proposed that the potent influence of religion on individuals' health and well-being (see Miller & Kelley, Chapter 25, and Oman & Thoresen, Chapter 24, this volume) may be in large part due to its provision of meaning (George, Ellison, & Larson, 2002), although this hypothesis has not yet been put to the test. The aim of this chapter is to describe this relationship between religion and meaning.

ORGANIZATION OF THIS CHAPTER

While research examining "meaning" has recently proliferated, the lack of standard definitions or conceptual frameworks has hampered advancement of our understanding of meaning. That is, researchers often use the same term to refer to different phenomena and different terms to refer to the same phenomenon, and there is, as yet, no widely accepted model of meaning. In an attempt to bring some clarity to this issue, this chapter begins by establishing what "meaning" means, presenting a conceptual model of meaning, and defining terms such as "meaning in life" and "meaning making." While not the main purpose of this chapter, a consideration of concepts and terminology is necessary prior to discussing the material that does constitute the central focus of this chapter, namely, the relations between religion and meaning. After defining terms and presenting a model of meaning and meaning making, this chapter describes how religiousness is involved in global meaning in terms of beliefs, goals, and the subjective sense of meaning, and then discusses the issue of religion and making meaning from stressful or traumatic life situations. The chapter concludes with speculation regarding future research on religion and meaning.

CONCEPTUALIZING MEANING

As Spilka et al. (2003) noted, "Though there is a kind of scientific vagueness to the idea of 'meaning,' no other word seems to capture as well its inherent significance" (p. 15). Defining *meaning* is difficult, perhaps because the very act of definition implies the use of meaning (Baumeister, 1991). In spite of this difficulty, however, a number of psychologists have proffered definitions or descriptions of meaning. Klinger (1998) noted that meaning has two related definitions, to intend (e.g., to aim) and to signify (e.g., the denotation [or connotation] of a word or sentence). Spilka et al. (2003) defined meaning as "the cognitive significance of sensory and perceptual stimulation and information to us" (p. 16), while Baumeister (1991) proposed "shared mental representations of possible relationships among things, events, and relationships," emphasizing that meaning "connects things" (p. 16).

Many authors have described the central role that meaning has in human life. In his book *Meanings of Life*, Baumeister (1991) considered at great length the pervasive nature of meaning, describing how it allows people to predict and control their personal and social environments, and in the process transforms human experience. "Meaning is a tool for adaptation, for controlling the world, for self-regulation, and for belongingness. Indeed, it is the best all-purpose tool on the planet" (Baumeister, 1991, pp. 357–358).

Earlier, Frankl (1969) had described the "will to meaning" as the primary and basic human motive, arguing that the main goal in life is not to gain pleasure or power, but to find meaning and value in life. Further, this meaning is not inherent in life, but must be actively created by each individual. Baumeister (1991) expanded on Frankl's ideas, noting that individuals actively construct the meaning of their lives on a daily basis, and that meaning is part of every action and thought. Baumeister went so far as to describe the human need for meaning as a craving, a desire, even an addiction (complete with tolerance and withdrawal).

Meaning, then, is central to human existence. In this chapter, two basic aspects of meaning are considered, *global meaning* and *meaning making* in crises or difficult circumstances. Figure 16.1 presents a model of the components of global meaning and illustrates how global meaning can be expressed in daily life. The lower part of Figure 16.1 presents the meaning-making process.

"Global meaning" (Park & Folkman, 1997) refers to general meaning in life, and consists of three aspects: beliefs, goals, and subjective feelings (cf. Reker & Wong's [1988] tripartite model of personal meaning, consisting of cognitive, motivational, and affective components). Global meaning is important both in general patterns of everyday life and in situations of adversity (Silberman, 2005). Global beliefs (also called "assumptive worlds," "personal theories," or "worldviews"; see Silberman, 2005; Janoff-Bulman, 1989) are widely encompassing beliefs such as fairness, justice, luck, control, predictability, coherence, benevolence, and personal vulnerability. These beliefs form the core schemas through which people interpret their experiences of the world (Janoff-Bulman & Frantz, 1997).

"Global goals" refer to those ideals, states, or objects that people hold most important in life, those that they work toward being or achieving or maintaining (Karoly, 1999). Goals are nested in hierarchies, with lower level goals leading to higher level goals (Vallacher & Wegner, 1987), and inform plans, activities, and behaviors (Silberman, 2005). Common global life goals include relationships, work, wealth, knowledge, and achievement (Emmons, 1999). Important goals can also include the converse of obtaining something, such as avoiding states that one fears or rejects (e.g., Silberman, 2005; Emmons, 1999). Further—although often overlooked—a central aspect of global goals involves maintaining objects or states that one already has, such as health or relationships with loved ones (Klinger, 1998).

Although, ideally, people live according to a series of short-term, concrete goals that lead to the achievement of their higher level goals, individuals' behavior often does not

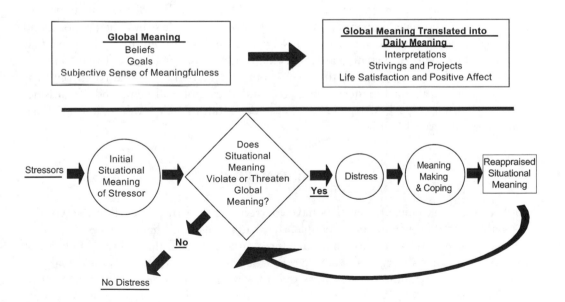

Note: Religion is often part of global meaning (beliefs, goals, and subjective sense of meaningfulness).

FIGURE 16.1. Model of life meaning.

closely match their expressed goals (Baumeister, 1991). Therefore, rather than asking directly about global goals, researchers sometimes infer them through indicators such as the amount of time, energy, resources, or money spent in their pursuit (e.g., Mahoney et al., in press).

A subjective "sense of meaning" refers to feelings of "meaningfulness," that is, a sense of meaning or purpose in life (Reker & Wong, 1988). Klinger (1977) described meaningfulness as feeling that one has purpose or direction, as in having plans and intentions. He noted that it is "very subjective, a pervasive quality of a person's whole inner life . . . experienced both as ideas and as emotions" (1977, p. 10). This sense of meaningfulness is derived from seeing one's actions as oriented toward a desired future state or goal. Importantly, those states or goals do not ever have to be realized or achieved in order to experience meaningfulness; the sense of being headed in the direction of, rather than actually achieving, ultimate goals creates the sense of meaningfulness (Baumeister, 1991). This construct of meaningfulness is often the focus of researchers who purportedly measure "meaning in life," but more accurately are measuring participants' *sense* of meaning in life or of goal-directedness (Baumeister, 1991), typically using measures such as the Life Regard Index (Debats, 1998) or the Purpose in Life Test (Crumbaugh & Maholick, 1964). Using items such as "I feel that I am living fully" (Debats, 1998), these scales aim to assess the amount of this subjective feeling that one's life has meaning.

Global meaning systems are usually constructed unwittingly, acquired from the surrounding culture (including parents, media, and other cultural agents) and through accumulated personal experiences (Baumeister, 1991; Singer & Salovey, 1991), and tend to remain outside of people's awareness (Baumeister, 1991; Silberman, 2005). If asked to directly focus on and report on their global beliefs and goals, people may be able to, but generally they are engaged in the daily business and busyness of life and do not reflect deeply on this level of their existence (Klinger, 1998). Regardless of their awareness of global meaning, however, it exerts powerful influences on people's thoughts, actions, and feelings, and gets translated into their daily lives through interpretations (the ways that they understand daily occurrences as well as major life events), strivings or personal projects (smaller, more concrete goals that people pursue on a daily basis, derived from their longer term, more abstract higher order goals), and a sense of well-being and life satisfaction (e.g., Emmons, 1999; Wong, 1998). These powerful influences of religion on global meaning are described below.

MEANING MAKING

People typically have beliefs that they have control over their own lives, that the world is reasonably fair, that they are good people, that bad things don't happen to good people, and that God is good and is looking after them and protecting them (Janoff-Bulman & Frantz, 1997). They also typically have a sense that they are on track with their goal pursuits, getting and maintaining the things that they want or hold most important in their lives (Baumeister, 1991). When something traumatic occurs, such as a diagnosis of cancer or the death of a child, both global beliefs (such as fairness or invulnerability) and global goals (such as continued health or a continued relationship with one's child) are violated, and people may experience a sense of meaninglessness (Baumeister, 1991). When these violations occur, people may become more aware of their global meaning systems, while their daily concerns fade into the background (Silberman, 2005).

Meaning making, in contrast to meaning in life, refers to a *process* of working to restore global life meaning when it has been disrupted or violated, typically by some major unpleasant or terrible life event. A number of stress and trauma theories emphasize that distress arises when something occurs that violates a person's global beliefs and goals (e.g., Janoff-Bulman, 1989; see Park & Folkman, 1997, for a review). Traumatic events can precipitate crises of meaning by raising questions about the purpose of life and the nature of suffering and justice in the world, leaving people struggling to understand why the events occurred and what the implications will be for their future (Lazarus, 1993). When individuals encounter stressful events, they appraise the meaning of the event (i.e., "What has happened?") and then determine the extent to which this appraised meaning is discrepant from their global meaning. The extent of this discrepancy (i.e., the extent to which the appraised meaning violates an individual's basic beliefs and goals) determines the level of distress that the events cause (Park & Folkman, 1997; see lower part of Figure 16.1).

Discrepancies between appraised and global meaning create a very unpleasant state, involving a sense of loss of control, predictability, or comprehensibility of the world. People tend to be quite motivated to reduce this discrepancy (Janoff-Bulman & Frantz, 1997; see Park & Folkman, 1997, for a review). "Meaning making" refers to the process of coming to see the situation in a different way and reviewing and reforming one's beliefs and goals in order to regain consistency among them. The processes through which people reduce this discrepancy involve changing the appraised meaning of the situation (i.e., reappraisal), changing their global beliefs and goals, or both, to achieve integration of the appraised (or eventually reappraised) meaning of the event into their global meaning system (Klinger, 1998; Parkes, 1996).

RELIGION AND GLOBAL MEANING

Religion is often invoked when discussing meaning in life. Religion, which can be defined as "a search for significance in ways related to the sacred"(Pargament, 1997, p. 32; see Zinnbauer & Pargament, Chapter 2, this volume), is central to the global meaning systems of many people, although its importance varies greatly among individuals. But does religion give rise to a need for meaning? Or does the need for meaning give rise to religion? Many have argued that, in fact, religion grows out of the need to understand or to find something comprehensible in the existential problems that humans face (Baumeister, 1991; Kotarba, 1983). Geertz (1966) asserted that religions provide possibilities that beneath the surface of the vicissitudes of life that seem beyond understanding, such as suffering and death, there is a basic pattern or rationale of order and purpose.

Regardless of whether religion arises specifically out of this need for meaning or simply helps to establish it for people who embrace religion for other reasons, many lines of research yield evidence for the wide-ranging and often central involvement of religion in global life meaning, as will be discussed below. The extensive, nearly universal, reliance on religious meaning systems may be due to that fact that, compared to secular meaning systems, religion is typically more comprehensive (Spilka, Shaver, & Kirkpatrick, 1995) and more existentially satisfactory (Emmons, 1999; Pargament, Ano, & Wachholtz,

Chapter 26, this volume). Further, religious meaning systems tend to be relatively immune from disconfirmation (Emmons, 1999). Pargament and his colleagues noted: "The
language of religion—faith, hope, transcendence, surrender, forbearance, meaning—
speaks to the limits of human powers. When life appears out of control, and there seems
to be no rational explanation for events—beliefs and practices oriented to the sacred
seem to have a special ability to provide ultimate meaning, order, and safety in place of
human questions, chaos, and fear" (Pargament et al., 2005).

RELIGION AND GLOBAL BELIEFS

Religious belief systems can provide individuals with comprehensive and integrated
frameworks of meaning that enable them to explain events in the world in highly satisfactory ways (Spilka et al., 2003). These frameworks of meaning are particularly important
in interpreting and responding to the most challenging aspects of life, such as suffering,
death, tragedy, and injustice (e.g., Pargament, 1997), but religion provides a way of un
derstanding mundane occurrences as well as extraordinary ones (e.g., Geyer & Baumeister,
Chapter 23, this volume; Spilka et al., 2003).

In addition to explicitly religious beliefs, such as the existence of God and the possibility of an afterlife, religion can inform and influence other global beliefs that are less explicitly religious, such as beliefs in fairness, control, coherence, benevolence of the world
and other people, and vulnerability (Pargament, 1997). For example, in describing the
just world theory (Lerner, 1980), Janoff-Bulman and Frantz (1997) noted that "theories
of deservingness generally encompass many religious perspectives, which enable believers
to perceive meaning through the expectations of rewards and punishments that may be
considerably delayed, such as one's fate after death" (p. 93). The influence of religion on
global beliefs is far-reaching. When religion is incorporated into people's global meaning
systems, their understanding of God or of the divine (e.g., as loving and benevolent, as
wrathful) are connected to beliefs about the nature of people (e.g., inherent goodness,
made in God's image, sinful human nature), of the self (e.g., as unworthy of God, as chosen), and of this world (e.g., the coming apocalypse, the illusory nature of reality) as well
as, perhaps, the next (e.g., Heaven, reincarnation) (McIntosh, 1995; Silberman, 2005).

RELIGION AND GLOBAL GOALS

Regarding global goals, religion is central to the life purposes of many people, providing
their ultimate motivation and primary goals for living as well as prescriptions and guidelines for achieving those goals (e.g., Baumeister, 1991; Pargament, 1997). Ultimate goals
can include connecting with or adhering to the sacred; living a life full of benevolence,
forgiveness, or altruism; achieving enlightenment; finding salvation; knowing God or experiencing the transcendent (Emmons, 1999; Pargament et al., 2005). Other goals can be
derived from these superordinate ones, including having peace of mind, working for
peace and justice in the world, devoting oneself to one's family, or finding deep intimacy
with others. Of course, it must be noted, people often embrace negative goals, such as
achieving supremacy and promoting destruction, in the name of religion as well (see
Silberman, Chapter 29, this volume). While some goals are explicitly religious or spiritual, each and every goal that an individual holds may become connected to the sacred

through the process of sanctification (e.g., Mahoney et al., in press). *Sanctification* is the act of assigning spiritual significance and character to secular objects (Mahoney et al., 1999). Therefore, any goal can take on religious value if the individual ties it to his or her conceptualization of the sacred (Pargament et al., 2005).

Related to goals are *values*, the guidelines that individuals use to determine worth, importance, or correctness (Schwartz & Bilsky, 1990). Religion is an extremely potent source of values for individuals as well as for entire cultures (Baumeister, 1991). Religion supplies a framework for determining what is right and good and to be sought after, and for determining what is wrong and bad and to be avoided. Since divine will can be considered the ultimate arbiter of right and wrong (Baumeister, 1991; Emmons, 1999), religions are in an unusually esteemed position to be able to determine or establish these criteria of right and wrong and good and bad; they may, in fact, be the most powerful source of values in many cultures (Baumeister, 1991).

Very little research has directly examined religion and values. Examining values cross-culturally, Schwartz and Huismans (1995) found that in those countries in which people reported highly valuing certainty, self-restraint, and submission over superior external truths, the people were more religious in general, while citizens in countries valuing openness to change and free self-expression were less religious.

RELIGION AND THE SUBJECTIVE SENSE OF MEANING IN LIFE

While the connections between religion and meaning in life may seem obvious, surprisingly few studies have specifically documented these connections, and most of the research has examined bivariate relations of fairly simple measures of religion and sense of purpose. Religiousness does seem to be related to a sense of meaning in life (Donahue, 1985; Tomer & Eliason, 2000), but the strength of these relations is modest (e.g., Chamberlain & Zika, 1988, 1992). It appears that religion is more strongly related to a sense of life meaning in the elderly (Ardelt, 2003; Krause, 2003), and that it is stronger for older black adults as compared to older white adults (Krause, 2003). Further, it may be that only some aspects of religion are related to a sense of meaning in life. Intrinsic religiousness was found to be more strongly positively related to meaning in life than was extrinsic religiousness in studies of both undergraduates (Bolt, 1975) and community-dwelling elders (Ardelt, 2003); in fact, Ardelt's (2003) study found that extrinsic religiousness was inversely related to a sense of meaning in life.

While higher levels of religion appear to be related to higher levels of life meaning, studies have also found that people often report that they derive their meaning in life from other sources (Delbridge, Headey, & Wearing, 1994). These studies suggest that those who are less religious may achieve a subjective sense of meaningfulness via the pursuit of other valued aspects of life, such as achievement, relationships with family and friends, intimacy, acceptance, and social justice (Delbridge et al., 1994; Wong, 1998).

RELIGION AND GLOBAL MEANING TRANSLATED INTO DAILY LIFE

Religion is pervasively present in the global meaning of many individuals, and they experience religious influences on a continual basis through their interpretations of daily events, the structure and motivations of their daily lives, and their general levels of mood and life satisfaction. For example, beliefs in salvation can influence an individual's understanding of his or her life, provide guidance regarding which goals to pursue and which decisions to make, and infuse life with a deep sense of purpose. Further, people may find great and ongoing comfort in notions of salvation for the just and ultimate punishment (i.e., the deprivation of eternal life) for the unjust (Hall & Johnson, 2001).

Interpretations

Religious aspects of global beliefs can be central to how one views daily experiences. Baumeister (1991) noted that religions offer their adherents "a set of doctrines about natural and supernatural reality that enable people to understand their broader, ultimate context. Religion guarantees that whatever happens to the individual, no matter how good or bad, will make sense. Thus religious beliefs provide a framework for perceiving, understanding and evaluating daily events, experiencing them as part of a broader pattern" (p. 184). These global religious beliefs continuously influence perceptions and interpretations (Silberman, 2005).

Causal attributions, people's understandings of why a given event occurred, can be of a naturalistic or a religious type (Spilka et al., 2003). For example, naturalistic explanations for illnesses can include stress, injury, pathogens, and weakened immune systems, while religious attributions could include God's efforts to teach, challenge, or punish the afflicted or to teach a lesson to others (Spilka et al., 2003)—although it is quite common for individuals to make naturalistic attributions for the immediate cause of the event but still invoke religious or metaphysical explanations for the more distal attributions (see Park & Folkman, 1997). The likelihood that an individual will make religious or nonreligious attributions for particular experiences or encounter depends, in large part, on the relative availability of global religious and naturalistic beliefs (Spilka et al., 2003) as well as the extent to which the explanatory power of each type of attribution is satisfactory (Spilka et al., 2003). Further, Spilka et al. speculate that religious explanations are most likely to be made in situations of high ambiguity and threat. Some scholars have proposed that the increased options for making benign interpretations and attributions provided by religion may account for its link with well-being, noted below (e.g., Silberman, 2005).

Strivings

As noted above, religion can create goals and prescribe behaviors to achieve these goals. Global goals are pursued through a variety of lower level, more concrete goals. Personal strivings refer to the recurrent or ongoing goals that a person characteristically tries to attain or maintain. Research has established that religion often informs these strivings or personal projects, and that their religious or sacred nature influences individuals' well-being (Emmons, 1999; Emmons, 2005).

According to Emmons (in press), spiritual strivings refer to goals that involve self-transcendence and that concern ultimate questions of meaning and existence. Prototypical of these types of strivings are those that reflect increasing knowledge of a God or a higher power (e.g., reading the Bible on a daily basis) or concern tending to one's ongoing relationship with God or a higher power (e.g., saying daily prayers).

In addition to strivings or personal projects that are explicitly religious or spiritual in nature, Mahoney and her colleagues have recently suggested that virtually any personal striving could be perceived by its owner as having spiritual significance and character (Mahoney et al., in press). In other words, they argue that a wide range of personal strivings may be invested with spiritual meaning, rather than only strivings that expressly discuss God, spiritual activities, or values that have been espoused in religious literature. In their study of a community sample of adults, Mahoney and her colleagues (in press) found that people often considered their strivings to be sacred even when they were not explicitly spiritual or religious. However, they found that participants rated strivings that explicitly involved religious and spiritual issues as more highly sanctified than their other strivings. They concluded that personal strivings that are concerned with things beyond the self are more likely to be characterized in sacred, transcendent terms than are strivings that are focused on the self or on material possessions.

The types of goals that people pursue have been related to general levels of well-being (see Emmons, 1999, for a review). Religious and sacred goals appear to be related to higher levels of well-being and psychological adjustment. Emmons, Cheung, and Tehrani (1998) found that people whose strivings made explicit reference to God or a higher power had higher levels of life satisfaction and marital satisfaction and lower levels of depression. The study of spiritual strivings by Mahoney et al. (in press) yielded a more complex picture. Consistent with their expectations, the more that participants rated their personal strivings as reflecting the spiritual realm (i.e., sanctified), the more they reported deriving happiness and a sense of meaning in their pursuit. However, greater sanctification of strivings was not consistently related to mental or physical well-being or life satisfaction. According to their interpretation of these results, pursuing self-transcendent and sacred goals involves considerable effort and sacrifice such that individuals may find a high sense of fulfillment in sacred strivings but they may encounter many challenges and difficulties in their pursuit.

Religion and Subjective Well-Being

In both large-scale surveys and more in-depth studies in the United States and worldwide, positive associations are typically found between religiosity and general well-being (Delbridge et al., 1994; Silberman, 2005), particularly for older adults (e.g., Chamberlain & Zika, 1988; Willits & Crider, 1988). It is important to note, however, that the results of large-scale surveys indicate relations between various aspects of religion and life satisfaction are quite modest. For example, Diener and Clifton (2002) cite results of a national U.S. survey of over 50,000 people that found small correlations between religiosity and life satisfaction ($r =. 08$) and between religiosity and happiness ($r =.06$). These correlations were highly statistically significant given the large sample size.

Several different explanations for this consistent positive relation between religiousness and well-being have been proposed. Some argue that religion's association with life satisfaction may be mediated through a sense of meaning in life (Ardelt, 2003; Chamberlain & Zika, 1992). Others have contended that religion may, on a continual basis, lead to the assignment of more positive meanings to ordinary daily events (Geyer & Baumeister, Chapter 23, this volume), which may, in turn, generate positive emotions such as joy, serenity, awe, gratitude, and hope (Frederick, 2002). For example, a belief about a loving personal God, particularly one with whom an individual has an intimate relationship, may have a general salutary effect on emotional well-being (Silberman, 2005). Religious or sacred goal pursuits, as noted above, may lead to general feelings of satisfaction and fulfillment, in part because they comprise more comprehensive and integrated patterns of goals (Emmons, 1999). Finally, religiousness can provide a sense of having ultimate control, through either primary or secondary means, such as through prayer, that is strongly related to general well-being (Rothbaum, Weisz, & Snyder, 1982; Spilka et al., 2003).

Some scholars have noted that, in spite of the general positive relations between religion and well-being, religiousness can also exert damaging or negative influences on well-being. For example, some forms of religiousness encourage a surrender of control and a placement of control in powerful others, while other forms espouse very negative views of humans (e.g., as wicked and sinful) that may lead to self-devaluation, particularly if one does not strictly follow the tenets of one's religion (Exline, 2002).

Crises, Religion, and the Making of Meaning

The previous section describes religion and meaning as applied primarily to life "in general," or under conditions that are typically considered to comprise the "status quo." In addition to these general influences of religion, there are the very potent influences of religion in those life situations that are beyond the ordinary, involving great stress or loss, challenging individuals' most deeply held beliefs and purposes. Crises trigger processes of meaning making through which individuals struggle to reduce the discrepancy between their appraised meaning of a particular stressful event and their global beliefs and goals (Baumeister & Vohs, 2002; Park & Folkman, 1997).

Pargament (1997) described the power of religion to transform the meaning of events in this way: "When the sacred is seen working its will in life's events, what first seems random, nonsensical and tragic is changed into something else—an opportunity to appreciate life more fully, a chance to be with God, a challenge to help others grow, or a loving act meant to prevent something worse from taking place" (p. 223). It is in these times of greatest stress and of searching for meaning that religion seems to exert its most pronounced influence (McIntosh, Silver, & Wortman., 1993; Pargament, 1997). There are at least two reasons for religion's prominence in times of crisis: (1) because, for most people, religion is part of their global beliefs and goals, which may be threatened or violated by traumatic events, and (2) because most religions provide ways of understanding, reinterpreting, and adding value to difficulties and suffering as well as ways to see the work of a loving God (Park, 2005). For people experiencing injustice, suffering, or trauma, a religious belief system and its associated goals may be the most unfailing way to make meaning from their experiences.

As noted above, religion as a framework for understanding experience can strongly influence individuals' initial appraisals, or assignment of meaning to particular events. Following those events determined to be highly stressful, individuals have a number of ways of meaning-making coping, involving changing the appraised meaning of the events by understanding them in a different and less stressful way (e.g., by understanding the suffering as having redeeming value, or by searching for positive aspects of the event; Baumeister, 1991), or by changing the global beliefs and goals that were violated to bring them more in line with their current understanding of what has happened (Pargament, 1997; Park & Folkman, 1997). Finally, religion can be highly involved in the positive changes that individuals report following stressful experiences (Park, 2004). The following sections describe how religion is involved in meaning making through the processes of initial appraisals, meaning-making coping (both changing appraised meaning and changing global meaning), and outcomes of the meaning-making process, including adjustment and stress-related growth.

Initial Appraisals

The same event can be viewed quite differently depending on individuals' specific views, including their religious beliefs. Religious beliefs provide many options for understanding the meaning of an event, including the notions that there is a larger plan, that events are not random, or that personal growth can arise from struggle. Some individuals may believe that God would not harm them or visit upon them more than they could handle, whereas others may believe that God is trying to communicate something important through the event, or that the event is a punishment from God (Furnham & Brown, 1992). For example, a study of hospice caregivers found that some caregivers appraised their situation as part of God's plan or as a way to gain strength or understanding from God, while others viewed their situation as a punishment from God (Mickley, Pargament, Brandt, & Hipp, 1998). Specific religious beliefs can lead directly to understandings of particular events. For example, Benore and Park (2004) described how death could be appraised very differently—and bereavement experienced very differently—depending on beliefs about the afterlife. Many people believe that the deceased continue to exist, that they will be reunited with the deceased after death, and even that they can continue to interact with the deceased currently, albeit in a different way. One prospective study of bereaved elders in Japan found that those with positive afterlife beliefs reported lower blood pressure (Krause et al., 2002). Some denominations have specific views on death that influence adherents' understandings of it. In a study of bereavement, a sample of Spiritualists and Christian Scientists completely denied the importance of death, noted that the situation did not call for grief, and claimed that they did not experience grief (Gorer, 1965, cited in McIntosh, 1995).

Religion and Meaning-Making Coping

If an event is determined to be discrepant with one's global beliefs and goals, attempts at meaning-making coping—the process of reappraising a situation and thinking through its implications—will follow. The eventual outcomes of this meaning-making coping are changes in appraised meaning of the stressful event, and sometimes changes in global meaning. Because religious beliefs, like other basic beliefs, tend to be relatively stable, people confronting crises are more likely to reappraise their perceptions of situations to fit their preexisting beliefs than to change their religious beliefs (Pargament, 1997). Once meaning has been made (i.e., the event is integrated satisfactorily into one's global meaning system), the distress will be alleviated (Baumeister, 1991; Janoff-Bulman & Frantz, 1997).

Changes in Appraised Meaning

Religion can be involved in reappraisals, or changes in situational meaning, by offering additional possibilities for causal attributions and by illuminating other aspects of stressful situations. While, theoretically, reappraisals can be either positive or negative, the motivation to reduce stress generally leads to placing stressful situations in more positive contexts by giving them a more acceptable meaning, one more consistent with global beliefs and goals. As reviewed below, numerous lines of research suggest that religion is often involved in these attempts to make more benign attributions and to facilitate the perception of positive aspects of stressful situations.

Religious Reattributions

As noted above, attributions involve the understanding of *why* an event occurred. Although initial attributions may be made following a trauma or crisis, a search for more acceptable reasons for the event's occurrence in the months following it is common (Davis, Nolen-Hoeksema, & Larson, 1998). People often make reattributions that help to alleviate their initial distress (Park & Folkman, 1997). For example, people may initially feel that God neglected to care for them or even deliberately and unjustly caused their trauma. Over time, however, people often come to see the stressful event as the will of a loving or purposeful God, even if it is a God who is inscrutable and beyond human understanding (Spilka et al., 2003).

Religion offers many avenues for making positive reattributions, and is frequently invoked in the search for a more acceptable reason why an event occurred than what one may have originally made, attributions that are more consistent with the individuals' global beliefs and goals. For example, people can come to see the stressful event as a spiritual opportunity, as the result of a punishing God, or as the result of human sinfulness (Pargament, 1997). Baumister (1991) wrote of the "attributional blank check" that many religions have, that possibility of believing that God many have higher purposes that humans cannot understand, so that one may remain convinced that events that seem highly aversive may, in fact, be serving desirable ends, even if one is unable to guess what these ends might be. Thus, religious explanations can allow religious individuals to trust that every event, regardless of its initial appearance and painfulness, is part of God's plan (Baumeister, 1991).

The meaning-making reattributions for stressful encounters that help to sustain global religious beliefs may appear to use somewhat convoluted reasoning. For example, in a study examining the attributions that bereaved college students made for their friends' deaths approximately 7 months after the deaths, one participant explained that her friend, who had been killed by a drunken driver who ran over the curb and struck her on the sidewalk, was entirely responsible for her own death and that God was not at all responsible. Another student explained that her friend, who had been severely disabled, was not at all responsible for her own death, a suicide, because God had made her the way she was and had given her no other options (Park & Cohen, 1992, cited in Park, 2005). These reattributions illustrate some of the powerful ways that people can manipulate their understandings of events in the service of sustaining their religious beliefs in the face of events that challenge them.

Religion and Positive Reinterpretation

Positive reinterpretation involves identifying and focusing on the benefits or positive implications that may follow from stressful encounters. Positive reinterpretation is a very common, and generally very adaptive, coping response (Aldwin, in press). Many religious traditions emphasize the necessity of, and possible good outcomes of, enduring the difficulties in life (Aldwin, in press). For example, Christian Scripture states, "Not only so, but we also rejoice in our sufferings, because we know that suffering produces perseverance; perseverance, character; and character, hope. And hope does not disappoint us, because God has poured out his love into our hearts by the Holy Spirit, whom he has given us" (Romans 5:3–5).

While few psychologists of religion have studied the concept of theodicy, this area seems to hold great promise for understanding how people come to withstand life's difficulties, even severely traumatic events. *Theodicy* refers to the explanations for human suffering, "philosophical/theological attempts to reconcile the presence of evil and suffering in the world with the idea of an all-powerful and good creator God" (Hall & Johnson, 2001, p. 5).

Hall and Johnson (2001) discussed how individuals can hold only two of the following three propositions simultaneously: God is all powerful, God is all good, and evil exists. They note that people struggle to find some way to believe that these three statements are not logically incompatible or to defend the plausibility of God's existence in the light of these seemingly contradictory propositions. Such struggle to make meaning or to hold onto one's beliefs in a powerful and loving God when one has personally experienced evil or severe negative trauma can be great (Kushner, 1981; Pargament, 1997).

Several solutions to this dilemma can be found that avoid having to alter one's global meaning system. Hall and Johnson (2001) note that one influential Christian viewpoint holds that goodness can occur only in a world where evil also exists, particularly those virtues that an individual comes to practice only through suffering because of evil, such as patience, mercy, forgiveness, endurance, faith, courage, and compassion. Under this meaning system, one can come to see one's traumatic or stressful experience as an opportunity to grow through one's suffering (e.g., to build one's soul, to become more Christ-like, to grow in agape love; Hall & Johnson, 2001). Another solution may be to view one's suffering as necessary for reaching future events, such as one's ultimate goal of salvation (Baumeister, 1991).

Alterations in the appraised meaning of a crisis or trauma usually allow the individual to view the stressful situation in a less distressing way. Religion clearly commonly plays an important role in reappraisals of the meaning of the situation. Although religion commonly facilitates the making of more positive meanings, religious reinterpretations are not always positive. For example, people sometimes come to believe that God harmed them, either through deliberate action or through passivity and neglect. These negative results of the meaning-making process can lead to mistrust, anger, hurt, and disappointment toward God, or even to doubt regarding God's existence (Exline & Rose, Chapter 17, this volume).

Religion and Changes in Global Meaning

Although less common than reappraisals of the particular stressor, traumatic events are sometimes so discrepant with global meaning that no amount of situational reappraisal will restore a sense of congruence with the individual's preexisting global meaning. In these instances, individuals may reduce the discrepancy between their understanding of an event and their global meaning by changing their fundamental global beliefs or goals. Thus, following traumatic events, people sometimes dramatically alter their beliefs about God, themselves, and the world (McCullough, Bono, & Root, Chapter 22, this volume). For example, sometimes those with faith may come to view God as less powerful (Kushner, 1981), or cease to believe in God altogether. Others may come to believe that they are unable to comprehend everything that happens in the world or God's reasoning for it, while others may become convinced of their own sinful nature (Exline & Rose, Chapter 17, this volume; Pargament, 1997). Individuals may change or reprioritize their global goals by, for example, rededicating themselves to their religious commitments or pledging to be more devout (Emmons, Colby, & Kaiser, 1998).

Periods of extreme stress and subsequent difficulties in making meaning from them appear to sometimes lead to instances of the phenomenon of religious conversion, that is, of radical religious transformation (Spilka et al., 2003). Within their new denomination or religion, converts may find alternative systems of purposes and goals that help them answer their difficult questions and solve their life problems (Pargament, 1997; Zinnbauer & Pargament, 1998; see Paloutzian, Chapter 18, this volume, for a review).

Outcomes of the Meaning-Making Process

Adjustment Outcomes

Research suggests that negative events are easier to bear when understood within a benevolent religious framework, and attributions of death, illness, and other major losses to the will of God or to a loving God are generally linked with better outcomes (Pargament, 1997). In a study of adjustment following a major personal loss, making a renewed commitment to spiritual and religious goals, including pleasing God, achieving salvation, and engaging in religious traditions, was strongly related to recovery (Emmons et al., 1998). Another study dramatically illustrates the possibility of negative outcomes of religious meaning-making coping: elderly medical inpatients' negative religious interpretations of their illness (e.g., seeing their illness as the work of the devil or a result of God's abandonment) were related to higher rates of subsequent mortality, even after controlling for sociodemographic variables and physical and mental health (Pargament, Koenig, Tarakeshwar, & Hahn, 2001).

As Exline and Rose (Chapter 17, this volume) note, religious reinterpretations are not always positive, and these negative reinterpretations can lead to more distress and negative outcomes. For example, in the study of caregivers of terminally ill patients mentioned earlier, Mickley et al. (1998) found that some caregivers viewed their situation as unfair punishment from God or as desertion by God, which was related to negative psychological adjustment. In general, however, the bulk of available research on the meaning-making process suggests that regaining a consistent worldview is an important part of recovery, although some individuals may develop or maintain negative beliefs about the nature of God and the world.

Few studies have explicitly examined the links between religion, meaning making, and adjustment. A handful of studies of religion and bereavement indicate that religion is involved in complex ways in making meaning following loss. A study of bereaved parents of infants who died from sudden infant death syndrome (SIDS) found that parents' ratings of the importance of religion was positively related to their reports of engaging in searching for meaning shortly after the death, which was related to better adjustment 18 months later (McIntosh et al., 1993). These findings suggest that having strong religious beliefs may sometimes be related to more initial distress, as the devout individuals' positive worldviews are shattered by their sudden and inexplicable loss, yet to eventually achieve better adjustment as the stressful event is integrated into their global meaning through meaning-making coping.

A study of college students coping with the death of a significant other found that religion appeared to be initially related to higher levels of disruption of global beliefs and goals (Park, 2005). Further, religion was associated with more meaning-making coping for those earlier in the bereavement experience, as reflected in higher levels of intrusive thoughts and avoidance. For people whose bereavement had occurred a year earlier, these effects disappeared or even reversed, suggesting a positive association between religion and longer term adjustment.

Taken together, these results are consistent with prior research showing that those higher in religion may experience more initial disruption following bereavement (Park & Cohen, 1993), but indicate that, over time, religion may be associated with better long-term adjustment to trauma and tragedy. However, very little research has addressed these issues of religion, meaning making, and adjustment to traumatic experiences over time, and much more remains to be known.

Stress-Related Growth and Transformation

In addition to the typically assessed adjustment outcomes such as depression and well-being (Aldwin, in press), the possibility of stress-related growth as an outcome of meaning-making coping has recently begun to receive intense empirical attention (Tedeschi & Calhoun, in press; Park, 2004). Some of the changes people report are profound, involving totally reorienting their lives and rededicating themselves to their reconsidered priorities, while others involve smaller changes, such as being more intimate with their loved ones, handling stress in better ways, taking better care of themselves, seeing their own identities more clearly, feeling closer to God, appreciating more the everyday aspects of life, and having the courage to try new things (Park, 2004). Growth appears to come from looking for positive aspects of negative events and identifying some redeeming features of the experience (Park & Fenster, 2004).

The notion that positive changes or transformation can arise from difficult and traumatic experiences is common to many religions (Aldwin, in press). Many religious traditions, such as Buddhism, Judaism, and Christianity contend that spiritual growth occurs primarily during times of suffering. Through suffering, humans develop character, coping skills, and a base of life experience that may enable them to manage future struggles more successfully. Many religions also attempt to cultivate virtues such as compassion, which make people more attuned to the suffering of others (Exline, 2002).

In fact, one of the most consistent findings regarding predictors of positive life change following life stressors or trauma is that religiousness, measured variously as intrinsic religiousness, religious attributions, and religious coping, is a strong predictor of reports of growth. Religiousness has been shown to be related to growth in individuals dealing with a variety of stressful life events, including bereavement (Park & Cohen, 1993), raising an autistic child (Tarakeshwar & Pargament, 2001), being diagnosed with cancer (Tomich & Helgeson, 2004), sexual assault (Frazier, Tashiro, Berman, Steger, & Long, 2004), and testing positive for HIV (Siegel & Schrimshaw, 2000). It has been hypothesized that having a religious framework for understanding, and perhaps also the presence of religious social support, helps individuals to make more meaning from their situation, including identifying positive aspects of the stressful encounter, although this hypothesis awaits empirical examination (Park, 2004).

Further, this growth is often of a religious nature. Growth following stressful encounters generally involves increased coping skills, increased social support and relationships, and deepened or renewed perspectives and philosophies of life (Schaefer & Moos, 1992), and religion can be an element of each of these. Research has found, for example, that following a stressful encounter, many people report feeling closer to God, more sure in their faith, and more religious; they often report using more religious coping and increasing their commitment to their religion and their involvement in their religious community (Emmons et al., 1998; Pargament, 1997).

CLINICAL IMPLICATIONS

Although clinicians and researchers have only very recently begun to focus on the integration of religious and spiritual issues in psychopathology and psychotherapy, this area is currently very popular (see Miller & Kelley, Chapter 25, this volume). Regarding psychopathology, some researchers have been focusing intensely on the role of meaning in producing and maintaining distress, such as in posttraumatic stress disorder. For example, Foa, Ehlers, Clark, Tolin, and Orsillo (1999) emphasize how trauma can violate world assumptions and thereby maintain ongoing distress. However, religious worldviews or assumptions have not been incorporated into this work.

A similar situation exists regarding psychotherapeutic interventions. While many writers have been focusing on incorporating religious and spiritual issues in psychotherapy (e.g., Shafranske, Chapter 27, this volume), very few focus explicitly on issues of meaning and meaning making in their work, although meaning is often implicit. On the other hand, there is a long tradition of incorporating aspects of meaning into psychotherapeutic work (e.g., Frankl, 1969) that remains a vital area of psychotherapy (e.g., Neimeyer, 2001), although religion is not typically addressed in meaning-focused therapies. One of the implications of this chapter is that religion and meaning have much to offer in explicating psychopathology and in conducting psychotherapy.

RECOMMENDATIONS FOR FUTURE RESEARCH ON RELIGION AND MEANING

This chapter has presented a conceptual framework of meaning, including the terminology and constructs that comprise elements of both global and situational meaning, and then described some of the ways that religion is implicated—and indeed pervasive—in the various components of this framework. Taken together, there is a substantial amount of research on religiousness and meaning, but the research to date seems to raise more questions than it answers, and much remains to be learned. Following are some recommendations for future research that follow from the framework presented and the research on religion and meaning that has been conducted to date.

Much more needs to be learned about how religion influences—or comprises—aspects of global meaning. While it is clear that religion can influence global beliefs, goals, and a subjective sense of well-being, the specific forms of these influences is poorly understood. Similarly, it is important to examine the roles that religion and meaning play when individuals encounter traumas or major stressors. Little is known about how religiousness influences the process of dealing with and recovering from highly stressful circumstances or how religious meaning changes through it. Evidence to date suggests that religious meaning can exert both positive and negative influences on coping with highly stressful circumstances, but longitudinal research that tracks these cognitive and affective processes is needed. Further, it is important to examine the directions of the relationships between religion and adjustment. For example, it may be that those who are better off psychologically use more religious meaning-making coping; prospective research is needed to disentangle these relationships. The robust connection between religiousness and positive life changes and growth following stressful situations needs to be examined in further depth. Although assessing veridical positive change is difficult (Park, 2004), it is likely that understanding religious meaning in this context will yield insights into the human capacity for resilience and growth.

In conducting their studies, researchers must remain aware of the strong influences that culture exerts on the global meaning systems of individuals, including their religious meanings (e.g., Tarakeshwar, Stanton, & Pargament, 2003). Further, even within a specific culture, people are influenced by the particular theology, doctrines, and rituals of their own denomination or faith tradition. While some researchers have examined these teachings in the context of health behaviors (see George et al., 2002), the influence of specific theologies, doctrines, and other teachings of various groups on the goals and beliefs, and subsequently sense of well-being, of their adherents (or even those raised in particular traditions), has remained virtually unaddressed (Donahue, 1989). A focus on the specific teachings regarding beliefs (e.g., human nature, sin, the afterlife) and goals (e.g., what is desirable, worthwhile, right) will yield a far richer knowledge of religion and meaning. Further, examining how theodicies influence people's responses to the suffering they observe in the world and the suffering they experience is critical to understanding how people make meaning in those highly stressful times (Hall & Johnson, 2001). Finally, it will be important for future research to grapple with the meaning systems and meaning making of those who define themselves as "spiritual but not religious," as well as those who define themselves as nonspiritual and nonreligious or atheistic (Park, 2005).

REFERENCES

Aldwin, C. M. (in press). *Stress, coping, and development* (2nd ed.). New York: Guilford Press.

Ardelt, M. (2003). Effects of religion and purpose in life on elders' subjective well-being and attitudes toward death. *Journal of Religious Gerontology, 14,* 55–77.

Baumeister, R. F. (1991). *Meanings of life.* New York: Guilford Press.

Baumeister, R. F., & Vohs, K. D. (2002). The pursuit of meaningfulness in life. In C. R. Snyder & S. J. Lopez (Eds.), *The handbook of positive psychology* (pp. 608–618). New York: Oxford University Press.

Benore, E., & Park, C. L. (2004). Death-specific religious beliefs and bereavement: Belief in an afterlife and continued attachment. *The International Journal for the Psychology of Religion, 14,* 1–22.

Bolt, M. (1975). Purpose in life and religious orientation. *Journal of Psychology and Theology, 3,* 116–118.

Chamberlain, K., & Zika, S. (1988). Religiosity, life meaning and well-being: Some relationships in a sample of women. *Journal for the Scientific Study of Religion, 27,* 411–420.

Chamberlain, K., & Zika, S. (1992). Religiosity, meaning in life, and psychological well-being. In J. F. Schumaker (Ed.), *Religion and mental health* (pp. 138–148). New York: Oxford University Press.

Crumbaugh, J. C., & Maholick, L. T. (1964). An experimental study in existentialism: The psychometric approach to Frankl's concept of noogenic neurosis. *Journal of Clinical Psychology, 20,* 200–207.

Davis, C. G., Nolen-Hoeksema, S., & Larson, J. (1998). Making sense of loss and benefiting from the experience: Two construals of meaning. *Journal of Personality and Social Psychology, 75,* 561–574.

Debats, D. L. (1998). Measurement of personal meaning: The psychometric properties of the Life Regard Index. In P. T. P. Wong & P. S. Fry (Eds.), *The human quest for meaning* (pp. 237–259). Mahwah, NJ: Erlbaum.

Debats, D. L. (2000). An inquiry into existential meaning: Theoretical, clinical, and phenomenal perspectives. In G. T. Reker & K. Chamberlain (Eds.), *Exploring existential meaning: Optimizing human development across the life span* (pp. 93–106). Thousand Oaks, CA: Sage.

Delbridge, J., Headey, B., & Wearing, A. J. (1994). Happiness and religious belief. In L. B. Brown (Ed.), *Religion, personality, and mental health* (pp. 50–68). New York: Springer-Verlag.

Diener, E., & Clifton, D. (2002). Life satisfaction and religiosity in broad probability samples. *Psychological Inquiry, 13,* 206–209.

Donahue, M. J. (1985). Intrinsic and extrinsic religiousness: Review and meta-analysis. *Journal of Personality and Social Psychology, 48,* 400–419.

Donahue, M. J. (1989). Disregarding theology in the psychology of religion: Some examples. *Journal of Psychology and Theology, 17,* 329–335.

Emmons, R. A. (1999). *The psychology of ultimate concerns.* New York: Guilford Press.

Emmons, R. A. (2005). Striving for the sacred: Personal goals, life meaning and religion. *Journal of Social Issues, 61*(4).

Emmons, R. A., Cheung, C., & Tehrani, K. (1998). Assessing spirituality through personal goals: Implications for research on religion and subjective well-being. *Social Indicators Research, 45,* 391–422.

Emmons, R. A., Colby, P. M, & Kaiser, H. A. (1998). When losses lead to gains: Personal goals and the recovery of meaning. In P. T. P. Wong & P. S. Fry (Eds.), *The human quest for meaning* (pp. 163–178). Mahwah, NJ: Erlbaum.

Exline, J. J. (2002). Stumbling blocks on the religious road: Fractured relationships, nagging vices, and the inner struggle to believe. *Psychological Inquiry, 13,* 182–189.

Foa, E. B., Ehlers, A., Clark, D. M., Tolin, D. F., & Orsillo, S. M. (1999). The Posttraumatic Cognitions Inventory (PTCI): Development and validation. *Psychological Assessment, 11,* 303–314.

Frankl, V. E. (1969). *The will to meaning.* New York: New American Library.

Frazier, P., Tashiro, T., Berman, M., Steger, M., & Long, J. (2004). Correlates of levels and patterns of positive life changes following sexual assault. *Journal of Consulting and Clinical Psychology, 72,* 19–30.

Frederickson, B. (2002). How does religion benefit health and well-being?: Are positive emotions active ingredients? *Psychological Inquiry, 13,* 209–213.

Furnham, A., & Brown, L. B. (1992). Theodicy: A neglected aspect of the psychology of religion. *The International Journal for the Psychology of Religion, 2,* 37–45.

Geertz, C. (1966). Religion as a cultural system. In M. Banton (Ed.), *Anthropological approaches to the study of religion* (pp. 1–46). London: Tavistock.

George L., Ellison, C. G., & Larson, D. (2002). Explaining the relationships between religious involvement and health. *Psychological Inquiry, 13,* 190–200.

Hall, M. E. L., & Johnson, E. L. (2001). Theodicy and therapy: Philosophical/ethological contributions to the problem of suffering. *Journal of Psychology and Christianity, 20,* 5–17.

Janoff-Bulman, R. (1989). Assumptive worlds and the stress of traumatic events: Applications of the schema construct. *Social Cognition, 7,* 113–136.

Janoff-Bulman, R., & Frantz, C. M. (1997). The impact of trauma on meaning: From meaningless world to meaningful life. In M. Power & C.R. Brewin (Eds.), *The transformation of meaning in psychological therapies* (pp. 91–106). New York: Wiley.

Karoly, P. (1999). A goal systems-self-regulatory perspective on personality, psychopathology, and change. *Review of General Psychology, 3,* 264–291.

Kenyon, G. (2000). Philosophical foundations of existential meaning. In G. T. Reker & K. Chamberlain (Eds.), *Exploring existential meaning* (pp. 7–22). Thousand Oaks, CA: Sage.

Klinger, E. (1977). *Meaning and void*. Minneapolis: University of Minnesota Press.

Klinger, E. (1998). The search for meaning in evolutionary perspective and its clinical implications. In P. T. P. Wong & P. S. Fry (Eds.), *The human quest for meaning* (pp. 27–50). Mahwah, NJ: Erlbaum.

Kotarba, J. A. (1983). Perceptions of death, belief systems, and the process of coping with chronic illness. *Social Science and Medicine, 17,* 681–689.

Krause, N. (2003). Religious meaning and subjective well-being in late life. *Journal of Gerontology: Social Science, 58B,* S160–S170.

Krause, N., Liang, J., Shaw, B. A., Sugisawa, H., Kim, H., & Sugihara, Y. (2002). Religion, death of a loved one, and hypertension among older adults in Japan. *Journals of Gerontology: Psychological Sciences and Social Sciences, 57B,* S96–S107.

Kushner, H. S. (1981). *When bad things happen to good people*. New York: Schocken Books.

Lazarus, R. S. (1993). Coping theory and research: Past, present, and future. *Psychosomatic Medicine, 55,* 234–237.

Lerner, M. J. (1980). *The belief in a just world: A fundamental delusion*. New York: Plenum.

Mahoney, A., Pargament, K. I., Cole, B., Jewell, T., Magyar, G. M., Tarakeshwar, N., & Murray-Swank, N. (in press). A higher purpose: The sanctification of strivings. *The International Journal of the Psychology of Religion*.

McIntosh, D. N. (1995). Religion-as-schema, with implications for the relation between religion and coping. *The International Journal for the Psychology of Religion, 5,* 1–16.

McIntosh, D. N., Silver, R. C., & Wortman, C. B. (1993). Religion's role in adjustment to a negative life event: Coping with the loss of a child. *Journal of Personality and Social Psychology, 65,* 812–821.

Mickley, J. R., Pargament, K. I., Brandt, C. R., & Hipp, K. M. (1998). God and the search for meaning among hospice caregivers. *Hospice Journal, 13,* 1–18.

Neimeyer, R. A. (2001). The language of loss: Grief therapy as a process of meaning reconstruction. In R. A. Neimeyer (Ed.), *Meaning reconstruction and the experience of loss* (pp. 261–292). Washington, DC: American Psychological Association.

Paloutzian R. F., & Silberman, I. (2003). Religion and the meaning of social behavior: Concepts and issues. In P. Roelofsma, J. Corvelyn, & J. van Saane (Eds.), *One hundred years of psychology and religion* (pp. 155–167). Amsterdam, The Netherlands: VU University Press.

Pargament, K. I. (1997). *The psychology of religion and coping*. New York: Guilford Press.

Pargament, K. I., Koenig, H. G., Tarakeshwar, N., & Hahn, J. (2001). Religious struggle as a predictor of mortality among medically ill elderly patients: A two-year longitudinal study. *Archives of Internal Medicine, 161,* 1881–1885.

Pargament, K. I., Magyar, G. M., & Murray-Swank, N. (2005). The sacred and the search for significance: Religion as a unique process. *Journal of Social Issues, 61*(4).

Park, C. L. (2004). The notion of stress-related growth: Problems and prospects. *Psychological Inquiry, 15,* 69–76.

Park, C. L. (2005). Religion as a meaning-making framework in coping with life stress. *Journal of Social Issues, 61*(4).

Park, C. L., & Cohen, L. H. (1993). Religious and non-religious coping with the death of a friend. *Cognitive Therapy and Research, 17,* 561–577.

Park, C. L., & Fenster, J. R. (2004). Stress-related growth: Predictors of occurrence and correlates with psychological adjustment. *Journal of Social and Clinical Psychology, 23,* 195–215.

Park, C. L., & Folkman, S. (1997). Meaning in the context of stress and coping. *General Review of Psychology, 1,* 115–144.

Parkes, C. M. (1996). *Bereavement: Studies of grief in adultlife* (3rd ed.). London: Routledge.

Reker, G. T., & Wong, P. T. P. (1988). Aging as an individual process: Toward a theory of personal meaning. In J. E. Birren & V. L. Bengston (Eds.), *Emergent theories of aging* (pp. 214–246). New York: Springer.

Rothbaum, F., Weisz, J. R., & Snyder, S. S. (1982). Changing the world or changing the self: A two-process model of perceived control. *Journal of Personality and Social Psychology, 42,* 5–37.

Schaefer, J. A., & Moos, R. (1992). Life crises and personal growth. In B. Carpenter (Ed.), *Personal coping: Theory, research, and application* (pp. 149–170). Westport, CT: Praeger.

Schwartz, S. H., & Bilsky, W. (1990). Toward a theory of the universal content and structure of values. *Journal of Personality and Social Psychology, 58,* 878–891.

Schwartz, S. H., & Huismans, S. (1995). Value priorities and religiosity in four Western religions. *Social Psychology Quarterly, 58,* 88–107.

Siegel, K., & Schrimshaw, E. W. (2000). Perceiving benefits in adversity: Stress-related growth in women living with HIV/AIDS. *Social Science and Medicine, 51,* 1543–1554.

Silberman, I. (2005). Religion as a meaning system: Implications for the new millennium. *Journal of Social Issues, 61*(4).

Singer, J. L., & Salovey, P. (1991). Organized knowledge structures and personality: Person schemas, self schemas, prototypes, and scripts. In M. Horowitz (Ed.), *Person schemas and maladaptive interpersonal patterns* (pp. 33–79). Chicago: University of Chicago Press.

Spilka, B., Hood, R. W., Jr., Hunsberger, B., & Gorsuch, R. (2003). *The psychology of religion: An empirical approach* (3rd ed.). New York: Guilford Press.

Spilka, B., Shaver, P. P., & Kirkpatrick, L. A. (1997). A general attribution theory for the psychology of religion. In B. Spilka & D. N. McIntosh (Eds.), *The psychology of religion: Theoretical approaches* (pp. 153–170). Boulder, CO: Westview Press.

Tarakeshwar, N., & Pargament, K. I. (2001). Religious coping in families of children with autism. *Focus on Autism and Other Developmental Disabilities, 16,* 247–260.

Tarakeshwar, N., Stanton, J., & Pargament, K. I. (2003). Religion: An overlooked dimension in cross-cultural psychology. *Journal of Cross-Cultural Psychology, 34,* 377–394.

Tedeschi, R. G., & Calhoun, L. (Eds.). (in press). *Handbook of post-traumatic growth*. Mahwah, NJ: Erlbaum.

Tomer, A., & Eliason, G. (2000). Beliefs about self, life, and death: Testing aspects of a comprehensive model of death anxiety and death attitudes. In A. Tomer (Ed.), *Death attitudes and the older adult* (pp. 137–153). Philadelphia: Brunner-Routledge.

Tomich, P. L., & Helgeson, V. S. (2004). Is finding something good in the bad always good?: Benefit finding among women with breast cancer. *Health Psychology, 23,* 16–23.

Vallacher, R. R., & Wegner, D. M. (1987). What do people think they're doing?: Action identification and human behavior. *Psychological Review, 94,* 3–15.

Willits, F. K., & Crider, D. M. (1988). Religion and well-being: Men and women in the middle years. *Review of Religious Research, 29,* 281–294.

Wong, P. T. P. (1998). Implicit theories of meaningful life and the development of the Personal Meaning Profile. In P. T. P. Wong & P. S. Fry (Eds.), *The human quest for meaning* (pp. 111–140). Mahwah, NJ: Erlbaum.

Wong, P. T. P., & Fry, P. S. (1998). *The human quest for meaning*. Mahwah, NJ: Erlbaum.

Zinnbauer, B. J., & Pargament, K. I. (1998). Spiritual conversion: A study of religious change among college students. *Journal for the Scientific Study of Religion, 37,* 161–180.

17

Religious and Spiritual Struggles

Julie Juola Exline
Ephraim Rose

Any core dimension of human existence has the power to yield both joy and sorrow, and the spiritual side of life is no exception. Religion and spirituality provide potent sources of comfort, direction, and meaning for many people, but they can also be sources of strain and struggle. Individuals sometimes feel angry toward God, or they feel unforgiven by God. They suffer hurts from fellow believers or witness hypocrisy among their leaders. They strive to cultivate virtue in accordance with their beliefs, but sometimes these same belief systems prompt them to condemn themselves when they fall short. Some believers see themselves as victims of supernatural attack.

The idea of religious and spiritual strain is certainly not new to theologians, clergy, spiritual directors, and religious counselors, who have a long history of expertise in these areas. Although empirically oriented psychologists are relative newcomers to this interdisciplinary conversation, their interest seems to be growing. During the past decade, scholars have turned attention to topics such as religious conflict (e.g., Nielsen, 1998; Nielsen & Fultz, 1995), negative religious coping (Pargament, Ano, & Wachholtz, Chapter 26, this volume; Pargament, Koenig, & Perez, 2000; Pargament, Smith, Koenig, & Perez, 1998; Pargament, Zinnbauer, et al., 1998), spiritual struggles and concerns (e.g., Johnson & Hayes, 2003; Murray-Swank, 2003; Pargament, 2002; Pargament, Koenig, Tarakeshwar, & Hahn, 2001; Pargament, Murray-Swank, Magyar, & Ano, 2004), religious strain (Exline, 2002; Exline, Yali, & Sanderson, 2000), spiritual risk (e.g., Fitchett, 1999a, 1999b), and spiritual injury (Lawson, Drebing, Berg, Vincellette, & Penk, 1998). This chapter highlights a few specific struggles and discuss some key challenges that each one presents.

WHY STUDY RELIGIOUS AND SPIRITUAL STRUGGLE?

Within the past several decades, researchers have produced a wealth of new studies documenting potential benefits of religious involvement for health and well-being (for reviews, see George, Ellison, & Larson, 2002; Koenig, McCullough, & Larson, 2001; McCullough, Hoyt, Larson, Koenig, & Thoresen, 2000). This pioneering research has helped to bring religiosity onto the radar screen of mainstream empiricists as a viable topic for study, and it has also prompted development of interventions that are sensitive to faith issues (e.g., Miller, 1999; Richards & Bergin, 2000; Shafranske, 1996). These represent major advances for the psychology of religion.

Yet this emphasis on religion's benefits introduces a potential problem. Casual consumers of this research might embrace a simplistic view of religion or spirituality as a panacea for life's troubles. But although people typically report more comfort than strain in their religious lives, strain is common (Exline et al., 2000; Johnson & Hayes, 2003; Pargament, Smith, et al., 1998). One study of 5,472 university students (Johnson & Hayes, 2003) revealed spiritual distress in over 25% of the sample. Furthermore, spiritual distress predicted suicidal ideation and confusion about values. A 2-year longitudinal study revealed that spiritual struggles predicted higher mortality rates in medically ill elderly patients (Pargament et al., 2001). Anger toward God has been linked with poorer recovery in medical rehabilitation settings, even with other social, psychological, and physical factors controlled (Fitchett, Rybarczyk, DeMarco, & Nicholas, 1999). Spiritual crises can also lead to shaken faith, as shown in studies of religious doubt (Altemeyer & Hunsberger, 1997; Brenner, 1980; Hunsberger, Pratt, & Pancer, 2002), apostasy (Altemeyer & Hunsberger, 1997; Holmes, 2001), and anger at God (Kampani & Exline, 2002).

According to James (1902/2002), a spiritual orientation focusing only on positive themes is incomplete, as it fails to address evil and suffering (Pargament et al., 2004). We agree, and we contend that scholarly attention to spiritual struggles is timely. It will provide greater balance to the empirical literature, and it will increase understanding of everyday spirituality. Knowledge of potential struggles may even help to inoculate seekers against later disenchantment.

Another reason to study religious and spiritual struggle is an optimistic one: such struggles may, paradoxically, enhance people's lives. Growth often occurs through suffering (e.g., Tedeschi, Park, & Calhoun, 1998). As such, neglecting problems of suffering might cause us to overlook vital sources of spiritual transformation and development (Paloutzian, Chapter 18, this volume). Within positive psychology, recent research suggests that life satisfaction is poorly predicted by simple pleasures but well predicted by engagement and meaning (Seligman, 2003). Questions about meaning arise in religious contexts, but they also arise in response to suffering (Park, Chapter 16, this volume; Park & Folkman, 1997). Responses to spiritual suffering can act as turning points, places in which faith can wither or bloom afresh. In keeping with a view of struggles as potential turning points, we suggest some key challenges associated with each type of struggle, along with ways in which interventions might address them.

FOUR TYPES OF RELIGIOUS AND SPIRITUAL STRUGGLE

Our aim is to pique interest in the struggles surrounding religious and spiritual life. Because space constraints prevent an exhaustive overview, we hold the more modest aim of discussing four types of struggles: those involving suffering, virtuous striving, perception of supernatural evil, and social strain. Also, although we include references to various cultures and religious systems, we readily acknowledge that many of our ideas and references reflect a Western, Judeo-Christian bias. This bias reflects oversampling of Western populations in research to date, and it also stems in part from our personal faith commitments and experiences. Rather than trying to be all-inclusive and risking misrepresentation of other faiths, we thought it prudent to focus primarily on the Judeo-Christian traditions about which we are most knowledgeable.

Is God to Blame?: The Challenge of Suffering

All human beings face the problem of suffering. Loved ones die. Floods and tornadoes destroy homes. Accidents, crime, and serious illness shatter the illusion of invulnerability. Acts of abuse steal childhood innocence. Yet suffering is not limited to cases of trauma. People also suffer when they experience garden-variety disappointments—when their prayers seem unanswered or when life events fail to conform to their desires. The ubiquity of suffering is well reflected in traditions such as Buddhism, where it is framed as a core part of human experience.

When faced with suffering, a natural response is to conduct an *attributional search* (Wong & Weiner, 1981), an attempt to pinpoint the source of suffering and the reasons behind it. Sometimes people attribute responsibility to God, in which they believe that God either caused or allowed the suffering. They may hold God partly responsible for suffering even when a human perpetrator exists, as in cases of parental divorce or abandonment, abuse, and romantic infidelity (Exline & Martin, in press). It seems likely that such attributions to God would occur primarily in faith traditions involving a personal, relational God who actively engages with individuals. It would seem more difficult (though not impossible) to attribute suffering to God if God is viewed as an impersonal energy force or an abstract figure far removed from human affairs.

Anger toward God

Attributions to God can provide consolation, particularly if people see the suffering as part of a good plan by God. But people sometimes believe that God deliberately harmed them, failed to heed their requests, or passively allowed their undeserved suffering. In such cases, people can develop intense anger and mistrust toward God (Exline & Martin, in press; Exline, Yali, & Lobel, 1999; Fitchett et al., 1999; Murray-Swank, 2003; Novotni & Petersen, 2001; Pargament, Smith, et al., 1998; Pargament, Zinnbauer, et al., 1998).

Anger toward God seems to be common, at least in the Western world. In the 1988 General Social Survey, 63% of Americans sampled reported that they sometimes felt anger toward God. When undergraduates in a recent study recalled negative events in which they believed God played a role, 50% reported that the event prompted negative feelings toward God (Exline & Bushman, 2004). Confusion and mistrust arose frequently among the students, often accompanying a conviction that God's actions were illogical or unfair (Exline & Martin, in press). These preliminary data come exclusively from U.S. samples, where Judeo-Christian beliefs continue to predominate. We are not aware of any data on the frequency of anger toward God (or gods) in samples focusing on other cultural groups or faith traditions.

Although occasional, transient anger toward God seems common, more prolonged or frequent anger has been linked with global indices of distress and poor adjustment. For example, frequent or unresolved anger toward God has been linked with low self-esteem (Pargament, Zinnbauer, et al., 1998), depression (Exline et al., 1999), anxiety (Pargament, Zinnbauer, et al., 1998), trait anger (Exline et al., 1999), poor problem-solving skills (Pargament, Zinnbauer, et al., 1998), and insecure attachment (Exline & Martin, in press; see also Hall & Edwards, 2002). Also, people are more likely to feel offended by God if they have an inflated, narcissistic sense of personal entitlement—that is, if they see themselves as better than others and believe that their superiority entitles them to special treatment (Exline & Bushman, 2004).

Some evidence suggests that religiosity and perceived closeness to God may protect against anger toward God (Exline & Bushman, 2004). However, this same study also suggested that religiosity is associated with greater belief that anger toward God is morally wrong. This raises the question of whether individuals—perhaps especially devout believers—might be afraid to report feelings of religious doubt or anger toward God. Clinical accounts suggest that not only might people balk at admitting to others that they feel anger toward God; they might be wary about admitting such feelings to God or even to themselves (Novotni & Petersen, 2001).

Holding God responsible for negative events might not only lead to anger and distress; in some cases, such attributions may shake basic beliefs about God's existence. Problems of evil and suffering constitute a major source of religious doubt (Altemeyer & Hunsberger, 1997). In a recent study of college students, 21% of those who previously believed in God reported that their belief in God's existence decreased in the wake of a major negative life event attributed to God (Kampani & Exline, 2002). Such responses were often transient, but not always. Nine percent of students in this sample indicated that they resolved their anger by deciding that God did not exist (Exline & Martin, in press). Further analyses identified a group of *conflicted unbelievers*, individuals who reported strong negative emotions toward God but were not certain whether to believe in God (Kampani & Exline, 2002). These data corroborate clinical accounts of *emotional atheism* (Novotni & Petersen, 2001), in which people who feel wounded by God decide that God does not exist. Even those who maintain belief may experience spiritual dryness or distress. They may see God as hidden from them (e.g., Cooke, 1998; Howard-Snyder & Moser, 2001; Yancey, 1988), leading to what Saint John of the Cross termed a "dark night of the soul" (Coe, 2000).

Possible Interventions

The ability to recover from an episode of disappointment with God has been framed as an index of healthy spiritual development (Hall & Edwards, 2002). Although empirical research on this topic is sparse, anecdotal accounts suggest that people may benefit from first acknowledging—and perhaps communicating—their negative feelings toward God (Novotni & Petersen, 2001). This might be accomplished through techniques such as prayer, writing a letter to God (Exline, 2003), or an empty chair technique (Smith, 1997). To facilitate this process of "crying out to God," those from Judeo-Christian traditions might also find it useful to meditate on holy writings written by fellow sufferers such as the Hebrew Psalmists (see Zornow, 2001, for an intervention). Before attempting such steps, however, individuals will need to decide whether they find it morally appropriate to express negative feelings toward God.

For those seeking a close relationship with God, steps may be needed to resolve negative feelings and to rebuild trust (see Murray-Swank, 2003, for an application to sexual abuse survivors). To facilitate closeness, individuals may need to reattribute events so that they are not seen as the actions of a malevolent, condemning deity (Exline & Martin, in press; Kushner, 1981). This may be a difficult task, particularly for those who have long-standing negative images of God. Tools to rebuild trust and intimacy might include prayer, imagery, and meditation on texts emphasizing positive attributes of God. Other tools may be social. Therapeutic bonds or expressions of encouragement, love, or blessing from others could help to heal spiritual wounds (Smalley & Trent, 1993). Also, to the extent that God images reflect parental images (Rizzuto, 1979), forgiving one's parents could facilitate resolution of anger toward God (Bliss, 2003).

What if the problem is not negative feelings per se, but rather a sense of God as distant, hidden, or silent? Although such perceptions might not trouble individuals who see God as an abstract force, they could greatly disturb those who desire an intimate, personal relationship with God. The sense of distance could prove distressing in itself, and it might also spread to other problems such as spiritual dryness and difficulty discerning God's will about specific situations.

When people experience distress around a sense that God is distant or hidden, they face a challenge about how to resolve or manage this sense of disconnection (see Coe, 2000). Some might benefit from experiential techniques designed to facilitate a sense of interaction with God. For example, one Christian intervention focuses on prayer as a two-way conversation, one in which individuals train themselves not only to speak to God, but also to use imagery, journaling, or reading of holy texts to "listen" to what God might say in response (Virkler & Virkler, 1986). Within Judaism, Nachman of Breslov began a practice known as *hitbodedut*, which encourages supplicants to speak to God as though God were one's closest friend (Shulman, 1993). Some might also choose to deepen relationships with others in their spiritual communities, with the notion that strengthening these bonds might help to facilitate a sense of connection with God as well. Another option might be to consider periods of dryness or distance as normal seasons of spiritual life, times in which people can grow in faith, character, and wisdom even when they do not feel the presence of God (Cooke, 1998). Where possible, normalizing periods of hiddenness might comfort those experiencing spiritual dryness, especially if the alternative is to believe that God has turned away from them.

Sin, Sacrifice, and Self-Forgiveness: The Challenge of Cultivating Virtue

Virtually all religious systems denote certain rules to obey, sins to avoid, and virtues to cultivate. In some cases religious rules and rituals become an end unto themselves, blocking the personal or experiential aspects of spiritual life. In fact, many people associate the term "religion" with empty, mindless, or compulsive motivated adherence to rules and rituals that have been externally imposed by religious institutions (Hill et al., 2000; Zinnbauer, Pargament, & Scott, 1999). One reaction to this negative view of religion would be to fashion a more personal form of spirituality or ethics, a practice that is common today. Personalized forms of spirituality allow people to use their own values and preferences as a guide. They may generate their own private belief systems and ethical codes, or they might draw from established religious traditions while keeping only selected parts (Exline, 2002). Another option would be to identify with a single faith but to focus on a personal relationship with God as opposed to rules and rituals. Any of these approaches could provide some freedom from externally imposed religious laws. Yet even the most personal systems of ethics or spirituality are likely to involve moral guidelines of some sort. As such, we contend that most forms of committed religiosity or spirituality entail self-discipline as people strive to follow their guiding principles.

Surrender

Attempts to cultivate virtue can translate into hard self-regulatory work as people strive to perform virtuous acts while avoiding indulgence in forbidden (but tempting) passions (Baumeister & Exline, 1999). Within theistic systems, one central struggle involves surrender or willingness to submit to God's authority (see Wallace, 2002, for a transpersonal perspective). Because surrender works directly against basic human desires for personal control, self-reliance, and freedom of choice, some will view it as a sign of weakness. Yet researchers have begun to discuss surrender as a potentially adaptive coping style (Cole & Pargament, 1999; Speer & Reinert, 1998; Wong-McDonald & Gorsuch, 2000). The challenges of surrender are well documented in the literature on 12-step groups (e.g., Hart & Huggett, 2003; Kurtz & Ketcham, 1992; Speer & Reinert, 1998). Because of its emphasis on dependence, self-sacrifice, and limited personal control, surrender is likely to be an ongoing source of struggle within theistic belief systems. Even after initial acts of surrender, committed followers may encounter continued challenges to self-interest as they continue to grow in their faith and to cultivate virtue.

Facing One's Sins

In any belief system that entails virtuous striving, people have to deal with times when they fall short. An initial challenge is simply being willing to acknowledge one's shortfalls and sins. Doing so would seem to require a sense of humility, which involves a nondefensive willingness to see the self accurately (for reviews, see Exline et al., 2004; Tangney, 2000). Religious involvement could arguably work for or against humility. On the one hand, success at cultivating virtue or adhering to the surface rules of one's religion could lead to a self-righteous pride that is the very opposite of humility (Rowatt, Ottenbreit, Nesselroade, & Cunningham, 2002). On the other hand, most major world religions denounce individualistic pride while promoting humility as a virtue (Tangney, 2000). Regardless of whether they explicitly promote humility, religious and spiritual systems often include experiences of transcendence and awe that help people to see themselves as part of a larger picture—thus fostering a sense of humility (Exline et al., 2004). Yet even with spiritual help, cultivation of humility is likely to be a struggle. Scholars list pride as one of the most deadly and insidious sins (e.g., Schimmel, 1997), one ready to rear its head whenever people are doing well in other areas.

Individuals seeking deeper spiritual commitment may also experience conflict between different parts of the self, in which a part seen as redeemed or divine wrestles against another part seen as sinful or merely human. For devout persons who strive to align their behavior with God's will, with deeply held principles, or with transcendent aspects of the self (e.g., the redeemed soul; the divine inner man), knowledge that one has sinned could yield intense pain and guilt (Kook, as referenced in Bokser, 1978). Such suffering might be heightened if people do not see any hope of doing better in the future—if they have a low sense of what we might term *spiritual self-efficacy*. To the extent that depression, shame, or low self-esteem could intensify such hopelessness, treatment focused on these problems could prove helpful. Another suggestion appears within Christian teaching: once people have experienced the saving grace of God through Christ, those who feel overwhelmed by their dark sides might find hope by focusing on God's power to transform them—as opposed to relying totally on themselves to perform all of the work.

For most people, simply coming to terms with their ongoing potential for sin will be difficult. But how should people respond in the wake of specific sins? On the one hand, from a moral or religious perspective, it seems crucial to accept responsibility where appropriate. Indeed, accepting responsibility is framed as one of the traditional steps to repentance within Judaism and other traditions (e.g., Schimmel, 2002). Taking responsibility for misdeeds is likely to entail feelings of sorrow, regret, and guilt, and these feelings may facilitate acts of repentance to repair damage (e.g., Baumeister, Stillwell, & Heatherton, 1994; Tangney & Dearing, 2002). If people simply shrug off their misdeeds without suffering distress or making amends, one might conclude that they are not taking their offenses seriously (e.g., Fisher & Exline, 2003; Holmgren, 1998). Yet the other extreme might pose problems as well. Even if they have made sincere attempts at making amends, some people engage in prolonged self-flagellation and rumination about their sins (Bassett et al., 1990). Those who are unable or unwilling to resolve punitive feelings toward themselves often suffer from low self-esteem, anxiety, and depression (e.g., Mauger et al., 1992). Such individuals might benefit from interventions to facilitate self-forgiveness.

For those committed to maintaining a personal relationship with God, a central goal in dealing with one's own sin might be to receive God's love and forgiveness—a process that has been empirically linked with self-forgiveness (Cafaro & Exline, 2003) and with unconditional forgiveness of others (Krause & Ellison, 2003). People might encounter a number of barriers when seeking God's forgiveness. Some barriers are purely psychological, such as perfectionism or negative self-views. Others might be more specific to religion. For example, some individuals might be unable to seek God's forgiveness—or to experientially receive it—because they believe that they have committed an unforgivable sin (Virkler, 1999). Others may see God as punitive and harsh (e.g., Benson & Spilka, 1973), which would make them reluctant to expect forgiveness from God. Seeing God as severe might lead to terror about breaking religious rules, which could lead to joyless, inhibited faith or obsessive–compulsive patterns of scrupulosity (Abramowitz, Huppert, Cohen, Tolin, & Cahill, 2002; Ciarrocchi, 1995; Greenberg, Witztum, & Pisante, 1987).

Possible Interventions

What interventions might help people receive God's forgiveness? Possible tools might include written or spoken confession (Martin & Exline, 2004; Murray-Swank & Pargament, 2001, 2003), reading holy texts about God's forgiveness, or the use of imagery or other means to listen for God's voice (Martin & Exline, 2004; Virkler & Virkler, 1986). Traditional rituals of repentance and atonement might also be helpful. For example, Roman Catholics might choose to fast, confess their sins to a priest, or recite the rosary. Jewish penitents might express repentance through the rites of Yom Kippur, the symbolic casting of sins into the river on Rosh Hashanah, or the traditional *mikvah* ritual involving immersion in fresh water. Penitent individuals might also make amends to those they have harmed, as in 12-step programs. However, one prior study suggests that if people believe that they have offended God, confession and making amends to others may actually not predict belief that God has forgiven the self (Cafaro & Exline, 2003). Although this finding awaits replication, it raises the possibility that atonement alone might not be sufficient. To be most effective, interventions may need to include some means by which people can find assurance of God's forgiveness.

It seems likely that desires to make peace with God will be especially relevant for those considering their own mortality. Mortality primes lead people to seek reassurance and affirmation of their value, as suggested by terror management studies (e.g., Greenberg, Solomon, & Pyszczynski, 1997). If a happy afterlife is believed to depend on God's forgiveness, desires for peace with God should become urgent when the prospect of death is made salient.

Perceived Attacks from the Spiritual Realm: The Challenge of Supernatural Evil

For most people, the term *spiritual experience* is likely to prompt images of sacred encounters: ecstatic visions, miracles, or moments when people feel united with God or the universe. Granted, most self-reports of spiritual experience are positive (Hardy, 1979). However, this is not always the case. Many believe that people can suffer attack, oppression, or even possession by evil forces such as Satan, demons, or evil spirits. Stark (1965) used the term *diabolical causation* to refer to these attributions in his taxonomy of religious experience. Since that time, psychologists have paid scant attention to this particular dark alley of spiritual life.

Possession

A review of the literature reveals many case studies discussing the possibility of possession by evil spirits, often using a cross-cultural, ethnographic framework (e.g., Al-Subaie & Alhamad, 2000; Brockman, 2000; Chiu, 2000). Professionals from diverse fields (e.g., medicine, anthropology, pastoral care, and mental health care) have documented strange, frightening behaviors sometimes interpreted as demonic possession. Common symptoms include a dramatic personality shift that includes bodily contortions and marked changes in behavior, facial expression, voice tone, and speech content (MacNutt, 1995). Speech might refer to the self as a specific demon or spirit, and it might include self-references using the plural term "we" instead of the singular "I." People in this state often show sacrilegious or sexual behavior that is grossly out of character. These syndromes are not entirely bound by culture, nor are they limited to persons with psychological disorders or impaired reality testing—although they do occur in psychiatric populations (see Wilson, 1998). Anecdotal accounts suggest that possession-like states may even occur in sacred settings, such as prayer sessions and religious retreats (MacNutt, 1995).

Diabolical Attributions

Regardless of whether they believe in demonic possession, many people do believe that supernatural forces of evil are active in the modern world. Some people attribute human suffering and sin to these forces. Although diabolical attributions are common among psychotic persons (Wilson, 1998) and those with other psychological disorders (Pfeifer, 1999), they are by no means limited to the mentally ill. One recent study revealed that although attributions to Satan were rare, they did sometimes occur for life-altering events with negative consequences (Lupfer, Tolliver, & Jackson, 1996). Other studies provide complementary results, suggesting that demonic and satanic appraisals correlate reliably with other indices of spiritual distress in nonclinical samples (e.g., Exline et al., 2000; Pargament, Smith, et al., 1998).

Controversy about Intervention

When people believe that evil forces are attacking them, the obvious challenge is to somehow find freedom from the torment. However, there is little agreement about how to accomplish this aim. First of all, individuals disagree sharply about whether supernatural evil forces exist. Sixty-five percent of Americans in the 1999 General Social Survey reported belief in the Devil (cited in Spilka, Hood, Hunsberger, & Gorsuch, 2003, p. 152). Even among those who do believe in the Devil, specific beliefs diverge considerably. Some view the Devil as an abstract evil force or a symbolic representation of human nature's dark side, while others see the Devil as a literal, active being who is deliberately wreaking havoc in the modern world (e.g., Wilson & Huff, 2001). Even those who share a belief in a literal Devil may disagree in their beliefs about the existence or power of lesser evil spirits.

Some individuals view demonic attributions or possession-like states as the result of physical processes or psychological phenomena such as somatization (Houran, Kumar, Thalbourne, & Lavertue, 2002), internalization of a bad paternal object (Ivey, 1993), or attempts to disavow responsibility (Spanos, 1989). If people believe that possession-like states can be explained through psychological or physical causes, their preferred treatments will focus on those routes. For example, if diabolical causation beliefs are seen as delusional or otherwise misguided, a likely aim would be to pinpoint social or psychological functions served by such beliefs.

On the other hand, some clinicians view demonic oppression or attack as an authentic source of emotional distress, and they argue for the importance of being able to distinguish demonically caused symptoms from more general psychological symptoms (e.g., Bufford, 1989; Friesen, 1992; Isaacs, 1987). Those who view demonic possession or attribution as authentic are likely to favor approaches focused on the spiritual realm itself. For example, people in some cultures attempt to appease evil or ancestral spirits through rituals involving sacrifice, dance, or trance states (e.g., Somer & Saadon, 2000). If they see themselves as victims of curses, they might try to mobilize supernatural forces in their favor, perhaps using magical spells or curses in the service of self-defense or counterattack. Some may even choose to side with evil forces in order to secure power for themselves, as reported in cases of Satan worship (Ivey, 1993).

In sharp contrast to the above perspectives, another approach involves viewing demons as mortal foes that must be cast out or "bound" (i.e., silenced or weakened by being subjected to God's authority). Casting out demons is the central focus of exorcism or deliverance rituals. Such rituals currently take place in many world religions, including some segments of Christianity (e.g., Rosik, 1997), Islam (e.g., Al-Subaie & Alhamad, 2000), and Judaism (e.g., Goodwin, Hill, & Attias, 1990). Although literature remains sparse, dramatic positive effects of exorcism appear in single-case accounts (Barlow, Abel, & Blanchard, 1977; MacNutt, 1995) and some empirical work on dissociative disorders (e.g., Bull, Ellason, & Ross, 1998). Yet these procedures do carry risks. For example, exorcisms are often used to treat mental illness in the Arab world, sometimes with dangerous effects (e.g., Younis, 2000). Negative outcomes have also been reported with use of exorcism in multiple personality disorder patients (Bowman, 1993; Fraser, 1993).

Even within circles that believe in supernatural evil, controversy surrounds the issue of whether deliverance ministries are an appropriate response (e.g., Rosik, 2003). Within Christianity, there is more agreement about other tools of *spiritual warfare*, such as using the "armor of God" to defend against Satan (Ephesians 6:11–18). This spiritual armor includes elements such as faith, righteousness, peace, and truth, with the Bible being the primary offensive weapon. To date, we are not aware of any empirical studies focusing on these techniques.

From the Supernatural to the All-Too-Natural: Challenges of Religious Community

Clearly, religious struggle does not always center on people's relationships with God or their battles against supernatural evil. In everyday life, religious problems often take more mundane forms, centering on the difficulties of interacting with other people.

Strife and Sin within Religious Communities

Individuals hurt and offend one another within religious communities just as they do in other domains of life. Some examples are dramatic, such as publicized cases of sexual abuse or financial corruption by religious authorities. Overt displays of hypocrisy, prejudice, violence, and abuse of power are likely to lead to distaste and reluctance to identify oneself with such a contaminated system. Such blatant offenses might even lead some followers to doubt the value of religion more generally (Altemeyer & Hunsberger, 1997).

In the shadows of these sensational crimes lurk ordinary ones that nonetheless do serious damage. As shown in recent studies (e.g., Krause, Chatters, Meltzer, & Morgan, 2000; Krause, Ellison, & Wulff, 1998), religious communities are not immune from the usual human tendencies toward gossip, greed, petty jealousies, turf battles, and the like. Members often disagree on central doctrines and on fine points about worship style and dress code. People may feel judged or scrutinized and can even become targets of hostility or prejudice from religious peers or leaders—a problem often reported by gays and lesbians (Schuck & Liddle, 2001).

Given the many potential areas for conflict, people in religious communities are likely to face the same challenges of "getting along" that they face in their other close relationships. They need to learn how to forgive and repent, when to trust others and when to protect themselves, and how to curb their own selfish or aggressive impulses. Furthermore, they may feel a strong need to maintain harmonious relationships with others in their religious communities because of their shared belief system. These prospects can be daunting, and the associated disagreements have been documented as a major source of religious struggle (e.g., Exline et al., 2000; Nielsen, 1998; Nielsen & Fultz, 1995; Pargament, Smith, et al., 1998; Pargament, Zinnbauer, et al., 1998).

Outgroup Issues

The issues just raised are *ingroup* problems—problems within communities. But what about cases involving *outgroups*, in which people do not see themselves as members of the same community? Disagreement may continue in spite of efforts on both sides, a problem that often occurs in interfaith marriages (Lehrer & Chiswick, 1993) or families in which children diverge from the faith of their upbringing (Altemeyer & Hunsberger, 1997).

Although religions vary in their degree of exclusivity, greater identification with a religious system often highlights differences between one's own group and other outgroups. Social-psychological studies suggest that these ingroup/outgroup distinctions often lead to biases favoring the ingroup (e.g., Tajfel, 1982) that may, in turn, lead to acts of discrimination or even violence. Also, to the extent that they see their group as correct, members of religious groups risk social conflict by trying to convert others (Langone, 1985).

Social-psychological research suggests that to avoid such problems, groups should focus on transcendent, common aims or beliefs in order to foster cooperation (e.g., Sherif, 1966). Yet a focus on shared beliefs might seem difficult or even misguided if one's religious system holds central tenets that oppose those of the other group. Religious affiliates might not want to compromise the purity of their faith by joining with outsiders. Also, if they believe that their fate in the afterlife is tied to ingroup membership, they may believe that they would ultimately harm outsiders by focusing on common ground rather than conversion.

Finally, people may suffer persecution if they hold unpopular religious beliefs. Persecution can take dramatic forms such as imprisonment or torture. But persecution also occurs in daily life, as when teens suffer teasing or ostracism from peers because of their religious beliefs or practices. Rejection is a powerful social force, as shown in recent research (e.g., Twenge, Catanese, & Baumeister, 2002). Some may manage threats of rejection by conforming with a majority group, while others reaffirm a sense of self-worth or belonging in other ways—perhaps by focusing on their strengths or by drawing closer to God or to like-minded others.

CONCLUDING THOUGHTS

In their discussion of *amazing apostates*, Altemeyer and Hunsberger (1997) suggest that some people from religious homes turn away from their faith because, having been raised to value truth, they find their religious systems lacking in the very quality they were raised to value. Perhaps for some of these youth, disenchantment results from seeing dissonance between rosy, idealized images of religious life and the personal struggles they face. In actuality, suffering is an integral part of all major world religions. Yet in the search for converts, it may be tempting to sugarcoat the religious experience in an effort to avoid alienating potential followers. Ironically, a willingness to discuss spiritual struggles might actually help to increase commitment, as people see their spiritual concerns acknowledged and addressed in a forthright manner.

The notion that suffering may expose hidden wellsprings of strength is expressed in the writings of Samson Raphael Hirsch, an Orthodox Jewish rabbi who writes of the role of suffering in personal development: "Suffering forces a man back upon himself and into himself, and because he is deprived of all external help, every spark of strength which slumbers in him is called forth, all those latent resources of his nature are awakened" (Hirsch, 1837/1962, p. 38). In a world without suffering, humans have no barriers against which to press, and they risk becoming weak through their complacency. Perhaps, then, the opportunity for struggle is actually one of the greatest gifts that religion and spirituality have to offer.

REFERENCES

Abramowitz, J. S., Huppert, J. D., Cohen, A. B., Tolin, D. F., & Cahill, S. P. (2002). Religious obsessions and compulsions in a non-clinical sample: The Penn Inventory of Scrupulosity (PIOS). *Behaviour Research and Therapy, 40*, 824–838.

Al-Subaie, A., & Alhamad, A. (2000). Psychiatry in Saudi Arabia. In I. Al-Issa (Ed.), *Al-Junun:*

Mental illness in the Islamic world (pp. 205–233). Madison, CT: International Universities Press.

Altemeyer, B., & Hunsberger, B. (1997). *Amazing conversions: Why some turn to faith and others abandon religion.* Amherst, NY: Prometheus.

Barlow, D. H., Abel, G. G., & Blanchard, E. B. (1977). Gender identity change in a transsexual: An exorcism. *Archives of Sexual Behavior, 6,* 387–395.

Bassett, R. L., Hill, P. C., Pogel, M. C., Lee, M., Hughes, R., & Masci, J. (1990). Comparing psychological guilt and Godly sorrow: Do Christians recognize the difference? *Journal of Psychology and Theology, 18,* 244–254.

Baumeister, R. F., & Exline, J. J. (1999). Virtue, personality, and social relations: Self-control as the moral muscle. *Journal of Personality, 67,* 1165–1194.

Baumeister, R. F., Stillwell, A. M., & Heatherton, T. F. (1994). Guilt: An interpersonal approach. *Psychological Bulletin, 115,* 243–267.

Benson, P. L., & Spilka, B. (1973). God image as a function of self-esteem and locus of control. *Journal for the Scientific Study of Religion, 13,* 297–310.

Bliss, P. (2003). *Debt-canceling: Form on forgiveness.* Unpublished workshop materials, The City Mission, Cleveland, OH.

Bokser, B. Z. (1978). *Abraham Isaac Kook: The lights of penitence, the moral principles, lights of holiness, essay, letters, and poems.* Mahwah, NJ: Paulist Press.

Bowman, E. S. (1993). Clinical and spiritual effects of exorcism in fifteen patients with multiple personality disorder. *Dissociation: Progress in the Dissociative Disorders, 6,* 222–238.

Brenner, R. R. (1980). *The faith and doubt of Holocaust survivors.* New York: Free Press.

Brockman, R. (2000). Possession and medicine in south central India. *Journal of Applied Psychoanalytic Studies, 2,* 299–312.

Bufford, R. K. (1989). Demonic influence and mental disorders. *Journal of Psychology and Christianity, 8,* 35–48.

Bull, D. L., Ellason, J. W., & Ross, C. A. (1998). Exorcism revisited: Positive outcomes with dissociative identity disorder. *Journal of Psychology and Theology, 26,* 188–196.

Cafaro, A. M., & Exline, J. J. (2003, March). *Correlates of self-forgiveness after offending God.* Poster presented at the Mid-Winter Conference on Religion and Spirituality, Timonium, MD.

Chiu, S. N. (2000). Historical, religious and medical perspectives of possession phenomenon. *Hong Kong Journal of Psychiatry, 10,* 14–18.

Ciarrocchi, J. W. (1995). *The doubting disease: Help for scrupulosity and religious compulsions.* Mahwah, NJ: Paulist Press.

Coe, J. H. (2000). Musings on the dark night of the soul: Insights from St. John of the Cross on a developmental spirituality. *Journal of Psychology and Theology, 28,* 293–307.

Cole, B. S., & Pargament, K. I. (1999). Spiritual surrender: A paradoxical path to control. In W. R. Miller (Ed.), *Integrating spirituality into treatment: Resources for practitioners* (pp. 179–198). Washington, DC: American Psychological Association.

Cooke, G. (1998, August). Flowing with the anointing. *Spread the Fire Magazine, 4*(4). Available online at www.tacf.org/stf/archive/4-4/feature1.html.

Exline, J. J. (2002). Stumbling blocks on the religious road: Fractured relationships, nagging vices, and the inner struggle to believe. *Psychological Inquiry, 13,* 182–189.

Exline, J. J. (2003). [Letter writing: A tool to reduce anger toward God?]. Unpublished raw data.

Exline, J. J., & Bushman, B. J. (2004). *Anger toward others versus God: A comparison of predictors, consequences, and means of resolution.* Manuscript in preparation.

Exline, J. J., Campbell, W. K., Baumeister, R. F., Joiner, T., Krueger, J., & Kachorek, L. V. (2004). Humility and modesty. In C. Peterson & M. E. P. Seligman (Eds.), *Character strengths and virtues: A handbook and classification* (pp. 461–475). New York: Oxford University Press.

Exline, J. J., & Martin, A. (in press). Anger toward God: A new frontier in forgiveness research. In E. L. Worthington, Jr. (Ed.), *Handbook of forgiveness research.* New York: Guilford Press.

Exline, J. J., Yali, A. M., & Lobel, M. (1999). When God disappoints: Difficulty forgiving God and its role in negative emotion. *Journal of Health Psychology, 4,* 365–379.

Exline, J. J., Yali, A. M., & Sanderson, W. C. (2000). Guilt, discord, and alienation: The role of religious strain in depression and suicidality. *Journal of Clinical Psychology, 56,* 1481–1496.

Fisher, M., & Exline, J. J. (2003). *Self-forgiveness: Virtue or vice?* Manuscript in preparation.

Fitchett, G. (1999a). Screening for spiritual risk. *Chaplaincy Today, 15*(1), 2–12.

Fitchett, G. (1999b). Selected resources for screening for spiritual risk. *Chaplaincy Today, 15*(1), 13–26.

Fitchett, G., Rybarczyk, B. D., DeMarco, G. A., & Nicholas, J. J. (1999). The role of religion in medical rehabilitation outcomes: A longitudinal study. *Rehabilitation Psychology, 44,* 1–22.

Fraser, G. A. (1993). Exorcism rituals: Effects on multiple personality disorder patients. *Dissociation: Progress in the Dissociative Disorders, 6,* 239–244.

Friesen, J. G. (1992). Ego-dystonic or ego-alien: Alternate personality or evil spirit? *Journal of Psychology and Theology, 20,* 197–200.

George, L. K., Ellison, C. G., & Larson, D. B. (2002). Explaining the relationships between religious involvement and health. *Psychological Inquiry, 13,* 190–200.

Goodwin, J., Hill, S., & Attias, R. (1990). Historical and folk techniques of exorcism: Applications to the treatment of dissociative disorders. *Dissociation: Progress in the Dissociative Disorders, 3,* 94–101.

Greenberg, D., Witztum, E., & Pisante, J. (1987). Scrupulosity: Religious attitudes and clinical presentations. *British Journal of Medical Psychology, 60,* 29–37.

Greenberg, J., Solomon, S., & Pyszczynski, T. (1997). Terror management theory of self-esteem and cultural worldviews: Empirical assessments and conceptual refinements. *Advances in Experimental Social Psychology, 29,* 61–139.

Hall, T. W., & Edwards, K. J. (2002). The Spiritual Assessment Inventory: A theistic model and measure for assessing spiritual development. *Journal for the Scientific Study of Religion, 41,* 341–357.

Hardy, A. (1979). *The spiritual nature of man: A study of contemporary religious experience.* Oxford, UK: Clarendon Press.

Hart, K. E., & Huggett, C. (2003). *Lack of humility as a barrier to surrendering to the spiritual aspect of Alcoholics Anonymous.* Manuscript submitted for publication.

Hill, P. C., Pargament, K. I., Hood, R. W., Jr., McCullough, M. E., Swyers, J. P., Larson, D. B., & Zinnbauer, B. J. (2000). Conceptualizing religion and spirituality: Points of commonality, points of departure. *Journal for the Theory of Social Behaviour, 30,* 51–77.

Hirsch, S. R. (1962). *Horeb: A philosophy of Jewish laws and observance* (I. G. Dayan, Trans.). London: Sencino Press. (Original work published 1837)

Holmes, E. R. (2001). A therapeutic model for amazing apostasy. *Dissertation Abstracts International: Section B: The Sciences and Engineering, 62*(3-B), 1579.

Holmgren, M. R. (1998). Self-forgiveness and responsible moral agency. *Journal of Value Inquiry, 32,* 75–91.

Houran, J., Kumar, V. K., Thalbourne, M. A., & Lavertue, N. E. (2002). Haunted by somatic tendencies: Spirit infestation as psychogenic illness. *Mental Health, Religion and Culture, 5,* 119–133.

Howard-Snyder, D., & Moser, P. (Eds.). (2001). *Divine hiddenness: New essays.* Cambridge, UK: Cambridge University Press.

Hunsberger, B., Pratt, M., & Pancer, S. M. (2002). A longitudinal study of religious doubts in high school and beyond: Relationships, stability, and searching for answers. *Journal for the Scientific Study of Religion, 41,* 255–266.

Isaacs, T. C. (1987). The possessive states disorder: The diagnosis of demon possession. *Pastoral Psychology, 35,* 263–273.

Ivey, G. (1993). Psychodynamic aspects of demonic possession and Satan worship. *South African Journal of Psychology, 23,* 186–194.

James, W. (2002). *The varieties of religious experience.* Amherst, NY: Prometheus Books. (Original work published 1902)

Johnson, C. V., & Hayes, J. A. (2003). Troubled spirits: Prevalence and predictors of religious and spiritual concerns among university students and counseling center clients. *Journal of Counseling Psychology, 50,* 409–419.

Kampani, S., & Exline, J. J. (2002, August). *Can unbelievers be angry at God?* Presentation at the annual meeting of the American Psychological Association, Chicago, IL.

Koenig, H. G., McCullough, M. E., & Larson, D. B. (2001). *Handbook of religion and health.* New York: Oxford University Press.

Krause, N., Chatters, L. M., Meltzer, T., & Morgan, D. L. (2000). Negative interaction in the church: Insights from focus groups with older adults. *Review of Religious Research, 41,* 510–533.

Krause, N., & Ellison, C. G. (2003). Forgiveness by God, forgiveness of others, and psychological well-being in late life. *Journal for the Scientific Study of Religion, 42,* 77–93.

Krause, N., Ellison, C. G., & Wulff, K. M. (1998). Church-based support, negative interaction, and psychological well-being: Findings from a national sample of Presbyterians. *Journal for the Scientific Study of Religion, 37,* 725–741.

Kurtz, E., & Ketcham, K. (1992). *The spirituality of imperfection: Storytelling and the search for meaning.* New York: Bantam Books.

Kushner, H. S. (1981). *When bad things happen to good people.* New York: Avon Books.

Langone, M. D. (1985). Cults, evangelicals, and the ethics of social influence. *Cultic Studies Journal, 2,* 371–388.

Lawson, R., Drebing, C., Berg, G., Vincellette, A., & Penk, W. (1998). The long term impact of child abuse on religious behavior and spirituality in men. *Child Abuse and Neglect, 22,* 369–380.

Lehrer, E. L., & Chiswick, C. U. (1993). Religion as a determinant of marital stability. *Demography, 30,* 385–403.

Lupfer, M. B., Tolliver, D., & Jackson, M. (1996). Explaining life-altering occurrences: A test of the "God-of-the-gaps" hypothesis. *Journal for the Scientific Study of Religion, 35,* 379–391.

MacNutt, F. (1995). *Deliverance from evil spirits: A practical manual.* Grand Rapids, MI: Chosen Books.

Martin, A. M., & Exline, J. J. (2004). *Facilitating self-forgiveness through religiously oriented interventions.* Manuscript in preparation.

Mauger, P. A., Perry, J. E., Freeman, T., Grove, D. C., McBride, A. G., & McKinney, K. E. (1992). The measurement of forgiveness: Preliminary research. *Journal of Psychology and Christianity, 11,* 170–180.

McCullough, M. E., Hoyt, W. T., Larson, D. B., Koenig, H. G., & Thoresen, C. (2000). Religious involvement and mortality: A meta-analytic review. *Health Psychology, 19,* 211–222.

Miller, W. R. (Ed.). (1999). *Integrating spirituality into treatment: Resources for practitioners.* Washington, DC: American Psychological Association.

Murray-Swank, A., & Pargament, K. I. (2001, October). *Spiritual confession: An integrative review of the psychological literature and spiritual perspectives.* Paper presented at the annual meeting of the Society for the Scientific Study of Religion, Columbus, OH.

Murray-Swank, A., & Pargament, K. I. (2003). [An experimental study of spiritual confession]. Unpublished raw data.

Murray-Swank, N. A. (2003). *Solace for the soul: An evaluation of a psycho-spiritual intervention for female survivors of sexual abuse.* Unpublished doctoral dissertation, Bowling Green State University, Bowling Green, OH.

Nielsen, M. E. (1998). An assessment of religious conflicts and their resolutions. *Journal for the Scientific Study of Religion, 37,* 181–190.

Nielsen, M. E., & Fultz, J. (1995). Further examination of the relationships of religious orientation to religious conflict. *Review of Religious Research, 36,* 369–381.

Novotni, M., & Petersen, R. (2001). *Angry with God.* Colorado Springs, CO: Piñon.

Pargament, K. I. (2002). The bitter and the sweet: An evaluation of the costs and benefits of religiousness. *Psychological Inquiry, 13,* 168–181.

Pargament, K. I., Koenig, H. G., & Perez, L. M. (2000). The many methods of religious coping: Development and initial validation of the RCOPE. *Journal of Clinical Psychology, 56,* 519–543.

Pargament, K. I., Koenig, H. G., Tarakeshwar, N., & Hahn, J. (2001). Religious struggle as a predictor of mortality among medically ill elderly patients: A two-year longitudinal study. *Archives of Internal Medicine, 161,* 1881–1885.

Pargament, K. I., Murray-Swank, N., Magyar, G. M., & Ano, G. G. (2004). Spiritual struggle: A phenomenon of interest to psychology and religion. In W. R. Miller & H. Delaney (Eds.), *Judeo-Christian perspectives in psychology: Human nature, motivation, and change* (pp. 245–268). Washington, DC: APA Books.

Pargament, K. I., Smith, B. W., Koenig, H. G., & Perez, L. (1998). Patterns of positive and negative religious coping with major life stressors. *Journal for the Scientific Study of Religion, 37,* 710–724.

Pargament, K. I., Zinnbauer, B. J., Scott, A. B., Butter, E. M., Zerowin, J., & Stanik, P. (1998). Red flags and religious coping: Identifying some religious warning signs among people in crisis. *Journal of Clinical Psychology, 54,* 77–89.

Park, C. L., & Folkman, S. (1997). Meaning in the context of stress and coping. *Review of General Psychology, 1,* 115–144.

Pfeifer, S. (1999). Demonic attributions in nondelusional disorders. *Psychopathology, 32,* 252–259.

Richards, P. S., & Bergin, A. E. (Eds.). (2000). *Handbook of psychotherapy and religious diversity.* Washington, DC: American Psychological Association.

Rizzuto, A. M. (1979). *The birth of the living god: A psychoanalytic study.* Chicago: University of Chicago Press.

Rosik, C. H. (2003). Critical issues in the dissociative disorders field: Six perspectives from religiously sensitive practitioners. *Journal of Psychology and Theology, 31,* 113–128.

Rowatt, W. C., Ottenbreit, A., Nesselroade, K. P., & Cunningham, P. A. (2002). On being holier-than-thou or humbler-than-thee: A social-psychological perspective on religiousness and humility. *Journal for the Scientific Study of Religion, 41,* 227–237.

Schimmel, S. (1997). *Seven deadly sins: Jewish, Christian, and classical reflections on human nature.* New York: Oxford University Press.

Schimmel, S. (2002). *Wounds not healed by time: The power of repentance and forgiveness.* New York: Oxford University Press.

Schuck, K. D., & Liddle, B. J. (2001). Religious conflicts experienced by lesbian, gay, and bisexual individuals. *Journal of Gay and Lesbian Psychotherapy, 5,* 63–82.

Seligman, M. E. P. (2003, October). *Positive psychology.* Keynote address at the conference Scientific Findings about Forgiveness, Atlanta, GA.

Shafranske, E. P. (Ed.). (1996). *Religion and the clinical practice of psychology.* Washington, DC: American Psychological Association.

Sherif, M. (1966). *In common predicament: Social psychology of intergroup conflict and cooperation.* Boston: Houghton Mifflin.

Shulman, Y. D. (1993). *The chambers of the palace: Teachings of Rabbi Nachman of Bratslav.* Northvale, NJ: Aronson.

Smalley, G., & Trent, J. (1993). *The gift of the blessing.* Nashville, TN: Nelson.

Smith, R. F., Jr. (1998). *Sit down, God . . . I'm angry.* Valley Forge, PA: Judson Press.

Somer, E., & Saadon, M. (2000). Stambali: Dissociative possession and trance in a Tunisian healing dance. *Transcultural Psychiatry, 37,* 580–600.

Spanos, N. P. (1989). Hypnosis, demonic possession, and multiple personality: Strategic enactments and disavowals of responsibility for actions. In C. A. Ward (Ed.), *Altered states of consciousness and mental health: A cross-cultural perspective* (pp. 96–124). Thousand Oaks, CA: Sage.

Speer, R. P., & Reinert, D. F. (1998). Surrender and recovery. *Alcoholism Treatment Quarterly, 16,* 21–29.

Spilka, B., Hood, R. W., Jr., Hunsberger, B., & Gorsuch, R. (2003). *The psychology of religion: An empirical approach* (3rd ed.). New York: Guilford Press.

Stark, R. A. (1965). A taxonomy of religious experience. *Journal for the Scientific Study of Religion,* 5, 97–116.

Tajfel, H. (1982). Social psychology of intergroup relations. *Annual Review of Psychology, 33,* 1–39.

Tangney, J. (2000). Humility: Theoretical perspectives, empirical findings and directions for future research. *Journal of Social and Clinical Psychology, 19,* 70–82.

Tangney, J. P., & Dearing, R. L. (2002). *Shame and guilt.* New York: Guilford Press.

Tedeschi, R.G., Park, C. L., & Calhoun, R. G. (Eds.). (1998). *Posttraumatic growth: Positive changes in the aftermath of crisis.* Mahwah, NJ: Erlbaum.

Twenge, J. M., Catanese, K. R., & Baumeister, R. F. (2002). Social exclusion causes self-defeating behavior. *Journal of Personality and Social Psychology, 83,* 606–615.

Virkler, H. A. (1999). Allaying fears about the unpardonable sin. *Journal of Psychology and Christianity, 18,* 254–269.

Virkler, M., & Virkler, P. (1986). *Dialogue with God.* Gainesville, FL: Bridge-Logos.

Wallace, G. C. M. (2002). Dying to be born: A meditation on transformative surrender within spiritual and depth psychological experiences. *Dissertation Abstracts International: Section B: The Sciences and Engineering, 63*(2-B), 1054.

Wilson, K. M., & Huff, J. L. (2001). Scaling Satan. *Journal of Psychology, 135,* 292–300.

Wilson, W. P. (1998). Religion and psychoses. In H. G. Koenig (Ed.), *Handbook of religion and mental health* (pp. 161–173). San Diego, CA: Academic Press.

Wong, P. T., & Weiner, B. (1981). When people ask "why" questions, and the heuristics of attributional search. *Journal of Personality and Social Psychology, 40,* 650–663.

Wong-McDonald, A., & Gorsuch, R. L. (2000). Surrender to God: An additional coping style? *Journal of Psychology and Theology, 28,* 149–161.

Yancey, P. (1988). *Disappointment with God: Three questions no one asks aloud.* New York: Harper Collins.

Younis, Y. O. (2000). Possession and exorcism: An illustrative case. *Arab Journal of Psychiatry, 11,* 56–59.

Zinnbauer, B. J., Pargament, K. I., & Scott, A. B. (1999). The emerging meanings of religiousness and spirituality: Problems and prospects. *Journal of Personality, 67,* 889–919.

Zornow, G. B. (2001). *Crying out to God: Prayer in the midst of suffering.* Unpublished manuscript, Evangelical Lutheran Church in America.

18

Religious Conversion and Spiritual Transformation

A Meaning-System Analysis

RAYMOND F. PALOUTZIAN

Learning about the processes that mediate religious conversion and spiritual transformation is a goal central to the heart and soul of the discipline of psychology. This is because much of psychology is concerned with learning how human beings change and/or developing effective methods to change them. Indeed, the study of learning, development, attitudes and persuasion, motivation, psychotherapy, and much else within the scope of basic psychology subdisciplines is in one way or another at the core concerned with some aspect of human change. It is understandable, therefore, that the study of the particular change called "religious conversion" was one of the first psychological topics ever studied scientifically (Starbuck, 1899). However, in contrast to learning, development, and maturation—all of which assume long-term continuity to the process—conversion is a more distinct process by which a person goes from believing, adhering to, and/or practicing one set of religious teachings or spiritual values to believing, adhering to, and/or practicing a different set. The transformative process in conversion may take variable amounts of time, ranging from a few moments to several years, but it is the distinctiveness of the change that is its central identifying element (Beit-Hallahmi & Argyle, 1997; Paloutzian, 1996; Paloutzian, Richardson, & Rambo, 1999; Rambo, 1993; Spilka, Hood, Hunsberger, & Gorsuch, 2003). In contrast to someone arriving at a point of belief through the process of socialization and other developmental mechanisms, the convert can identify a time before which the religion was not accepted and after which it was accepted. This is a unique kind of change that has yet to be explained by a powerful model.

FROM RELIGIOUS CONVERSION TO MEANING-SYSTEM CHANGE

Until now the search for a model broad enough to accommodate the body of research on conversion came up empty-handed. Each individual piece of research occasionally was guided by and lent support to a particular theoretical orientation (e.g., Ullman, 1982, 1989, reports findings consistent with a psychodynamic approach; Paloutzian, 1981, reports findings consistent with a social-cognitive approach; Richardson, 1985, 1995, reports findings consistent with a sociological approach), but these interpretative frameworks were for the most part insulated from one other and what few efforts there were to integrate them did not last. The one comprehensive review of the research on religious conversion (Paloutzian et al., 1999) did succeed in organizing the research around one core question, namely, "Does religious conversion cause personality change?" Although this degree of synthesis of the findings is good as far as it goes in answering one outcome question, it was not done within a framework that can explain the findings in an integrated way. The need for an intellectual device that could do this has been a glaring one since the first empirical study of conversion over 100 years ago. Fortunately, the recent introduction to this area of research of the concept of spiritual transformation, construed here as a superset of religious conversion, and the integrative capability of the model of religion as a meaning system (Park & Folkman, 1997; Park, Chapter 16, this volume; Silberman, 2005b), may together emerge as the intellectual device that has been needed.

The review by Paloutzian et al. (1999) concluded that some aspects of personality seem to change following religious conversion and some do not. The data do not support the idea that a religions conversion results in an overall change of the whole person. In particular, there is little evidence that core personality traits such as those subsumed within the Big Five (see Piedmont, Chapter 14, this volume) are different because a person changes from one religion to another or from no religion to a religion. Instead, core traits remain fairly stable throughout adulthood (Costa & McCrae, 1994) so that what changes following a religious conversion is the particular form that expression of the traits will take (i.e., in a way consistent with the new religion), not the traits themselves.

However, something changes in religious conversion. The data suggest that it is midlevel and more global-level aspects of personality that are affected by conversion (Paloutzian et al., 1999). Midlevel personality functions that often change following religious conversion include such factors as the broader or narrower purposes toward which one strives (e.g., to minister to other people in order to bring them into this family of faith), specific goals (e.g., to do my job well as an evidence of faith), or values and attitudes expressed as new ways that one may wish to be (e.g., I want to be a good Muslim) (see Emmons, 1999, for examples). Global-level functions that may change with conversion include overarching life guides such as self-definition and identity (e.g., before I was a Christian, now I am a Jew), overall purpose (e.g., to fulfill God's mission), a new life narrative that highlights the importance of this turning point in the story and its consequences, and that which serves as the ultimate concern (e.g., God or other supreme entity).

The finding that it is a person's purposes, goals, values, attitudes and beliefs, identity, and focus of ultimate concern that change, and not his or her core traits, means that what becomes different about a person who converts are those expressions of the new religion that reflect what the new religion means to him or her, not "what the person is like" in some basic sense. Those aspects of the whole person through which conversion shows its effects are those that relate to whatever is transcendent to the person—that is, what is spiritual relative to him or her (Emmons, 1999, 2000; Pargament, 1997). For this reason, a religious conversion can be properly understood as one type of a larger category of phenomena called "spiritual transformations."

There is correspondence between the aspects of a person that show change from before to after religious conversion and spiritual transformation and the elements within the person's social-cognitive system that together reflect what the person is committed to. These elements would reflect whatever is spiritual for that person, and their arrangement and relative weights and positive or negative valences would make up a unique system of meaning. This means that because religion is about meaning (Paloutzian & Park, Chapter 1, this volume; Park, Chapter 16, this volume; Silberman, 2005a), the thing that undergoes transformation in a religious conversion is the person's meaning system.

Let us explore the implications of this idea by examining the research on religious conversion within the framework of the meaning-system model. A meaning-system analysis of research on religious conversion both integrates the known outcomes of conversion and allows for more refined specification of the relation between inputs that put pressure on the system to change and the characteristics of the output responses that are the evidence that an internal change has happened.

RELIGIOUSNESS AND SPIRITUALITY:
FUNCTIONAL EQUIVALENCE IN THE CHANGE PROCESS

In a substantial portion of the literature, the concept of spirituality has increased in use in recent years but has not replaced the concept of religion. Zinnbauer and Pargament (Chapter 2, this volume) suggest that the concepts of religion and spirituality overlap but are not synonymous. Religion often but not necessarily connotes a belief in a faith system, whereas spirituality connotes those values, ideas, or goals and purposes that transcend a person and to which he or she is committed. Both religion and spirituality involve commitment to something that transcends the individual person. At a psychological functional level, each one seems to imply the other and there may be little difference between them other than personal preference for which language (and its connotations) one uses to describe transcendent values and ultimate concerns (Paloutzian & Park, Chapter 1, this volume). Whichever terminology one employs, the functional dynamics among the components of the meaning system seem to be the same.

People have individual preferences for which terminology they prefer. A sizeable proportion of the people prefer to call themselves *spiritual* but not *religious* (Zinnbauer & Pargament, Chapter 2, this volume), and in the population as a whole a number of interesting combinations of *spiritual* and *religious* are used to represent an individual's own orientation (Paloutzian & Park, Chapter 1, this volume). For the purposes of psychological analysis, it is more parsimonious to proceed on the assumption that even though people may use either or both of these terms to describe their own orientation, there is nevertheless a common psychological process by which they function (Paloutzian & Park, Chapter 1, this volume). In fact, this assumption would be the only legitimate basis for expanding the accumulated research on religious conversion to overlap with and be subsumed within the topic of spiritual transformation of a meaning system.

The argument of this chapter is based on the idea that spiritual transformations occur, that a model for the process mediating such transformations can be described and tested empirically, that spiritual transformation partially overlaps with religious conversion, and that a spiritual transformation constitutes a change in the meaning system that a person holds as a basis for self-definition, the interpretation of life, and overarching purposes and ultimate concerns (Park, Chapter 16, this volume; Silberman, 2005b). That is, religious conversions constitute one variety of spiritual transformation and are so described because traditional language and concepts are used. However, other life changes occur that are based on the same fundamental psychological mechanisms but are not necessarily couched in traditional religious language (Park, Chapter 16, this volume). These changes may invoke the alternative terminology of spiritual transformation.

Some implications of this argument are that (1) there must be pressures on the system—doubts, cracks, breaks, or strains of some kind—prompted by the discrepancies or discontinuities between the implicit or intended expectancies about how an aspect of meaning would be expressed or a need associated with it would be met, (2) the traditional type of spiritual transformation that has been studied in the psychology of religion has been religious conversion, (3) the concept of spiritual transformation is broader than the concept of religious conversion because people can be spiritual in ways that they do not regard as religious (Zinnbauer & Pargament, Chapter 2, this volume), and (4) spiritual transformation constitutes a change in the person's meaning system (Park, Chapter 16, this volume; Silberman, 2005b). Therefore, this chapter takes the approach that religious conversion and spiritual transformation are functionally equivalent and that religious conversion is one among a larger category of phenomena called spiritual transformation. In order to explore the ramifications of this model to its limits, it will be helpful to:

1. Present a working model of religious conversion as spiritual transformation.
2. Identify research on religious doubts, strain, and other pressures on the system in order to illustrate how they may contribute to the process of transformation.
3. Briefly summarize research on religious conversion with a particular emphasis on recasting it into the meaning-system model as a framework for understanding spiritual transformation.
4. Assess how well the existing research fits the model, and set the agenda for future research and theory.

The overall process can be summarized thus: spiritual transformations, religious and otherwise, occur because people are confronted with discrepancies in life that require them to construct a new meaning system because the old one no longer works. Some changes in a meaning system may be partial and may not result in objectively identifiable outcomes, since some changes in people are not expressed in overt behavior. However, when spiritual transformations occur in their fullest form there will be measurable changes in self-perception and identity, life purpose, attitudes and values, goals, sensitivities, ultimate concerns, and behavior.

A WORKING MODEL

Components of a Meaning System

A number of elements are subject to change in a meaning system. This presentation synthesizes the key elements of the concept of meaning system as described with some variations by Baumeister (1991), Park (Chapter 16, this volume), and Silberman (2005b). Silberman (2005b) has explained how religion and (by implication) spirituality constitute a meaning system that is in some ways unique. She suggests that its uniqueness is due to its connection to that which is perceived as sacred (Pargament, 1997). As represented within the present framework, this connection is made evident through goals, attitudes and beliefs, overall purposes, values, self-definition, and ultimate concern that comprise the meaning system. These may find expression through emotions and actions.

The components of a meaning system and their expression can be illustrated in many ways (see Park, Chapter 6, this volume, and Silberman, 2005a, for variations of this idea). First, for example, a person's religiousness or spirituality may include conceptions about an ultimate concern such as the nature of the sacred being (e.g., the attributes of God) and its relation to people, the self, other aspects of this world, and whatever there may be beyond this world (Zinnbauer & Pargament, Chapter 2, this volume; Silberman, 2005b). Variations of such notions may say that this being is forgiving versus vengeful, caring versus uncaring, personal versus impersonal, and so on. Second, such conceptions are unavoidably tied to strong conscious and unconscious emotions (Emmons, Chapter 13, this volume). For example, belief that God is loving and caring may prompt feelings of safety and security, whereas belief in a strict and punitive God may prompt fear or even terror. Third, although meaning systems exist within people's cognitive structures (Paloutzian & Silberman, 2003), they do not exist in a behavioral vacuum. They instead prescribe actions (Park, Chapter 16, this volume; Silberman, 2005b). A religion may prescribe a certain form of ritual, song, prayer, or worship behavior or sacrifice (Spilka, Chapter 20, this volume). A form of spirituality that is not traditionally religious may likewise prescribe its rituals, musical expressions, and foci of awe or gratitude (Emmons & McCullough, 2004), and encourage special ways of relating to the world or treating other people. Fourth, this implies that meaning systems include the notion of goal direction that is an expression of values and more global, overall purposes. The goals may be near, intermediate, or distant, but would, in one way or another, be in the service of overall purposes connected to the ultimate concern (Emmons, 1999, 2000) that takes the functional role of the sacred in the person's life. All of these thus feed and are fed by the person's identity and self-definition. A total spiritual transformation, therefore, would constitute a change in all aspects of a meaning system.

Meaning System and Faith

The meaning-system construct integrates cognitive, affective, motivational, and behavioral elements (Park, Chapter 6, this volume; Silberman, 2005b). Ultimately, whatever serves the function of ultimate concern for a person is in the end an article of faith. This means that a meaning system is a psychological construct of a dynamic set of mental processes whose operation cannot be understood as independent from some element of faith. The components of a meaning system interact with each other in a dynamic way to affect an individual's whole character within the context of that faith. In his classic treatise on faith development, James Fowler (1981) put it this way: "Faith, classically understood, is not a separate dimension of life, a compartmentalized specialty. Faith is an orientation of the total person, giving purpose and goal to one's hopes and strivings, thoughts, and actions" (p. 14), so that ". . . as such, faith is an integral part of one's character or personality" (p. 92).

Change of a Meaning System

The process of spiritual transformation can be conceptualized as a series of three steps in which (1) input pressures prompt (2) internal change in one or more components of the meaning system that (3) shows expression as altered outcomes that are connected to those internal components of the meaning system that have been affected. Overall, as people go through life they come to a point of equilibrium between the components of their meaning system, and these remain in a balanced state unless some pressure is brought to bear on the system. Such pressure would force it to change. The kinds of forces that prompt the particular change called religious conversion have been studied and are well documented elsewhere (Beit-Hallahmi & Argyle, 1997; Paloutzian, 1996; Paloutzian et al., 1999; Rambo, 1993; Spilka et al., 2003). Summaries of conversion research from an attachment theory perspective have recently been added to the literature (Granqvist & Kirkpatrick, 2004; Kirkpatrick, 2005; Oksanen, 1994). These helpful, up-to-date references make it unnecessary to merely redocument this research. Instead, the need now is to extrapolate the argument that the psychological processes involved in religious conversions apply to all kinds of spiritual transformations, religious and otherwise. That is, it will be useful to (1) examine the findings on religious conversion within the meaning-system framework in order to assess the adequacy of the meaning-system model to accommodate the existing body of knowledge, (2) examine the degree to which the existing data match the components and predictions of the model, and (3) identify lines of research that are needed. Similarly, it does little to merely restate the components of a meaning system. Instead, the present focus is on the process of how a person's meaning system becomes different from what it once was.

A key element to any conversion or transformation process must be some element of doubt, pressure, or motivation to change: there is no reason to change one's belief system or worldview if one has no doubts whatsoever about them or if life circumstances have not confronted the person's religious beliefs or practices sufficient for them to be called into question. The term *doubt* is used here in its broadest sense as general unease, an unpleasant cognitive and/or emotional process, whether experienced primarily as intellectual discrepancies between what one understands or believes and what actually happens, or primarily as the loss of an emotional base and sense of security, safety, trust, or continuity because of such a discrepancy, or both (see Hill, 2002; Hunsberger, Alisat, Pancer, & Pratt, 1966; Hunsberger, McKinzie, Pratt, & Pancer, 1993; Hunsberger, Pratt, & Pancer, 2002). Doubts broadly construed in this way need not be openly expressed and may in fact be matters that an individual has kept secret and never discussed with another person (Altemeyer, 1988). Doubts occur because life circumstances happen that are inconsistent with deeply held beliefs, wants, expectations, or predictions. Thus stress and strain that is connected with one's religiousness (Exline, chapter 17, this volume) may contribute to the process of change. Doubts set the process of questing in motion (Allport, 1950; Batson, Schoenrade, & Ventis, 1993; Rambo, 1993). For example, a parent may believe that God will protect his or her child, yet the child may fall victim to a terminal illness or be fatally injured. Such circumstances automatically confront deeply held beliefs and may start the process of transformation (see, e.g., Cook & Wimberley, 1983). Overall, doubts understood in the broad (not necessarily intellectualized) way can be a consequence of crises (not necessarily catastrophic) of purpose, value, efficacy, or self-worth (Hill, 2002) or any other discrepancy or discontinuity between what one wants or expects and what one gets or what happens, so long as the person implicitly or explicitly connects those outcomes to the ultimate concern.

A blend of theoretical underpinnings is at the basis of the notion that these ideas can be integrated into a cohesive understanding of the process of spiritual transformation. Each one reflects a different way of conceptualizing the changes that take place in the human mind. The model assumes that confrontation between these two things sets the process of spiritual transformation in motion. Both emotional and cognitive aspects of the process are central to this model, but the process works because of the essential element of *discrepancy* between the *ought* and the *is* of a person's life (Hill, 2002).

For example, this can be a discrepancy between the belief that a person will live if prayed for, and the subsequent death of that person. If a parent deeply believes that the prayers he or she offers for his or her sick child will allow the child to live but the child dies, then this parent is faced with a discrepancy between what ought to have happened based on his or her firmly held beliefs and what actually happened. In cognitive developmental models of religiousness, this would be called the "creation of disequilibrium," which requires some sort of problem solving in order to return to a state of balance (Oser, 1991; Oser & Gmunder, 1991; Oser, Reich, & Bucher, 1994; Reich, 1991). In cognitive consistency terms derived from social psychology, this could be, for example, dissonance generated by the confrontation between the belief that God is good and takes care of individual persons when asked to do so, and the suffering and death of that person (Festinger, 1957). Feelings of stress and strain in relation to God or erosion of trust in God (Exline, Chapter 17, this volume) would seem likely to follow. Such circumstances would set in motion those social, cognitive, and emotional processes that prompt a person to make attributions for the cause of what happened and perhaps for its purpose (Spilka et al., 2003; Spilka, Shaver, & Kirkpatrick, 1985). Also, a person may experience doubts in a more formal, intellectual sense, such as those based on science, hypocrisy among clergy, a specific event, shortcomings of organized religion, or personal reactance (Hunsberger et al., 1993). All such discrepancy or discontinuity models raise questions about how people respond when life hands them a negative event. In the example noted above, the parents who lost their child are faced with a dilemma. Their religious beliefs taught them that a particular outcome would occur, but that outcome did not occur. How do they cope with or resolve the discrepancy between their beliefs, their desires concerning what should happen, and what actually happened? Such confrontations set the stage for spiritual transformations.

Clinically we know that such events have to be dealt with (Miller & Kelley, Chapter 25, and Pargament, Ano, & Wachholtz, Chapter 26, this volume), but the focus of the proposed model of spiritual transformation in this chapter does not have clinical or mental health outcomes nor coping as its central component. Instead, the model concerns how spiritual transformations occur. The basic orientation of the model assumes a social cognition approach that postulates that spiritual transformations are a matter of a new construction of meaning due to the requirements that negative life events or the perception of inadequately met needs make on a person's cognitively constructed meaning system. The more that the elements of a person's meaning system are under pressure due to such events or unmet needs, the greater the disequilibrium and the greater the possibility of change (Park, Chapter 6, this volume; Silberman, 2005b).

This model is consistent with the more descriptive model of religious conversion elaborated by Rambo (1993), but unlike it, this new model is explicit about the psychological processes. It is assumed that spiritual transformations include, but are not limited to, changes from no religion to a religion, from one religion to another religion, from one level of commitment to a religion to either a deeper level or a more shallow level of commitment to the same religion, from one orientation to a religion to a different interpretation or application of the same religion to one's life, or turning from a religious to an areligious or an antireligious point of view. Other varieties of spiritual transformations are possible that do not necessarily involve religion but that nevertheless include changes in values, goals, higher purposes, or whatever else an individual might regard as ultimately meaningful or of ultimate concern (Park, Chapter 16, this volume).

Exhausting the Limits of a Meaning System

A total spiritual transformation represents the complete turning over of a previously held spirituality in favor of a new version that more thoroughly encompasses and makes sense of the "data." In the spiritual and religious realm, the "data" that may most vividly illustrate the areas of deficiency in an existing religious framework could be a dramatic life event such as the death of a loved one or a natural disaster, especially when seen from the perspective of one who assumes a loving and all-powerful supreme being who takes care of people's physical needs and protects them from harm (e.g., see Kushner, 1981). When these pieces of information begin adding up, it may become clear that the existing spiritual understanding of the meaning of life is not adequate. If the realization of this inadequacy is compelling, the religious or spiritual beliefs may be overturned. New, more consistent ideas replace the former views that proved deficient.

Changes in the system can occur in different ways. When doubts accumulate in sufficient number or when one doubt emerges in a major life area, a strain on the system is set in motion to prompt movement at some level (Hill, 2002). For example, people can increase in the strength of adherence to the same belief, they can decrease in the strength of adherence within the same belief system, they can go from being nonreligious to being religious, or they can set aside or outgrow formal religions in favor of some alternative, more personally meaningful, kind of spirituality. Furthermore, such changes can be partial or total, and aspects of them can in principle occur in combination. For example, a person might become stronger in the belief that there is a God, while no longer holding to traditionally taught doctrines in favor of new interpretation.

Possible Characteristics of Outputs

Given that the meaning system as a whole exists as an interlocking set of elements that can be independently identified and yet also interact dynamically with each other, and given that confrontations to the system can flow through a number of channels, we can predict that whenever spiritual transformations occur, they need not occur in a total sense. In fact, as I show in the literature review below, the research on religious conversion suggests that most changes do not involve a total overhaul of the whole system of meaning but instead are identified as changes in strength or type of one or more specific elements of the system. For example, a transformation might be identified as (1) either an increase or a decrease in adherence to the same religion or worldview, (2) a change of religion or worldview from one to a completely different one, (3) a change in a specific element within the same religion or worldview (e.g., belief that God cannot intervene to cure diseases; see Kushner, 1981), (4) the adoption of different overall purposes or specific goals even though one maintains the same religion or worldview, (5) a modified view of self or change in self-definition, and (6) the selection of new items that fill the need for ultimate concern and that direct or define life purpose in the most global sense. In sum, a religious conversion may properly be called a spiritual transformation even if it is identifiable as a modification of only one of these elements. Of course, it is in principle possible that all elements of the system change. This would be the most extravagant or dramatic type of conversion and could be what Miller and C'deBaca (1994, 2001) meant by "quantum change" or what Altemeyer and Hunsberger (1997) meant by "amazing conversions," and, as the research shows, also probably the least common type.

It should be possible to identify the nature of the output changes that would occur due to certain confrontations that put stress on the meaning system. Also, we should be able to predict that the stronger the confrontations and the more channels through which they are bearing on the system, the greater will be the transformative effects in strength and number. For example, information that causes an individual to doubt the truth of his or her beliefs puts strain on one channel of the system. In the simplest case of this, two outcomes seem possible. First, the person may decrease the strength of belief. Second, the person may actually increase strength of belief following awareness of information that raises doubts—an outcome consistent with research stemming from dissonance theory and its intellectual descendents (Batson, 1975; Festinger, Rieken, & Schachter, 1956). Which response occurs is dependent upon other factors including the strength and configuration of other elements of the person's meaning system, the person's personality (Paloutzian et al., 1999), whether the person uses an open versus a closed cognitive style (Batson, Schoenrade, & Ventis, 1993), degree of fundamentalistic mind-set (Altemeyer & Hunsberger, 1992), group context (Galanter, 1989), and larger cultural milieu (Rambo, 1993). Given this list of factors that are not part of the meaning system itself but that are part of a larger network of elements with which the meaning system is interconnected, it would seem that a meaning system, once established, is relatively durable and not easy to change. This is because it exists in a web in which its parts are relatively tightly fit together. It would not be realistic to expect, therefore, that just because one element of a meaning has been affected, that the whole system would be transformed. Stereotypes of dramatic transformations aside, most changes in a meaning system are partial and graded, not total and abrupt. Whether or not a change occurs depends upon the complex interaction of the one or more confrontational elements with the whole array of extra-meaning-system factors noted above. In fact, much of the traditional research on religious conversion has focused solely on these factors, such as whether personality affects conversion, whether group influences induce conversion, and so on (Galanter, 1989; Paloutzian, 1996; Paloutzian et al., 1999; Spilka et al., 2003).

The above illustration of one single confrontation through the channel of doubt can be extrapolated to include any subset or even all elements of the system. In general, a greater number and strength of confrontations tends to result in more measurable outcomes.

COMPONENT ANALYSIS OF RESEARCH

Given the above description of the meaning-system model and the processes through which it would change, it is now useful to find out the degree to which the data in the religious conversion research literature fit it. This will enable us not only to assess how much conversion research has actually focused on meaning-system components, but also will shed light on which components have been of greatest interest, which sorts of research were focused on which element(s) of a meaning system, and what sorts of output behaviors would serve as a satisfactory criteria for change. Especially helpful as a guide to future research within the meaning-system framework is to find out whether past research has investigated the combined effects of simultaneous input pressures on more than one component of the system, and if so, whether those combinations of forces produce outcomes not explainable as the sum of the individual input pressures.

Attitudes and Beliefs

Attitudes are evaluative components of social cognition (broadly construed) that are comprised of cognitive, affective, and behavioral tendency components, and beliefs are intimately connected to them (Eagly & Chaiken, 1993; Fishbein & Ajzen, 1975; Petty & Cacioppo, 1981). Simple connections between attitudes and beliefs are illustrated by the observation that people who believe in the truth claims of a particular religion (e.g., that the Qu'ran is the written word of God) are more likely to have a positive attitude about the religion of Islam and its teachings, and are less likely to hold those same attitudes about Christians, Jews, and atheists. However, the connections can be bidirectional, that is, accepting a belief can lead to attitudes consistent with it, and holding a particular attitude is likely to function as a perceptual set to prepare a person to accept certain beliefs as foundations of the preheld attitudes. For example, studies of converts to new religious movements have shown that a person who is a member of a religious group often accepted its system of belief after, not before, participating in the group and developing a positive attitude toward it (Richardson, 1985, 1995); in such cases, belief followed attitude acquisition in the context of behavior in the group. Similarly, research on a stage model of Jewish conversion found that as acceptance of Jewish Orthodox practices and commitment to the Jewish people increased, scores on a Christian belief scale decreased (Bockian, Glenwick, & Bernstein, 2005). Participating in the group and developing a positive attitude toward it and its members, although often done to satisfy personal needs (Galanter, 1989; Paloutzian et al., 1999; Richardson, 1995), would nevertheless be sufficiently different from what the person would have anticipated that he or she would do that the subsequent accepting of the belief as true serves the dual purpose of reducing dissonance and justifying having joined the group. In general, there is a strain toward consistency among the components of attitudes and beliefs, and these may or may not conflict with other components of the meaning system.

Overall, the knowledge that comes from social psychology about the nature of attitudes and beliefs, their acquisition and change, and their relation to other aspects of human functioning can be validly applied to the understanding of religious conversion as a spiritual transformation within the context of the meaning-system model. For example, Hill and Bassett (1992) straightforwardly adapted the elaboration likelihood model of attitude change (Petty & Cacioppo, 1981), which posits that attempts to persuade someone for which the message is processed centrally are more likely to result in durable change in attitude and belief than attempts for which the message is processed peripherally, to religious conversion. It would seem, therefore, to have adaptability to the understanding of the spiritual transformation of a meaning system.

Values and Value Change

Values function as overall guides for setting priorities and for making attitudinal and behavioral choices; thus attitudes and behaviors can be regarded as expressions of values. It is also possible that values and the conflicts that can arise among them be manifestations of religious beliefs. In the context of a religious or spiritual meaning system, for example, a person may hold a positive attitude toward and belief in a particular religion—for example, Judaism or Christianity—and therefore positively value those principles expressed in the Ten Commandments in the book of Exodus. If so, then the person would likely positively value both life and property, both represented in the Ten Commandments (i.e., "Thou shall not kill" and "Thou shall not steal," respectively). It is possible, as well, for values within the same meaning system to conflict with one another. For example, the well-known Heinz Dilemma that illustrates the most influential line of research on the development of how a person makes moral judgments (Kohlberg, 1969) pits two ancient, biblical values against each other: the value of life and love of spouse versus the value of respecting others' property. In essence, moral developmental research has emphasized the value component of a meaning system by pitting two or more values against one another in a storyline called a moral dilemma. How the research participant decides among the alternatives is an indication of the person's level of reasoning about conflicts between those values inherent in that dilemma.

Research has shown that a general sense of valuing can be more prominent in religious converts. For example, Paloutzian (1981) found that college students who had experienced conversion to Christianity had a greater tendency to value all 36 items (18 terminal values, 18 instrumental values) on the Rokeach Value Survey (Rokeach, 1973). Zinnbauer and Pargament (1998) likewise found a greater sense of value change in spiritual converts. In additionally, converts may change in the relative positioning of specific values. In people who joined a religious cooperative village (Rosén & Nordquist, 1980) had elevated rankings of Rokeach's values of *loving, forgiving, helpful,* and *cheerful.* Similarly, Paloutzian (1981) found that people who scored high on purpose in life (associated with being a convert) had increased relative emphasis on Rokeach's values of *salvation* and *being clean,* and that people who scored low on purpose in life (associated with being a nonconvert) had increased relative emphasis on *comfort, happiness, freedom,* and *mature love.* Research of this general sort needs to be extended to incorporate the more recent value model and research methods of Schwartz (see, e.g., Fontaine, Duriez, Luyten, Corveleyn, & Hutsebaut, 2005; Schwartz, 1992; Schwartz & Huismans, 1995). Also, theoretically, to the degree that a person's values are tied to the object of ultimate concern, they occupy a position in the meaning system that would be superordinate to attitudes and specific goals while being subordinate to the ultimate concern, and perhaps on an equal plane with the person's sense of self and identity and with overall purposes. The utility of this sort of arrangement of the components of a meaning system, especially in the context of what makes for greater or lesser transformation of it, has yet to be researched.

Goals and Goal Redefinition

A meaning system would be incomplete unless it included an ability to be manifested in behavior. The component of a meaning most closely connected to behavior is that which contains the goals toward which people aspire. Emmons (1996, 1997, 1999) has cogently argued how the relation between meaning and goals is bidirectional. That is, the goals that people strive to achieve express meanings within the system, and they also serve to construct or concretize meanings through the very process of enacting them. Emmons uses the term *personal strivings* to refer to this process. Goals may range in scope from the narrow and specific to the global and abstract. Personal goals and strivings are defined as "what a person is typically or characteristically trying to do" (Emmons, 1999, p. 92). Examples of strivings that reflect global aspects of meaning include such things as "seek out new ways of bettering my spiritual growth, attitudes, behavior," "deepen my relationship to God," and "express to people that I love them." Examples of more specific goals and strivings include such things as "look well groomed and clean cut," "look attentive and not bored in class," and "keep my room clean" (Emmons, 1999).

Do goals and personal strivings, or, more concretely, does behavior change when a religious spiritual transformation has occurred? The answer depends upon what behaviors are in question and what their roots are. Paloutzian et al.'s (1999) review of the literature bearing upon the question of whether religious conversion caused personality change found that there was little evidence that core traits—and by implication those patterns of behavior that would be characteristic of them—were different following a person's acceptance of a different religious belief or joining a different religious group. However, the data did show that behaviors and goals consistent with Emmons's notion of personal strivings can change. For example, converts to some new and traditional religions have been reported to show changes in behaviors that were causing them trouble (e.g., addictions, use of tobacco, involvement in sexual activity) that they wanted to change, and joining a religion was occasionally a method used by these persons to overcome these behaviors that they saw as problems (Muffler, Langrod, Richardson, & Ruiz, 1997). Robbins and Anthony (1982) report that termination of illicit drug use, renewed vocational interest, and an increase in a sense of social compassion and responsibility have been shown to occur in persons who have participated in new religious movements. Starbuck (1899) reported an increase in the sense of altruism in converts. Barker (1984) reported that people who joined the Unification Church often were looking for a setting in which they could realize their ideals, that is, more fully accomplish their spiritual strivings.

Overall Purpose

Whether of a global or a specific nature, the things toward which a person strives are elements of a meaning system because they reflect the overall purposes and spiritual values to which a person adheres. Whatever a person values and strives to fulfill at a higher and more encompassing level is part of that person's spirituality. Because of this, Emmons's (1999, 2000) concept of spiritual intelligence may be invoked as a model of the cognitive, affective, and motivational cluster of elements that enable people to sustain behavior with a high degree of self-efficacy in pursuit of long-term or higher purposes. Thus even mundane, daily tasks such as washing clothes and preparing food may be imbued with a sense of meaning in someone who performs them for a higher purpose such as a service to God or whatever is the person's ultimate concern.

A variety of studies provide data on sense of purpose in life in relation to religious conversion. The findings for conversion to Christianity (Paloutzian, 1981) and to new religious movements (Kilbourne & Richardson, 1984) suggest that sense of purpose in life increases with conversion, a finding consistent with the proposal that a crisis of purpose is among the forces motivating it (Hill, 2002). In addition, however, much of the research that has assessed changes in the self with conversion shows that people's reports of self-changes are often made in terms that imply changes in their sense of purpose. Changes in self and changes in purpose seem to be highly interconnected, an observation consistent with a meaning-system analysis.

Self-Definition

Traditional literature on religious conversion placed great emphasis on the idea conversion involves a change in the self. James (1902/1958) said that a "hitherto divided" self becomes unified. Pargament (1997) documents that other writers referred to "a transcending self," a change in the "core identity construct," and a change in "identity consolidation" to describe what a religious conversion is. Such terminology places the emphasis on self-transformation at the core of the process. The general pattern of research is consistent with this and shows changes in aspects of self in a number of ways. For example, Ullman (1982, 1989) found that converts to Judaism, Catholicism, Bahai, and Hare Krishna showed that sense of self increased and perception of stress decreased with conversion. Zinnbauer and Pargament (1998) found that self-definition changed in converts as evidenced by reports of greater personal competence, lower postconversion stress, and more spiritual experiences. Much of the research done within the framework of attachment theory (Granqvist & Kirkpatrick, 2004) found that converts report a perception of a new relationship with God, a sense of a different identity, and a feeling that a solid base of love and sense of security has been found.

Ultimate Concerns

A change in the focus of ultimate concern would constitute a transformation of the most global, encompassing aspect of a person's meaning system and would likely be the most difficult element to alter. This implies that the dramatic, total, or radical conversion that serves as a stereotype of conversion is actually the least common form of conversion. Radical, dramatic conversions remain as our stereotype precisely because of their vividness due to their low base rate combined with their status as exemplars. Hill (2002) points out that although most people do not show dramatic conversions or total spiritual transformations, James (1902/1958) nevertheless chose them as his main interest. In general, the greater the difference between the religious-laden context of an individual's past life and the newly adopted religion, the more the change to the new focus of ultimate concern can be regarded as total or extreme. The British converts to Islam reported by Köse and Loewenthal (2000) may fit this category.

CONCLUSION AND DIRECTIONS

It is clear that some research on religious conversion has focused on each element of a meaning system. The concept of spiritual transformation within a meaning-system framework seems to be useful for describing past research on religious conversion and as a conceptual framework to guide future research.

Many things are not clear, however, and each of them points directly to one or more research hypotheses. For example, we do not know how tightly each element of a meaning system is connected to each of the others, how many of them must be under pressure of what amount(s) and of what specific nature(s), or for how long and within what social or environmental context this must occur for a spiritual transformation to happen. To some degree we can intuit, but do not know based upon solid data, what the relative strengths of positions of the elements are in a system of priority. To what degree might some of them be on an equal plane in a hierarchy of components of a meaning system? To what degree do they show interaction effects? Does a meaning system have an upper limit of endurance, beyond which all of them are susceptible to manipulation by others and below which a transformation is unlikely?

So far, each piece of research was done in order to focus primarily on one facet of the change process. No research has been done that would assess changes in all or even most of the components of a meaning system, nor to assess combinations of them. The most frequently studied component of a meaning system in the context of religious conversion has been the self, either self-definition or perceptions of various aspects of self-functioning and well-being. The potential to widen this research domain within the meaning-system framework seems great.

ACKNOWLEDGMENTS

Preparation of this chapter was supported by a faculty development grant from Westmont College. I wish to express my thanks to Kenneth Pargament for his helpful review of the rough draft, and to Perrine Leung and Erica Swenson for their help as my research assistants.

REFERENCES

Allport, G. W. (1950). *The individual and his religion*. New York: Macmillan.

Altemeyer, B. (1988). *Enemies of freedom*. San Francisco: Jossey-Bass.

Altemeyer, B., & Hunsberger, B. (1992). Authoritarianism, religious fundamentalism, quest and prejudice. *The International Journal for the Psychology of Religion, 2*, 113–133.

Altemeyer, B., & Hunsberger, B. (1997). *Amazing conversions: Why some turn to faith and others abandon religion*. Amherst, NY: Prometheus Press.

Barker, E. (1984). *The making of a Moonie: Choice or brainwashing?* Oxford, UK: Blackwell.

Batson, C. D. (1975). Rational processing or rationalization?: The effect of disconfirming information on a stated religious belief. *Journal of Personality and Social Psychology, 32*, 176–184.

Batson, C. D., Schoenrade, P., & Ventis, W. L. (1993). *Religion and the individual: A social psychological perspective*. London: Oxford University Press.

Baumeister, R. F. (1991). *Meanings of life*. New York: Guilford Press.

Beit-Hallahmi, B., & Argyle, M. (1997). *The psychology of religious behaviour, belief and experience*. New York: Routledge.

Bockian, M. J., Glenwick, D. S., & Bernstein, D. P. (2005). The applicability of the stages of change model to Jewish conversion. *The International Journal for the Psychology of Religion, 15*(1), 35–50.

Cook, J. A., & Wimberley, D. W. (1983). If I should die before I wake: Religious commitment and adjustment to the death of a child. *Journal for the Scientific Study of Religion, 22*(3), 222–238.

Costa, P. T., Jr., & McCrae, R. R. (1994). Set like plaster?: Evidence for the stability of adult personality. In T. F. Heatherton & J. L. Weinberger (Eds.), *Can personality change?* (pp. 21–40). Washington, DC: American Psychological Association.

Eagly, A. H., & Chaiken, S. (1993). *The psychology of attitudes*. New York: Harcourt.

Emmons, R. A. (1996). Striving and feeling: Personal goals and subjective well-being. In P. M. Gollwitzer & J. A. Bargh (Eds.), *The psychology of action: Linking cognition and motivation to behavior* (pp. 313–337). New York: Guilford Press.

Emmons, R. A. (1997). Motives and life goals. In R. Hogan, J. Johnson, & S. Briggs (Eds.), *Handbook of personality psychology* (pp. 485–512). San Diego: Academic Press.

Emmons, R. A. (1999). *The psychology of ultimate concerns: Motivation and spirituality in personality*. New York: Guilford Press.

Emmons, R. A. (2000). Is spirituality an intelligence?: Motivation, cognition, and the psychology of ultimate concern. *The International Journal for the Psychology of Religion, 10*, 3–26.

Emmons, R. A., & McCullough, M. E. (Eds.). (2004). *The psychology of gratitude*. Oxford, UK: Oxford University Press.

Emmons, R. A., & Paloutzian, R. F. (2003). The psychology of religion. *Annual Review of Psychology, 54*, 377–402.

Festinger, L. (1957). *A theory of cognitive dissonance*. Stanford, CA: Stanford University Press.

Festinger, L., Riecken, H. W., & Schachter, S. (1956). *When prophecy fails*. Stanford, CA.: Stanford University Press.

Fishbein, M., & Ajzen, I. (1975). *Belief, attitude, intention and behavior: An introduction to theory and research*. Reading, MA: Addison-Wesley.

Fontaine, J. R., Duriez, B., Luyten, P., Corveleyn, J., & Hutsebaut, D. (2005). Consequences of a multidimentional approach to religion for the relationship between religiosity and value priorities. *The International Journal for the Psychology of Religion, 15*(2), 123–143.

Fowler, J. W. (1981). *Stages of faith: The psychology of human development and the quest for meaning*. San Francisco: Harper & Row.

Galanter, M. (1989). *Cults: Faith, healing, and coercion*. New York: Oxford University Press.

Granqvist, P., & Kirkpatrick, L. A. (2004). Religious conversion and perceived childhood attachment: A meta-analysis. *The International Journal for the Psychology of Religion, 14*(4), 223–250.

Hill, P. C. (2002). Spiritual transformation: Forming the habitual center of personal energy. *Research in the Social Scientific Study of Religion, 13*, 87–108.

Hill, P. C., & Bassett, R. L. (1992). Getting to the heart of the matter: What the social-psychological study of attitudes has to offer psychology of religion. In M. Lynn & D. Moberg (Eds.), *Research in the social scientific study of religion* (Vol. 4, pp. 159–182). Greenwich, CT: JAI Press.

Hunsberger, B., Alisat, S., Pancer, S. M., & Pratt, M. (1996). Religious fundamentalism and religious doubts: Content, connections, and complexity of thinking. *The International Journal for the Psychology of Religion, 6*, 201–220.

Hunsberger, B., McKinzie, B., Pratt, M., & Pancer, S. M. (1993). Religious doubt: A social psychological analysis. In M. Lynn & D. Moberg (Eds.), *Research in the social scientific study of religion* (Vol. 5, pp. 27–51.) Greenwich, CT: JAI Press.

Hunsberger, B., Pratt, M., & Pancer, S. M. (2002). A longitudinal study of religious doubts in high school and beyond: Relationships, stability, and searching for answers. *Journal for the Scientific Study of Religion, 41*, 255–266.

James, W. (1958). *Varieties of religious experience*. New York: Mentor Books. (Original work published 1902)

Kilbourne, B., & Richardson, J. T. (1984). Psychotherapy and new religions in a pluralistic society. *American Psychologist, 39*(3), 237–251.

Kirkpatrick, L. A. (2005). *Attachment, evolution, and the psychology of religion*. New York: Guilford Press.

Kohlberg, L. (1969). Stage and sequence: The cognitive developmental approach to socialization. In D. A. Goslin (Ed.), *Handbook of socialization theory and research* (pp. 347–480). Chicago: Rand-McNally.

Köse, A., & Loewenthal, K. M. (2000). Conversion motifs among British converts to Islam. *The International Journal for the Psychology of Religion, 10*, 101–110.

Kushner, H. S. (1981). *When bad things happen to good people*. New York: Avon Books.

Miller, W. R., & C'deBaca, J. (1994). Quantum change: Toward a psychology of transformation. In T. F. Heatherton & J. L. Weinberger (Eds.), *Can personality change?* (pp. 253–280). Washington, DC: American Psychological Association.

Miller, W. R., & C'deBaca, J. (2001). *Quantum change: When epiphanies and sudden insights transform ordinary lives*. New York: Guilford Press.

Muffler, J., Langrod, J., Richardson, J., & Ruiz, P. (1997). Religion. In J. Lowinson, P. Ruiz, R. Millman, & J. Langrod (Eds.), *Substance abuse* (pp. 492–499). Baltimore: Williams & Wilkins.

Oksanen, A. (1994). *Religious conversion: A meta-analytical study*. Lund, Sweden: Lund University Press.

Oser, F. K. (1991). The development of religious judgement. In F. K. Oser & W. G. Scarlett (Eds.), *Religious development in childhood and adolescence* (pp. 5–25). San Francisco: Jossey-Bass.

Oser, F. K., & Gmunder, P. (1991). *Religious judgement: A developmental perspective*. Birmingham, AL: Religious Education Press.

Oser, F. K., Reich, K. H., & Bucher, A. A. (1994). Development of belief and unbelief in childhood and adolescence. In J. Corveleyn & D. Hutsebaut (Eds.), *Belief and unbelief: Psychological perspectives* (Vol. 3, pp. 39–62). Atlanta, GA: Rodopi.

Paloutzian, R. F. (1981). Purpose in life and value changes following conversion. *Journal of Personality and Social Psychology, 41*, 1153–1160.

Paloutzian, R. F. (1996). *Invitation to the psychology of religion* (2nd ed.). Boston: Allyn & Bacon.

Paloutzian, R. F., Richardson, J. R., & Rambo, L. R. (1999). Religious conversion and personality change. *Journal of Personality, 67*, 1047–1079.

Paloutzian, R. F., & Silberman, I. (2003). Religion and the meaning of social behavior: Concepts and issues. In P. Roelofsma, J. Corveleyn, & J. van Saane (Eds.), *One hundred years of psychology and religion: Issues and trends in a century long quest* (pp. 155–167). Amsterdam, The Netherlands: VU University Press.

Pargament, K. I. (1997). *The psychology of religion and coping*. New York: Guilford Press.

Park, C. L., & Folkman, S. (1997). Meaning in the context of stress and coping. *Review of General Psychology, 1*, 115–144.

Petty, R. E., & Cacioppo, J. T. (1981). *Attitudes and persuasion: Classic and contemporary approaches*. Dubuque, IA: Brown.

Rambo, L. R. (1993). *Understanding religious conversions*. New Haven, CT: Yale University Press.

Reich, K. H. (1991). The role of complementarity reasoning in religious development. In F. K. Oser & W. G. Scarlett (Eds.), *Religion's development in childhood and adolescence* (pp. 77–89). San Francisco: Jossey-Bass.

Richardson, J. T. (1985). The active vs. passive convert: Paradigm conflict in conversion/recruitment research. *Journal for the Scientific Study of Religion, 24*(2), 119–236.

Richardson, J. T. (1995). Clinical and personality assessment of participants in new religions. *The International Journal for the Psychology of Religion, 5*(3), 145–170.

Robbins, T., & Anthony, D. (1982). Deprogramming, brainwashing, and the medicalization of deviant religious groups. *Social Problems, 29*, 283–297.

Rokeach, M. (1973). *The nature of human values*. New York: Free Press.

Rosén, A.-S., & Nordquist, T. A. (1980). Ego developmental level and values in a yogic community. *Journal of Personality and Social Psychology, 39*(6), 1152–1160.

Schwartz, S. H. (1992). Universals in the content and structure of values: Theoretical advances and empirical tests in 20 countries. In M. P. Zanna (Ed.), *Advances in experimental social psychology* (Vol. 25, pp. 1–65). San Diego: Academic Press.

Schwartz, S. H., & Huismans, S. (1995). Value priorities and religiosity in four Western religions. *Social Psychology Quarterly, 58*, 88–107.

Silberman, I. (2005a). Religion as a meaning system. *Journal of Social Issues* [special issue], *61*(4).

Silberman, I. (2005b). Religion as a meaning system: Implications for the new millennium. *Journal of Social Issues, 61*(4).

Spilka, B., Hood, R. W., Jr., Hunsberger, B., & Gorsuch, R. (2003). *The psychology of religion: An empirical approach* (3rd ed.). New York: Guilford Press.

Spilka, B., Shaver, P., & Kirkpatrick, L. A. (1985). A general attribution theory for the psychology of religion. *Journal for the Scientific Study of Religion, 24,* 1–20.

Starbuck, E. D. (1899). *The psychology of religion.* London: Walter Scott.

Ullman, C. (1982). Cognitive and emotional antecedents of religious conversion. *Journal of Personality and Social Psychology, 43,* 183–192.

Ullman, C. (1989). *The transformed self: The psychology of religious conversion.* New York: Plenum Press.

Zinnbauer, B. J., & Pargament, K. I. (1998). Spiritual conversion: A study of religious change among college students. *Journal for the Scientific Study of Religion, 37*(1), 161–180.

19

Mystical, Spiritual, and Religious Experiences

RALPH W. HOOD, JR.

The one undisputed classic in the field of psychology of religion is *The Varieties of Religious Experience* (James, 1902/1985), a text that Miller and Thorensen (1999, p. 7) say might be titled *The Varieties of Spiritual Experience* if published today. It is worth emphasizing that the subtitle of this classic is "A Study in Human Nature" and that James claimed that the "root and centre" of personal religion is in mystical states of consciousness (1902/1985, p. 301). Thus psychologists ought to be interested in mystical, spiritual, and religious experiences insofar as they are part of human nature. Since there are major current reviews of the research on both mysticism (Hood, 2002b; Spilka, Hood, Hunsberger, & Gorsuch, 2003, Chap. 10; Wulff, 2000) and spiritual and religious experience (Hood, 1995a; Spilka et al., 2003, Chap. 9), we shall be selective in our evaluation of the literature. Our focus is framed within the proposal for a new *multilevel interdisciplinary paradigm* (Emmons & Paloutzian, 2003, p. 395, emphasis in original) as we reconsider some of the material in the reviews noted above.

THE RELIGION/SPIRITUALITY DEBATE
AND ITS EMPIRICAL CONSEQUENCES FOR EXPERIENCE

A dominant theme both conceptually and empirically within the psychology of religion is whether religion and spirituality can or ought to be differentiated. Reviews of this debate are readily available (see Zinnabauer & Pargament, Chapter 2, this volume). While investigators may vary in their personal commitment to transcendence, they share a consensus that scientific definitions of both spirituality and religion must include a sense of, a belief in, or a search for the transcendent (Hill et al., 2000). However, scholars continue to debate whether or not the transcendent is "vertical," implying a sense of the divine, essentially a code expression for a supernatural being or beings. Those who accept a "vertical" transcendence identify it with religion in the sense of a shared community of believers that identifies, labels, or even constructs its ultimate reality (Beit-Hallahmi, 2003; Hood, 2003b). As a community of affirmation, religion necessarily excludes competing claims to reality. Thus, in this sense, "religion" is a more narrow term than the term "spirituality." While most religious persons define themselves as spiritual, there is an emerging group of people in the United States who define themselves as spiritual but not religious (Hood, 2003b). Some social scientists have argued that the diversity of belief and experiences of these people make spirituality a "fuzzy" concept (Spilka, 1993). We explore this claim shortly, but for now it is worth noting that when religion is defined so broadly as to exclude the necessity for a sense of the divine the term loses its analytical power, as both psychologists (Beit-Hallahmi, 2003) and sociologists (Stark, 2001) have noted. If religion is defined to necessitate the supernatural, the psychological consequence is that those who identify themselves as both religious *and* spiritual will define experiences within the language forms of a particular faith tradition. An individual experiences the realities of his or her faith, labeled or constructed accordingly. Even mystical experiences are faith-specific (Katz, 1977).

Experiences of Being Both Religious and Spiritual

The majority of persons identify themselves as *both* religious and spiritual. While predominantly U.S. Protestant college students have been sampled, the findings are consistent for U.S. culture as a whole (Hood, 2003a; Zinnbauer et al., 1999). For these persons, being spiritual identifies a largely experiential component of their faith. Field studies have been particularly useful in identifying both the normative constraints and the social support that legitimate particular religious experiences. For instance, Apolito (1998) has used direct testimony to explore how complex social and psychological processes interacted to result in the acceptance of the apparition of the Virgin Mary that appeared to children at Oliveto Citra, Spain. Likewise, Carroll (1986) has provided an empirically based interpretation of the psychodynamics involved in Marian apparitions. Quasi-experimental techniques support Carroll's thesis among Protestants males unfamiliar with the Catholic tradition (Hood, Morris, & Watson, 1991).

Hufford (1982, p. xv) has proposed the useful term "phenomenography," paralleling the term "ethnography," while demanding that social scientists pay careful attention to the richness of experience to see precisely what aspects of experience their theories can and cannot explain. His own empirical work on the "Old Hag" phenomenon common in Scandinavian culture and Wiebe's (1997, 2000, 2004) phenomenological studies of historical and contemporary visions of Christ indicate that such experiences cannot be adequately explained by contemporary psychological theories. The new paradigm is useful in suggesting ways in which partial theoretical explanations of such experiences can be used to compliment one another to provide a more complete and adequate explanation than any one theory can provide by itself.

Sectarian Experiences of Being Both Religious and Spiritual

Consistent with the new paradigm are a series of studies using both field and quasi-experimental methods to understand the conditions under which sectarian forms of experiencing religion occur. Historical, narrative, ethnographic, and quasi-experimental studies supplement one another to provide an enhanced understanding of less normatively accepted religious practices. A term gaining acceptance that unites all these approaches is "reflexive ethnography" (Davies, 1999). It tends to focus upon the "lived religion" of everyday experience (Hall, 1997). For instance, Poloma's (1989) participant observation study of The Assemblies of God and her more recent study of the Toronto Blessing (2003) documents the shift in Pentecostalism from an emphasis on glossolalia to other gifts of the spirit (such as holy laughter) that serve to revitalize religious feelings suppressed by institutionalization. Likewise, Hood and his colleagues have used a wide variety of methodologies to explore the contemporary serpent handlers of Appalachia (see Hood & Belzen, Chapter 4, this volume).

Experiences of Being Spiritual but Not Religious

The persistent finding that about 25–30% of individuals in U.S. culture identify themselves as spiritual but not religious has been explored by qualitative methods (Hood, 2003b). Qualitative studies by both psychologists (Day, 1994) and sociologists (Roof, 1993) indicate that this minority is likely to be vociferously antireligious. For some, spirituality is a fierce rejection of religion.

The recent rediscovery by psychologists of a spirituality opposed to religion has been well established in more sociologically oriented literatures and is an integral aspect of the church–sect–mysticism theory proposed by Troeltsch (Hood, 2003b). Vernon (1968) noted over a quarter of a century ago that those who answered "none" when asked about their religious preference nevertheless had experiences that those with a religious preference would identify as experiences of religion. For instance, reviews of the empirical literature indicate that those who identify themselves as spiritual but not religious have high rates of spiritual experiences, including mystical experiences (Hood, 2003a, 2003b). However, they are reluctant to describe these experiences in explicitly religious language. Thus, the social construction of experience for "spiritual but not religious" persons is not framed within the language of a specific faith tradition.

The common complaint made by psychologists of religion that spirituality is a "fuzzy" concept is misleading. The application of the term "fuzzy" to spirituality was first made by Bernard Spilka (1993) and then was given wide play by Zinnbauer et al. (1999). However, paying careful attention to the qualitative analyses of respondents' descriptions reveals that rather than being "fuzzy" spirituality is a fluid term allowing for a wide range of genuinely spiritual experiences that many conservative religious traditions reject (Hood, 2003a, 2003b).

Another issue in the "spiritual but not religious" worldview is the possibility that transcendence can be "horizontal" as opposed to "vertical." For instance, the sociologist Mathew's (2003) typology of the sacred explicitly *excludes* restricting the sacred to the supernatural. Likewise the psychologist Elkins (2001) has proposed a humanistic model of the sacred focusing upon its more secular (horizontal) psychological expressions. The psychologist Emmons (1999) allows for both a "vertical" and a "horizontal" axis of spiritual striving. Finally, McClenon (1994), working from an experience-centered approach that is quite akin to reflexive ethnography, reminds us that what he terms "wondrous events" can occur in cultures and traditions that have no term for the supernatural (such as Tibetan Buddhism). Thus, while wondrous events may stimulate religious explanations, they need not do so. Hufford (1982) and Spickard (1993) make the same claim for paranormal experiences. We next explore two controversial but persistently identified areas of paranormal experiences that are often identified as spiritual but not religious experiences: reports of alien abduction and experiences triggered by specific chemicals.

PARANORMAL CLAIMS OF UFOs AND ALIEN ABDUCTIONS

Psychologists of religion have avoided the study of paranormal experiences, tending to classify them as neither religious nor spiritual. Earlier investigators labeled paranormal experiences as anomalous, attributing them to erroneous ("magical") thinking (Zusne & Jones, 1989). However, more recent work keeps open the possibility of nonreductionist views even regarding the more extreme among anomalous experiences. A recent edited work published by the American Psychological Association defines *anomalous experiences* as those that while common are nevertheless believed to deviate from ordinary experience or from the usually accepted definitions of reality (Cardeña, Lynn, & Krippner, 2000a, p. 4). Examples include hallucinations, near-death, past-life, mystical, and paranormal experiences. The religious and spiritual relevance of these experiences is that they often gain added meaning when they are embedded in sectarian discourse, whether religious or scientific, that both explains and legitimates them in opposition to more culturally accepted knowledge systems (Cardeña, Lynn, & Krippner, 2000b; McClenon, 1994). As Truzzi (1971) notes, anomalous experiences contradict institutionalized knowledge, *both* scientific and religious.

Alien abduction experiences are beginning to gain significant subcultural support, granting believers in these abductions a form of social legitimation that refutes the claim that such experiences are delusional (Appelle, Lynn, & Newman, 2000; Skal, 1998, pp. 195–229; Williams & Fallconer, 1994). It is less profitable to ask what causes these experiences than to try to understand the experience of the world from within a deviant subculture that validates and finds meaningful what others can only describe as anomalous experiences from within their own perspective. Some define paranormal events in a fashion that denies them religious importance (Spickard, 1993). However, as Kelsey (1972, p. 21) notes, "The Bible is a mine of information on ESP or psi phenomena. Nearly every book of the Bible shows the belief that human beings have contact with more than just the physical world and that there are ways of influencing the world and people besides the physical senses." Poloma (1989) created a Charismatic Experience Index (CHAREX) that rates what she defines as paranormal powers, including praying in tongues, receiving answers to prayers, prophecying, being slain in the spirit, and receiving personal confirmation of scriptural truths (p. 12). Based upon her participant observation study of the Assemblies of God tradition, Poloma's data are consistent with Kelsey's (1972) claim. For many Pentecostals the experience of the paranormal is "normal" (Poloma, 1989, p. 2).

Studies employing survey data reveal that reports of paranormal experiences have similar antecedents and structures as reports of other ecstatic experiences commonly accepted as religious (Fox, 1992; Hood, 1989b; Yamane & Polzer, 1994). Among paranormal experiences, the perception of UFOs and their more recent elaboration into "alien abduction experiences" (AAE) have begun to generate a considerable body of scientific study. Jung (1958/1964, p. 315) referred to the citing of UFOs as "visionary" experiences and cautioned that psychology alone could not exhaust their explanation. Recently, investigators such as Strassman (2001) have suggested that certain chemicals that effect receptor cites for serotonin may elicit awareness of dimensions of reality in which reports of alien abduction become possible as actual events. However, as with many religious experiences, psychologists are more likely to be comfortable with explanations that are more within the mainstream of realities psychologists accept. For instance, Skal (1998) has noted that the term "flying saucer" came into vogue only after June 1947 when newspapers reported that a Boise, Idaho, pilot named Kenneth Arnold saw nine strange objects flying near Mt. Rainer and described them as moving "like a saucer if you skipped it across the water" (p. 204). Thus, first came newspaper headlines referring to "flying saucers," and only then did individuals began to report sightings of them. Thus, cultural expectations based upon journalistic headlines that actually were in error might have played a role in shaping what have become common sightings of "UFOs." Instead of moving "like saucers" skipping across the water, they became identified as "flying saucers." This social construction became the template for perception of flying saucers within U.S. culture.

Apparently even less plausible than the existence of UFOs are claims to AAE that include being captured, taken aboard a UFO, and then being subjected to physical, mental, and spiritual examinations before being returned to earth (Bullard, 1987). Other more extreme claims may include the taking of tissue samples, body implants, and even the birth of alien–human hybrid babies (Jacobs, 1992). As fantastic as these claims appear, researchers must accept the fact that the reports of such experiences are no more frequent among the mentally ill than among normals (Berenbaum, Kerns, & Raghavan, 2000; Jacobson & Bruno, 1994; Parnell & Sprinkle, 1990). Thus, pathological processes cannot explain the experience, however curious, nor is it necessarily delusional (Williams & Fallconer, 1994).

Among the most plausible and least controversial explanations for these reports are fantasy-proneness or boundary deficits caused by using cultural available scenarios derived from film and other media sources; confusing subjective experiences with objectively real events; suggestibility and hypnosis (especially when such reports are "recovered" in therapeutic encounters using hypnosis); sleep disorders; and various possible psychoses in at least a minority of cases (Appelle et al., 2000). However, the fact that often AAEs contain theophanies (the receipt of explicit religious or spiritual messages) links AAEs to other experiences more common within mainstream faith traditions. Lest skeptics too quickly consider these experiences to be simply bizarre manifestations exhaustively explainable by the social sciences, they might be cautioned that those who have studied these experiences in depth have found that the dismissal of their veridicality, as with many claims to more mainstream religious experiences, is more difficult than one might at first think (Appelle, 1996; Skal, 1998; Strassman, 2001). The fact that psychology of religion is confronted with the power of alien abduction claims in such groups as Heaven's Gate is but a recent example. Despite the popular press descriptions of a suicide cult, the cult's own framing of their acts was made in religious terms. For instance, the cult's official website referred to the "willful leaving of the body." It noted the sacrifices of the Jews at Mazada in 73A.D. and claimed the willingness of the cult members to avoid "true suicide" by not refusing to prepare to enter the Kingdom of Heaven by means of the Hale–Bopp Comet.[1] The linking of images of inhabitants of the Kingdom of Heaven with aliens associated with UFOs aided Heaven Gate's claims to religious legitimacy. Bader (2003) has empirically documented that the demographics of members of Heaven's Gate parallels those for members attracted to new religious movements that mix the therapeutic and the spiritual. Finally, Zeller (2003) notes how the cult opposed both the supernatural claims of religion and the purely natural scientific epistemologies in favor of its own "scientific religion." It has been more than half a century since Jung said of UFOs that "if military authorities have felt compelled to set up bureaus for collecting and evaluating UFO reports, then psychology, too, has not only the right but also the duty to do what it can to shed light on this dark problem" (1958/1964, p. 416). The new paradigm is ideally suited to guide research in this area.

PSYCHEDELICS OR ENTHEOGENS

A controversial area of empirical research is the study of entheogens, the preferred term (instead of psychedelics) for those who argue that drugs can facilitate spiritual and religious experiences (Forte, 1997). It has long been recognized that many religions employ various naturally occurring mind-altering substances in their religious rituals. However, until the discovery of psychedelic drugs psychologists of religion rather arrogantly assumed that concern with the facilitation of religious or spiritual experience by drugs was the domain of anthropology and sister disciplines concerned with less "advanced" religions. In a new and controversial discipline with the cumbersome name *archaeopsychopharmacology*, researchers combine study of ancient texts and artifacts with examination of contemporary groups that use naturally occurring psychedelic substances to speculate on the origins of religions (see Spilka et al., 2003, pp. 283–284). They combine speculation with experimental studies to elicit primary religious experiences. While the speculative theories of achaeopsychopharmacology cannot be easily empirically confirmed, its proponents have raised a crucial issue for the social-scientific study of religion: Can entheogens facilitate or produce religious experiences?

The literature on the psychology of entheogens is immense, easily running to several thousand studies. Much of the U.S. research has stopped or has been drastically curtailed due to legislation against these drugs. Rätach (1990) concluded that "since the beginning of the 1970s, there has been little new research into psychedelic substances" (p. 2). However, Rätach's claim must be qualified, given the significant current research by anthropologists and ethnobotanists with naturally occurring plant substances and the study of entheogens in European countries where laws are more flexible. There is a continually growing body of research on these drugs (Lukoff, Zanger, & Lu, 1990; Roberts & Hruby, 1995).

Curiously, very few studies have been conducted using religious variables or directly assessing the religious importance of entheogens. This is curious since it has long been noted that there is an obvious similarity between various religious experiences and some chemically facilitated experiences. Back in the late 19th century this similarity was used by Leuba (1896) as evidence to argue that religious experience in advanced traditions should be invalidated because it was similar to drug-induced states in less advanced traditions. The essentials of Leuba's argument have been more recently advanced by Zaehner (1957), who argues that if a mystical experiences is drug-induced it cannot be genuinely religious in the manner of those that occur spontaneously or by means of disciplined religious practice. These largely conceptually based debates do little to advance a scientific understanding of the possible religious importance of psychedelic drugs. Since James's (1902/1985, pp. 20–21) discussion of "medical materialism," it has been obvious that one can no more invalidate an experience because its physiology is known than one can invalidate physiology because its biochemistry has been identified. As Weil (1986) has emphasized, the similarity of psychedelic substances found within plants, animals and the human brain suggests that any simple distinction between natural and artificially induced brain states is arbitrary. Empirical studies indicate that more dogmatic persons will reject as "genuine" religious experiences triggered by drugs, despite the fact that outside of mainstream religious one of the most commonly cited triggers of mystical experience is entheogens (see Hood, 2002b).

The term "psychedelic," the most common precursor to entheogen, has a controversial history (Stevens, 1987). Debates over the common name for the class of drugs we are discussing ranges from "hallucinogenic," to "psychotomimetic," to "psychedelic," to "entheogen." Ironically, "hallucinogenic" is the most inadequate term because hallucination is one of the least common responses to psychedelic drugs (Barber, 1970). While these drugs do produce various visual and imagery effects, both with eyes open and with eyes closed, they do not produce false perceptions mistaken as real (i.e., hallucinations). "Psychotomimetic" was the term favored by early researchers who thought this class of drugs produced psychoses or psychotic-like states. Given the cultural evaluation of psychoses, the negative connotations of "psychotomimetic" are obvious. However, it is well established that the ability of psychedelics to elicit sudden psychoses in otherwise normal persons is highly exaggerated (Barr, Langs, Holt, Goldberger, & Klein, 1972). Ironically, "psychedelic" was the term most favored by those who favored the "mind-manifesting" aspect of these drugs. It is the most common term in use today, despite its association with the illicit street drug culture (Stevens, 1987). As noted above, those who prefer to focus upon the religious significance of these plant and chemical substances prefer the term "entheogen."

For well-established physiological reasons, entheogens can be expected to produce reliable alterations in visual and imagery phenomena, which to informed and stable participants are interesting objects of conscious exploration (Shanon, 2002; Strassman, 2001). Meaningful images that occur under the influence of these substances when a person's eyes are closed are not typically attributed to the object expected to exist in the world in the sense that if one opened one's eyes the object would be in physical reality. Likewise, when a person's eyes are open, he or she notes alterations in his or her perception of objects as *perceptual* alterations of real existing objects, not as changes in the actual physical objects themselves or as the perception of objects that are in fact not real. However, the ability to interpret perceptions in terms of a meaningful frame can transform a person's perception of the world. With an appropriate religious set and setting, psychedelic drugs can facilitate religious experiences insofar as someone under the influence of these drugs may for the first time see the world in terms appropriate to a particular system of meaning. In this sense the "otherworldly" property of entheogens is well established and suggests that they elicit wondrous or anomalous experiences. In a classic study Masters and Houston (1966) found that religious imagery was quite common, even when many participants did not identify themselves as having a "religious" drug experience. For instance, religious architecture was one of the most common imageries reported, but Masters and Houston (1966, pp. 265–266) claim that this occurred more out of a sense of aesthetic appreciation, not as a manifestation of a genuine religious interest.

The frequent report of religious imagery is likely to be a function of set and setting, long known to be major determinants of the content of imagery elicited by entheogens (Barber, 1970; Barr et al., 1972). It would be naive to claim that religious experiences are drug-specific effects. Rather, the power of entheogens to facilitate religious experience is the extent to which states of consciousness, altered by chemical substances, are seen as relevant in religious terms. Within U.S. culture the ironic fact is that mainstream religions send mixed signals relative to religious experiences—often encouraging and validating experiences when they are interpreted as originating in God, but discouraging and invalidating experiences known to be chemically facilitated, as has been empirically demonstrated (see Spilka et al., 2003, Chap. 10). The fact that many participants in studies using entheogens experience religious imagery and use religious language to describe otherwise secular imagery (e.g., cosmological events) is difficult to assess. Masters and Houston (1966, p. 260) noted that the use of sacramental or religious metaphors was a common practice for participants even though "genuine" religious experiences may have been rare. Grof (1980) has argued that the therapeutic use of entheogens often provides a set and setting that encourages the report of religious and spiritual experiences, many of which he interpreted in terms of Jungian theory. Jungian theory is particularly favorable to describing religious imagery, but it has been ignored by measurement-oriented psychologists. Leary (1964) demonstrated that religious imagery in LSD psychotherapy sessions is common and increases if the set and setting are made even more explicitly religious—for instance, by having religious symbols in the therapeutic room. Furthermore, Leary, Metzner, and Alpert (1964) utilized a religious classic (*The Tibetian Book of the Dead*) as a cartography for psychedelic-induced mental states. More recently the Dali Lama has favored Thurman's (1994) translation of this classic text, also known as *The Book of Liberation through Understanding in the Between* (Dali Lama, 1994, p. xxi). The phrase "in the between" focuses upon states of consciousness and not death. Once it is recognized that reincarnation is taken for granted in Tibetan culture, the ontological relevance of states of consciousness, drug-facilitated or not, meshes nicely with the new proposed paradigm for the psychology of religion.

Stevens (1987) has documented the history of the original "psychedelic movement" and its failed effort to have "psychedelic" drugs accepted for sacramental use within a religious frame. However, two exceptions are the Native American Church in the United States (Bergman, 1971; LaBarre, 1969) and the Church of Santo Daime in Brazil (Shanon, 2002). Both these churches have a history of the sacramental use of entheogens that demonstrate that drugs can be incorporated into religious frameworks and used to facilitate experiences whose meaning is accepted as religious (Bergman, 1971; LaBarre, 1969).

The cultural bias against entheogens has not only affected serious study of these chemicals, but it has also made it difficult to arrive at a balanced view of the range of their effects (Forte, 1997). Furthermore, several reviewers have argued that typical double-blind studies are particularly inappropriate ways to investigate entheogens, especially since those who are in the control conditions are likely to be immediately aware of this fact (Bakalar & Greenspoon, 1989; Yensen, 1990). Many researchers have supported the view that ingestion of psychedelic substances on the part of researchers is a valid and (some claim) necessary method of study. The provocative studies of ayahuasca (a psychoactive brew consumed throughout the upper Amazon region) by the cognitive psychologist Benny Shanon (2001) carefully compare his own numerous experiences with this brew with those reported by others to develop a nonreductive assessment of the phenomenology of the ayahuasca experience. Interestingly, it has both been incorporated into a religious tradition (the Church of Santo Daime, a mixture of indigenous traditions with Catholicism) and cultivated by those who refuse to interpret the experience in specific religious language.

The examples cited above suggest that within the new paradigm, truly multilevel interdisciplinary approaches extend the range of material that psychologists must consider as they explore the conditions under which individuals experience their religion or spirituality. However, to explore another option within this paradigm we shall look at the possibility of mystical, religious, or spiritual experiences that do not simply get absorbed into a social constructionist paradigm.

MYSTICAL, SPIRITUAL, AND RELIGIOUS EXPERIENCES

Spickard has identified different approaches to the study of religious experiences, which he notes sociologists (and we add psychologists) have not comprehended well (1993, p. 115). For this review we simply note that we can collapse Spickard's constructionist and labeling models as similar. Both these approaches emphasize the role of language and social process in identifying experiences of religion, spirituality, or mysticism within the confines of language, tradition, and culture in what we have termed experiences of religion, spirituality, or mysticism. Spickard also identifies a Jamesean "overbelief" model (1993, p. 111) in which the distinction between experience and interpretation is maintained but the focus is upon experience and not the language in which it is expressed ("overbelief"). Thus we prefer to talk of social expression, rather than of construction, and leave it an open conceptual and empirical possibility that there are fundamental experiences that are inherently mystical, religious, or spiritual and that become only partially expressed through language. More than one scholar of religion has claimed that such experiences are always a response to a reality not reducible to simple sensory terms (Hick, 1989, pp. 252–261; Jones, 1986, p. 225). As we focus upon mystical, religious, or spiritual experiences, it behooves us to define such experiences as including recognition of and response to what might be inherently sacred realities. Two candidates are the numinous and the mystical.

Numinous and Mystical Experiences

Many scholars have contrasted numinous experience with mystical experience. A *numinous experience* is an awareness of a holy other beyond nature and a sense that one is in communion with this holy other. Typically, this experience is identified with the classic work of Otto (1917/1958) whose phenomenological analysis illuminates the human response to the transcendent. Elkins's (2001, p. 208) humanistic model includes a response to the numinous, meaning that there is a divine component to his model. Thus, introducing the numinous back into empirical psychology is congruent with the nonreductive nature of the new multilevel paradigm. Otto's phenomenology of religious experience includes the essential fact that for him religious experience includes a nonrational component that is characterized psychologically by a numinous consciousness. Otto's translator noted that the emphasis on a response to the divine that characterizes numinous consciousness is the sensing of a "beyond" that gradually is realized "within," whether obscurely or clearly (Harvey, 1958, p. xv). This goes far to correct Schleiermacher's emphasis on a primary feeling of dependence that Proudfoot (1985) criticized as demanding a cognitive framework to experience. As social scientists, we can study the response to the numinous by noting that from the believer's perspective it is a response to a transcendent object experienced as real. Numinous experiences allow the realization of a personal transcendent object, often referred to as God, Allah, or Yahweh. Obviously, religious traditions assert the reality of this object, refusing to accept reductive interpretations of the numinous.

The numinous consciousness is both compelled to seek out and explore this transcendent object (*mysterium fascinans*) and to be repelled in the face of the majesty and awfulness of this object in whose presence one's creatureness is accentuated (*mysterium tremendum*). Efforts to rationally confront the feelings of *tremendum* are articulated in personal conceptualizations of a holy other such as God or Allah or Yahweh. The *fascinans* is explicated in rational concepts such as grace, in which the inadequacy of personal analogies to conceptualize the holy other are revealed. The *fascinans* thus has a mystical element insofar as the personal analog revealed in the *tremendum* is found to be inadequate and an impersonal language is sought to describe it. Not surprisingly, Stace's (1960) categories of introvertive and extrovertive mysticism are derived from Otto's (1932) mysticism of introspection and unifying vision, respectively. Thus, while it is possible to separate the numinous and the mystical as two poles of religious experience, they are ultimately united. Mystical experiences of unity (variously expressed) can be numinous as well, eliciting the *mysterium fascinans* when the object is experienced in impersonal terms and the *mysterium tremendum* when the object is experienced in personal terms. Hick (1989, pp. 252–296) has articulated this duality as the *personae* and *impersonae* of the Real. Hood (1995b, 2002a) has emphasized that William James accepted both impersonal (the Absolute) and personal (God) interpretations as compatible with the facts of mystical experience. Empirical studies use measurements that tend to emphasize either experiences of a sense of presence favoring numinous experiences or a sense of unity favoring mystical experiences.

Numinous Experiences as a Sense of Presence

The empirical study of numinous experiences has largely focused upon responses to surveys and questionnaires. Pafford (1973) had university and grammar-school students read selections from an autobiography that described a numinous experience and then asked them to write about an experience of their own similar to the one they had just read. He found that the most common word used to describe such experiences was "awesome." He suggested that children have an innate capacity to experience the numinous that gradually dissipates as they become more involved in the secular world. A study done in Sweden in the mid-1940s but not published until 1959 collected reports from 630 children who responded to the phrase "Once when I thought about God. . . . " Of the 630 compositions, 566 contained reports of religious experiences, including a felt sense of an invisible presence (Klingberg, 1959, p. 213). Tamiminen (1991) utilized a question first proposed by Glock and Stark (1965) to assess the experiential dimension of their model of religion. They had found that in a survey sample of almost 3,000, 72% of respondents answered "yes" to the question "Have you ever as an adult had the feeling that you were somehow in the presence of God?" (Glock & Stark, 1965, p. 157). Using this question with children (dropping "as an adult"), Tamiminen showed a gradual decline of affirmative responses across grade level in a longitudinal study of Scandinavian youth. Thus, in more secular cultures one could argue that an innate ability to experience the numinous is possible but is likely to decline without cultural support. Hoffman's (1992) collection of spiritual and inspirational experiences in childhood also supports his claim (also see Boyatzis, Chapter 7, this volume).

Also in support of this claim are numerous survey studies conducted in the United States and the United Kingdom asking respondents if they have ever had an experience that is a numinous one. Reviews of these studies show consistently high rates of response despite variations in the wording of questions (see Spilka et al., 2003, pp. 307–312). Hence, the empirical point is simply that both children and adults report numinous experiences whether they identify themselves as religious and spiritual or simply as spiritual but not religious. The former data is inferred from obtained religious identifications and the latter from the fact noted above that even people whose religious self-identification is "none" report such experiences. The fact that such experiences are so readily reported means that psychologists who take the new paradigm seriously should construct measures compatible with the already considerable phenomenological and survey work illuminating the nature of such experiences. Keitner and Haidt (2003) have created a measure of awe that may reference, but need not reference, a vertical dimension. The cautionary note here is that measures that do not include explicit indices of the transcendent miss connecting to the large literatures in phenomenology and religious studies (Sundararajan, 2002). They also are less likely to empirically identify additional unique or uniquely interactive variance explained by measures that are explicitly linked to a sense of the divine. In this sense the measure of awe proposed by Williamson and Froese (2001) is promising as it is directly based upon Otto's work and thus links the empirical study of awe to classic works in the phenomenology of awe.

Mystical Experiences

Mystical experience has long been a central topic both in the psychology of religion and in the field of religious studies. Two current empirical approaches can be contrasted, that of Hood and his colleagues and that of Thalbourne and his colleagues.

Hood based his measure of mysticism on the phenomenological work of Stace (1960). Reviews of this work are readily available (see Hood, 2002b; Spilka et al., 2003, Chap. 10). Here we focus only upon the claim that mystical experience has a common core that is universal despite variations in the language in which this experience is expressed. This position is identified as the "unity thesis." Stace's work has been central in the philosophical and religious studies literatures, inspiring an entire volume of critical responses to his common core or unity thesis (Katz, 1977). Thus Hood's research links the empirical study of mysticism to these largely conceptual literatures in the spirit of the new paradigm (Hood, 2002b).

Stace's (1960) phenomenology of mysticism identifies *introvertive* (an undifferentiated unity), *extrovertive* (unity amid multiplicity), and *interpretative* factors. Hood argues that the common unity factors are possibly inherent in the nature of the experience (and perhaps reality), while the interpretation factor (whether noetic, religious, etc.) can vary. In a series of factor-analytic studies Hood has essentially replicated Stace's phenomenology. Most recently, in a cross-cultural study comparing U.S. and Iranian subjects, confirmatory factor analysis supported Hood's three-factor model over various alternatives (Hood et al., 2001).

Hood's work has included the facilitation of mystical experiences in a series of quasi-experimental studies (Hood, 1995a). This links to earlier research on entheogens in which set and setting were manipulated to enhance mystical experiences assessed by means of Stace's criteria for mysticism. The well-known Good Friday experiment in which subjects who had taken psilocybin produced higher mysticism scores than those who took a placebo has been found to be significant for its participants even in a 25-year follow-up study (see Spilka et al., 2003, pp. 321–322). Further, as noted above, the fact that Leary and his colleagues (1964) found *The Tibetan Book of the Dead* relevant to psychedelic experiences returns us to the study of achaeopsychopharmacology but now with the focus on the elicitation of mystical experiences in individuals who in Jamesean fashion have original experiences and not simply a "second-hand religious life" (James, 1902/1985, p. 15).

Thalbourne has developed a measure of mysticism based partly upon his own experiences that heavily correlates with Hood's measure (Thalbourne & Delin, 1999, p. 53). In a series of studies, he and his colleagues have suggested that mysticism is best identified by a single factor associated with other phenomena such as creativity, belief in the paranormal, and psychopathology (especially bipolar disorder). He and his colleagues have long championed the concept of *transliminality* as a concept to describe the ability, likely genetically based, to attend to inner psychological states and processes (Thalbourne, 1998; Thalbourne, Bartemucci, Delin, Fox, & Nofi, 1997; Thalbourne & Delin, 1994).

Much of Thalbourne's work has been published in journals of parapsychology that are often ignored by mainstream psychologists. However, it is significant for two reasons. First, it counters Hood's view that suggests that the phenomenology of mysticism developed by Stace is in fact an experience central to both religion (when interpreted within a specific faith tradition) and spirituality (when interpreted outside the claims of any dogma). Hood's claim that mysticism is a universal experience with ontological ramifications is countered by the research agenda of Thalbourne and his colleagues which suggests that mysticism is part of a purely natural psychology rooted in the tendency to be sensitive to internally generated states of consciousness, including a tendency to pathology. Thalbourne has noted that it remains to be seen if transliminality is "nothing more than schizotpy" (Thalbourne et al., 1997, p. 327). Still, Thalbourne is willing to consider that not only does the eruption into consciousness produced by high transliminality appear to some to be miraculous or to derive from the Godhead, but that in fact it may be so (Thalbourne & Delin, 1999, p. 59).

Second, both Hood and Thalbourne reintroduce the fact that mystical experiences are associated with reports of paranormal phenomena. The frequency of the report of paranormal phenomena in survey studies parallels that of the report of mystical and numinous experiences, and the same predictors of the report of this experience are associated with the predictors of the reports of paranormal phenomena (Fox, 1992; Yamane, 2000). For instance, using survey data from Canadians, Orenstein (2002) has shown that when controlled for unconventional religious beliefs, church attendance is strongly associated with lower paranormal belief. Using the same data set, McKinnon (2002) has suggested belief in the paranormal and church attendance is correlated only for those who do not attend church regularly. Thus, mainstream religion tends to counter belief in the paranormal while those outside mainstream religions, including those who practice sectarian forms of religion that remain "spiritual but not religious," likely account for the substantial proportion of believers. A recent review of the issue by Targ, Schlitz, and Irwin (2000) concluded that paranormal experiences are reported by over half the population in all countries where samples have been taken.

This review of experiences often ignored in mainstream psychology documents that the field of the psychology of religion has a tumultuous history. This history can serve to remind us of the state of the field when it began. As Coon (1992) notes, North American psychologists fought hard to differentiate methodologically sound, scientific psychology from "pop psychology" which supported and validated dubious spiritual (as in "spiritualism") and psychic phenomena. Perhaps the study of mystical, spiritual, and religious experiences within the spirit of the proposed new paradigm will serve to shed what light science can and leave others to ponder what ultimate meanings may remain.

NOTE

1. See www.wave.net/upg/gate/letter.htm.

REFERENCES

Apolito, P. (1998). *Apparitions of the Madonna at Oliveto Citra: Local visions and cosmic drama* (W. Christian, Jr., Trans.). University Park, PA: University of Pennsylvania Press.

Appelle, S. (1996). The abduction experience: A critical evaluation of theory and evidence. *Journal of UFO Studies, 6*, 29–79.

Appelle, S., Lynn, S. J., & Newman, L. (2000). Alien abduction experiences. In E. Cardeña, S. J. Lynn, & S. Krippner (Eds.), *Varieties of anomalous experience: Examining the scientific evidence* (pp. 253–282). Washington, DC: American Psychological Association.

Bader, C. D. (2003). Supernatural support groups: Who are the UFO abductees and ritual-abuse survivors? *Journal for the Scientific Study of Religion, 42*, 669–678.

Bakalar, J., & Greenspoon, L. (1989). Testing psychotherapies and drug therapies: The case of psychedelic drugs. In S. Peroutka (Ed.), *Ecstasy: The clinical, pharmacological and neurotoxicological effect of the drug MDMAS.* Norwell, MA: Kluwer Academic.

Barber, T. X. (1970). *LSD, marijuana, yoga and hypnosis.* Chicago: Aldine Press.

Barr, H. L., Langs, R. J., Holt, R. R., Goldberger, L. & Klein, C. S. (1972). *LSD, personality and experience.* New York: Wiley.

Beit-Hallahmi, B. (2003). In debt to William James: The *Varieties* as inspiration and blueprint. In H.M. P. Roelfsma, J. M. T. Corveleyn, & J. W. van Saane (Eds.), *One hundred years of psychology and religion: Issues and trends in a century long quest* (pp. 83–104). Amsterdam, The Netherlands: VU University Press.

Berenbaum, H., Kerns, J., & Raghavan, C. (2000). Anomalous experiences, peculiarity, and psychopathology. In E. Cardeña, S. J. Lynn, & S. Krippner (Eds.), *Varieties of anomalous experience: Examining the scientific evidence* (pp. 25–46). Washington, DC: American Psychological Association.

Bergman, R. L. (1971). Navajo peyote use: Its apparent safety. *American Journal of Psychiatry, 128*, 695–699.

Bullard, T. E. (1987). *UFO abductions: The measure of a mystery.* Mount Rainer, MD: Fund for UFO Research.

Cardeña, E., Lynn, S. J., & Krippner, S. (2000a). Introduction: Varieties of anomalous experience. In E. Cardeña, S. J. Lynn, & S. Krippner (Eds.), *Varieties of anomalous experience: Examining the scientific evidence* (pp. 3–21). Washington, DC: American Psychological Association.

Cardeña, E., Lynn, S. J., & Krippner, S. (Eds.). (2000b). *Varieties of anomalous experience: Examining the scientific evidence.* Washington, DC: American Psychological Association.

Carroll, M. P. (1986). *The cult of the Virgin Mary: Psychological origins.* Princeton, NJ: Princeton University Press.

Coon, D. J. (1992). Testing the limits of sense and science: American experimental psychologists combat spiritualism, 1880–1920. *American Psychologist, 47*, 143–151.

Dali Lama. (1994). Foreword. In R. A. F. Thurman (Trans.), *The Tibetan book of the dead* (pp. xxi–xxii). New York: Doubleday Dell.

Davies, C. A. (1999). *Reflexive ethnography: A guide to researching ourselves*. New York: Routledge.

Day, J. M. (1994). Moral development, belief and unbelief: Young adults' accounts of religion in the process of moral growth. In J. Corveleyn & D. Hustebaut (Eds.), *Belief and unbelief: Psychological perspectives* (pp. 155–173). Amsterdam, The Netherlands: Rodopi.

Elkins, D. N. (2001). Beyond religions: Toward a humanist spirituality. In K. J. Schneider, J. T. Bugental, & J. F. Pierson (Eds.), *The handbook of humanistic psychology: Leading edges in theory, research, and practice* (pp. 201–212). Thousand Oaks, CA: Sage.

Emmons, R. A. (1999). *The psychology of ultimate concerns: Motivation and spirituality in personality*. New York: Guilford Press.

Emmons, R. A., & Paloutzian, R. F. (2003). The psychology of religion. *Annual Review of Psychology, 54*, 377–402.

Forte, R. (Ed.). (1997). *Entheogens and the future of religion*. San Francisco: Council on Spiritual Practices.

Fox, J. W. (1992). The structure, stability, and social antecedents of reported paranormal experiences. *Sociological Analysis, 53*, 417–431.

Glock, C. Y., & Stark, R. (1965). *Religion and society in tension*. Chicago: Rand McNally.

Grof, S. (1980). *LSD psychotherapy*. Pomona, CA: Hunter House.

Hall, D. D. (Ed.). (1997). *Lived religion in America*. Princeton, NJ: Princeton University Press.

Harvey, J. W. (1958). Translator's preface. In R. Otto, *The idea of the holy* (rev. ed., pp. ix–xix). London: Oxford University Press.

Hick, J. (1989). *An interpretation of religion*. New Haven, CT: Yale University Press.

Hill, P. C., Pargament, K. I., Hood, R. W., Jr., McCullough, M. E., Sawyers, J. P., Larson, D. B., & Zinbauer, B. (2000). Conceptualizing religiosity and spirituality: Points of commonality. *Journal for the Theory of Social Behavior, 30*, 50–77.

Hoffman, E. (1992). *Visions of innocence: Spiritual and inspirational experiences of childhood*. Boston: Shambahla Press.

Hood, R. W., Jr. (1989a). Mysticism, the unity thesis, and the paranormal. In G. K. Zollschan, J. F. Schumaker, & G. F. Walsh (Eds.), *Exploring the paranormal: Perspectives on belief and experience* (pp. 117–130). New York: Avery.

Hood, R. W., Jr. (1989b). The relevance of theologies for religious experiencing. *Journal of Psychology and Theology, 17*, 336–342.

Hood, R. W., Jr. (1995a). The facilitation of religious experience. In R. W. Hood, Jr. (Ed.), *The handbook of religious experience* (pp. 569–597). Birmingham, AL: Religious Education Press.

Hood, R. W., Jr. (1995b). The soulful self of William James. In D. W. Capps & J. L. Jacobs (Eds.), *The struggle for life: A companion to William James'* The varieties of religious experience (Society for the Scientific Study of Religion Monograph Series, Whole No., 9, pp. 209–219). West Lafayette, IN: Society for the Scientific Study of Religion.

Hood, R. W., Jr. (2002a). The mystical self: Lost and found. *The International Journal for the Psychology of Religion, 12*, 1–14.

Hood, R. W., Jr. (2002b). *Dimensions of mystical experience: Empirical studies and psychological links*. Amsterdam, The Netherlands: Rhodopi.

Hood, R. W., Jr. (2003a). Conceptual and empirical consequences of the unity thesis. In J. Belzen (Ed.), *Mysticism: Some psychological considerations* (pp. 17–54). Amsterdam, The Netherlands: Rodopi

Hood, R. W., Jr. (2003b). The relationship between religion and spirituality. In A. L. Griel & D. G. Bromley (Eds.), *Religion and the social order: Vol. 10. Defining religion: Investigating the boundaries between the sacred and the secular* (pp. 241–264). Oxford, UK: JAI/Elsevier Science.

Hood, R. W., Jr., Ghorbani, N., Watson, P. J., Ghramalleki, A. F., Bing, M. B., Davison, H. R., Morris, P. J., & Williamson, P. W. (2001). Dimensions of the Mysticism Scale: Confirming the three-factor structure in the U.S. and Iran. *Journal for the Scientific Study of Religion, 40*, 691–705.

Hood, R. W., Jr., Morris, R. J., & Watson, P. J. (1991). Male commitment to the cult of the Virgin Mary and the Passion of Christ as a function of early maternal bonding. *International Journal for the Psychology of Religion*, 1, 221–231.

Hufford, D. (1982). *The terror that comes in the night. An experience-centered study of supernatural assault traditions*. Philadelphia: University of Pennsylvania Press.

Jacobs, D. M. (1992). *Secret life: First-hand accounts of UFO abductions*. New York: Simon & Schuster.

Jacobson, E., & Bruno, J. (1994). Narrative variants and major psychiatric illnesses in close encounter and abduction narrators. In A. Pritchard, D. E. Pritchard, J. E. Mack, P. Kasey, & C. Yapp (Eds.), *Alien discussions: Proceedings of the Abduction Study Conference, MIT* (pp. 304–309). Cambridge, MA: North Cambridge Press.

James, W. (1985). *The varieties of religious experience*. Cambridge, MA: Harvard University Press. (Original work published 1902)

Jones, R. H. (1986). *Science and mysticism*. London: Associated Universities Press.

Jung, C. G. (1964). Flying saucers: A modern myth of things seen in the skies. In H. Read, M. Fordham, & G. Adler (Eds.) & R.F.C. Hull (Trans.), *The collected works of C. G. Jung* (2nd ed., Vol. 10, pp. 309–433). Princeton, NJ: Princeton University Press. (Original work published 1958)

Katz, S. (1977). *Mysticism and philosophical analysis*. New York: Oxford University Press.

Keitner, D., & Haidt, J. (2003). Approaching awe: A moral, spiritual, and aesthetic emotion. *Cognition and Emotion*, 17, 297–314.

Kelsey, M. T. (1972). *Encounter with God*. Minneapolis, MN: Bethany Fellowship.

Klingberg, G. (1959). A study of religious experience in children from nine to thirteen years of age. *Religious Education*, 54, 211–216.

LaBarre, W. (1969). *The peyote cult* (rev. ed.). New York: Schoken Books.

Leary, T. (1964). Religious experience: Its production and interpretation. *Psychedelic Review*, 1, 324–346.

Leary, T., Metzner, R., & Alpert, R. (1964). *The psychedelic experience: A manual based on* The Tibetan book of the dead. New York: Citadal Press.

Leuba, D. (1896). A study on the psychology of religious phenomena. *American Journal of Psychology*, 7, 309–385.

Lukoff, D., Zanger, R., & Lu, F. (1990). Transpersonal psychology research review: Psychoactive substances and transpersonal states. *Journal of Transpersonal Psychology*, 22, 107–148.

Masters, R. E. L., & Houston, J. (1966). *The varieties of psychedelic experience*. New York: Delta.

Mathew, T. E. (2003). The sacred: Differentiating, clarifying, and extending concepts. *Review of Religious Research*, 45, 32–47.

McClenon, J. (1994). *Wondrous events: Foundations of religious belief*. Philadelphia: University of Pennsylvania Press.

McKinnon, A. M. (2003). The religious, the paranormal, and church attendance: A response to Orenstein. *Journal for the Scientific Study of Religion*, 42, 299–303.

Miller, W. R., & Thorensen, L. E. (1999). Spirituality and health. In W. R. Miller (Ed.), *Integrating spirituality into treatment* (pp. 3–18). Washington, DC: American Psychological Association.

Orenstein, A. (2002). Religion and paranormal belief. *Journal for the Scientific Study of Religion*, 41, 301–311.

Otto, R. (1932). *Mysticism east and west* (B. L. Bracey & R. C. Paynes, Trans.). New York: Macmillan.

Otto, R. (1958). *The idea of the holy* (rev. ed., J. W. Harvey, Trans.). London: Oxford University Press. (Original work published 1917)

Pafford, M. (1973). *Inglorious Wordsworths: A study in some transcendental experiences in childhood and adolescence*. London: Hodder & Stoughton.

Parnell, J. O., & Sprinkle, R. L. (1990). Personality characteristics of persons who claim UFO experiences. *Journal of UFO Studies*, 2, 105–137.

Poloma, M. M. (1989). *The Assembles of God at the crossroads*. Knoxville: University of Tennessee Press.

Poloma, M. M. (2003). *Main street mystics: The Toronto Blessing and revitalizing Pentecostalism*. Walnut Creek, CA: Altamira Press.

Proudfoot, W. (1985). *Religious experience*. Berkeley, CA: University of California Press.

Rätach, C. (Ed.). (1990). *Gateway to inner space: Sacred plants, mysticism and psychotherapy*. Dorset, UK: Prism Press.

Roberts, T. B., & Hruby, P. J. (1995). *Religion and psychoactive sacraments: A bibliographic guide*. San Franscisco: Council on Spiritual Practices.

Roof, W. C. (1993). *A generation of seekers: The spiritual journeys of the boom generation*. San Francisco: Harper.

Shanon, B. (2002). *The antipodes of the mind: Charting the phenomenology of the ayahuasca experience*. New York: Oxford University Press.

Skal, D. J. (1998). *Screams of reason*. New York: Norton.

Spickard, J. V. (1993). For a sociology of religious experience. In W. H. Swatos, Jr. (Ed.), *A future for religion?: New paradigms for social analysis* (pp. 109–127). Thousand Oaks, CA: Sage.

Spilka, B. (1993). *Spirituality: Problems and directions in operalizing a fuzzy concept*. Paper presented at the annual conference of the American Psychological Association, Toronto, Canada.

Spilka, B., Hood, R. W., Jr., Hunsberger, B., & Gorsuch, R. (2003). *The psychology of religion: An empirical approach* (3rd ed.). New York: Guilford Press.

Stace, W. (1960). *Mysticism and philosophy*. Philadelphia: Lippincott.

Stark, R. (2001). Reconceptualizing religion, magic, and science. *Review of Religious Research, 43*, 101–120.

Stassman, R. (2001). *DMT: The spirit molecule*. Rochester, VT: Park Street Press.

Stevens, J. (1987). *Storming heaven: LSD and the American dream*. New York: Harper & Row.

Sundararajan, L. (2002). Religious awe: Potential contributions of negative theology to psychology, "positive" or otherwise. *Journal of Theoretical and Philosophical Psychology, 22*, 174–197.

Tamiminen, K. (1991). *Religious development in childhood and youth: An empirical study*. Helsinki, Finland: Soumalainen Tiedeakatemia.

Targ, E., Schlitz, M., & Irwin, H. J. (2000). Psi-related experiences. In E. Cardeña, S. J. Lynn, & S. Krippner (Eds.), *Varieties of anomalous experience: Examining the scientific evidence* (pp. 219–252). Washington, DC: American Psychological Association.

Thalbourne, M. A. (1998). Transliminality: Further correlates and a short measure. *Journal of the American Society for Psychical Research, 92*, 402–419.

Thalbourne, M. A., Bartemucci, L., Delin, P. S., Fox, B., & Nofi, O. (1997). Transliminality: Its nature and correlates. *Journal of the American Society for Psychical Research, 91*, 305–331.

Thalbourne, M. A., & Delin, P. S. (1994). A common thread underlying belief in the paranormal, creative personality, mystical experience and psychopathology. *Journal of Parapsychology, 58*, 3–38.

Thalbourne, M. A., & Delin, P. S. (1999). Transliminality: Its relation to dream life, religiosity, and mystical experience. *The International Journal for the Psychology of Religion, 9*, 35–43.

Truzzi, M. (1971). Definition and dimensions of the occult: Toward a sociological perspective. *Journal of Popular Culture, 5*, 635–646.

Vernon, G. M. (1968). The religious "nones": A neglected category. *Journal for the Scientific Study of Religion, 7*, 219–229.

Weil, A. (1986). *The natural mind* (rev. ed.). Boston: Houghton Mifflin.

Wiebe, P. H. (1997). *Visions of Jesus: Direct encounter from the New Testament to today*. New York: Oxford University Press.

Wiebe, P. H. (2000). Critical reflections on Christic visions. In J. Andresen & R. K. Forman (Eds.), *Cognitive models and spiritual maps: Interdisciplinary explorations of religious experience* (pp. 119–141). Bowling Green, OH: Imprint Academic.

Wiebe, P. H. (2004). Degrees of hallucinatoriness and Christic visions. *Archiv für Religionpsychologie, 26*, 201–222.

Williams, R. N., & Fallconer, J. E. (1994). Religion and mental health: A hermeneutical consideration. *Review of Religious Research*, *35*, 335–349.

Williamson, W. P., & Froese, A. D. (2001, April). *Preliminary scale construction: Toward a measure of reported religious experience based on Otto's Idea of the Holy.* Poster paper presented at the annual meeting of the Southwestern Psychological Association, Houston, TX.

Wulff, D. M. (2000). Mystical experience. In E. Cardeña, S. J. Lynn, & S. Krippner (Eds.), *Varieties of anomalous experience: Examining the scientific evidence* (pp. 397–440). Washington, DC: American Psychological Association.

Yamane, D. (2000). Narrative and religious experience. *Sociology of Religion*, *61*, 171–189.

Yamane, D., & Polzer, M. (1994). Ways of seeing ecstasy in modern society: Experimental-expressive and cultural-linguistic views. *Sociology of Religion*, *61*, 171–189.

Yensen, R. (1990). LSD and psychotherapy. *Journal of Psychoactive Drugs*, *17*, 267, 277.

Zaehner, R. C. (1957). *Mysticism, sacred and profane: An inquiry into some varieties of praenatural experience.* London: Oxford University Press.

Zeller, B. (2003, November). *Gatekeepers of (Ir) religion: The scientific religion of Heaven's Gate.* Paper presented at the annual meeting of the American Academy of Religion, Atlanta, GA.

Zinnbauer, B. J., Pargament, K. I., Cole, B., Rye, M. S., Butter, E. M., Belavich, T. G., Hipp, K. M., Scott, A. B., & Kadar, J. K. (1999). Religion and spirituality: Unfuzzying the fuzzy. *Journal for the Scientific Study of Religion*, *36*, 549–584.

Zusne, L., & Jones, W. H. (1989). *Anomalistic thinking: A study of magical thinking* (2nd ed.). Hillsdale, NJ: Erlbaum.

20

Religious Practice, Ritual, and Prayer

BERNARD SPILKA

Religious practice and prayer are basically forms of ritual. In order to understand these religiospiritual expressions from a social-scientific and behavioral perspective, one must first comprehend the nature of ritual. After recognizing the special character of religious ritual, I examine religious practices and worship as collective forms of ritual. Prayer is then treated as individualized ritual.

THE NATURE AND SIGNIFICANCE OF RITUAL

The inability of social scientists to define religion comprehensively and satisfactorily amply testifies to its complexity. When one, however, attempts to delineate religion, three major components are usually identified: belief, experience, and behavior. Our concern is with the last, namely, the practice of one's faith, which is basically ritual. It has been called "the single most important characteristic of any living religiousness" (Pilgrim, 1978, p. 64). Hargrove (1971) claims that "there is a universal tendency for religion to become ritualized, to involve highly predictable patterns of behavior" (p. 30). Wiebe's (cited in Anttonen, 2002) recommended that a scientific approach to religion stresses the significance of religious practices. In other words, the essence of religion is ritual performance.

Ritual is fundamentally a prescribed pattern of behavior, hence behavior that is structured, otherwise it will not be considered effective for whatever purpose is intended. Some rituals, particularly public and religious ones, are often rigidly patterned. Invariably these rites are also repetitive, but according to a formula that clearly denotes how many times the various responses are to be enacted in specific situations.

Speaking almost exclusively of religious ceremonies, Pruyser (1968) states that the outstanding feature of ritual acts is that "they are measured, precise, specified in great detail, highly stereotyped, and often very repetitive" (p. 185). He further stresses that ritual is "antispontaneous; it distrusts impulsivity. It capitalizes on inhibition, delay, and various other control devices" (p. 186).

The above specification of ritual reinforces the erroneous notion that ritual is a unique and relatively rare form of behavior. In reality, it is surprisingly common. Roberts (1984) poignantly observes that that there is "a great attraction of humans to ritual experience" (p. 100). Think, for example, of the routine one goes through when meeting another person, starting a conversation, responding to a phone call, or getting up in the morning and preparing for the day. We are surrounded by ritual, practice it compulsively, and then take it for granted, usually failing to recognize its presence. Popularly, the word and the concept appear to be reserved for special occasions (Fulghum, 1995).

Apparently there are no cultures without ritual (Helman, 1994). This does not constitute proof of evolutionary or genetic origins, but it does suggest a potentially useful research direction (Mead, 1966/1972). The literal omnipresence of ritual in a broad spectrum of animals, invertebrates and vertebrates, including humans, is well illustrated by Huxley (1966).

The Functions of Ritual

According to Lorenz (1966), "human rituals serve the same function as animal ritualization-communicating" (Wulff, 1997, p. 155). This, of course presupposes relationships with whatever is the object of communication, whether the self, others, deities, nature, or something else. Ritual, however, also performs other individual and social functions. Lorenz (1963, 1966) and Pruyser (1968) both note that ritual is manifested when there is a need to control and direct emotion, and it also plays roles of considerable importance in religion. With regard to the latter, public ceremonies, in particular, manage, reduce, and/ or focus aggression. This binds people together, enhances social organization, and creates a sense of community (Lorenz, 1963). Needless to say, these are also prime goals for institutional faith.

All of the above imply individual and social control mechanisms. These are evident in the statement of a Navajo physician who describes the purposes of Navaho ritual as one of building community: "Ceremonies in my tribe are events of power and healing . Ceremony invites change, it prays for growth, harmony, order, balance" (quoted in Alvord, 1999, p. 12). In like manner, we read an insightful fictional account of how ritual brought family members together following the death of a mother. They jointly engaged in a personally constructed ritual. One states that "It wasn't so much participating in the rituals themselves as it was the feeling of being part of a tribe, of feeling for the first time that I was involved in something authentic. . . . This was my place. These were my people. My culture" (Ragen, 1998, p. 278).

Ritual, Coping, and Adaptation

Evidence demonstrating the adaptive and coping significance of ritual is overwhelming. Virtually all rituals connote control of self and/or environment. Psychologically, they reduce anxiety and uncertainty (Benson & Stark, 1996; Hinde, 1999; Pruyser, 1968). Erikson (1966) avers that "in man the overcoming of ambivalence as well as of ambiguity is one of the prime functions of ritualization" (p. 339). Uncertainty means unpredictability, discomfort, and threat, implying a lack of power. Emphasizing the discrepancy between reality and ideal over which one frequently lacks control, Smith (1982/1996) claims that ritual indicates the way things ought to be. Ceremonial participation confirms the individual's identification with the ideal, establishing a sense of mastery and certainty.

Erikson (1966) also speaks of a ritualized affirmation that increases one's sense of safety and security. This enhances meaning; reduces stress, anxiety, and impulsivity; facilitates social bonding; and channels destructive and extreme emotions into controllable forms (Benson & Stark, 1996; Pargament, 1997; Pruyser, 1968). Jacobs (1992) goes a step further, noting that rituals appears to counter mental disturbance.

RELIGION, SPIRITUALITY, AND RITUAL

There is broad agreement that religious ceremonies are a distinctive and special form of ritual. First, they involve a unique group of referents, what Lawson and McCauley (2002a, 2002b) term "culturally postulated superhuman" (CPS) agents. Second, the aim of those who practice religious rituals is to contact, identify with, and/or influence the CPS. Third, when the rite in question has been completed, the sequence of enabling actions ends. This means that the next step is up to the CPS. Fourth, religious rituals can only be undertaken by members of a specific religious body: outsiders are not part of the sacred circle. Fifth, frequently, the ritual must be exercised through special religious figures (e.g., clergy). For further detailed analysis of ritual, the reader is referred to the excellent writings of Lawson and McCauley on religious ritual (1990, 2002a, 2002b). Recently, McClenon (1997) proposed a theory of the origin of religion by invoking ritual to produce altered states of consciousness that relate to hypnosis and the role of shamans. These convey to group members impressive images of power and supernatural connection. Becker (1973) feels that "the thing that has to be explained in human relations is precisely the fascination of the person who holds or symbolizes power" (p. 127). This "fascination" (p. 128) possesses a shamanic quality that Freud and other analytic thinkers assert "has the elements of an intense love affair" (p. 128–129) that equally affects both sexes. Freud, Ferenczi, and Fenichel analogized this to hypnosis, all of which they claimed is based upon a desire to return to the protection of the family (Becker, 1973). These encounters include the features of religious experiences: sublime feelings, mystification, and identification with ultimate power. In essence, psychologically and anthropologically, this is religion: common explanatory and justifying beliefs and myths that represent a religious perspective. The central figure in the production of such a system is the shaman who occupies a very privileged place in society. In modern society, clergy may play similar roles.

Ritual appears to be inextricably interwoven with myth, and both are essential to religion. Kluckhohn (1942) ties all three together by succinctly claiming that "those realms of behavior and of experience which man finds beyond rational and technological control . . . are capable of manipulation through symbols. . . . The myth is a system of word symbols, whereas ritual is a system of object and act symbols" (p. 58).

Even though spirituality has most often been affiliated with religious and mystical experience, the manner in which one engages in public and private worship and prayer is an essential part of the larger expression of personal spirituality. Where experience is frequently not under the conscious control of religious seekers, religious practices are under such control even if it is not exercised. Such actions are taught and learned in an orderly manner. As noted, public ritualistic controls vary little in expression. As a rule, religious institutions may establish how, when, and where various public services are offered and articulated. Thus far ritual has been treated as a collective phenomenon. This must be supplemented with recognition that the human craving for ritual results in the production of individualized, self-generated ceremonial expressions. Not infrequently traditional group forms have "gaps," and do not always meet personal needs. People therefore are not averse to creating their own idiosyncratic rites that more accurately express their feelings and desires (Hine, 1981). Ritual is clearly an endemic feature of humanity.

Since we are dealing with a topic that spans both the humanities and the sciences, our emphasis on psychological theory and research largely restricts us to Western religions, particularly Christianity and Judaism, as the overwhelming majority of studies have been conducted with members of these faiths. The language of religious practice further suggests the necessity of focus and selection since religion is involved in virtually every major human activity from birth to death. Are we to analyze in depth the meanings of life transition ceremonies, such as baptisms, circumcisions, confirmations, bar and bat mitzvahs, wedding ceremonies, and funeral and death rites? What about daily family observances and healing services? There are also the religiospiritual facets of civil religion: services for special holidays and events, celebrations, graduations, the induction of people into organizations or high office, the giving of awards and honors, and a host of other notable events. The principles underlying the role of religion in all of these activities are quite similar, and at the heart of these religious rituals one invariably finds elements of worship and prayer.

The role of ritual in ceremony and prayer cannot be minimized, for it is a means of communicating both with the supernatural and concurrently with oneself and others. It is often a call for vicarious aid and comfort by a deity when a supplicant is unable to exercise mastery (Brown, 1994). This is detailed by Tremmel (1984) who identifies three major functions for religious ritual. The first is a metatechnological function in which ritual brings supernatural power into the natural world via magic, miracles, or forces that are designed to support people in everyday life. A second function is termed "sacramental." Divine power is called upon to help the individual buttress self-control and offer protection against death and threats to life. The third, or experiential, function fosters identification with one's God, and insinuates divine power into life; the person is renewed and reborn. Recognizing in this last function a place for worship, Pruyser (1968) claims that the purpose of ritual worship is to stimulate religious experience.

The cognitive-structural approach to religious ritual offered by Lawson and McCauley (1990) is primarily concerned with the symbolic organization and significance of ritual. These scholars stress the themes of control, power and change. According to Lawson and McCauley, "Religious rituals always do something to some thing or somebody. Participants perform rituals in order to bring about changes in the religious world" (p. 125). This is largely a way station to effect alterations in the real world. In other words, power and control needs are a fundamental source of ritual.

Clearly, ritual involves reification. Animism is one outcome of this process. Von Bertalanffy connotes such action a primeval but beneficial effort to achieve environmental control (LaViolette, 1981). One can easily argue that religious ritual is a mechanism for enhancing mastery over oneself and one's personal world. Its use is strengthened by reinforcement, particularly of a social nature.

Ritual control in social life has also been called "a practical instrument of ethics" that serves to "coalesce the individual into the group which would be fragmented by his uncurbed impulses. . . . When effective it not only curbs, but also helps to create the desire to serve the community in an extension of the service that ritual calls for" (Ostow & Scharfstein, 1954, pp. 100–101). In other words, ritual is a conservative cultural force that preserves the status quo. Ritual therefore supports expectations of how others will or should react. This pattern extends into religion, suggesting that our responses ought to elicit certain actions on the part of our deity.

The Dark Side of Religious Ritual

Unhappily, the positive and constructive roles of ceremony have their counterparts in a pathology of ritual. Normal uses of ritual can shade into obsession, compulsivity, and a dogmatic rigidity that takes over one's daily life. One tragic manifestation is an excessive preoccupation with sin. The disorder of scrupulosity is an extreme example in which the individual suffers from severe doubts as to whether he or she has sinned or not (Spilka, Hood, Hunsberger, & Gorsuch, 2003). Rituals are developed to counter such thoughts and also to atone for possible sinning. St. Ignatius of Loyola, who had such concerns, created a substitute set of rituals to offset his obsessions (Gomez, 2001). Similar difficulties apparently affected a number of saints, often resulting in their bizarre attempts to treat personal problems (McGinley, 1969).

Another negative connotation for religious ritual has come from the association of this concept with the notion of "ritual child abuse" (Victor, 1992). Though fairly widely believed, it has been used to justify a search for "satanist abusers." This fantasy may have been invented by some troubled religious moral crusaders, and appears to have no substance.

RELIGIOUS PRACTICE AND RITUAL

The foregoing describes the core of religious practice relative to worship and prayer in a general ritualistic sense. Prayer and worship clearly overlap. A widely employed framework denotes worship as a group and public function while prayer is a corresponding private expression. Both are viewed as efforts to communicate with CPS agents. To understand both worship and prayer, we can do no better than accept William James's (1902) view that prayer refers to "every kind of inward communion or conversation with the power recognized as divine" (p. 464). This clearly also covers worship.

Worship

Worship is socioculturally circumscribed ritual that is sometimes referred to as "corporate prayer." The public nature of worship makes it highly dependent on objectified cultural signs and symbols that convey common meanings to large numbers of people. By functioning in this manner common experiences are created that weld participants into a community of worshippers (Whitley, 1964). Another factor uniting worshippers is the belief that the rituals established by religious institutions are either directly or indirectly mandated by God, and further that divine power and authority is vested in the officials who conduct worship services. An additional feature that heightens attachment to both the ceremonies and their organizational sponsors is the aesthetic character of many worship rites. These usually involve group singing, choral offerings, and the use of musical instruments, particularly the organ.

Technological progress has brought church worship services to television (Goethals, 2000; Wolff, 1999). Though ritual is present in both settings, it is much more influential in a church service. To most people, this form of devotion is personally more real and satisfying than watching a television presentation. Contemporary megachurches frequently televise their services. When these are watched, usually in the home, the observers are concurrently often involved in various household activities. Total dedication to the ongoing worship is commonly lacking. As might be expected, the absence of other worshippers means the communal effects of the ritual are also absent, as is the presence of the divine that is usually experienced when one attends a regular service (Wolff, 1999). Some parishioners claim that a personal quality of engagement is lacking in television presentations. Apparently in-church participation in worship rituals is more likely to elicit an experiential richness than passively watching a television service. For some congregants, Wolff (1999) suggests, "whereas church provides security, television is perceived as dangerous" (p. 232). Nevertheless, for those who are unable to attend church, TV offerings may provide a much-desired contact with a religiospiritual setting and activity.

The second half of the 20th century saw the development of what Hadden and Swann (1981) call "the rising power of televangelism" (p. iii). Though presenting some of the trappings of an evangelical church service, this is also a way for impressive clerical speakers to present sermons that advertise themselves and their ministries plus religiously and politically conservative positions. Appeals for funds are common, and in some well-known instances the misuse of these tele-pulpits to amass personal wealth has been publicized (Wills, 1990).

Much of the foregoing comes under the heading of charismatic worship in which exceptional personalities dominate (Benson, 1960). Figures such as Billy Graham have exercised a major influence for many years. Their basic goal is to stress the utility and significance of traditional religious and scriptural values. Such "revivalist" worship is designed to organize the audience, to create a group whose implicit power will move dissenting individuals into line.

On the level of the individual, worship increases commitment to one's faith. A well-known finding in psychology is that attitudes follow behavior (Festinger, 1954). This is amply demonstrated by repetitive worship. Muslim worship occurs five times a day, and participants explain their behavior ideologically and experientially. In like manner, in the Judeo-Christian tradition, specific worship times for annual holy days (e.g., midnight mass for Christmas) and established fast days are based on the same principle. Not only must worshippers justify to themselves why they engage in these rituals, but their faith and its theology provides virtually all the reasons needed for such observance.

Berger (1967) suggests that people forget, need to be reminded, and "religious ritual has been a crucial instrument of this process of 'reminding' "(p. 40). Psychologically, this is known as reinforcement, a repetitive strengthening of commitment to the religious system via ritual.

There is, however, much more to worship than ritual as reinforcement. It is especially meaningful when it supports courage in times of stress (Klausner, 1961). We might also add personal strength as one result of group appeals to a higher power that are manifest in organizations such as Alcoholics Anonymous (Benson, 1960).

Considering these potential benefits from worship, it comes as no surprise that enterprising clergy and pastoral counselors have found ways of using worship in pastoral care. Roberts (1995) shows how this might alleviate the negative effects of family problems, divorce, life crises, bereavement, and aging and retirement difficulties among other possibilities.

The argument has been advanced that worship itself is both humanizing and therapeutic (Empereur, 1987). The worshipper, however, needs to understand the church service as ritualistic communication with him- or herself, others, and God. Aune (1993) also feels that worship basically makes the interrelatedness of humans explicit.

In the traditional explanation of ritual as fundamentally communication, both worship and prayer are viewed as coping mechanisms that maintain connections between people and their god. Treating worship and prayer as adaptive, Pruyser (1968) describes their outcome as bolstering courage, lifting spirits, promoting confidence, invigorating the worshipper, releasing tensions, correcting attitudes, boosting morale, and so on.

Prayer

Prayer is simply individualized ritual (Janssen, de Hart, & den Draak, 1990). Even though each person develops his or her own style of prayer or prayers depending on the situation or its acknowledged purpose, we can briefly analyze each prayer into three parts: an introduction, a goal-directed middle, and a conclusion (Buttrick, 1942; Heiler, 1932; Magee, 1957). A conventional opening involves glorification of the Deity, for some supplicants possibly an effort at ingratiation (Jones, 1964). This practice is commonly found in inspirational prayer books (Army and Navy Commission of the Protestant Episcopal Church, 1941; Bartlett, 1947; Cushman, 1941). Magee (1957) explicitly ritualizes prayer by offering a sequence that begins the actual prayer with adoration, which is clearly glorification. He follows this with confession, a baring of one's soul to show a true need for God's help. Now comes the main purpose of the chosen prayer: usually petition, but there are other needs as well, such as intercession. Harkness (1948) adds time to the ritual: "The most important times of private prayer are upon waking, at bedtime, before meals, at irregular intervals through the day, and in a regular, uninterrupted unhurried period which can be fixed" (p. 118). Finally, the prayer ends, but usually with another humble endorsement of the power of the Deity. This general formula for prayer ritual is very much personalized as far as content is concerned. Elements from public worship or new creations by the person praying may be habitually used.

The Purpose and Effects of Prayer as Ritual

The communicative purpose of ritual enunciated earlier has been recognized by students of prayer. Proposals for theories and models of prayer as communication that deal with relatedness to a deity and also oneself have been proposed (Benson, 1960; Childs, 1983; Crocker, 1984; Ellens, 1977). In other words, there is a reflexive aspect to prayer. The tension reduction results of ritual behavior have also been replicated with prayer (Elkins, Anchor, & Sandler, 1979).

Some Beneficial Aspects of Prayer

Prayer has beneficial consequences for the individual (Duke & Johnson, 1984). This parallels similar observations for the practice of ritual, particularly religious ritual (Benson & Stark, 1996; Hinde, 1999; Pruyser, 1968; Tremmel, 1984).

The desirable effects and/or correlates of prayer both match and extend the favorable outcomes of ritual. Prayer relates negatively to health concern (e.g., hypochondria), aids emotional adjustment to arthritis (Laird, 1991), opposes depressive feelings (Parker & Brown, 1986), and helps individuals cope with the stress of cardiac surgery (Saudia, Kinney, Brown, & Young-Ward, 1991), kidney transplantation (Sutton &

Murphy, 1989), and being on hemodialysis (Baldree, Murphy, & Powers, 1982). It also counters the use of alcohol and drugs among homeless women (Shuler, Gelberg, & Brown, 1994). The positive outcomes of praying almost seem legion. Just as it is an aid in dealing with the hopefully transitory stressors of life, it is an important support in the long-term coping efforts of the aged (Gibson, 1982; Koenig, George, & Siegler, 1988; Manfredi & Pickett, 1987; Shaw, 1992) and parents who care for children with disabilities (Bennett, Deluca, & Allen, 1995). It even contributes to marital adjustment (Gruner, 1985).

Focusing on prayer must not make us fail to recognize its broader identification with religion. In other words, it is religious practice in toto that needs to be examined relative to these findings. When, however, prayer is specifically researched in relation to such broad variables as life satisfaction, quality of life, general well-being, and purpose in life positive relationships are again found (Cox, 2000; Francis & Burton, 1994; Poloma, 1993; Poloma & Gallup, 1990; Poloma & Pendleton, 1989, 1991). We may infer that prayer as ritual is a very significant aid in coping with life.

As we continue to study the role and place of prayer in life, it is shocking to realize how much psychological speculation has been devoted to prayer over the last century, and how little empirical work has been undertaken in this area. In all likelihood well over 90% of the latter has occurred within the last two decades; an even shorter span of time has witnessed attempts to assess the complexity of this domain.

The Multiform Nature of Prayer

Thus far prayer has been discussed as a single, unitary concept. In actuality, it is multidimensional and rather complex. Much of the research cited has not dealt with it in this manner. A few studies report findings that appear specific to certain kinds of prayer (Cox, 2000; Poloma & Pendleton, 1989). Unfortunately, researchers and theorists do not always agree on what the various prayer forms are.

Conceptualizing Prayer Forms

Probably for as far back as people have contemplated prayer, its complexity has been evident. Religionists have offered a variety of theoretical schemes that have not yet been psychometrically evaluated. A recent rather comprehensive proposal by Foster (1992) is worthy of such investigation. He suggests 21 different forms of prayer, and discusses these inspirationally and theologically. This approach is generally true of all religiously knowledgeable authors who write for a relatively well-informed audience, but few show Foster's sensitivity and sophistication. Most focus on a few types of prayer, such as prayers of adoration, thanksgiving, confession, petition, and intercession (Harkness, 1948). Puglisi (1929) speaks of eudaemonistic prayer, which is fundamentally petitionary, but also denotes variants like aesthetic, noetic, and ethical prayer. Puglisi, however, expands his list to include "prayers of invocation, of lamentation, of appeal, of petition, of sacrifice, of offering, of persuasion, of trust, of devotion, of submission, of dependence, of thanksgiving, etc." (p. 150). Such schemes become almost endless as their inspired writers consider the human condition plus all of the situations in which prayers may be offered. For example, Richards and Hildebrand (1990) detail over 100 categories of prayer. In addition, one specific kind of prayer, such as the intercessory form, may be analyzed to reveal that a surprising complexity underlies what often initially appears to be a simple concept (Vennard, 1995).

Empirically Dimensionalizing Prayer

Notwithstanding the fertility of the theological and inspirational mind-set, the decade of the 1990s witnessed an outpouring of research on the multidimensionality of prayer. Poloma and Gallup (1991) initiated this trend in their significant volume, *Varieties of Prayer*. They distinguished four forms: colloquial, petitionary, ritual, and meditative. Colloquial prayer is conversational in nature and may include other types such as prayers of intercession, confession, and thanksgiving. It can become a basket category depending on the items used to measure it. Petitionary prayer is the most widely used of all forms, simply being a request for God to provide whatever the supplicant wants (Capps, 1982). Intercession for others and self-aggrandizement can unite under such a heading. Ritual prayer stresses the ceremonial quality of order and regularity in prayer pattern and content. Last, meditative prayer focuses on the desire for experiential communication with the deity. Laird (1991) theorized five kinds of prayer, and then selected 18 items to evaluate these domains. Using factor analysis, he constructed five reliable scales to assess prayers of adoration (praising God), supplication (petition), confession (admitting negative qualities and actions), thanksgiving (gratitude expressions), and reception (openness to experience, knowledge, guidance).

Also utilizing factor analytic methods with 71 prayer items, David, Ladd, and Spilka (1992) created scales to measure eight kinds of prayer: confession, petition, thanksgiving, ritual, meditation, self-improvement, intercession, and habit. These forms were further studied in relation to religious orientations, globalization indices, a variety of control measures, and well-being (Beck, Spilka, David, & Mason, 1992; Carlson, Friedman, & Spilka, 1991; David et al., 1992; Navrot et al., 1992).

A series of follow-up studies with different combinations of items and samples totaling almost 1000 respondents from different universities, a conservative Protestant seminary, and cancer patients resulted in new versions of the above scales (Luckow, 1997; Luckow, McIntosh, Spilka, & Ladd, 2000; Luckow et al., 1996). Some of these instruments have been termed egocentric petition, material petition, and compassionate petition (a fusion of intercessory and thanksgiving prayers). Additional possibilities such as prayers indicating confessional desires, personal ritualism, meditation, self-improvement, and simply habit were also proposed.

Using similar methodology, Hood and his associates created four prayer scales they named petitional, contemplative, liturgical, and material (like petition) (Hood, Morris, & Harvey, 1993; Williamson, Morris, & Hood, 1995). These were studied in relationship to mystical experience and well-being. Multidimensional analytic procedures such as factor analysis often resulted in overlapping but not identical findings. This variation may be a function of the nature of the samples employed and their size, differences in factor extraction procedures, rotations utilized, and, of course, the items assessed. More work is needed to resolve discrepancies among the various proposed frameworks.

As already noted, prayer as either a unitary or multiform construct has been extensively studied, and often found to relate positively to a broad spectrum of psychological and physical benefits. Even though negative relationships with these same variables are rarely found, in most instances no relationships have been observed (Pargament, 1997).

With regard to religious rituals in general, only slightly more positive associations than nonsignificant ones were noted (Pargament, 1997). Clearly, these contradictions are a call for more exacting research.

SUMMARY AND CONCLUSION

I have barely touched on an extremely complex pattern of relationships among ritual, worship, and prayer. Though the basic content of these realms has been identified, one needs to distinguish the benefits of religious practice from those of ritual and understand the relative contributions of each. The biological and anthropological aspects of ritual imply the potential of natural selection advantages that are probably not true for the nonritualistic components of worship and prayer. In the latter, consciousness, learning, cognition, and personal choice enter the picture. There is much more to the foundations of religious practice than is commonly recognized. Individually and collectively, the intermingled strands of ritual, worship, and prayer have yet to be distinguished.

By no means does the research on prayer cited thus far tell the entire story. Efforts have also been directed at the development of prayer in children and others (Francis & Astley, 2001). Brown (1994) extensively details the considerable conceptual and empirical work that psychologists and other social scientists have conducted in order to understand how and why prayer is important to most people. Multidimensional approaches have opened up new research vistas, and some very contentious issues such as the effectiveness of intercessory prayer have yet to be resolved (Spilka et al., 2003). In more than a few ways, interest in prayer is an old concern in the psychology of religion, yet contemporary research suggests it is a topic that has become increasingly attractive and significant to the current generation of researchers.

REFERENCES

Alvord, L. (1999, December). New beginnings. *Dartmouth Alumni Magazine*, p. 12.

Anttonen, V. (2002). Identifying the generative mechanisms of religion: The issue of origin revisited. In I. Pyysiainen & V. Anttonen (Eds.), *Current approaches in the cognitive science of religion* (pp. 14–37). New York: Continuum.

Army and Navy Commission of the Protestant Episcopal Church. (1941). *A prayer book for soldiers and sailors*. New York: The Church Pension Fund.

Aune, M. B. (1993). "But only say the word": Another look at Christian worship as therapeutic. *Pastoral Psychology, 41*, 145–157.

Baldree, K. S., Murphy, S. P., & Powers, M. J. (1982). Stress identification and coping patterns in patients on hemodialysis. *Nursing Research, 31*, 107–112.

Bartlett, R. M. (1947). *Boy's prayers: The ascending trail*. New York: Association Press.

Beck, J. R., Spilka, B., David, J. P., & Mason, R. (1992). *Prayer in religious and social perspective: A study of a seminary sample*. Paper presented at the annual meeting of the American Psychological Association, Washington, DC.

Becker, E. (1973). *The denial of death*. New York: Free Press.

Bennett, T., Deluca, D. A., & Allen, R. W. (1995). Religion and children with disabilities. *Journal of Religion and Health, 34*, 301–312.

Benson, H., & Stark, M. (1996). *Timeless healing: The power and biology of belief*. New York: Scribner.

Benson, P. H. (1960). *Religion in contemporary culture.* New York: Harper & Brothers.

Berger, P. L. (1967). *The sacred canopy.* Garden City, NY: Doubleday.

Brown, L. B. (1994). *The human side of prayer.* Birmingham, AL: Religious Education Press.

Buttrick, G. A. (1942). *Prayer.* New York: Abingdon-Cokesbury.

Capps, D. (1982). The psychology of petitionary prayer. *Theology Today, 39,* 130–141.

Carlson, C., Friedman, S., & Spilka, B. (1991). *The structure of prayer and well-being.* Paper presented at the meeting of the Rocky Mountain Psychological Association, Denver, CO.

Childs, B. H. (1983). The possible connection between "private speech" and prayer. *Pastoral Psychology, 32,* 24–33.

Cox, R. J. (2000). *Relating different types of Christian prayer to religious and psychological measures of well-being.* Unpublished doctoral dissertation, Boston University, Boston, MA.

Crocker, S. F. (1984). Prayer as a model of communication. *Pastoral Psychology, 33,* 83–92.

Cushman, R. S. (1941). *A pocket prayer book and devotional guide.* Nashville, TN: The Upper Room.

David, J., Ladd, K., & Spilka, B. (1992). *The multidimensionality of prayer and its role as a source of secondary control.* Paper presented at the annual meeting of the American Psychological Association, Washington, DC.

Duke, J. T., & Johnson, B. L. (1984). Spiritual well-being and the consequential dimension of religiosity. *Review of Religious Research, 26,* 59–72.

Elkins, D., Anchor, K. N., & Sandler, H. M. (1979). Relaxation training and prayer behavior as tension reduction techniques. *Behavioral Engineering, 6,* 81–87.

Ellens, J. H. (1977). Communication theory and petitionary prayer. *Journal of Psychology and Theology, 5,* 48–54.

Empereur, J. L. (1987). Liturgy as humanizing or as sacred. In J. L. Empereur (Ed.), *Worship: Exploring the sacred* (pp. 85–96). Washington, DC: Pastoral Press.

Erikson, E. H. (1966). Ontogeny of ritualization in man. In J. Huxley (Ed.), *A discussion on ritualization of behavior in animals and man. Philosophical Transactions of the Royal Society of London, Series B, Biological Sciences, 251,* 337–349.

Festinger, L. (1954). *A theory of cognitive dissonance.* Stanford, CA: Stanford University Press.

Foster, R. J. (1992). *Prayer: Finding the heart's true home.* San Francisco: Harper.

Francis, L. J., & Astley, J. (Eds.). (2001). *Psychological perspectives on prayer.* Leominster, Herefordshire, UK: Gracewing.

Francis, L. J., & Burton, L. (1994). The influence of personal prayer on purpose in life among Catholic adolescents. *Journal of Beliefs and Values, 15,* 6–9.

Fulghum, R. (1995). *From beginning to end: The rituals of our lives.* New York: Fawcett Columbine.

Gibson, R. C. (1982). Blacks at middle and late life: Resources and coping. *Annals of the American Academy of Political and Social Science, 464,* 79–90.

Goethals, G. (2000). The electronic Golden Calf: Transforming ritual and icon. In B. F. Forbes & J. H. Macon (Eds.), *Religion and popular culture in America* (pp. 125–144). Berkeley, CA: University of California Press.

Gomez, L. O. (2001). When is religion a mental disorder?: The disease of ritual. In D. Jonte-Pace & W. B. Parsons (Eds.), *Religion and psychology: Mapping the terrain* (pp. 202–226). New York: Routledge.

Gruner, L. (1985). The correlation of private, religious devotional practices and marital adjustment. *Journal of Comparative Family Studies, 16,* 47–59.

Hadden, J. K., & Swann, C. E. (1981). *Prime time preachers.* Reading, MA: Addison-Wesley.

Hargrove, B. W. (1971). *Reformation of the holy.* Philadelphia: F. A. Davis.

Harkness, G. (1948). *Prayer and the common life.* New York: Abingdon-Cokesbury.

Heiler, F. (1932). *Prayer: A study in the history and psychology of religion.* New York: Oxford University Press.

Helman, C. G. (1994). *Culture, health and illness* (3rd ed.). Oxford, UK: Butterworth Heineman.

Hinde, R. A. (1999). *Why Gods persist: A scientific approach to religion.* London: Routledge.

Hine, V. H. (1981). Self-generated ritual: Trend or fad? *Worship, 55,* 404–419.

Hood, R. W., Jr., Morris, R. J., & Harvey, D. (1993). *Religiosity, prayer, and their relationship to mystical experience*. Paper presented at the annual meeting of the Religious Research Association, Raleigh, NC.

Huxley, J. (1966). A discussion on ritualization of behavior in animals and man: Introduction. In J. Huxley (Ed.), *A discussion on ritualization of behavior in animals and man. Philosophical Transactions of the Royal Society of London, Series B, Biological Sciences, 251,* 249–272.

Jacobs, J. L. (1992). Religious ritual and mental health. In J. F. Schumaker (Ed.), *Religion and mental health* (pp. 291–299). New York: Oxford University Press.

James, W. (1902). *Varieties of religious experience*. New York: Longmans, Green.

Janssen, J., de Hart, J., & den Draak, C. (1990). Praying as individualized ritual. In H.-G. Heimbrock & H. B. Boudewijnse (Eds.), *Current studies on rituals: Perspectives for the psychology of religion* (pp. 71–85). Amsterdam: Rodopi.

Jones, E. E. (1964). *Ingratiation: A social psychological analysis*. New York: Appleton-Century-Crofts.

Klausner, S. Z. (1961). The social psychology of courage. *Review of Religious Research, 3,* 63–72.

Kluckhohn, C. (1942). Myths and rituals: A general theory. *Harvard Theological Review, 35,* 45–79.

Koenig, H. G., George, L. K., & Siegler, I. C. (1988). The use of religion and other emotion-regulating coping strategies among older adults. *The Gerontologist, 28,* 303–310.

Laird, S. P. (1991). *A preliminary investigation into the role of prayer as a coping technique for adult patients with arthritis*. Unpublished doctoral dissertation, University of Kansas, Lawrence, KS.

LaViolette, P. A. (Ed.). (1981). *A systems view of man: Ludwig von Bertalanffy*. Boulder, CO: Westview Press.

Lawson, E. T., & McCauley, R. N. (1990). *Rethinking religion: Connecting cognition and culture*. Cambridge, UK: Cambridge University Press.

Lawson, E. T., & McCauley, R. N. (2002a). The cognitive representation of religious ritual form: A theory of participants' competence with religious ritual systems. In I. Pyysiainen & V. Anttonen (Eds.), *Cognitive approaches in the cognitive science of religion* (pp. 153–176). New York: Continuum.

Lawson, E. T., & McCauley, R. N. (2002b). *Bringing ritual to mind*. Cambridge, UK: Cambridge University Press.

Lorenz, K. (1963). *On aggression*. New York: Harcourt, Brace & World.

Lorenz, K. S. (1966). Evolution of ritualization in the biological and cultural spheres. In J. Huxley (Ed.), *A discussion on ritualization of behavior in animals and man*. Philosophical Transactions of the Royal Society of London, Series B, *Biological Sciences, 251,* 273–284.

Luckow, A. (1997). *The structure of prayer: Exploratory and confirmatory analyses*. Unpublished master's thesis, University of Denver, Denver, CO.

Luckow, A., Ladd, K. L., Spilka, B., McIntosh, D. N., Poloma, M., Parks, C., & LaForett, D. (1996, August 11). *The structure of prayer: Explorations and confirmations*. Paper presented at the convention of the American Psychological Association, Toronto, Canada.

Luckow, A., McIntosh, D. N., Spilka, B., & Ladd, K. (2000, February). *The multidimensionality of prayer*. Paper presented at the annual convention of the Society for Personality and Social Psychology, Nashville, TN.

Magee, J. (1957). *Reality and prayer: A guide to the meaning and practice of prayer*. New York: Harper & Brothers.

Manfredi, C., & Pickett, M. (1987). Perceived stressful situations and coping strategies utilized by the elderly. *Journal of Community Mental Health Nursing, 4,* 99–110.

McClenon, J. (1997). Shamanic healing, human evolution, and the origin of religion. *Journal for the Scientific Study of Religion, 36,* 345–354.

McGinley, P. (1969). *Saint-watching*. New York: Viking Press.

Mead, M. (1972). Ritual expression of the cosmic sense. In M. Mead (Ed.), *Twentieth century faith* (pp. 153–160). New York: Harper & Row. (Original work published 1966)

Navrot, A., Richardson, A., Marrocco, C., Dashosh, D., Kvern, K., Yang, J., Fairchild, D., Rotschild,

M., Ladd, K., & Spilka, B. (1995, April). *Prayer and the sense of control: A multidimensional approach*. Paper presented at the convention of the Rocky Mountain Psychological Association, Boulder, CO.

Ostow, M., & Scharfstein, B.-A. (1954). *The need to believe*. New York: International Universities Press.

Pargament, K. I. (1997). *The psychology of religion and coping*. New York: Guilford Press.

Parker, G. B., & Brown, L. B. (1982). Coping behaviors that mediate between life events and depression. *Archives of General Psychiatry, 39*, 1386–1391.

Pilgrim, R. B. (1978). Ritual. In T. W. Hall (Ed.), *Introduction to the study of religion* (pp. 64–84). New York: Harper & Row.

Poloma, M. M. (1993, January). The effects of prayer on mental well-being. *Second Opinion, 18*, 37–51.

Poloma, M. M., & Gallup, G. H., Jr. (1990, November). *Religiosity, forgiveness and life satisfaction: An exploratory study*. Paper presented at the convention of the Society for the Scientific Study of Religion, Virginia Beach, VA.

Poloma, M. M., & Gallup, G. H., Jr. (1991). *Varieties of prayer: A survey report*. Philadelphia: Trinity Press International.

Poloma, M. M., & Pendleton, B. F. (1989). Exploring types of prayer and quality of life: A research note. *Review of Religious Research, 31*, 46–53.

Poloma, M. M., & Pendleton, B. (1991). The effects of prayer and prayer experiences on measures of general well- being. *Journal of Psychology and Theology, 19*, 71–83.

Pruyser, P. (1968). *A dynamic psychology of religion*. New York: Harper & Row.

Puglisi, M. (1929). *Prayer*. New York: Macmillan.

Ragen, N. (1998). *The ghost of Hannah Mendes*. New York: Simon & Schuster.

Richards, C., & Hildebrand, L. (1990). *Prayers that prevail*. Tulsa, OK: Victory House.

Roberts, H. W. (1995). *Pastoral care through worship*. Macon, GA: Smith & Helwys.

Roberts, K. A. (1984). *Religion in sociological perspective*. Homewood, Il: Dorsey.

Saudia, T. L., Kinney, M. R., Brown, K. C., & Young-Ward, L. (1991). Health locus of control and helpfulness of prayer. *Heart and Lung, 20*, 60–65.

Shaw, R. J. (1992). Coping effectiveness in nursing home residents. *Journal of Aging and Health, 4*, 551–563.

Shuler, P. A., Gelberg, L., & Brown, M. (1994). The effects of spiritual/religious practices on psychological well-being among inner city homeless women. *Nurse Practicioner Forum, 5*, 106–113.

Smith, J. Z. (1996). The bare facts of ritual. In R. L. Grimes (Ed.), *Readings in ritual studies* (pp. 473–483). Upper Saddle River, NJ: Prentice-Hall. (Original work published 1982)

Spilka, B., Hood, R. W., Jr., Hunsberger, B., & Gorsuch, R. L. (2003). *The psychology of religion: An empirical approach* (3rd ed.). New York: Guilford Press.

Sutton, T. D., & Murphy, S. P. (1989). Stressors and patterns of coping in renal transplant patients. *Nursing Research, 38*, 46–49.

Tremmel, W. C. (1984). *Religion: What is it?* New York: Holt, Rinehart, & Winston.

Vennard, J. E. (1995). *Praying for friends and enemies*. Minneapolis, MN: Augsburg.

Victor, J. S. (1992). Ritual abuse and the moral crusade against satanism. *Journal of Psychology and Theology, 20*, 248–253.

Whitley, R. (1964). *Religious behavior*. Englewood Cliffs, NJ: Prentice-Hall.

Williamson, W. P., Morris, R. J., & Hood, R. W., Jr. (1995, October). *Prayer as a predictor of spiritual and existential well-being*. Paper presented at the convention of the Society for the Scientific Study of Religion, St. Louis, MO.

Wills, G. (1990). *Under God: Religion and American politics*. New York: Simon & Schuster.

Wolff, R. F. (1999). A phenomenological study of in-church and televised worship. *Journal for the Scientific Study of Religion, 38*, 219–235.

Wulff, D. (1997). *Psychology of religion: Classic and contemporary views* (2nd ed.). New York: Wiley.

21

Fundamentalism and Authoritarianism

BOB ALTEMEYER
BRUCE HUNSBERGER

FUNDAMENTALISM

Religious fundamentalism can be traced back to a series of 80 pamphlets collectively called "The Fundamentals" (n.d.) that were published in the United States between 1910 and 1915. Written mostly by scholars and clergymen and distributed in great numbers around the world, the pamphlets presented a response to the "Higher Criticism" of the Bible that had become prominent during the second half of the 19th century. This criticism cast strong doubt on the divine origins of the Bible. "The Fundamentals" refuted this school of textual religious research and set out to present "the essential doctrines of [Protestant] Christianity that should not in any way be set aside or tampered with" (Introduction to "The Fundamentals Homepage," available online at www.xmission.com).

Most of the initial pamphlets focused on Scripture, but eventually other essential beliefs were covered such as the existence of God, the divinity of Jesus, the virgin birth, the Resurrection, salvation by grace, and "Satan and his kingdom." One searches in vain for a composite list of what exactly the fundamental doctrines of Christianity might be, such as one finds in a creed, and toward the end the essays were advocating evangelism, battling "The Decadence of Darwinism," and attacking "Romanism," Christian Science, Mormonism, and socialism. But the notion that basic principles of the Christian faith exist that could never be modified goes back to "The Fundamentals," and persons who preached these writings came to be called "fundamentalists."

Today "Fundamentalists" in the Christian context are sometimes differentiated from "Pentecostals" and "Evangelicals." (See Hood, Hill, & Williamson, 2005, for an alternate expanded discussion of these matters.) Furthermore, one hears of "Muslim fundamentalists" and "Hindu fundamentalists" as well as Christian ones these days. And one can speak of theological fundamentalists, cultural fundamentalists, and maybe even vegetarian fundamentalists. So the term has many meanings, and arises in many contexts.

The Religious Fundamentalism Scale

We are social psychologists, and have advanced a definition of *religious fundamentalism* that to some degree mirrors the spirit of "The Fundamentals": the belief that there is one set of religious teachings that clearly contains the fundamental, basic, intrinsic, essential, inerrant truth about humanity and deity; that this essential truth is fundamentally opposed by forces of evil which must be vigorously fought; that this truth must be followed today according to the fundamental, unchangeable practices of the past; and that those who believe and follow these fundamental teachings have a special relationship with the deity (Altemeyer & Hunsberger, 1992, p. 118). Of course, this definition makes no mention of Christianity; indeed, it could apply to many religions. So we have (purposely) defined fundamentalism not as a particular set of doctrines, but as an *attitude* about those beliefs, whatever the tenets may be.

We developed an attitude scale to measure our concept of religious fundamentalism that we adroitly named the Religious Fundamentalism (RF) Scale. Originally 20 items long, it has recently been retooled and shortened to the 12 items shown in Figure 21.1 (Altemeyer & Hunsberger, 2004). Customarily people give their responses on a –4 ("Very strongly disagree") to +4 ("Very strongly agree") basis. The scoring is reversed for the con-trait items (e.g., No. 2) where the fundamentalist answer is to disagree. The total score on the scale is obtained by summing the scores obtained from the 12 responses.

Like many scales dealing with religion, the RF Scale parades a relatively high degree of internal consistency, with mean interitem correlations routinely running over .35 for the original 20-statement version, and over .45 for the new, shorter one. This cohesiveness among the answers means that the scale has almost always produced an alpha coefficient of reliability over .90. Factor analyses show that it essentially measures just one thing, and we hope the reader will agree that that "one thing" is the concept of fundamentalism contained in our definition.

Who scores highly on the RF Scale? It has mostly been administered to introductory psychology students at the University of Manitoba and their parents,[1] and to similar students at Wilfrid Laurier University. The vast majority of these samples come from Christian backgrounds. One can find members of all Christian denominations in the top 25% scorers on the measure. But year after year, about three times as many "fundamentalist Protestants"—for example, Baptists, Evangelicals, Pentecostals, Jehovah's Witnesses, Alliance Church members, and Salvation Army affiliates—appear among the high RF scorers as one would expect from their proportion of the overall sample. Mennonites show up about twice as often as their numbers would seemingly warrant. Catholics and Lutherans appear in accordance with their overall frequency. "Liberal" Protestant denominations (the United Church—an amalgamation of Congregationalist, Methodist, and some Presbyterian churches—and the Anglican Church) are substantially *under*represented. (Jews score low as a group, while Muslims score high.)

Demographically, high fundamentalists are slightly more likely to be females than males. Looking at the parent samples, they went to school a little less than the rest of the parents, and tend to favor "conservative" political parties more than most parents do. But their most notable distinction involves church attendance: they go to church much more often than most people do.

This survey is part of an investigation of general public opinion concerning a variety of social issues. You will probably find that you *agree* with some of the statements, and *disagree* with others, to varying extents. Please indicate your reaction to each statement by blackening a bubble in SECTION 1 of the bubble sheet, according to the following scale:

Blacken the bubble labeled

-4 if you *very strongly disagree* with the statement.
-3 if you *strongly disagree* with the statement.
-2 if you *moderately disagree* with the statement
-1 if you *slightly disagree* with the statement.

Blacken the bubble labeled

+1 if you *slightly agree* with the statement.
+2 if you *moderately agree* with the statement.
+3 if you *strongly agree* with the statement.
+4 if you *very strongly agree* with the statement.

If you feel exactly and precisely *neutral* about an item, blacken the "0" bubble.

You may find that you sometimes have different reactions to different parts of a statement. For example, you might very strongly disagree ("-4") with one idea in a statement, but slightly agree ("+1") with another idea in the same item. When this happens, please combine your reactions, and write down how you feel on balance (a "-3" in this case).

1. God has given humanity a complete, unfailing guide to happiness and salvation, which must be totally followed.
2. No single book of religious teachings contains all the intrinsic, fundamental truths about life.*
3. The basic cause of evil in this world is Satan, who is still constantly and ferociously fighting against God.
4. It is more important to be a good person than to believe in God and the right religion.*
5. There is a particular set of religious teachings in this world that are so true, you can't go any "deeper" because they are the basic, bedrock message that God has given humanity.
6. When you get right down to it, there are basically only two kinds of people in the world: the Righteous, who will be rewarded by God; and the rest, who will not.
7. Scriptures may contain general truths, but they should NOT be considered completely, literally true from beginning to end.*
8. To lead the best, most meaningful life, one must belong to the one, fundamentally true religion.
9. "Satan" is just the name people give to their own bad impulses. There really is *no such thing* as a diabolical "Prince of Darkness" who tempts us.*
10. Whenever science and sacred scripture conflict, *science* is probably right.*
11. The fundamentals of God's religion should never be tampered with, or compromised with others' beliefs.
12. *All* of the religions in the world have flaws and wrong teachings. There is *no* perfectly true, right religion.*

FIGURE 21.1. The revised 12-item Religious Fundamentalism Scale. * Indicates item is worded in the con-trait direction, for which the scoring key is reversed.

Religious Beliefs

No one will be surprised to learn that persons who score highly on the RF Scale believe in God. In one study (Hunsberger & Altemeyer, in press) students and parents were asked if they believed in a God who was almighty, eternal, constantly aware of us, all loving and all good, and so on. Seven different attributes were presented; complete-and-total belief would have earned a score of 7. High fundamentalists averaged 6.8, which means nearly all of them got a perfect 7. (In comparison, atheists from the same samples averaged 0.4, meaning a solid majority of them got a perfectly *non*believing 0.)

The beliefs extend far beyond the divinity, of course. Fullerton and Hunsberger (1982) presented a 24-item Christian Orthodoxy Scale, based on the Nicene Creed, that measures belief in the central tenets of Christianity such as the divinity of Jesus, the virgin birth, the miracles reported in the Gospels, and Jesus' Resurrection. RF scores correlate .66–.74 with Christian Orthodoxy Scale beliefs. (The correlation would be higher yet except for some respondents who have little personal involvement in religion, yet endorse the beliefs seemingly on a cultural basis.)

Fundamentalists believe in other things just as strongly. Over 800 parents recently answered a 12-item scale that measured acceptance of "creation science" explanations of the origin of the world and its species, as opposed to the theory of evolution. RF scores correlated .71 with belief in creation science.

Fundamentalists' beliefs are usually highly important to them. We once asked a sample of parents to indicate, in 16 different ways, how much traditional religious beliefs brought them happiness, joy, and comfort—for example, "They tell me the purpose of my life," "They help me deal with personal pain and suffering," and "They take away the fear of dying." RF scores correlated .68 with these responses. On the other hand, fundamentalists proved relatively *un*likely to say that logic and science brought them such rewards as "They bring me the joy of discovery" and "They serve as a check on my own biases and wrong ideas" ($r = -.33$) (Altemeyer & Hunsberger, 1997).

Proselytizing

Few readers would probably disagree with the observation that religious fundamentalists tend to proselytize their beliefs. To test this perception, we asked some parents what they would do if a teenager came to them for advice about religion: "S/he had been raised in a nonreligious family as an atheist, but now this person is thinking about becoming much more religious, and wants your advice on what to do. What would you say?" Eighty-eight percent of highly fundamentalist parents said they would tell this teen that atheism was wrong and that their religion was right; 96% said they would want this teen to adopt their beliefs; and 98% said they would try to lead the teen to join their faith (Hunsberger & Altemeyer, in press).

Well, would atheists similarly advocate atheism? No, actually. Presented with a mirror-image case in which a teen raised religiously began to have doubts and came to them for advice, only 11% of atheist parents said they would say religion was wrong and atheism was right. Most (86%) said they would instead advise the teen to "search among alternative beliefs and decide for yourself." Only 40% of the atheists said they would want the teen to believe what they believed. Only 18% said they would try to lead the questioning youth to atheism (Hunsberger & Altemeyer, in press).

What did the fundamentalist parents say when asked if they wanted their own children to have the same religious beliefs that they have? Ninety-four percent said yes, they would, while only 6% checked off, "I wanted them to search and make up their own minds." Among atheist parents, however, the figures were almost exactly the opposite. Four percent answered, "Yes, I wanted them to be atheists," and the other 96% answered, "I wanted them to search and make up their own minds" (Hunsberger & Altemeyer, in press).

In the 1990s we developed a Zealot's Scale to measure how fired up people were about whatever they most believed in. How enthused were they about their beliefs, their causes? It did not have to be religion. It could be a philosophy, a social perspective, a scientific orientation, feminism, capitalism, environmentalism, whatever. But how much did this outlook color and shape almost everything they did in life? How much did they try to explain this outlook to others at every opportunity? How much were they learning everything they could about this outlook? And so on, for 12 different ways of being zealous. At the end of the scale, the participants were asked to indicate what exactly their "most important outlook" was.

Religious fundamentalism correlated .44–.55 among students and parents with being zealous. While that is not as big as the other findings we have encountered thus far, we have to remember that nonreligious people could also be zealous about their philosophy or outlook. The fact is, however, that most of the people who were zealous about anything were fundamentalists who were zealous about their religion. You just do not find many socialists, capitalists, feminists, environmentalists, or atheists as excited about their beliefs as fundamentalists are burning with zeal about their religion (Altemeyer, 1996).

This explains what happened when highly fundamentalist parents were asked how they would react if born-again Christianity were taught in the public schools in Canada: "Suppose a law were passed requiring the strenuous teaching of religion in public schools. Beginning in kindergarten, all children would be taught to believe in God, pray together in school several times each day, memorize the Ten Commandments and other parts of the Bible, learn the principles of Christian morality, and eventually be encouraged to accept Jesus Christ as their personal savior." Nearly all (84%) of the fundamentalist parents said that would be a good law (Hunsberger & Altemeyer, in press).

Would atheists be just as interested in promoting atheism in the school system? We asked a sample of atheist parents how they would react if "a law were passed requiring strenuous teaching in public schools *against* belief in God and religion. Beginning in kindergarten, all children would be taught that belief in God is unsupported by logic and science, and that traditional religions are based on unreliable scriptures and outdated principles. All children would eventually be encouraged to become atheists or agnostics." *All* of the atheists said this would be a bad law, and that "no particular kind of religious beliefs should be taught in public schools"—not even their own (Hunsberger & Altemeyer, in press).

Dogmatism

Dogmatism, defined as relatively unchangeable, unjustified certainty, is measured by a 20-item DOG Scale containing such statements as "The things I believe in are so completely true, I could never doubt them," "There are no discoveries or facts that could possibly make me change my mind about the things that matter most in life," and "I am so sure I am right about the important things in life, there is no evidence that could convince me otherwise" (Altemeyer, 1996). As was true with zealotry, people with many different philosophies and belief systems can be highly dogmatic. The DOG scale says nothing about religion. Yet religious fundamentalism has correlated .57–.78 with DOG scores in studies thus far, and as with zealotry, most of the highly dogmatic people one finds in a sample are religious fundamentalists.

How would Christian fundamentalists react if an archeological discovery cast the strongest doubt that Jesus had ever existed? Suppose, it was hypothesized, excavations in the Near East uncovered a set of parchments, scientifically established to predate Jesus' era, that told the story of a Greek man-god, Attis. Suppose further that the story had so many of the Gospel accounts of Jesus' background, life, teachings, death and resurrection, and that the authenticity of the scrolls became so well verified, that scholars concluded that the myth of Attis was adapted by a group of Jewish reformers during the Roman occupation of Palestine, and Jesus of Nazareth never existed.

When asked whether this discovery would affect their belief in the divinity of Jesus, 93% of a group of highly fundamentalist parents said no, they would continue to believe just as strongly as they did before—which was usually to the maximum. In comparison, only 53% of a sample of atheist parents presented with a hypothetical mirror-image discovery of the "Roman file" on Jesus of Nazareth that strongly *backed up* the story of the Gospels said they would remain unaffected. The other 47% said they would shift their beliefs toward Jesus' divinity at least to some degree (Hunsberger & Altemeyer, in press).

These same samples were also asked if there was anything, *any* kind of event or evidence, that could cause them to change their beliefs about God. *All* of the fundamentalists said no, that there was no conceivable way they would ever change their minds about God. In comparison, 43% of the atheists said they *could* think of things that, were they to happen, would make them believe in the traditional Judeo-Christian God. They had strong beliefs to the contrary, but their minds could be changed.

Finally, many samples of students and their parents have been asked to answer a 20-item Religious Doubts Scale. It asks people to indicate how much they have had doubts about religion because of such things as the evil and unfair suffering in the world, the bad things religions did in the past, and the death of a loved one (Altemeyer & Hunsberger, 1997). Religious fundamentalism scores have correlated −.40 to −.59 with such doubts, meaning the higher the RF score, the fewer the doubts.

Relationships with Prejudice

Religious fundamentalists tend to be highly ethnocentric when it comes to religion. When we have administered a 16-item scale that has such items on it as "All people may be entitled to their own religious beliefs, but I don't want to associate with people whose views are quite different from my own," "I would be against letting some other, different religion use my church for its services when we were not using it," and "If it were possible, I'd rather have a job where I worked with people with the same religious views I have rather than with people with different views," RF scores correlate .70–.82 with summed religious ethnocentrism (Altemeyer, 2003).

Fundamentalists also tend to be hostile toward homosexuals, as measured by a 12-item scale that contains such items as "I won't associate with known homosexuals if I can help it," "Homosexuals should be locked up to protect society," and "In many ways, the AIDS disease currently killing homosexuals is just what they deserve" (Altemeyer, 1996). Many studies of university students and their parents have found correlations ranging from .42 to .61 with scores on this Attitude Toward Homosexuals Scale.

(Interestingly, fundamentalist opposition to laws protecting homosexuals appears to backfire in the long run. Attitudes toward homosexuals have softened remarkably in Canada in a short period of time, and when asked why, both students and parents say—more than anything else—they have changed their views because they have gotten to know homosexuals personally. But the reason cited second-most by the parents, and third-most by the students was "I have been turned off by *anti*-homosexual people" [Altemeyer, 2001].)

We have used the Attitudes Toward Homosexuals Scale in several studies that tested the RF Scale's reliability and validity in non-Christian samples. Hindus, Muslims, and Jews living in Toronto were contacted by mail and asked to complete a questionnaire that contained the RF and Attitudes Toward Homosexuals Scales. (They had no way of knowing they were contacted because of their religious affiliation.) Answers to the fundamentalism measure showed good internal consistency in all three samples, producing alpha coefficients ranging from .85 to .94. So the RF Scale *does* seem to measure fundamentalist attitudes in a variety of faiths. And as with our many Christian samples, the higher the person's RF score, the more likely he or she was hostile toward homosexuals, with correlations ranging from .42 to .65 (Altemeyer, 1996). Similar results were obtained among Muslims in Ghana, with the RF Scale posting an alpha of .87 and correlating .78 with Attitudes Toward Homosexuals scores (Hunsberger, Owusu, & Duck, 1999).

Fundamentalists' religious ethnocentrism is understandable, given how important religion is to them and how less important it is to many others. And the hostile attitudes toward homosexuals would not surprise many who have heard fundamentalists citing Leviticus and Paul's Letter to the Romans. (Indeed, some have argued that the faith-based rejections of others should not be called prejudice; however, it seems to us that prejudice based on religious belief still qualifies as prejudice.) But how does one explain the connection between white people's RF scores and their degree of racial and ethnic prejudice, which has appeared in numerous studies using the Manitoba Ethnocentrism Scale? This measure seeks reactions to statements such as "Certain races of people clearly do NOT have the natural intelligence and 'get up and go' of the white race," "As a group Indians are naturally lazy, promiscuous and irresponsible," and "Black people as a rule are, by their nature, more violent than white people are." The RF–racism correlations have never been large, ranging from .17 to .33 in our student and parent studies. But they have been consistently *positive*, when one might expect persons who follow Jesus to be among the less prejudiced, not the more prejudiced, one can find.

How Do People Become Fundamentalists?

The most obvious hypothesis, fundamentalists come from fundamentalist parents, turns out to be only partly true. University students' RF scores correlate about .50–.65 with their parents' RF answers, which is substantial, but still leaves some explaining to be done. Similarly, scores on a Religious Emphasis Scale that asks questions about how much the family religion was emphasized when the respondent was a child, in terms of going to church, praying before meals, reading Scripture, and so on, correlate .54–.69 with adult RF scores. Which again explains a lot, but not everything.

Part of the reason these correlations fall short of perfection can be traced to the fact that parents do not always succeed in transferring the family religion to the next generation, no matter how hard they try. Data on over 5,000 Canadian men and women, nearly 50 years old on the average, reveal that only 64% still consider themselves members of the religion in which they were raised. (The big winner among those who shifted is "None.") The fundamentalist Protestant sects, which have higher Religious Emphasis scores than any other Christian faith, actually do a little poorer than average at retaining their youth, holding onto only 56% of their next generation (Altemeyer, 2004). So the RF correlation between generations "only" lands in the .50s and .60s partly because some of the seed falls on shallow soil.

Another reason will please fundamentalists more: they make up their "in-house" losses through conversions from other faiths, and then some. In those same "home religion versus present religion" data, fundamentalists started off with 314 youth and ended up with 372 adults—after losing 137 of their own! Our research indicates that the conversions come from at least three different sources. First, fundamentalist religions attract more than their share of disaffected youth who were raised in no religion (Altemeyer &

Hunsberger, 1997). While few in number, these "amazing believers" typically are going through some emotional crisis and are attracted to fundamentalist religions that offer love and community through their youth groups. Second, speaking of love, some adults join fundamentalist faiths when they get married. Fundamentalist (and Catholic) adults are more likely than most Christians to insist upon conversion as a condition of marriage. While such "shotgun conversions" do not always produce genuine or long-term commitment, they do increase the numbers of people who call themselves "Evangelicals," "Pentecostals," and so on. Third, speaking of genuine commitment, the fundamentalists gain a certain number of converts from more mainstream Christian faiths that have undergone "liberalization." These converts have many reasons for turning to fundamentalist religions, reporting such thing as: "A personal belief in Christ was stressed," "It teaches exclusively the Bible," and "The United Church was too liberal and wishy-washy, not committed to absolutes." Add up the flow from these three streams, and the fundamentalist groups are the only denominations that show a net *increase* from "home to dome" in our data.

Still, you may have been surprised by the raw numbers cited above, because the perception exists that the fundamentalist Protestant sects are growing like crazy. Actually, they are not; 372 is only a spoonful of the 5,488 adults in our study. Bibby (2002) has observed that the percentage of religious "conservatives" in Canada has remained about 8% since 1871. One finds far more in the United States, but the General Social Survey (Davis, Smith & Marsden, 2000) found that the number of Americans who call themselves "fundamentalist"—as opposed to "moderate" or "liberal" in their religious views—peaked at 36% in 1987, and had dropped down to 31% in 1998 and 2000. In the United States, as in Canada, the "None" category has shown the biggest recent gains. But one does not notice this decline, because the fundamentalist churches' parking lots can be seen to be full on Sundays—because of their high level of church attendance— while the Nones' cars are home in the garage.

Summary

Religious fundamentalism, defined as an attitude about one's religious beliefs, is measured by an essentially unidimensional RF Scale that has good reliability and seemingly strong validity. Some high scorers appear in all religions, but they are more concentrated in fundamentalist Protestant denominations. Fundamentalists have highly orthodox beliefs in God and in Christianity, and they embrace creation science. Their beliefs bring them great comfort and joy in life, which they do not particularly get from logic and science. They are given to intensive proselytizing. They would make strong efforts to convert a troubled teen raised as an atheist. They certainly raised their own children to believe as they do. They seem to be more zealous about their beliefs than just about any other group of people you can find. They unfortunately maintain some double standards about the separation of church and state because of their zealotry. They tend to be dogmatic. Scientific evidence that shows they are wrong would simply be ignored. They cannot conceive of anything that would lead them to change their belief in God. They admit to virtually no doubts about their religious beliefs. (In comparison, their opposite extremists in religiousness, atheists, prove substantially less proselytizing, zealous, and dogmatic.) Fundamentalists are highly ethnocentric about religion, and are generally hostile toward homosexuals. They also tend to be more racially prejudiced than most people are, if by small amounts. They emphasize the family religion a lot to their children, but do a poorer job than most faiths at retaining the next generation. However, they make up these losses, and often obtain a net gain, through conversions of troubled youth, through marriage, and by attracting persons disaffected by "liberalizing" religions. Their numbers do *not* appear to be growing, but their great activity may create the impression that they are.

One further observation should be made. Religious fundamentalism turns out to be a *powerful* predictor of many things. Nearly all the relationships described above involve correlations over .50, and sometimes reach into the lofty atmosphere of .70s where they approach the very reliability of the scales involved. At other times, we find that over 90% of highly fundamentalist people did this or said that. Sometimes it is 100%! And even when the relationships are smaller, they carry weight. The connection between fundamentalism and hostility toward homosexuals usually runs in the .50s, but RF scores are the second-best predictor of attitudes toward homosexuals we have ever found. And the RF correlation with racial prejudice may only run in the .20s, yet it raises one's eyebrows.

But, it turns out, religious fundamentalism is only part of a larger phenomenon, to which we now turn. It happens to be the best predictor of hostility toward homosexuals, and a whole lot more.

AUTHORITARIANISM

It may seem a complete non sequitur, but we shall now shift our analysis to the Nuremberg Rallies of the Nazi Party in the late 1930s. Films of those events still convey today the overwhelming image of a 100,000 ardent Nazis filling the stands and playing field of the sports stadium, adoring one of the most evil men in history. That adoration enabled Adolf Hitler to plunge the world into the most calamitous, destructive, murderous war of all time.

Even as the Nazi Party celebrated its existence and triumphs in Nuremberg each fall, social scientists wondered how this nightmare could be occurring, and whether it could reappear elsewhere—even in North America. An ambitious research program on "the authoritarian personality" accordingly began at the University of California at Berkeley during World War II under the guidance of Nevitt Sanford (Adorno, Frenkel-Brunswik, Levinson, & Sanford, 1950). Its watershed conclusions shaped research in personality and social psychology for decades.

Today we know that *two* kinds of authoritarian personalities exist. Authoritarian *leaders* tend to be social dominators. Felicia Pratto and Jim Sidanius's Social Dominance Orientation Scale elegantly measures these power hungry and amoral personalities (Pratto, Sidanius, Stallworth, & Malle, 1994). Authoritarian *followers*, the subjects of the Berkeley investigation, are today called right-wing authoritarians (Altemeyer, 1981, 1988, 1996). We have plenty of both kinds of authoritarian personalities among us today, wanna-be dominators and gladly following followers. The dominators do not, as you might guess, have many religious inclinations. But authoritarian followers tend to be religious, and religious fundamentalists in particular (Altemeyer, 1996).[2]

Right-Wing Authoritarianism

Right-wing authoritarianism is defined as the covariation of three attitudinal clusters in a person: authoritarian submission, authoritarian aggression, and conventionalism (Altemeyer, 1981). It is called "right-wing," not in a political sense, but in a social-psychological one, as the submission occurs to authorities who are perceived to be established and legitimate in society. You could have "left-wing" authoritarians too, persons who follow revolutionary authorities, as some North American students became "Maoists" in the early 1970s. But such left-wing authoritarians are very hard to come by nowadays, whereas one can find lots of right-wing ones (Altemeyer, 1996, 1998).

Right-wing authoritarianism is measured by an attitude scale inventively named the Right-Wing Authoritarianism (RWA) Scale. For most of its life it has been 30 items long, but like the RF Scale, it has recently been shortened to the 20 statements shown in Figure 21.2. Covering more ground that the RF Scale, it does not have as high an internal consistency among its responses. But its greater length gives it an alpha reliability of about .90. If you look at the items in Figure 21.2, you may agree that most of them cover at least two of the three defining elements, and some (such as No. 1) tap all three. Factor analyses indicate that the 20 items basically measure just one thing, which appears to be the *covariation* of authoritarian submission, authoritarian aggression, and conventionalism.

1. Our country desperately needs a mighty leader who will do what has to be done to destroy the radical new ways and sinfulness that are ruining us.
2. Gays and lesbians are just as healthy and moral as anybody else.*
3. It is always better to trust the judgment of the proper authorities in government and religion than to listen to the noisy rabble-rousers in our society who are trying to create doubt in people's minds.
4. Atheists and others who have rebelled against the established religions are no doubt every bit as good and virtuous as those who attend church regularly.*
5. The only way our country can get through the crisis ahead is to get back to our traditional values, put some tough leaders in power, and silence the troublemakers spreading bad ideas.
6. There is absolutely nothing wrong with nudist camps.*
7. Our country *needs* free thinkers who have the courage to defy traditional ways, even if this upsets many people.*
8. Our country will be destroyed someday if we do not smash the perversions eating away at our moral fibre and traditional beliefs.
9. Everyone should have their own lifestyle, religious beliefs, and sexual preferences, even if it makes them different from everyone else.*
10. The "old-fashioned ways" and the "old-fashioned values" still show the best way to live.
11. You have to admire those who challenged the law and the majority's view by protesting for women's abortion rights, for animal rights, or to abolish school prayer.*
12. What our country really needs is a strong, determined leader who will crush evil, and take us back to our true path.
13. Some of the best people in our country are those who are challenging our government, criticizing religion, and ignoring the "normal way things are supposed to be done."*
14. God's laws about abortion, pornography and marriage must be strictly followed before it is too late, and those who break them must be strongly punished.
15. There are many radical, immoral people in our country today, who are trying to ruin it for their own godless purposes, whom the authorities should put out of action.
16. A "woman's place" should be wherever she wants to be. The days when women are submissive to their husbands and social conventions belong strictly in the past.*
17. Our country will be great if we honor the ways of our forefathers, do what the authorities tell us to do, and get rid of the "rotten apples" who are ruining everything.
18. There is no "ONE right way" to live life; everybody has to create their *own* way.*
19. Homosexuals and feminists should be praised for being brave enough to defy "traditional family values."*
20. This country would work a lot better if certain groups of troublemakers would just shut up and accept their group's traditional place in society.

FIGURE 21.2. The revised 20-item Right-Wing Authoritarianism Scale. *Indicates the item is worded in the con-trait direction, for which the scoring key is reversed.

Evidence for Validity

Nature has been good to the RWA Scale, as evidence of its validity has appeared quite consistently, and from far and wide (Altemeyer, 1996, 1998). Persons who score relatively highly on the measure trust and support established authorities stronger and longer than most do, as they did President Nixon during the Watergate scandal. They support unjust and illegal acts by governments. They support police who abuse their power. In emergent leadership situations, they do not emerge, but usually sit quietly and let others assume command. After viewing a film about Milgram's famous "obedience" experiments, they tended to blame the Teacher and the Learner for what happened more than most people do, but not the authority, the Experimenter.

In turn, they themselves aggress in laboratory experiments involving electric shock, when authority sanctions it. They harbor many prejudices against many minorities, accepting stereotypes uncritically. In fact, most highly prejudiced persons turn out to be either social dominators or right-wing authoritarians (Altemeyer, 1998). High RWAs strongly believe in punishment, and admit that they derive personal pleasure from administering it to "wrongdoers."

They also adopt the conventions of their society more than most do, especially those backed by established authority. For example, at the end of the cold war, persons in the Soviet Union who scored highly on the RWA Scale believed that their government had been the "good guys" during the struggle, and the United States had been the "bad guys." U.S. right-wing authoritarians felt just the opposite. The authoritarians would likely have exchanged positions if they had instead been raised in the other's country. High RWAs also have a mean-spirited streak when evaluating "immoral" behavior. They appear relatively likely to help governments persecute a wide variety of unconventional victims. They endorse traditional sex roles and conformity to traditional practices. They believe strongly in "group cohesiveness" and in following group norms. Simply discovering that their attitudes differ significantly from some group average causes them to shift toward the norm. They tend to have "right-wing" economic philosophies and to favor "conservative" political parties. In both U.S. and Canadian legislatures, RWA Scale scores almost always differentiate "liberal" from "conservative" caucuses (Altemeyer, 1996).

Personal Origins of Right-Wing Authoritarianism

How do people come to believe in authoritarian submission, authoritarian aggression, and conventionalism? Our first guess, "from their parents," again receives some support. Student RWA scores correlate about .40 with their parents' scores, which is some but not a whole lot. Most children probably start off being pretty authoritarian as they submit to authority far and wide in their early years. But by the time they get to university, many of them have become much less so. Why?

We can make fairly accurate estimates of how highly university students will score on the RWA Scale if we know the answers to 24 questions about their experiences thus far in their lives. For example, have they ever found that authorities were unfair? Have they gotten to know members of minorities and unconventional people? Have they done unconventional things, and with what result? The more experiences such as these a person has had, the lower his or her RWA Scale score usually becomes. But some people just do not have many of these shaping experiences, and consequently they post high scores on the RWA Scale. For example, right-wing authoritarians tend to dislike homosexuals, but most of them have never known one—as far as they know (Altemeyer, 1988).

Cognitive Weaknesses

So while many people derive their opinions from their experiences in life, high RWAs tend to have relatively limited experiences and instead their opinions come from their authorities. This can produce many cognitive blind spots, for their beliefs have not necessarily been checked for consistency so much as they have been memorized as a package. Indeed, high RWAs hold many sets of inconsistent thoughts, such as "The trouble with democracy is that it usually represents the will of all the people, instead of just the best people" and "The trouble with democracy is that it seldom represents the will of the people." They are particularly likely to endorse slogans and cultural sayings even though they contradict each other.

A second problem can arise if you have not examined your ideas for consistency. You may use double standards in your thinking, and right-wing authoritarians do, over and over. They would sentence gay protestors who incite an attack on opponents to much longer prison terms than antigay protestors who commit the same crime. They would punish a "hippie" more than they would punish an accountant for the same crime. They would punish a prisoner for beating another prisoner in jail more than they would a chief of detectives who did the same thing. They believe in "majority rights" when they are in the majority, and "minority rights" when they are in the minority. They think unfair election practices are more serious when committed by a liberal party than when done by a conservative one. Well, does not everyone think out of both sides of his head as it suits his cause? No. Persons who score low on the RWA Scale do so much less.

You might also predict that, since they have not thought out their own ideas as much as most people have, right-wing authoritarians would rely more on social support to validate their opinions. If so, you would be right, for they show a heightened tendency to surround themselves with friends who tell them they are right. They tend to travel in "tight circles" of like-minded people. This makes them susceptible, however, to manipulators (such as social dominators) who tell them what they want to hear. Experiments have shown that high RWAs ignore background factors that might lower a speaker's credibility (e.g., a politician who has studied what the voters want him to say before he takes a stand) if he takes a stand they agree with. They are so ingroup-oriented, and so glad to have their opinions verified by someone new, that they believe people that prudent individuals would doubt.

Would you be surprised to learn that RWA Scale scores correlate solidly with dogmatism? It makes sense that they would, because if you are carrying around a lot of ideas that you copied as a package, as out of a catechism, but have not really scrutinized and given a good "shaking," they may be wrong for all *you* know. So you are vulnerable, and the easiest defense is erected by insistence that all of your ideas are perfectly right.

THE CONNECTION BETWEEN RIGHT-WING AUTHORITARIANISM AND RELIGIOUS FUNDAMENTALISM

RWA and RF scores generally correlate in the .70s, which means they share most of their variance. To put it another way, about two-thirds of persons who score highly on the measure of right-wing authoritarianism also score highly on the measure of religious fundamentalism. Some authoritarians are not fundamentalists, but most are. And some fundamentalists are not right-wing authoritarians, but most are.

You may have expected this from the moment you read over the items on the RWA Scale, since so many of them mention religion or bring up issues of morality, pushing such fundamentalist "hot buttons" as homosexuality, abortion, pornography, and school prayer. But these topics arise on the RWA Scale not so much because they follow from believing that God has one fundamentally true religion, but because they tap sentiments of authoritarian submission, authoritarian aggression, and conventionalism. So in an RWA Scale item such as No. 14 in Figure 21.2, "God's laws about abortion, pornography and marriage must be strictly followed before it is too late, and those who break them must be strongly punished," the issues are indeed "hot buttons," but the sentiments involve submission ("strictly followed"), aggression ("strongly punished"), and conventionalism ("God's laws"). If you look at the con-trait items Nos. 11 and 13, they also touch upon issues important to many fundamentalists, but the notion of admiring those who oppose fundamentalists, saying these opponents are some of the "best people," runs directly against the right-wing authoritarian's impulse to throttle them.

If religious fundamentalists score highly on the RWA Scale mainly because of the religion/morality topics it raises, then their responses to those items should correlate higher with RF scores than with the rest of the RWA Scale items. But if they score so highly on the RWA Scale because religious fundamentalists tend in the first place to be submissive to authority, aggressive in authority's name, and highly conventional, then items like No. 14 should correlate more highly with the rest of the RWA Scale. They should have stronger relationships with items about wanting a mighty leader, silencing troublemakers, upholding traditional ways, keeping women in their place, honoring forefathers, obeying authorities, and getting rid of "bad apples." The evidence has consistently supported the second hypothesis (Altemeyer & Hunsberger, 1992). Fundamentalists score highly on the RWA scale because fundamentalists strongly tend to be right-wing authoritarians.

Why are they so? Well, persons who grow up in fundamentalist families tend to be taught authoritarian submission, authoritarian aggression, and conventionalism. They report being taught that their religion's rules about morality were absolutely right and not to be questioned, that they had to strictly obey the commandments of an almighty God, and that the persons who acted as God's representatives, such as priests, ministers, pastors, or deacons, had to be obeyed. They learned that persons who tried to change the meaning of Scripture and religious laws were evil and doing the Devil's work, and unrepentant sinners would burn in hell for all eternity. It was stressed that they had to be good representatives of their faith, who acted the way a devout member of their religion was expected to act, that their religion was the center, the most important part of their lives, that it should fill their lives, that the deepest layers of Hell are set aside for those who abandon God's true religion (Altemeyer & Hunsberger, 1997). In short, obey the proper authorities, condemn the evildoers, follow the rules. Fundamentalist religions, indeed fundamentalist upbringings in many religions, directly teach the defining attributes of right-wing authoritarianism in many ways.

These teachings may have less than desirable side effects as well. Take that low but unsettling correlation between fundamentalism and religious prejudice. Research has discovered that a certain amount of prejudice arises from (1) fear, which instigates an aggressive reaction in some, that is then (2) released by self-righteousness. RF Scale scores correlate .44–.51 with scores on a Fear of a Dangerous World Scale, and .52–.54 with a measure of self-righteousness based on condemning people who have different social attitudes than fundamentalists have (Altemeyer, 1988). Is it hard to understand why fundamentalists, who have been taught that "Satan is everywhere," that their island of respectability is under constant attack by forces of immorality and degeneracy, and that the social fabric is being ripped apart, would see the world as dangerous? Is it hard to understand why persons who have been taught that they have a special relationship with God because they most honor God's teachings tend to be self-righteous? In a similar vein, fundamentalists may unwittingly teach their children to make sharper "Us versus Them" judgments in life by stressing the family's religious identity from a very early age. This training in ethnocentrism could create a template for later racial and ethnic ethnocentrism (Altemeyer, 2003).

Of course, not everyone raised in a fundamentalist religion, or in a fundamentalist way, remains a fundamentalist throughout life. As we saw, these religions may lose more than the usual share of their youth, and probably lose them because their "strayers" had experiences in life that made them less authoritarian. But those who remain faithful, the fundamentalist adults who were raised that way, have very high RWA Scale scores— usually higher than those who convert to fundamentalist religions as adults.

THE CHICKEN AND THE EGG AND THE APPREHENSION

When two variables each have strong relationships with many behaviors, are themselves highly correlated, and appear to have some common roots, one's mind naturally wonders which one is more important, which one is more basic, which one is the dog and which one is the tail. One can answer that question statistically by using partial correlation analyses, which show how much one variable (e.g., right-wing authoritarianism) can explain if you take away the influence of its fellow traveler (e.g., religious fundamentalism). Such analyses over the years yield a very consistent story: when it comes to explaining religious variables, such as church attendance, religious ethnocentrism, religious doubts, zealotry, and dogmatism, RF Scale scores can explain a lot more on their own when you take away the effect of RWA Scale scores than vice versa. But when it comes to nonreligious realms, such as racial prejudice, hostility toward women, economic philosophy, "militia" sentiments, political affiliation, belief in a dangerous world, and a host of cognitive inconsistencies, the fundamentalism scale gets whatever predictive power it has mostly because it is associated so strongly with right-wing authoritarianism. That is, RF rides piggy-back on RWA in these cases. And because right-wing authoritarianism offers such a wide range of explanations, one can say that as personality variables go, it is more fundamental than fundamentalism. "Fundamentalism can therefore usually be viewed as a religious manifestation of right-wing authoritarianism" (Altemeyer, 1996, p. 161).

The conclusion leads to a larger concern. Without followers, would-be tyrants like Hitler are just comical figures on a soapbox. But with millions of followers, they can pose a threat to everyone, including the nation they might well lead to rack and ruin. A social dominator's loyal legions are likely to be filled with submissive, aggressive, right-wing authoritarians, and a lot of those (in our samples at least) turn out to be religious fundamentalists. This analysis will shock fundamentalists, who see themselves as "the good people." But so did those who rushed to Hitler's banner.

IN REMEMBRANCE

Bruce Hunsberger, one of the leading researchers in the psychology of religion, died in October 2003 after a courageous and remarkably uncomplaining 11-year battle with leukemia. Besides being a steady research collaborator with Bob Altemeyer, Bruce was also Bob's best friend. Bruce lived long enough to enlighten thousands of students with his remarkable teaching and he made so many contributions to his field that he won the Gordon Allport Research Prize awarded by the American Psychological Association. But he would have done so much more, and our loss is great.

NOTES

1. The limitation may not be as great as it seems, as research based on these populations has a good record of replication elsewhere; see Altemeyer (1996, Chap. 1). Manitoba students and their parents certainly are not representative of Manitobans in general, much less Canadians, much less North Americans. But whatever differences may exist (say) between religiousness in Manitoba students and religiousness in Alabama or Pennsylvania or Wyoming students, the *relationships* between religiousness and other variables within each population may be similar. And the evidence suggests it will be (Altemeyer, 1981, Chap. 5).

2. If you can stand a little complication, a few people (about 8% of a sample) score highly on both the social dominance measure and the RWA Scale. These "double highs" turn out to be very dominant persons who have high RWA scores because they believe in authoritarian submission—*to them.* They are the most highly and deeply and widely prejudiced persons in our samples. They also have stronger religious backgrounds, beliefs, and practices than one ordinarily finds in a social dominator. But they are less religious than ordinary right-wing authoritarians and religious fundamentalists would be.

REFERENCES

Adorno, T. W., Frenkel-Brunswik, E., Levinson, D. J., & Sanford, R. N. (1950). *The authoritarian personality.* New York: Harper.

Altemeyer, B. (1981). *Right-wing authoritarianism.* Winnipeg, Canada: University of Manitoba Press.

Altemeyer, B. (1988). *Enemies of freedom.* San Francisco: Jossey-Bass.

Altemeyer, B. (1996). *The authoritarian specter.* Cambridge, MA: Harvard University Press.

Altemeyer, B. (1998). The other "authoritarian personality." In M. P. Zanna (Ed.), *Advances in Experimental Social Psychology* (Vol. 30). San Diego: Academic Press.

Altemeyer, B. (2001). Changes in attitudes toward homosexuals. *Journal of Homosexuality, 42,* 63–75.

Altemeyer, B. (2003). Why do religious fundamentalists tend to be prejudiced? *The International Journal for the Psychology of Religion, 13,* 17–28.

Altemeyer, B. (2004). The decline of organized religion in Western civilization. *The International Journal for the Psychology of Religion, 14,* 77–89.

Altemeyer, B., & Hunsberger, B. (1992). Authoritarianism, religious fundamentalism, quest and prejudice. *The International Journal for the Psychology of Religion, 2,* 113–133.

Altemeyer, B., & Hunsberger, B. (1997). *Amazing conversions: Why some turn to faith and others abandon religion.* Amherst, NY: Prometheus Press.

Altemeyer, B., & Hunsberger, B. (2004). A revised Religious Fundamentalism Scale: The short and sweet of it. *The International Journal for the Psychology of Religion, 14,* 47–54.

Bibby, R. W. (2002). *Restless gods: The renaissance of religion in Canada.* Toronto: Stoddart.

Davis, J. A., Smith, T. W., & Marsden, P. V. (2000). *General Social Survey.* Chicago: National Opinion Research Center.

Fullerton, J. T., & Hunsberger, B. (1982). A unidimensional measure of Christian orthodoxy. *Journal for the Scientific Study of Religion, 21,* 317–326.

The fundamentals: A testimony to the truth. (n.d.). Grand Rapids, MI: Baker Book House.

Hood, R. W., Jr., Hill, P. C., & Williamson, W. P. (2005). *The psychology of religious fundamentalism.* New York: Guilford Press.

Hunsberger, B., & Altemeyer, B. (in press). *Atheists!* Amherst, NY: Prometheus Press.

Hunsberger, B., Owusu, V., & Duck, R. (1999). Religion and prejudice in Ghana and Canada: Religious fundamentalism, right-wing authoritarianism, and attitudes toward homosexuals and women. *The International Journal for the Psychology of Religion, 9,* 181–194.

Pratto, F., Sidanius, J., Stallworth, L.M., & Malle, B.F. (1994). Social dominance orientation: A personality variable predicting social and political attitudes. *Journal of Personality and Social Psychology, 67,* 741–763.

22

Religion and Forgiveness

MICHAEL E. MCCULLOUGH
GIACOMO BONO
LINDSEY M. ROOT

The concept of forgiveness has gone from complete scientific obscurity as recently as 1980 to remarkable visibility in the first few years of the 21st century. The boom in forgiveness research can be appreciated by examining Figure 22.1, in which we have displayed the annual number of items catalogued in PsycINFO that include the word stem "forgiv*" in their abstracts (1980–2004). This figure clearly shows that whereas forgiveness was a psychological concept that received negligible empirical attention in the 1980s, social scientists have been producing scores of publications on the topic annually for the last several years.

Psychologists have given sustained attention to several aspects of forgiveness, including (1) the development of reasoning about forgiveness (e.g., Enright, Gassin, & Wu, 1992) (2) applications of forgiveness to counseling and psychotherapy (e.g., Enright, 2001; Worthington, 2001; Worthington & Wade, 1999); (3) social-psychological factors that facilitate or deter forgiveness (e.g., Finkel, Rusbult, Kumashiro, & Hannon, 2002; McCullough et al., 1998); (4) personality correlates of forgiveness (e.g., McCullough, 2001; McCullough & Hoyt, 2002); (5) the associations of forgiveness with measures of mental health, physiological functioning, and physical health (e.g., Karremans, Van Lange, & Ouwerkerk, 2003; Lawler et al., 2003; Witvliet, Ludwig, & Vander Laan, 2001); and (6) the religious contours of forgiveness (e.g., McCullough & Worthington, 1999; Tsang, McCullough, & Hoyt, 2005).

In this chapter, we focus specifically on the links between forgiveness and religious experience, belief, and behavior. We describe the relevance of forgiveness to the religious lives of individuals and communities, as well as the importance of religion in shaping how people understand and experience forgiveness. We also speculate about the relevance of forgiveness for understanding the relationships of religion to aging and health. We close by introducing some ideas drawn from evolutionary psychology that might provide direction for future interdisciplinary work in this area.

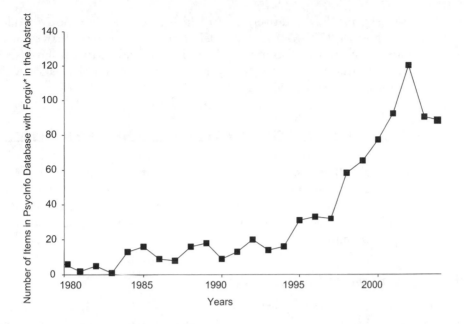

FIGURE 22.1. Number of items in PsychInfo database with "forgiv*" in the abstract, 1980–2004.

WHAT IS FORGIVENESS?

Psychologists seem to agree on several points about forgiveness. First, most concur with Enright and Coyle (1998) who argue that forgiveness should be distinguished from pardoning, condoning, excusing, forgetting, and denying. Most also concur that forgiveness should be distinguished from related concepts such as reconciliation. This is because reconciliation, which involves "the restoration of trust in an interpersonal relationship through mutually trustworthy behaviors" (Worthington & Drinkard, 2000), is not a prerequisite for forgiveness. For instance, people can forgive people with whom they cannot resume a relationship (e.g., someone who is in jail or is deceased) or with whom they do not wish to resume a relationship (e.g., an abusive partner).

But scholars continue to disagree somewhat about how forgiveness should be defined (Scobie & Scobie, 1998). Enright and colleagues (Enright & Coyle, 1998; Enright, Gassin, & Wu, 1992) defined "genuine forgiveness" according to philosopher J. North's (1987) proposal that forgiveness occurs when the target of an interpersonal transgression is able to "view the wrongdoer with compassion, benevolence, and love while recognizing that he has willfully abandoned his right to them" (p. 502). Worthington and colleagues (Berry & Worthington, 2001; Worthington & Wade, 1999) proposed that when one forgives, positive, love-based emotions (e.g., empathy, compassion, sympathy, and affection) replace the negative emotions he or she previously experienced regarding the transgressor (Worthington & Wade, 1999). McCullough and colleagues proposed that people forgive when they undergo a suite of motivational changes. Specifically, people come to experience forgiveness as they become less motivated to avoid and to seek revenge against a transgressor and simultaneously become more benevolent toward the transgressor (e.g., McCullough et al., 1998; McCullough & Hoyt, 2002). It is presumed that these motivational changes will increase the likelihood that a transgression recipient will, in turn, behave more positively and less negatively toward his or her transgressor. McCullough, Pargament, and Thoresen (2000) proposed a definition of forgiveness that emphasized the commonalities in the above conceptualizations. They suggested that forgiveness is an "intraindividual, prosocial change toward a perceived transgressor that is set within a specific interpersonal context" (p. 9).

IS THERE ANYTHING PARTICULARLY RELIGIOUS ABOUT FORGIVENESS?

Forgiveness is a deeply religious concept for people from many faiths and cultures, and therefore, we believe, an important topic of study for the psychology of religion. Issues of guilt, reconciliation, salvation, and redemption are common to many religions and many cultures, as are at least indirectly, questions about forgiveness and its place in the life of individuals and communities.

Forgiveness as a Universal Religious Concern

Anyone who peruses ethnographic studies of the world's cultures cannot help but note that forgiveness is a major religious concern. Consider this observation about the importance of forgiveness in the lives of people from the animistic Igbo culture of Nigeria:

> The offering of sacrifice is deemed to be essential only to those spirits which reside or operate outside the pale of human ken and control. The animist's life is permeated with the thought of their sinister power. All he can comprehend is that there are devastating forces at work in the world about him. He believes that, in some mysterious manner, these spirits can, and do, execute vengeance upon unprotected men. He may be unable to trace any definite reason for their antagonism, nevertheless, he is forced to conclude that punishment is meted out for some sin committed. Whether of omission or commission he may be unable to state: all he can do is to accept the verdict and meekly submit to whatever falls to his lot. In his distress, he appeals to the "dibia" and, either by his own endeavours, or by the services of the "dibia", he seeks a way of forgiveness by offering appropriate sacrifices in order to "drive away evil" ("ichu aja"), or to "drive out the devil" ("ichu Ogbonuke"). For this latter, a dog or a fowl is killed and left lying in the street, or outside the village, as an offering to the evil one." (Basden, 1966, p. 57)

Or consider De Laguna's (1972) description of how the Tlingit of southeastern Alaska would treat the remains of bears they killed on hunting expeditions:

> After the bear was killed, the hunter would pray to it for forgiveness, explaining why he needed to kill it. The head would be cut off and buried, facing the mountains. Sometimes it was covered with boughs, or it might be put in a mountain stream, or buried under a waterfall, so no birds could get at it. . . . "If they don't do that, the other bears would notice and get angry and get after the hunter." (De Laguna, 1972, pp. 365–366)

Even cultures that are better known for their vengefulness also have well-established rituals for effecting forgiveness among belligerents, and many of these rituals are made sensible by shared religious values among the belligerent parties. Consider Rovinskii's (1901) description of a ritual for reconciliation following a feud between two clans that have been locked in a cycle of blood revenge, which we have taken from Boehm's (1984) study of tribal Montenegrins:

> At the ceremony, the two clans stayed away from each other "like two hostile regiments." Rovinskii describes the ceremony in detail: A short moment of silence falls, and then a group of people steps out from the other side. The son of the murderer, in a single undergarment, barefoot and without a cap, creeps on all fours. And on his neck hangs a long gun on a strap (it is always a long gun, for a greater effect, even if the murder was just by pistol). . . . Seeing this, Zec hastily runs ahead in order to shorten this severe, humiliating scene. He runs to Bojković in order to raise him up more quickly, but at that very moment Bojković kisses him on the feet, the chest and the shoulder. Taking the gun off Bojković's neck, Zec addresses him with the following words: "First a brother, then a blood enemy, then a brother forever. Is this the rifle which took the life of my father?" And not waiting for a reply, he hands the gun back to Bojković, expressing by this the full forgiveness of the past, and they both kiss each other, embracing each other like brothers. (Rovinskii, 1901, p. 386, as cited in Boehm, 1984, p. 136)

This Montenegrin ritual of forgiveness and reconciliation was consummated by establishing 12 godfather relationships between members of the two clans, as well as 24 different blood-brother relationships (Boehm, 1984). It was their shared Orthodox Christian faith that made these kinship relationships possible in a culture in which vengeance was the normative response to homicide.

The roles of forgiveness in each of the above cultures reflect what may be a universal function of forgiveness for societies: its value for preserving stability in humans' relationships in the social world, the natural world, and the world of spirits.

Forgiveness as a Religious Concern in the United States

Closer to home and the present day, forgiveness is an acute religious concern in the Christian and Jewish traditions that form the mainstream of religious expression in the United States. According to data from a 1998 General Social Survey, over 80% of U. S. adults feel that their religious beliefs "often," "almost always," or "always" help them to forgive others, to forgive themselves, and to feel forgiven by God, respectively (Davis & Smith, 1999). Wuthnow (2000) studied a representative sample of U.S. adults involved in religiously oriented small groups (e.g., prayer groups, Bible study groups). Sixty-one percent of the sample reported that their group had helped them forgive someone and 71% of the sample reported that they had experienced healing in a relationship because of their group participation.

How Religion Promotes Forgiveness

Religious scholars have noted that all of the major world religions have structures that promote forgiveness (McCullough & Worthington, 1999; Rye et al., 2000). Tsang et al. (2005) noted that religions can promote forgiveness in several ways. Religious meaning systems can prescribe forgiveness as a value, encourage emotions such as compassion and empathy, and model forgiving actions through Scriptures and/or rituals. Religion can also sanctify forgiveness behavior by providing role models of forgiving behavior and presenting a worldview that allows individuals to interpret events and relationships in ways that facilitate forgiveness. Thus, religion is a concern that people bring to their thoughts, feel-ings, and behavior regarding forgiveness.

But perhaps the opposite is also true: Perhaps people also reformulate their religious convictions as a result of choices that they make about forgiveness. People may question or even redefine their religious convictions when confronted with difficult dilemmas of forgiving. Indeed, philosophers and psychologists have noted the potential of forgiveness to transform an individual's entire outlook on life (Enright & Coyle, 1998; North, 1987).

RELIGION AND THE PROPENSITY TO FORGIVE OTHERS

Because the teachings of many of the major religions promote forgiveness (McCullough & Worthington, 1999; Rye et al., 2000), it is worth considering how religion might influ-ence whether and how individuals forgive.

Religion and "Forgivingness"

For three decades, psychological research has consistently demonstrated that religious in-volvement is positively related to the disposition to forgive others—a trait that research-ers are now referring to as forgivingness (Roberts, 1995). In some of the earliest work on the topic, Rokeach (1973) found that people who reported greater church attendance, re-ligiousness, and intrinsic as well as extrinsic motivation for religious involvement placed "forgiveness" as a higher priority in their personal value systems than did people who scored lower on these religious indicators. Poloma and Gallup (1991) also found a posi-tive relationship between religious involvement and self-reports of people's tendency to forgive those who have harmed them. In a reanalysis of Poloma and Gallup's nationally representative data, Gorsuch and Hao (1993) found that, compared to nonreligious peo-ple, highly religious people reported having greater motivation to forgive, working harder to forgive, and harboring fewer reasons for getting even and staying resentful toward their transgressors. Others have reported similar findings (e.g., Bono, 2002; Mauger, Saxon, Hamill, & Pannell, 1996; Mullet et al., 2003).

The Religion–Forgiveness Discrepancy

The above-mentioned research on the links between religiousness and forgiving others is based on measures of people's valuing of forgiveness, their self-reported forgivingness re-garding typical or hypothetical transgressions, and their general reasoning about the pro-priety of forgiveness as a way of dealing with transgressions. However, research on the association of religious involvement with measures of forgiveness in response to specific, real-life transgressions has yielded less consistent evidence (McCullough & Worthington, 1999). McCullough and Worthington referred to this tendency for religiousness to be positively associated with people's self-reported tendencies to forgive others in general but only trivially associated with forgiveness responses to specific transgressions as the re-ligion-forgiveness discrepancy. Tsang et al. (2005) investigated the possibility that this discrepancy is caused by the fact that a single measure of behavior does not provide a good indicator of the dispositional or personality-based influences on that behavior be-cause of situation-specific error. Applying the aggregation principle (Fishbein & Ajzen, 1974), Tsang et al. (2005) found that, indeed, when self-reports of forgiveness were based on transgressions that were recalled under restrictive procedures (i.e., forcing participants to recall specific types of transgressions occurring within specific types of relationships) as well as aggregated across multiple transgressions, positive correlations emerged between religiousness and transgression-specific forgiveness. Measures of religiousness such as religious commitment and intrinsic religious motivation accounted for approximately 4% of the variance in people's typical tendencies to forgive across many transgressions committed by many relationship partners (e.g., friends, parents, and romantic partners). Therefore, studies with improved methods seem to support the proposition that religious individuals are, in general, slightly more forgiving than are less religious people, although this association is rather small.

Choosing Forgiveness-Oriented or Revenge-Oriented Aspects of Religious Belief Systems

The research we have reviewed above clearly suggests that people with high levels of religious participation, religious salience, or religious commitment tend to be more forgiving than are their less religious counterparts. However, the major world religions also condone revenge and retributive justice in some contexts. As Tsang et al. (2005) pointed out, support for the doctrine of *lex talionis* (equal and direct retribution) can be found in the Judaic Old Testament (e.g., "an eye for an eye, a tooth for a tooth, an arm for an arm, a life for a life"), the Christian New Testament (e.g., "God is just: He will pay back trouble to those who trouble you"; 2 Thessalonians 1:6, New Internation Version Bible), and the Islamic Qur'an (e.g., "O ye who believe! the law of equality is prescribed to you in cases of murder: the free for the free, the slave for the slave, the woman for the woman"; 2:178). The doctrine of karma in Buddhism and Hinduism can also be seen as an endorsement for retributive justice: all our actions, good and bad, will eventually bring proportional consequences. This availability of religious doctrines that promote retributive justice or belief in a just world—the belief that God's (or karmic) justice ensures that wrongdoers will ultimately get what they deserve (Lerner & Simmons, 1966)—may enable people to use their religious beliefs to justify their own vengeful stances toward transgressors.

Tsang et al. (2005) proposed that individuals who are actively motivated to seek revenge in response to a specific transgression might selectively employ religious beliefs that will justify their vengeful stances, presumably to maintain self-consistency. If so, people's religious beliefs and commitments may shift temporarily so that they can maintain self-concepts that are perceived to be in accordance with the mandates of their religious belief systems—a notion that is consistent with models of the self as flexible and subject to momentary shifts to accommodate social goals (e.g., Andersen & Chen, 2002).

To examine this possibility, Tsang et al. (2005) measured Christian university students' transgression-related interpersonal motivations (i.e., how avoidant, vengeful, and benevolent they felt) regarding a transgressor who harmed them within the last 7 days. Tsang et al.'s participants also completed two measures of religiousness to examine whether people who were highly vengeful toward a specific transgressor were using their religious beliefs to rationalize their unforgiving stances. First, participants indicated whether they endorsed a variety of religious sayings (some of which were from the Christian Scriptures and some of which sounded religious but were not from the Christian Scriptures) that were either forgiving or punitive in nature. Participants also indicated the extent to which a set of *justice*-related adjectives (e.g., "just," "fair"), a set of *forgiveness-*

related adjectives (e.g., "forgiving," "merciful"), and a set of *wrath/retribution*-relevant adjectives (e.g., "wrathful," "avenging") accurately described their concept of God (Gorsuch, 1968). There is a long tradition of research finding multidimensional and varied images of God; one reliable dimension is an image of God as a loving/forgiving entity versus a just/punishing entity (e.g., Gorsuch, 1968; Kunkel, Cook, Meshel, Daughtry, & Hauenstein, 1999). Research has shown that holding positive images of God and perceived relationships with God are related cross-sectionally to holding positive mental models of both self and others (Kirkpatrick, 1998), so Tsang et al. reasoned that individuals' working models of God might be related to their current interpersonal motivations vis-à-vis their transgressors.

In support of these ideas, Tsang at al. (2005) found that individuals who were, at the time of testing, motivated to avoid their transgressors were less likely to endorse forgiveness Scripture (e.g., "Forgive as the Lord forgave you"), whereas individuals who were high in benevolence (i.e., wishing goodwill toward their transgressor) were more likely to endorse the forgiveness Scripture and marginally less likely to endorse the retribution Scripture (e.g.,"Eye for an eye, tooth for a tooth, life for a life"). They also found that avoidance motivations were negatively correlated with forgiving images of God, and marginally negatively correlated with justice images of God, whereas benevolence was marginally positively related to forgiving images of God. These results suggest that people may selectively use retributive and forgiving themes inherent in religious meaning systems (whether they pertain to Scripture or conceptualizations of God) to rationalize their current vengeful or forgiving stances, rather than simply relying on their religious beliefs to shape their forgiveness- and revenge-related behavior.

RELIGION AND THE PROPENSITY TO SEEK FORGIVENESS FROM OTHERS

Confessing, repenting, and seeking forgiveness play important roles in many religious systems. In particular, the Scriptures of all of the Abrahamic religions place a strong emphasis on the importance of confession and contrition as a means of achieving forgiveness and relational wholeness. As a result, it seems likely that religion exerts an influence on whether and how people will seek forgiveness when they harm others.

Preliminary Work on Religion and Seeking Forgiveness

Sandage, Worthington, Hight, and Berry (2000) made the first attempt to define and empirically investigate seeking forgiveness. They defined seeking forgiveness as "a motivation to accept moral responsibility and to attempt interpersonal reparation following relational injury in which one is morally culpable" (p. 22). Sandage et al. found no relationship between participants' general religiousness and the extent to which they reported having sought forgiveness after committing a particular transgression. However, their failure to find a significant relationship may be due to some of the methodological factors that McCullough and Worthington (1999) invoked to explain why religiousness tends not to correlate with the extent to which people report having forgiven specific individuals who harmed them in the past.

Indeed, other research that obviates such methodological problems has yielded results that suggest that religiousness does indeed promote seeking forgiveness. In Meek, Albright, and McMinn's (1995) study, participants read a vignette in which they were to imagine that they had committed a dishonest act for personal satisfaction and then confessed for it. Participants then completed self-report measures of intrinsic and extrinsic religious motivation, along with single-item measures of how much they would feel forgiven by themselves, how much they would feel forgiven by God, and how likely they would be to confess, to feel good about confessing, to feel good for committing the act in the first place, and to repeat the offense. Individuals who were high in intrinsic religiousness reported being more prone to guilt, more likely to confess and to feel good about confessing, more likely to forgive themselves, and more likely to feel forgiven by God than individuals who were extrinsically religious. Moreover, Meek et al. found that guilt completely mediated the negative relationship between intrinsic religiosity and feeling good for committing the dishonest act. Guilt partially mediated the negative relationship between intrinsic religiosity and likelihood of repeating the offense (i.e., intrinsically religious people felt more guilty about their dishonest behavior, enjoyed the act less, and had a decreased likelihood of repeating the act in part because they felt more guilty). Although the validity of Meek et al.'s study was limited by studying people's hypothetical responses instead of their actual behavior, it nonetheless provides preliminary evidence that people who internalize religious values (in this case, within the Christian faith) may seek forgiveness more readily because of a stronger inclination to feel guilt for their transgressions.

Witvliet, Ludwig, and Bauer (2002) examined the physiological correlates of guilt and seeking forgiveness and consequently helped clarify the role that religion may play in seeking forgiveness. In this study, participants identified an incident from their past in which they were to blame for significantly hurting another person. Having recalled an appropriate incident, each participant engaged in five different types of imagery: (1) recalling the feelings associated with hurting the victim; (2) imagining seeking forgiveness from the victim; (3) imagining the victim responding in an unforgiving way; (4) imagining the victim responding in a forgiving way; and (5) imagining the victim responding with some appropriate form of reconciliation.

Witvliet et al. (2002) found that when people focused on recalling what they did and how it harmed the relationship partner, they felt more forgiveness from God, but *less* self-forgiveness, and less forgiveness from their victims, than when they imagined seeking forgiveness from the victim (i.e., confessing the wrong, apologizing, and asking forgiveness). This suggests that thinking about one's harmful behavior may lead to a sense of divine forgiveness, but it may deter one from engaging in interpersonal behaviors that would facilitate interpersonal forgiveness. Conversely, focusing on how one can repair the relational damage probably encourages one to seek forgiveness directly from the victim. Witvliet et al. also found that when participants focused on seeking forgiveness they experienced (1) increased hope; (2) reduced sadness, anger, guilt, and shame regarding the transgression; and (3) smaller increases in *corrugator* (brow) muscle tension, compared to when they simply thought about their harmful behavior. Together, these results suggest that seeking forgiveness directly from the victim may ultimately reduce negative affect, even though the prospect of seeking forgiveness itself is associated with some psychological stress in the short term (as shown by increased corrugator tension relative to baseline).

Religion and Humility: A Psychological Pathway to Seeking Forgiveness?

The above results suggest that intrinsically religious individuals are more likely to use interpersonal routes (e.g., confessing, seeking forgiveness from the people whom they injure) rather than strictly religious routes (e.g., seeking forgiveness exclusively from God) when they harm others, and that these interpersonal routes lead to the most enduring psychological and interpersonal benefits. Still, the act of seeking forgiveness is unpleasant and interpersonally risky. Religiousness might make people more willing to take this risk by fostering humility. Humility (i.e., a willingness to incorporate flattering as well as unflattering aspects of one's behavior into one's self-view, along with a realistic assessment of one's strengths and weaknesses relative to others; Emmons, 1999) has been empirically linked to religiousness (e.g., Cline & Richard, 1965). More recent research has shown that people who are high in quest religiousness (i.e., embracing the existential complexity inherent in religious questions, viewing religious doubt as positive, and remaining open to religious change) appear to be relatively humble (Rowatt, Ottenbreit, Nesselroade, & Cunningham, 2002). Although a link between humility and seeking forgiveness has yet to be established empirically, Sandage et al. (2000) found that narcissism—which might be thought of as the mirror opposite of humility—is negatively related to seeking forgiveness.

In summary, the work to date on the influence of religion on seeking forgiveness suggests that people who have high levels of intrinsic religious motivation tend to take more personal responsibility for their wrongdoings and are more inclined to undertake reparative action for them (Meek et al., 1995). On the other hand, studies of forgiveness seeking in the context of real-life transgressions suggest that religiousness does not influence forgiveness seeking (Sandage et al., 2000), or that religion may either encourage forgiveness seeking if people assume that they should focus on reconciling (i.e., confessing for the wrongdoing, apologizing, and asking for forgiveness) or discourage forgiveness seeking if people assume that they should focus exclusively on their relationship with God (Witvliet et al., 2002). To the extent that religions promote humility, they may also be successful in prompting people to seek forgiveness when they harm others.

RELIGION AND FORGIVING GOD

When Do People Deliberate about Forgiving God?

What do people mean by the notion of "forgiving God"? This is a third area in which the religious contours of forgiveness have been explored. Many religious people will disagree on theological or philosophical grounds that God can be forgiven, since forgiveness presupposes the ability to commit moral errors, which a perfect God, by definition, cannot possess. But philosophical or theological questions about whether God is a conceptually appropriate target for forgiveness aside, people do seem to feel a need to ask questions about forgiving God, especially when they have difficulty explaining life experiences that they perceive as highly painful or unfair.

The 1988 General Social Survey revealed that only 36% of respondents reported that they "never" felt angry toward God: anger toward God is common and may set the stage for people to ask questions about whether they need to "forgive" God to move on with their lives after they encounter great pain or tragedy. When people's suffering violates their own standards of justice or morality, they may feel disappointed, frustrated, or angry with God, and they may conclude that God has betrayed them. Indeed, undeserved suffering is a dominant theme in people's accounts of why they are unforgiving toward God (see Exline & Rose, Chapter 17, this volume).

Some of the events that can make people feel unforgiving toward God include negative experiences that seem to involve no direct human agency (e.g., innocents who suffer, evil acts that go unpunished, untimely death or illness, freak accidents, natural disasters); those that involve human agency but seem avoidable or preventable by God (e.g., murder, war atrocities, assault, sexual abuse, divorce, and betrayal); and even common misfortunes that simply seem ill-timed (e.g., rain on a wedding day; Exline, 2004).

Empirical research on forgiving God is scant and has focused on conditions in which these dilemmas arise (as described above) or the personality variables that are relevant to forgiving God. In a review of this literature, Exline (2004) described the main predictors of difficulty forgiving God and discovered that they largely mirror the predictors of anger and unforgiveness toward other people: (1) belief that God intentionally caused severe suffering; (2) an elevated sense of narcissistic entitlement; (3) less closeness to God or insecure attitudes toward religion prior to the negative event; (4) insecure attachment with one's parents or with other important relationship partners; and (5) a larger pattern of emotional and spiritual distress in one's life.

Forgiving God: Links with Well-Being

Exline (2004) also reviewed research on the outcomes of unforgiveness toward God. She noted correlational work suggesting that resentment toward God is associated with low spiritual well-being, which may lead to psychological distress more generally (see Pargament et al., 1998). Exline, Yali, and Lobel (1999) also conducted research on the negative outcomes of being unforgiving toward God. They administered self-report measures of negative emotion (i.e., depressed mood, anxious mood, and trait anger), religiousness (i.e., religious beliefs, religious participation, and feelings of alienation from God), and forgiveness (i.e., general difficulty forgiving God, forgiving God for a specific incident, and difficulty forgiving the self and others) to 200 people of various ethnicities and religions. They found that difficulty forgiving God was associated with higher levels of anxious and depressed mood and that difficulty forgiving God was distinct from difficulty forgiving the self or others in leading to these outcomes.

Exline et al.'s (1999) study provides preliminary evidence that dilemmas of forgiveness toward God are associated with low psychological well-being. They are also important because of their implications for religious functioning. Dilemmas of forgiveness toward God can be turning points where people question their faith in God and must resolve to make fundamental changes to their philosophy of life—for example, whether to seek ways to strengthen their belief in God or, on the other extreme, abandon their belief in God altogether (see Park, Chapter 16, this volume). More research on this topic would be extremely valuable for understanding religious means of coping with suffering and the implications of such means of coping for religious and psychological well-being.

RELIGION AND FEELING FORGIVEN BY GOD

As mentioned above, seeking God's forgiveness is a religious preoccupation for individuals from many religious faiths and cultures. Moreover, the extent to which God is viewed as loving and forgiving is a major dimension underlying people's images of God. However, the psychological dynamics of feeling forgiven by God (or other spiritual entities) has received relatively little empirical attention. Using nationally representative data, Toussaint, Williams, Musick, and Everson (2001) examined the experience of feeling forgiven by God (along with other aspects of forgiveness) among adults in three age groups: 18–44, 45–64, and 65+. Feeling forgiven by God was measured by agreement with two self-report items (i.e., "Knowing that I am forgiven for my sins gives me the strength to face my faults and be a better person" and "I know that God forgives me"). The investigators found that older adults were significantly more likely to feel forgiven by God than younger adults and marginally less likely to feel forgiven by God than middle-aged adults. Francis, Gibson, and Robbins (2001) also found that viewing God as loving/forgiving was correlated with self-worth among Scottish adolescents.

Krause and Ellison (2003) investigated in more detail the relationships between feeling forgiven by God and forgiving others. Using nationally representative data, they found that people who felt forgiven by God were less likely to expect people who had harmed them to perform acts of contrition than those who did not feel forgiven by God. This suggests an important relationship between one's sense of having received divine forgiveness and one's behavior toward one's own human transgressors.

ADDITIONAL AREAS OF RESEARCH IN THE STUDY OF RELIGION AND FORGIVENESS

Two additional areas of research related to the relationships of religion and forgiveness are worthy of attention in the present chapter. First, we comment on the interrelationships of religion, forgiveness, and aging. Second, we comment on the interrelationships of religion, forgiveness, and health.

Religion, Forgiveness, and Aging

Longitudinal studies have shown that as people in the United States age, they tend to become more religious (Argue, Johnson, & White, 1999; see also McFadden, Chapter 9, this volume). There is also good evidence that people who are older tend to be generally more forgiving and less vengeful than are younger people (e.g., Girard & Mullet, 1997; Mullet et al., 2003). For example, Mullet, Houdbine, Laumonier, and Girard (1998) found that two dimensions of a multidimensional construct they called "forgivingness" were positively associated with age in a sample of adults. Their findings also indicated that younger adults forgive because they tend to be motivated by personal and social considerations (e.g., their mood at the time, whether family or friends think they should forgive, or because the consequences of the harm have been canceled in some way) to a greater extent than is true for older adults. This is consistent with previous research that shows that older persons tend to forgive mainly out of strong convictions that forgiveness should be practiced unconditionally (Girard & Mullet, 1997).

Previously, we speculated that the common association of religiousness and forgiveness may come from the fact that as people age, they appear to become both more religious and more forgiving (McCullough & Bono, in press). Work by Carstensen and her colleagues (e.g., Carstensen, 1995; Carstensen, Isaacowitz, & Charles, 1999) helps to provide a theoretical account for why this might be so. According to Carstensen's socioemotional selectivity theory, as people age, their goals gradually shift away from future-oriented goals such as acquiring information, and toward more present-oriented goals such as being emotionally satisfied. With the recognition that the years of life they have remaining is becoming ever smaller, people become less motivated to maintain high numbers of interpersonal relationships irrespective of the quality of these relationships and turn instead to nurturing relatively few higher quality, emotionally satisfying relationships. Thus, as individuals pass through older adulthood, they choose social partners more and more for their emotional value, they regulate their social interactions in a way that optimizes emotionally gratifying outcomes, and they become more vested in the relationships they want to maintain.

In this light, religious concerns may become stronger in older adulthood not only to help people come to terms with their mortality, but also because the interpersonal contacts that are fostered by interaction in religious settings may be particularly satisfying and meaningful. Similarly, people may become more forgiving with age because forgiveness helps them to maintain important, emotionally satisfying relationships even though relational transgressions are probably inevitable. We therefore suspect that forgiveness and religiousness both play larger roles as people age precisely because they serve higher order goals of securing stable and supportive relationships. The relationships among religiousness, forgiveness, and aging have yet to be investigated jointly in empirical research, however.

Religion, Forgiveness, and Health

There is considerable evidence that religious involvement is positively associated with many indices of physical and mental health (e.g., Koenig, McCullough, & Larson, 2001; Oman & Thoresen, Chapter 24, this volume; Powell, Shahabi, & Thoresen, 2003). It is possible that religious people's tendency to forgive is one of the mechanisms by which religiousness obtains its associations with positive health outcomes (Koenig et al., 2001; Levin, 1996).

In support of this notion, researchers have found that unforgiving personality traits and/or acute unforgiving thoughts are associated with increases in cardiovascular arousal (Lawler et al., 2003; Witvliet et al., 2001) and increased cortisol secretion (Berry & Worthington, 2001). For example, Witvliet et al. instructed participants (undergraduate students) to engage in four types of thinking about a specific transgression they had incurred in the past: (1) thoughts about holding a grudge, (2) thoughts about revenge, (3) empathic thoughts about the transgressor, and (4) forgiving thoughts. They found that when participants engaged in grudge or revenge imagery, they exhibited increases in facial muscle tension, skin conductance, heart rate, and blood pressure compared to when they engaged in empathic or forgiving imagery regarding their transgressors. Not only did these physiological responses parallel participants' self-reported emotions (i.e., they felt more negative, aroused, angry, and sad, and less in control when engaging in the thoughts about grudges and revenge), but they also persisted into the postimagery recovery period. In other words, the psychophysiological effects of thinking about revenge and grudges persisted even after people had been instructed to stop thinking these thoughts. Based on these findings, Wivliet et al. argued that unforgiving responses to transgressions, if chronic, might erode physical health—particularly by increasing risk for cardiovascular diseases.

In addition, researchers have posited that forgiving one's transgressors has a positive effect on psychological well-being. Interventions designed to help people forgive have been shown to improve psychological well-being, yielding reduced anxiety and depressive symptoms, as well as increased self-esteem and hope (for a review, see Enright & Coyle, 1998). In addition, studies have demonstrated positive correlations between people's self-reported global tendencies to forgive and measures of psychological well-being (e.g., Maltby, Macaskill, & Day, 2001).

Given the empirically established links between religiousness and forgiveness, and their independent associations with measures of health and well-being, it seems plausible that some of the beneficial influence of religion on health and well-being occurs because religion encourages people to practice forgiveness in their relationships with friends and family. However, the research that directly explores the connections among these three concepts simultaneously has not yet been conducted.

SUMMARY AND CONCLUDING COMMENTS

Research has begun to show a clearer picture of how religion can influence people's seeking and granting of forgiveness in the interpersonal realm. In addition, research has begun to shed light on how people seek forgiveness from God and on the notion of "forgiving God." Although the proposition that God might be an appropriate target for forgiveness is theologically and philosophically problematic from some perspectives, it may nonetheless be experientially real for many people. In this chapter we have also described some promising connections between religion and forgiveness as they relate to aging, health, and well-being.

The concept of forgiveness appears to exist within most religions and most cultures (McCullough & Worthington, 1999; Rye et al., 2000), although each culture works out the specifics of forgiveness in unique ways (e.g., see Sandage, Hill, & Vang, 2003). In particular, religions provide norms, role models, and psychological resources that help people to forgive when they have been harmed by others. Religion also helps to identify what transgressions and transgressors can be forgiven, as well as when and under what circumstances those transactions can take place. In this vein, it is important to note that in many cultures, people often use religion to justify their decisions not to forgive. In some cultures, avenging one's family members who have been killed is even understood to be a solemn duty and a virtue that is readily justified by the dominant religious system (e.g., see Boehm, 1984). Similarly, religion appears to be an important force that shapes people's decisions about when they should seek forgiveness after harming others and when, conversely, they should feel justified in their harmful behavior toward other people.

Research on forgiveness has been growing rapidly, particularly during the last decade. If this progress continues, there is every reason to think that social science will reveal even more about how religion influences granting and seeking forgiveness in interpersonal relations, as well as how seeking forgiveness from God and perhaps forgiving God affect, and are affected by, other religious and nonreligious aspects of people's lives. Perhaps it will soon be time for social scientists who study religion to begin posing more fundamental questions about the relationships between religion and forgiveness: Why is forgiveness so common across cultures? Why does religion so often seem to be important for cultures' social constructions of forgiveness? Why is religion sometimes used to justify forgiveness, but on other occasions to justify revenge instead? Might forgiveness be such a common feature of religious and cultural systems because this concept helped our ancestors solve adaptive problems? Such questions might best be addressed by more explicitly incorporating evolutionary theory (e.g., Buss, 1995; Kenrick, Li, & Butner, 2003) into research and theorizing on religion and forgiveness. Contemporary psychological theorists have recently applied evolutionary thinking to many aspects of religion (e.g.,

Buss, 2002; Kirkpatrick, 1999; Wilson, 2002), and the religious contours of forgiveness also may be amenable to an evolutionary treatment (e.g., see Wilson, 2002). We close this chapter with some preliminary thoughts about how the religious contours of forgiveness might emerge through cultural evolution.

To remain intact, all cultures—especially large ones that are vulnerable to fissioning because of pressures exerted upon them by outside threats—must develop norms for socially acceptable behavior among their members, along with the means to enforce those norms. Recently, researchers have presented findings that suggest that belief in moralizing gods (i.e., gods who tell people what they should and should not do) is especially useful for this purpose (Roes & Raymond, 2003). Wherever societies face high degrees of external threat in the form of wars or droughts, for instance, belief in moralizing gods tends to arise. Belief in moralizing gods is useful in such contexts because the belief can be used to (1) explain why the norms exist in the first place; and (2) enforce the norms more efficiently because people can be convinced that they may receive spiritual sanctions (e.g., being haunted, illness, death, hell) if they violate the norms, and that they may receive spiritual rewards (e.g., wealth, fertility, safe passage to the next life) if they honor them.

However, because some individuals will inevitably violate the norms of these religiously prescribed moral systems, it seems likely that religious systems with moralizing gods will also need to provide adherents with means for seeking forgiveness from those spiritual forces, and by extension, from each other (Wilson, 2002). Without the possibility of forgiveness, after all, how is someone who violates the precepts established by a moralizing god (or gods) able to rejoin his or her community as a member in good standing? Religious systems with moralizing gods must be clear and strict in order to foster the desired level of group cohesion, to be sure, but they must also provide an outlet for reintegrating individuals whose behavior falls below the articulated standards. For some infractions, a community will decide that a permanent exclusion of a transgressor is warranted (i.e., that some sins are unforgivable), but for other infractions, it is more advantageous to rehabilitate the transgressor than to expel him or her through ostracizing or death. The possibility of forgiveness not only allows a reaffirmation of the culture's standards and the rehabilitation of the offending member, but may also make the offending member less self-centered than he or she might have been otherwise (for a nonreligious, modern-day example of this phenomenon in action, see Kelln & Ellard, 1999). Because the belief that people can be forgiven by their moralizing gods might have served this reintegrative function, we tentatively propose that the belief that people can be forgiven by their gods, given the proper demonstrations of contrition or sacrifice, will arise in any religious system in which belief in moralizing gods is also present, although the circumstances under which forgiveness is likely to be perceived to be available as a religious option will no doubt vary across cultures.

Although interpersonal (rather than divine) forgiveness no doubt served adaptive functions for our ancestors (e.g., fostering positive relations among close friends and family members, thereby maximizing inclusive fitness) quite apart from its connections to religion, it seems likely that many of people's ideas about seeking and granting forgiveness will be modeled upon their understandings of how their own forgiveness transactions with their god or gods are believed to occur. Specifically, when people are put in a position to forgive individuals who have harmed them, or to seek forgiveness from others, it seems likely that their religious systems will encourage them to model their own thoughts, feelings, and behaviors after the thoughts, feelings, and behaviors that their god or gods might experience. If so, then it seems likely that we can shed considerable light on contemporary differences in forgiveness across religions and cultures (e.g., the substantial differences between Jewish and Christian practices regarding forgiveness) by integrating research findings from modern psychological science with historical and anthropological research that provides a deeper view of particular religions and cultures.

The few paragraphs above are hardly a comprehensive evolutionary account of religious forgiveness. In presenting these ideas (which may turn out upon scientific scrutiny to be completely incorrect), we have merely tried to illustrate some of the issues that might be addressed by evolutionary theorizing. Incorporating an evolutionary paradigm for studying forgiveness, and in particular its religious contours, could provide the field with a better framework for making sense of what we already know about the religious contours of forgiveness. It might also inspire new questions that could lead to a deeper understanding of the many connections between religion and forgiveness.

ACKNOWLEDGMENT

This chapter was prepared with the support of a grant from the Campaign for Forgiveness Research.

REFERENCES

Andersen, S. M., & Chen, S. (2002). The relational self: An interpersonal social-cognitive theory. *Psychological Review, 109,* 619–645.

Argue, A., Johnson, D. R., & White, L. K. (1999). Age and religiosity: Evidence from a three-wave panel analysis. *Journal for the Scientific Study of Religion, 38,* 423–435.

Basden, G. T. (1966). *Niger Ibos: A description of the primitive life, customs and animistic beliefs, etc., of the Ibo people of Nigeria.* London: Cass.

Berry, J. W., & Worthington, E. L., Jr. (2001). Forgivingness, relationship quality, stress while imagining relationship events, and physical and mental health. *Journal of Counseling Psychology, 48,* 447–455.

Boehm, C. (1984). *Blood revenge: The anthropology of feuding in Montenegro and other tribal societies.* Lawrence: University of Kansas Press.

Bono, G. (2002). *Commonplace forgiveness among and between groups and cross-cultural perceptions of transgressors and transgressing.* Unpublished doctoral dissertation, Claremont Graduate University, Claremont, CA.

Buss, D. M. (1995). Evolutionary psychology: A new paradigm for psychological science. *Psychological Inquiry, 6,* 1–30.

Buss, D. M. (2002). Sex, marriage, and religion: What adaptive problems do religious phenomena solve? *Psychological Inquiry, 13,* 201–203.

Carstensen, L. L. (1995). Evidence for a life-span theory of socioemotional selectivity. *Current Directions in Psychological Science, 4,* 151–156.

Carstensen, L. L., Isaacowitz, D. M., & Charles, S. T. (1999). Taking time seriously: A theory of socioemotional selectivity. *American Psychologist, 54,* 165–181.

Cline, V. B., & Richard, J. M. (1965). A factor-analytic study of religious belief and behavior. *Journal of Personality and Social Psychology, 1,* 569–578.

Davis, J. A., & Smith, T. W. (1999). *General Social Survey.* Chicago: National Opinion Research Center, University of Chicago, 1999 [producer]. Ann Arbor, MI: Inter-University Consortium for Political and Social Research, 1999 [distributor]. Retrieved on May 7, 2004, from webapp.icpsr.umich.edu/gss.

De Laguna, F. (1972). *Under Mount Saint Elias: The history and culture of the Yakutat Tlingit.* Washington, DC: Smithsonian Institution Press.

Emmons, R. A. (1999). Is spirituality an intelligence?: Motivation, cognition, and the psychology of ultimate concern. *The International Journal for the Psychology of Religion, 10,* 3–26.

Enright, R. D. (2001). *Forgiveness is a choice.* Washington, DC: American Psychological Association.

Enright, R. D., & Coyle, C. T. (1998). Researching the process model of forgiveness within psychological interventions. In E. L. Worthington, Jr. (Ed.), *Dimensions of forgiveness: Psychological research and theological perspectives* (pp. 139–161). Philadelphia: Templeton Foundation Press.

Enright, R. D., Gassin, E. A., & Wu, C. (1992). Forgiveness: A developmental view. *Journal of Moral Development, 21,* 99–114.

Exline, J. J. (2004). Anger toward God: A brief overview of existing research. *Psychology of Religion Newsletter, 29*(1), 1–8.

Exline, J. H., Yali, A. M., & Lobel, M. (1999). When God disappoints: Difficulty forgiving God and its role in negative emotion. *Journal of Health Psychology, 4,* 365–379.

Finkel, E. J., Rusbult, C. E., Kumashiro, M., & Hannon, P. A. (2002). Dealing with a betrayal in close relationships: Does commitment promote forgiveness? *Journal of Personality and Social Psychology, 82,* 956–974.

Fishbein, M., & Ajzen, I. (1974). Attitude toward objects as predictive of single and multiple behavioral criteria. *Psychological Review, 81,* 59–74.

Francis, L. J., Gibson, H. M., & Robbins, M. (2001). God images and self-worth among adolescents in Scotland. *Mental Health, Religion, and Culture, 4,* 103–108.

Girard, M., & Mullet, É. (1997). Propensity to forgive in adolescents, young adults, older adults, and elderly people. *Journal of Adult Development, 4,* 209–220.

Gorsuch, R. L. (1968). The conceptualization of God as seen in adjective ratings. *Journal for the Scientific Study of Religion, 22,* 56–64.

Gorsuch, R. L., & Hao, J. Y. (1993). Forgiveness: An exploratory factor analysis and its relationship to religious variables. *Review of Religious Research, 34,* 333–347.

Karremans, J. C., Van Lange, P. A. M., & Ouwerkerk, J. W. (2003). When forgiving enhances psychological well-being: The role of interpersonal commitment. *Journal of Personality and Social Psychology, 84,* 1011–1026.

Kelln, B. R. C., & Ellard, J. H. (1999). An equity theory analysis of the impact of forgiveness and retribution on transgressor compliance. *Personality and Social Psychology Bulletin, 25,* 864–872.

Kenrick, D. T., Li, N. P., & Butner, J. (2003). Dynamical evolutionary psychology: Individual decision rules and emergent social norms. *Psychological Review, 110,* 3–28.

Kirkpatrick, L. A. (1998). God as a substitute attachment figure: A longitudinal study of adult attachment style and religious change in college students. *Personality and Social Psychology Bulletin, 24,* 961–973.

Kirkpatrick, L. A. (1999). Toward an evolutionary psychology of religion and personality. *Journal of Personality, 67,* 921–952.

Koenig, H. G., McCullough, M. E., & Larson, D. B. (2001). *Handbook of religion and health.* New York: Oxford University Press.

Krause, N., & Ellison, K. (2003). Forgiveness by God, forgiveness of others, and psychological well-being in late life. *Journal for the Scientific Study of Religion, 42,* 77–93.

Kunkel, M. A., Cook, S., Meshel, D. S., Daughtry, D., & Hauenstein, A. (1999). God images: A concept map. *Journal for the Scientific Study of Religion, 38,* 193–202.

Lawler, K. A., Younger, J. W., Piferi, R. L., Billington, E., Jobe, R., Edmondson, K., et al. (2003). A change of heart: Cardiovascular correlates of forgiveness in response to interpersonal conflict. *Journal of Behavioral Medicine, 26,* 373–393.

Lerner, M. J., & Simmons, C. H. (1966). Observer's reaction to the "innocent victim": Compassion or rejection? *Journal of Personality and Social Psychology, 4,* 203–210.

Levin, J. S. (1996). How religion influences morbidity and health: Reflections on natural history, salutogenesis, and host resistance. *Social Science and Medicine, 43,* 849–864.

Maltby, J., Macaskill, A., & Day, L. (2001). Failure to forgive self and others: A replication and extension of the relationship between forgiveness, personality, social desirability and general health. *Personality and Individual Differences, 30,* 881–885.

Mauger, P. A., Saxon, A., Hamill, C., & Pannell, M. (1996). *The relationship of forgiveness to interpersonal behavior.* Paper presented at the annual meeting of the Southeastern Psychological Association, Norfolk, VA.

McCullough, M. E. (2001). Forgiveness: Who does it and how do they do it? *Current Directions in Psychological Science, 10,* 194–197.

McCullough, M. E., & Bono, G. (in press). Religion, forgiveness, and adjustment in older adulthood. In K. W. Schaie, N. Krause, & A. Booth (Eds.), *Religious influences on health and well-being in the elderly.* New York: Springer.

McCullough, M. E., & Hoyt, W. T. (2002). Transgression-related motivational dispositions: Personality substrates of forgiveness and their links to the Big Five. *Personality and Social Psychology Bulletin, 28,* 1556–1573.

McCullough, M. E., Pargament, K. I., & Thoresen, C. E. (2000). The psychology of forgiveness: History, conceptual issues, and overview. In M. E. McCullough, K. I. Pargament, & C. E. Thoresen (Eds.), *Forgiveness: Theory, research, and practice* (pp. 1–14). New York: Guilford Press.

McCullough, M. E., Rachal, K. C., Sandage, S. J., Worthington, E. L., Jr., Brown, S. W., & Hight, T. L. (1998). Interpersonal forgiving in close relationships II: Theoretical elaboration and measurement. *Journal of Personality and Social Psychology, 75,* 1586–1603.

McCullough, M. E., & Worthington, E. L., Jr. (1999). Religion and the forgiving personality. *Journal of Personality, 67,* 1141–1164.

Meek, K. R., Albright, J. S., & McMinn, M. R. (1995). Religious orientation, guilt, confession, and forgiveness. *Journal of Psychology and Theology, 23,* 190–197.

Mullet, É., Barros, J., Frongia, L., Usai, V., Neto, F., & Shafihi, S. R. (2003). Religious involvement and the forgiving personality. *Journal of Personality, 71,* 1–19.

Mullet, É., Houdbine, A., Laumonier, S., & Girard, M. (1998). Forgivingness: Factorial structure in a sample of young, middle-aged, and elderly adults. *European Psychologist, 3,* 289–297.

North, J. (1987). Wrongdoing and forgiveness. *Philosophy, 62,* 499–508.

Pargament, K. I., Zinnbauer, B. J., Scott, A. B., Butter, E. M., Zerowin, J., & Stanik, P. (1998). Red flags and religious coping: Identifying some religious warning signs among people in crisis. *Journal of Clinical Psychology, 54,* 77–89.

Poloma, M. M., & Gallup, G. H. (1991). *Varieties of prayer.* Philadelphia: Trinity Press International.

Powell, L. H., Shahabi, L., & Thoresen, C. E. (2003). Religion and spirituality: Linkages to physical health. *American Psychologist, 58,* 36–52.

Roberts, R. C. (1995). Forgivingness. *American Philosophical Quarterly, 32,* 289–306.

Roes, F. L., & Raymond, M. (2003). Belief in moralizing gods. *Evolution and Human Behavior, 24,* 126–135.

Rokeach, M. (1973). *The nature of human values.* New York: Free Press.

Rovinskii, P. (1901). *Chrnogoriia v eia proshlom i nastoiashchem* [Montenegro in its past and present] (Vol. 2, pt. 2). St. Petersburg, Russia: Printing Office of the Imperial Academy of Sciences.

Rowatt, W. C., Ottenbreit, A., Nesselroade, K. P., & Cunningham, P. A. (2002). On being holier-than-thou or humbler-than-thee: A social psychological perspective on religiousness and humility. *Journal for the Scientific Study of Religion, 41,* 227–237.

Rye, M. S., Pargament, K. I., Ali, M. A., Beck, G. L., Dorff, E. N., Hallisey, C., et al. (2000). Religious perspectives on forgiveness. In M. E. McCullough, K. I. Pargament, & C. E. Thoresen (Eds.), *Forgiveness: Theory, research, and practice* (pp. 17–40). New York: Guilford Press.

Sandage, S. J., Hill, P. C., & Vang, H. C. (2003). Toward a multicultural positive psychology: Indigenous forgiveness and Hmong culture. *The Counseling Psychologist, 31,* 564–592.

Sandage, S. J., Worthington, E. L., Jr., Hight, T. L., & Berry, J. W. (2000). Seeking forgiveness: Theoretical context and an initial study. *Journal of Psychology and Theology, 28,* 21–35.

Scobie, E. D., & Scobie, G. E. W. (1998). Damaging events: The perceived need for forgiveness. *Journal for the Theory of Social Behaviour, 28,* 373–401.

Toussaint, L. L., Williams, D. R., Musick, M. A., & Everson, S. A. (2001). Forgiveness and health: Age differences in a U.S. probability sample. *Journal of Adult Development, 8,* 249–257.

Tsang, J., McCullough, M. E., & Hoyt, W. T. (2005). Psychometric and rationalization accounts for the religion–forgiveness discrepancy. *Journal of Social Issues, 61*(4).

Wilson, D. S. (2002). *Darwin's cathedral: Evolution, religion, and the nature of society.* Chicago: University of Chicago Press.

Witvliet, C. v. O., Ludwig, T. E., & Bauer, D. J. (2002). Please forgive me: Transgressors' emotions and physiology during imagery of seeking forgiveness and victim responses. *Journal of Psychology and Christianity, 21,* 219–233.

Witvliet, C. v. O., Ludwig, T. E., & Vander Laan, K. L. (2001). Granting forgiveness or harboring grudges: Implications for emotion, physiology, and health. *Psychological Science, 12,* 117–123.

Worthington, E. L., Jr. (2001). *Five steps to forgiveness: The art and science of forgiving.* New York: Crown.

Worthington, E. L., Jr., & Drinkard, D. T. (2000). Promoting reconciliation through psychoeducational and therapeutic interventions. *Journal of Marital and Family Therapy, 26,* 93–101.

Worthington, E. L., Jr., & Wade, N. G. (1999). The psychology of unforgiveness and forgiveness and the implications for clinical practice. *Journal of Social and Clinical Psychology, 18,* 385–418.

Wuthnow, R. (2000). How religious groups promote forgiving: A national study. *Journal for the Scientific Study of Religion, 39,* 125–139.

Religion, Morality, and Self-Control

Values, Virtues, and Vices

ANNE L. GEYER
ROY F. BAUMEISTER

All known societies have moral rules that identify certain classes of action as right or wrong. In general, these moral rules condemn selfish, impulsive, shortsighted actions and instead promote acts that provide benefits in larger perspectives—for example, by being good for society as a whole or by bringing long-term gains. The capacity to make such choices is rare in nature and arguably uniquely human. From an evolutionary perspective, the capacity for moral thought and moral action may be uniquely human, which suggests that that capacity is a recent addition onto a psyche that in other respects resembles that of other animals, including being selfish, impulsive, and shortsighted. Put another way, human beings may have many tendencies and impulses that are similar to what most other animals have, but humans have also developed a capacity to restrain and override those tendencies so as to act morally (Baumeister, 2005). That capacity is self-control.

In that perspective, self-control is a psychological capability for bringing one's behavior into line with meaningful rules and standards. It is hardly surprising that its success is incomplete. Probably everyone has occasionally failed to live up to his or her moral ideals at some point, and most people experience such failures throughout life. Self-control thus needs help. In this chapter, we examine the power of religion to promote morally virtuous behavior by means of improving self-control. More precisely, the goal of this chapter is to discuss how people are sometimes able to be virtuous and why they sometimes fail. We propose self-control as the master virtue and consequently focus our analysis on the operation of self-control. We intend to explore the relationship between religion and virtuous behavior, focusing on religion's potential contributions to people's attempts to control themselves and be virtuous. We will suggest ways in which religion may be a resource in the pursuit of virtue.

DEFINITIONS

The *Webster's* dictionary (7th edition) defines morality as "the set of rules, doctrines, and lessons pertaining to principles of rightness and wrongness in human behavior." At an individual, intrapsychic level of analysis, virtue refers to having the intention and the wherewithal to behave in a morally excellent way (Baumeister & Exline, 1999). Although a more refined analysis may be possible, for the purposes of this chapter, we simply use "vice" or "sin" to mean the opposite of virtue.

Religion has strong ties to morality, in that religions prescribe morality. Religious writings are replete with instructions on how people ought to live, such as the Ten Commandments in the Judeo-Christian tradition or the Eightfold Plan in the Buddhist tradition (Baumeister & Exline, 1999). Further, many religious persons believe that religion is the source of morality; they view morality as originating in the will of God.

In this chapter, we are taking a social functionalist approach, that is, we view morality as adapted by culture to facilitate social relations (see Hogan, 1973). This perspective focuses on the role of morality in society. Moral behavior helps society to function successfully; immoral behavior poses problems for society, such as causing violence and aggression (Baumeister & Boden, 1998). The social functionalist perspective defines *virtue* as that which promotes healthy, harmonious society and *sin* as that which causes interpersonal damage.

Self-control (also self-regulation) refers to the self's altering its own responses. Typically this is a matter of overriding one incipient response, thereby permitting an (often unspecified) alternative. Using self-control, one may resist temptation, refocus attention, alter a mood or emotional state, overcome fatigue, or in other ways change one's states or actions. As a capacity for altering responses, self-control contributes greatly to the flexibility and diversity of human behavior. If people did not have the capacity to alter their behavior, moral rules would be useless. At best, such rules might make people realize the wrongness of their actions, but they would be powerless to change those actions.

SELF-CONTROL AS THE MASTER VIRTUE

Self-control can be considered the master virtue, in that self-control is necessary for people to be able to behave virtuously and avoid vice or sin, Baumeister and Exline (1999, 2000) have argued. They pointed out how an analysis of some of the major virtues and vices illustrates the centrality of self-control to moral behavior. The famous "Seven Deadly Sins" (e.g., Lyman, 1978) provides a convenient taxonomy of vices to examine. The first, gluttony, refers to overeating and possibly engaging in other pleasures to excess. Failure to regulate eating behavior is a classic example of a lack of self-control. People also need self-control to overcome sloth, or laziness. Sloth involves the failure to override the impulse either to stop working or to continue doing something other than working. Greed, lust, and envy have to do with excessive striving after the inappropriate goals of money, sexual satisfaction, and the possessions or advantages of others. When the desire for these inappropriate goals arises, people must exert self-control in order to override the urge to act in pursuit of the goal. Similarly, self-control is required to override the impulse to act sinfully out of anger, such as aggressing. The mere experience or feeling of greed, lust, envy, and anger may also reflect failures of self-control. Finally, pride reflects failure to override the urge to think well of oneself. Thus, self-control failure seems likely to play a central role in each of these sins.

According to Baumeister and Exline (1999, 2000), just as vices exhibit a failure of self-control, many virtues stem from success at self-control. Their examination of Thomas Aquinas's list of cardinal virtues (Rickaby, 1896) demonstrates the connection between self-control and virtue. The first cardinal virtue, prudence, refers to weighing long-term implications and risks when making decisions or acting. Prudence is related to the ability to forego immediate gratification for the sake of a greater, delayed benefit. Ability to delay gratification has been studied as a classic example of self-control (e.g., Mischel, Shoda, & Peake, 1988). Self-control also seems essential to the virtue of justice, or doing what is morally right. Temperance refers to being moderate rather than excessive; the ability to refrain from excess also requires self-control. Fortitude is to remain resolute despite adversity, pain, or passion. This courage or firmness demands self-control to overcome the desire to compromise and thereby escape one's suffering. Each of these virtues thus seems to hinge upon the ability to control oneself.

A broader, social functionalist perspective also depicts self-control as crucial for virtuous behavior. The social functionalist perspective says that sometimes, though not always, the individual's interests are at odds with society's interests. When self-interest and the common good conflict, the virtuous course of action is for the individual to sacrifice his or her interests for the sake of society's good (Baumeister & Exline, 1999). To sacrifice one's own interests, one must override the automatic, selfish response. Both from an examination of common sins and virtues and from the social functionalist perspective, self-control consistently appears to be crucial to morality. In that sense, self-control can fairly be designated the "master" virtue.

OPERATION OF SELF-CONTROL

How do people act virtuously? Taking self-control to be the master virtue allows us to focus that question to "How does self-control operate?" Researchers have identified three main elements in the operation of self-control: standards, monitoring, and operations that alter the self (Baumeister & Heatherton, 1996; Baumeister, Heatherton, & Tice, 1994).

First, for self-control to be possible, people must have a standard, a conception of what they ought to do. Standards give direction to a person's self-control efforts. Problems can arise when a person either lacks standards or has conflicting standards, such as in a moral dilemma. In the face of conflicting standards, people may feel frustrated and confused. Research by Emmons and King (1988) suggests that having conflicting goals can stymie effective action because it tends to produce rumination.

Second, people must monitor their own behavior. They must be aware of what they are doing and how that compares to the standard. Self-monitoring is very similar to the concept of self-awareness, which also involves comparing the self against standards (Carver & Scheier, 1981). Self-control is more likely to fail when the person is not paying attention to his or her behavior; thus, factors that reduce self-awareness should also reduce self-control. In a state of deindividuation, for example, people are more likely to steal or lie (e.g., Diener, Fraser, Beaman, & Kalem, 1976). Similarly, consumption of alcohol, which impairs self-relevant cognitive processing (Hull, 1981), is associated with sexual misbehavior and violence (Baumeister, 1997; Baumeister, Heatherton, & Tice, 1994).

By contrast, factors that increase self-awareness should also enhance self-control. For example, people are less likely to cheat when in the presence of a mirror because mirrors focus attention on the self (Diener & Wallbom, 1976).

Finally, even if a person has a clear standard, he or she still has to be able to make him- or herself behave according to that standard. People must have the power to change their own behavior; without this capacity, standards and monitoring are useless. Thus, the third step involves the actual operations that alter the self.

The Strength Model and Ego Depletion

How does self-control operate? Recent findings suggests that it resembles a strength or energy supply (e.g., Baumeister, Bratslavsky, Muraven, & Tice, 1998; Muraven & Baumeister, 2000; Muraven, Tice, & Baumeister, 1998). Operations that alter the self all consume a single resource, which is similar to a muscle in that it is limited but renewable. Any time a person exercises self-control, overrides an impulse, or makes a conscious choice, the store of this resource is depleted. When the resource has been depleted, the person will attempt to conserve the limited remaining stores. Thus, using self-control will deplete this resource, causing subsequent self-control efforts to be impaired. We can think of this depletion as being analogous to a temporary state of muscle fatigue.

The predictions of this strength or muscle model were tested in a series of studies by Baumeister et al. (1998) and Muraven et al. (1998). In many of these studies, first some participants performed a task that would be expected to deplete their self-control resources, while some participants did not. Afterward, all participants completed a different task, but one that would also require self-control. The experimenters wanted to know how having either performed versus not performed the first task would affect participants' performance on the second task. Different self-control models would predict different outcomes in this situation. For example, if self-control is like a skill, then one would expect gradual improvement over repeated self-control attempts, but no improvement after just one attempt. Assuming a "constant capacity" model of self-control would also predict no change on the second task as a result of having performed the first task. If self-control operates like a cognitive construct, then one would expect the first task to prime self-control, causing self-control to be enhanced on the second-task. In contrast, if self-control depletes a single, limited resource like a form of strength, then one would expect that participants' performance on the second task would be impaired if they had already been required to perform a different self-control task earlier.

The results of many studies have generally conformed to the pattern predicted by the muscle model. Muraven et al. (1998) found that participants who were first asked to regulate their emotional response to an upsetting video subsequently performed worse on a hand-grip task. Thus, exerting control over their emotions impaired participants' later physical stamina. They replicated this effect using different tasks requiring self-control in other domains; for example, participants who were first required to suppress forbidden thoughts subsequently showed reduced persistence on an anagram-solving task. Subsequent persistence and performance are both impaired by depletion (Baumeister et al., 1998). Participants who first had to eat radishes while resisting the temptation to sample some freshly baked chocolate cookies subsequently persisted for a shorter time on a different task. Similarly, participants who were first asked to try to suppress their emotional response to funny and sad videos subsequently performed worse than a control group on solvable anagrams. In these studies, the effect of depletion carried across strikingly different domains of self-control, including regulating task performance, suppressing thoughts, and regulating emotional responses. This pattern of results is consistent with the muscle model's assumption that various forms of self-control all draw from the same, limited resource.

Acts of conscious choice also seem to draw upon the same limited resource that self-control attempts (such as resisting the temptation to eat chocolates) consume. Baumeister et al. (1998) found that participants who were required to make a meaningful personal choice in the first part of the study subsequently showed decrements on a task requiring self-control. Making a conscious choice thus appeared to have depleted the self's resources. They also found that participants who had first performed a different self-control task later showed a preference for a passive rather than an active response option. When the self's resources are depleted, active responding is reduced. Together, these findings suggest that acts of conscious choice and acts of self-control do indeed draw upon the same limited resource. Depletion effects appear to extend to all acts of volition, not only to self-control. Thus, they use the term "ego depletion" to refer to the "state of weakness and vulnerability that apparently ensues when the self has already engaged in some acts of deliberate choice, active responding, or effortful self-regulation."

Depletion of this resource also impairs certain cognitive processes, as research by Schmeichel, Vohs, and Baumeister (2003) indicates. They found that participants who had first performed a depleting task showed subsequent decrements in performance on complex cognitive tasks such as logic and reasoning, cognitive extrapolation, and answering thoughtful reading-comprehension questions. These cognitive operations all require some kind of executive supervision, in the sense that the conscious self controls the process of moving from one set of information to something quite different (such as by logical deduction or extrapolation). In contrast, ego depletion did not affect participants' performance on more straightforward and automatic cognitive tasks, such as answering questions about general knowledge, or rote memorization and recall of nonsense syllables. Such automatic tasks do not depend on conscious or executive supervision. Thus, when thinking requires effortful volition, it too is degraded under conditions of ego depletion (such as results from a recent act of self-control).

This body of evidence, in summary, suggests that all acts of volition—including conscious choice, self-regulation, and effortful reasoning—place demands upon the same limited resource. Thus, exercising self-control depletes the self's resources, causing a state of ego depletion. During a state of ego depletion, a person is more likely to experience impaired self-control. The operation of self-control can therefore be conceptualized according to a strength or muscle model.

Implications of the Strength Model

The fact that various self-control acts, as well as other acts of volition, all require the same limited resource directly affects the degree of success people experience in their self-control efforts. For example, because all acts of volition, including all forms of self-control, draw upon the same limited resource, self-control is likely to break down in multiple areas at once (Baumeister & Exline, 1999). Gottfredson and Hirshi (1990) reported that criminals exhibit a similar pattern: Most criminals are arrested repeatedly but for different crimes. In addition, criminals are more likely to smoke, drink, contribute to unplanned pregnancies, and have erratic attendance at school and work, all of which are legal but reflect further signs of chronically low self-control. A related implication of the limited resource assumption is that attempting too many different self-control projects at the same time, such as when people make ambitious lists of self-improvement "New Year resolutions," may be unwise (Baumeister & Exline, 2000). Since all of the self-control projects will be drawing upon the same limited resource, the resulting state of ego depletion will increase the likelihood of failure. Similarly, people may experience more success at a self-control project if they start it at a time when they are not under a lot of stress because coping with stress depletes the self's resources (Baumeister & Exline, 1999; Glass, Singer, & Friedman, 1969).

Making conscious choices depletes the self's resources. Consequently, tasks that involve many decisions will be more depleting and will also be more impaired by depletion than tasks that involve few decisions (Baumeister et al., 1998; Baumeister & Exline, 2000). The same holds true for tasks that require complex thought. When depleted, people may find it easier to exercise self-control in areas that will not require numerous decisions or an extensive amount of complex cognitive processing.

Another implication of the finding that effortful thought can be impaired by depletion is that moral reasoning is likely to be impaired under ego depletion, even though automatic moral responses such as gut reactions would not be affected. When the self's resources have been expended by acts of decision making or self-control, it should be less able to carry out moral-reasoning processes so as to resolve moral dilemmas in mature, sophisticated ways. Simple, deeply rooted moral reactions, such as revulsion against incest, would, however, most likely remain intact.

The formation of good habits may further ease self-control efforts. Controlled processes that are repeated again and again can eventually become at least somewhat automatic. Automatic processes do not deplete the self's resources as much as controlled processes do (Bargh, 1982). So, automatizing virtuous behavior should help to conserve the resource (Baumeister, Muraven, & Tice, 2000). If people regularly perform *virtuous behaviors*, eventually they will no longer have to make a decision each time about whether to perform the virtuous behavior, and they will have formed a *virtuous habit*. To the extent that they can do that, people's self-control should be less likely to suffer decrements during states of ego depletion.

The muscle analogy also implies that a person's self-control should grow stronger with regular exercise. William James, for example, recommended, "Keep the faculty of effort alive in you by a little gratuitous exercise every day. . . . The man who has daily inured himself to habits of concentrated attention, energetic volition, and self-denial in unnecessary things . . . will stand like a tower when everything rocks around him" (James, 1890/1950, p. 127). The idea that exercise may increase or build up people's self-control strength has been supported by findings by Muraven, Baumeister, and Tice (1999). They asked participants to perform self-control exercises (monitoring and improving posture, regulating mood, or monitoring and recording eating) for 2 weeks. After the 2 weeks, participants were asked to do first a thought suppression exercise and then a hand-grip task. Participants who had practiced their self-control exercises for 2 weeks persisted longer at the hand-grip task than a control group of participants who had not practiced the self-control exercises. Thus, the thought suppression exercise appears to have depleted the participants who exercised their self-control less than it depleted the participants who had not exercised their self-control for 2 weeks prior. Regular, long-term exercise may reduce a person's vulnerability to becoming quickly depleted and consequently experiencing decreased self-control.

Summary: Virtue, Self-Control, and Ego Depletion

According to a social functionalist perspective, virtue entails sacrificing self-interest for the sake of society when self-interest and society's interest conflict. Such sacrifice requires self-control because the person must override the natural, automatic tendency to act on the basis of self-interest. Baumeister and Exline (1999, 2000) noted that vices reflect a failure of self-control and that virtues depend on successful operation of self-control. On the basis of this consistent pattern, they concluded that self-control could be characterized as the master virtue. Thus, to understand virtuous behavior, we needed to examine how self-control operates. There are three basic ingredients to self-control: standards, monitoring, and operations that alter the self.

Research has indicated that self-control functions like a strength or muscle. After using self-control, subsequent uses of self-control will be impaired temporarily, as if self-control were a muscle that had become tired from exertion. Other acts of volition in general can deplete the same resource. Furthermore, states of depletion can cause impaired performance in any of the wide range of activities that involve acts of volition.

This model has many practical implications. For example, initiating too many new self-control projects at the same time sets oneself up for failure. Regular exercise of self-control should decrease one's vulnerability to becoming rapidly depleted by exertions of self-control. Automatizing behaviors, or forming virtuous habits, can conserve the self's resource and make it easier to maintain virtuous behavior when one is depleted.

RELIGION AND VIRTUE

Religious organizations, as an external source of discipline, can be very helpful to people's personal self-control endeavors (Baumeister, Heatherton, & Tice, 1994). This section focuses on some of the practical ways that religion may facilitate virtuous behavior. The preceding review of how self-control operates serves as the foundation for our exploration of religion's potentially supportive role in the operation of self-control.

We do not, of course, presume to assess the validity of religious beliefs about any supernatural processes here. We do not intend to imply anything about the possibility of religion providing supernatural help to self-control. Rather, we are concerned with how beliefs and behaviors commonly associated with religion may be helpful to people trying to exercise self-control. Thus we consider some specific religious beliefs and behaviors in the light of psychological research and theory about self-control.

Standards

The first way in which religion can facilitate self-control is by providing clear standards. Religions specify right and wrong. Religious traditions include direct commands about what people ought to do as well as moral exemplars for people to emulate. However, Baumeister and Exline (1999) noted certain cultural changes that may hamper the ability of religion to set forth clear standards.

One such cultural change is the adoption of a capitalist economy (Baumeister & Exline, 1999). Historically, virtue meant sacrificing self-interest for the sake of society when self-interest conflicted with society's interest. However, in a capitalist economy, if a person tries to make as much profit for him- or herself as possible, not only will this self-interested act not be harmful for society, but theoretically it should benefit the economy (and thus society) as a whole. Under capitalism there is no longer a simple, clear distinction between what is good for the individual and what is good for society. This shift is also reflected in the changed moral sensibilities of the Christian church: Whereas the early Christian church had taught that trying to make money qualified as the sin of greed, today most Christians have no moral qualms about seeking to maximize profits (Baumeister & Exline, 1999).

A second important cultural change is the elevation of selfhood into a value base (Baumeister, 1991; Baumeister & Exline, 1999). Habermas (1973) posited that society needs to have sources of value (such as tradition or God's will) that do not have to derive their value from any outside source, but rather are sources of value for other things. These "value bases" (as Baumeister, 1991, called them) are important moral resources for society. When a value base is destroyed, as occurred during the process of modernization, Habermas argued, society experiences a shortage of value, or a "legitimation crisis." Baumeister (1991) has theorized that when a society experiences a legitimation crisis, that society will turn to other sources of value and attempt to elevate them into value bases to fill the value gap. He suggested that society has attempted to do just this with the self. It is now considered acceptable, and perhaps even morally obligatory, to act in the best interest of one's self, whereas, traditionally, morality and religion have sought to restrain self-interested behavior. This essentially means almost a reversal of some moral norms. For example, in the past, society put pressure upon women to be willing to sacrifice a great deal for the sake of a marriage; now, women are often made to feel as though they have an obligation—to themselves!—to leave a marriage that does not satisfy them fully or allow them to pursue their own potential (Zube, 1972). People are exhorted to think of themselves first and are reminded, for example, "You've got to do what's best for you."

This development of the self into a value base puts morality in a strange position (Baumeister, 1991; Baumeister & Exline, 1999). Historically, a central and explicit goal of religion and morality in general has been to restrain the self and to override people's tendency to act out of self-interested motives. Now people must find a way to reconcile historical conceptions of morality with the recent formulation of the self as a source of value with inherently authoritative claims. Society may compromise between traditional morality and the newly elevated status of the self by, for example, approving a person's selfish actions except in those cases where the person deliberately tries to hurt someone else (Baumeister & Exline, 1999). Traditional morality and the newly elevated status of the self as a locus of entitlements and rights seem to be coexisting at best in an uneasy tension. Both of these cultural changes have contributed to the obscuring of moral standards and the lack of consensus on moral issues. Moral diversity, more so than demographic diversity, may pose problems for society (Haidt, Rosenberg, & Hom, 2003).

As one of culture's foremost promulgators of moral standards, religion can scarcely escape this cultural evolution unscathed. In response, some religious groups shift their moral stance to be more in line with the broader culture (Baumeister, 1991). This may occur either as part of a more or less deliberate attempt to maintain relevance and to "meet people where they're at," or simply as a result of the fact that religious groups are made up of people who are themselves part of the culture and are thus inevitably affected by the changes occurring in their culture. Some religious groups compromise by altering or deemphasizing their standards. They may be hesitant to insist upon their traditional moral standards out of fear of offending people's sense of autonomy or of alienating potential members. Some religious groups may also adapt by increasing their attention to values and services that are "friendly" to the self, such as positive self-worth, mental health, or recreation and leisure activities. Although such adaptations may help religious groups to meet the felt needs of people in society, they may do so at the cost of being able to provide guidance and clear standards for people who may be experiencing moral confusion.

Religious groups do not all make the same concessions; some groups may actually react against cultural trends by emphasizing their traditional standards even more stringently. This response, as well, may carry both advantages and disadvantages. Religious groups that do not compromise their moral stance are able to offer clearer and simpler rules to their members. As a result, their members may possess greater confidence that they understand what is right to do. Members of these groups may find the impression of permanence to be reassuring, as well. For example, some people may derive comfort from the idea that certain doctrines of the Catholic Church can never be changed. Furthermore, since acts of volition such as making a personal choice are depleting (Baumeister et al., 1998), people may feel relieved to be spared the burden of having to make a conscious personal choice on every moral issue. Being able to defer automatically to the moral ruling of their religious group may permit people to conserve their self-regulatory resources.

However, people may have more difficulty maintaining sincere faith in the teaching of their religion if that teaching diverges too sharply from the understanding of the surrounding culture. Even if a religious group offers clear standards, its members may still feel conflicted about those standards. For example, some Catholics, finding the Catholic Church's unwavering stance opposing birth control to be impractical, simply do not obey the rule. Such persons may resolve the resulting cognitive dissonance either by considering themselves to be "bad Catholics" for intentionally disobeying, or they may decide that they simply do not believe that the pope is infallible. If they decide they do not believe, this can erode or undermine their ability to accept the church's moral authority over their lives in general. Simple rules may be clear but rigid. Even if standards are clear, if those standards do not also allow for the flexibility, complexity, or nuance necessary to comprehend the evolution of culture, their usefulness for guiding people's virtuous strivings may be limited.

In summary, cultural changes such as the evolution of a capitalist economy and the elevation of the self to a value base may cause deficient or conflicting moral standards to become an increasingly common problem. This may be problematic for society in multiple ways; in particular, it deprives people of a clear standard to direct their self-control efforts. These cultural changes also may undermine the capacity of religion to serve as a source of moral standards the way it traditionally has done. Of course religion still does provide moral standards for many people; however, religion's standard-setting role is accompanied by additional challenges and complications due to these cultural shifts.

Motivation

A second way in which religion can contribute to self-control efforts is by supplying motivation. Self-control efforts are more likely to falter without sufficient motivation. Muraven and Slessareva (2003) manipulated participants' level of motivation. They found that highly motivated participants' performances were not impaired by depletion, whereas depletion did impair the performances of participants who were lower in motivation. This finding suggests that when people are more highly motivated, despite being depleted, they are able and/or willing to expend more of the self's resources. Motivation may help people to circumvent lapses of self-control.

Religion provides an array of compelling reasons for moral conduct. The belief that God wants you to behave in a certain way is the ultimate reason to do so (Baumeister, 1991; Emmons, 1999). Particularly motivating may be religious beliefs about salvation or enlightenment (Baumeister, 1991). Many religious people associate moral virtue with positive outcomes after death, such as with beliefs that moral behavior will earn or guarantee salvation. Thinking about this ultimate goal (i.e., salvation) can help people to transcend their immediate stimulus environment (Baumeister, Heatherton, & Tice, 1994). Rather than focusing on everything around them that makes them want to quit being good, they can remind themselves of their larger or more abstract goals, and base their behavior upon those. Some Jewish theology, for example, portrays life as a time for preparing oneself, through repentance and good deeds, for what will occur after death: "This world is like the vestibule before the world to come; prepare yourself in the vestibule so that you may be able to enter the banquet hall" (Hirsch, 1989).

Some religious people also associate immoral behavior with negative outcomes after death. The fear of eternal torment in hell can be highly motivating for some people. As an extreme example, consider the story told about a fourth-century "desert father" (i.e., an ascetic Christian who lived as a hermit). A woman arrived at his cell one night and begged for shelter. Determined to restrain his sexual desire, the hermit thought about "the judgment of God." When that thought alone failed to quench his burning lust, he reportedly said to himself, "Well, let's see whether you will be able to bear the flames of hell," and put his fingers into the flame of the lamp, burning them one by one until morning came and he could finally send the woman on her way (Merton, 1960). Thus, whereas the promise of ultimate fulfillment may motivate some people, others may be inspired to virtue more effectively by their desire to avoid the ultimate negative outcome.

Religion can provide other motivations for virtuous behavior as well, aside from concerns about what will happen after death. Many Protestant Christians, for example, believe that people are incapable of earning salvation by their moral behavior but that moral behavior is the appropriately grateful response to God's free gift of salvation. Such persons may be motivated to obey religious commands because they believe that their obedience will please or "bless" God, toward whom they feel gratitude and love. Others, for example, may obey religious commands because they believe that their moral behavior will bring glory to God; thus, they perceive themselves as having the opportunity to play a significant role in an unimaginably grand plan and purpose.

A variety of religious beliefs may serve effectively to motivate virtuous, self-controlled behavior. Religious beliefs have to do with the highest levels of meaning and the longest ranging time frames (Baumeister, 1991). Religious beliefs are ideal for facilitating transcendence because religion is abstract, provides long-term goals, and lays claim to ultimate value as well as the ultimate frame of reference (Emmons, 1999). Religion can imbue the most mundane of activities with meaning because it allows people to base their everyday behavior upon high-level principles. The ability to view one's activity in a larger meaningful context can help people to persist on aversive or dull tasks (Sansone, Weir, Harpster, & Morgan, 1992). Similarly, Berg, Janoff-Bulman, and Cotter (2001) suggested that people's type of motivation for doing something can affect outcomes. Their findings suggest that people may be more likely to reach their goals when their motivation is autonomous (i.e., because they "want to") rather than an obligation (i.e., because they "should"). Religious beliefs give people multiple angles for transforming externally imposed moral rules into intrinsically motivated personal values.

In short, religion offers people a range of potent motivations for moral behavior. Foremost among religious motivations may be the pursuit of ultimate fulfillment in the form of religious salvation. As MacIntyre (1981) has noted, without the framework of religion, people are often hard put to come up with compelling motivations for good behavior (also see Baumeister & Exline, 1999). Motivation is therefore a vital contribution that religion can make to people's self-control efforts.

Monitoring

Third, religion can facilitate people's monitoring of their own behavior. Monitoring is often crucial to the success of self-control efforts. Many religious groups have instituted periodic times for self-examination. For example, members may be expected to regularly attend religious meetings, at which they are reminded of standards and prompted to consider whether they are meeting those standards. Catholics follow the rite of confession, in which they confess their sins to a priest. In addition, religious groups often encourage people to engage in daily self-monitoring on their own time through prayer, meditation, reading, or keeping a "spiritual journal." Some religions remind adherents that God is also monitoring their behavior; for example, a Jewish saying counsels: "Consider three things and you will not fall into the grip of sin. Know what is above you: a seeing eye and a hearing ear, and that all your deeds are recorded in The Book" (Hirsch, 1989). This may furnish an additional incentive for accuracy in self-monitoring.

Managing Inappropriate Desires

Fourth, religion may help people to manage their nonvirtuous desires. There are two separate levels on which self-control may be required in order for a person to be virtuous: eliminating inappropriate desires and refraining from acting on those desires. This distinction relates to sins such as lust, envy, and anger, from the list of the Seven Deadly Sins. For example, many people believe that to be virtuous it is sufficient merely to refrain from acting on their lust. On the other hand, some people believe that it is also immoral merely to entertain lustful thoughts or feelings and may therefore attempt to suppress or eradicate the lustful desire itself. Even people who do not believe that having lustful desires is sinful may still wish to eradicate their desires, so as to be able to avoid acting out of lust. Their reasoning might follow along the lines of, "It would be a lot easier to be good if I didn't want so badly to be bad." However, is it possible to eradicate sinful desires?

Baumeister, Heatherton, and Tice (1994) have argued that attempting to control impulses is likely to prove futile. They summarized the way impulses arise in terms of the combination of a latent motivation and an activating impulse. People have a variety of latent motivations, or wants and needs. These motivations may be more or less automatic or biologically programmed. At any given time, these motivations, although present, may not be felt consciously if there is no activating cue or stimulus—either in the environment or naturally arising in the person (such as hunger). However, in the presence of the appropriate cue, the impulse to satisfy a particular motivation will arise. Because no conscious effort or choice is required for this impulse to arise, the impulse cannot be consciously controlled by mere force of will. Given a latent motivation and an activating cue, the impulse will automatically arise, whether a person wants it to or not. Thus, in managing one's desires, the impulse itself is not a productive target of control efforts. An easier and therefore more effective target of control may be the environment: To the extent that a person can purge his or her environment of activating cues, he or she may be able to prevent an impulse from arising. A secondary and less certain target of control may be the latent motivations themselves. Motivations that are biologically programmed would resist change, but it is possible that other motivations that are more a product of learning may be somewhat amenable to being unlearned.

In dealing with inappropriate desires, attention is the place to begin (Baumeister, Heatherton, & Tice, 1994). The most effective strategies are likely to be those that prevent a cue or stimulus from ever activating the latent motivation in the first place. The safest way to ensure that a cue does not capture one's attention may be to remove the cue from one's environment. For example, a person who is trying to avoid drinking alcohol would want to make sure that there is no alcohol in his home and may also wish to remove any Absolut Vodka posters and take down his neon Bud Lite sign left over from his college days.

Being a member of a religious group or living in a religious community permits even greater control over the tempting stimuli in the environment, because people can surround themselves with others who share similar moral standards. For example, some religious groups and orders seek to promote celibacy as a way of life. From our reading, very few of these favor mixed-gender living arrangements or fashionable clothing. Instead, to avoid activating sexual thoughts, they remove people from contact with sexually suggestive stimuli. Living in a cave or desert is one option. Another is to have the members live in same-gender groups with unflattering haircuts and concealing, unfashionable clothing.

However, suppose that a cue or stimulus does slip through the person's net. What can a person do once an impulse has arisen and the inappropriate motivation has made its existence felt? Some people may attempt to suppress their thoughts about the vice that is tempting them. Research by Wegner, Schneider, Carter, and White (1987) suggests that this strategy is likely to have at best limited success. They asked participants not to think about a white bear, and found that a rebound effect occurred: After the prohibition against white bear thoughts was lifted, those participants thought about white bears even more than participants who were instructed to think about white bears. Thus, while people's energy lasts or while people remember to monitor their thoughts, they may be able to at least reduce their thoughts about the temptation. However, when they run out of energy, or simply stop suppressing the thoughts, they may find themselves more obsessed with the temptation than they would have been had they not tried to control their thoughts at all.

However, Wegner et al. (1987) found that providing participants with a distraction—in this case, instructing them to think about a red Volkswagen instead of a white bear—enabled them to be much more successful at suppressing thoughts about the white bear. Distraction is another important aid to management of inappropriate desires. The effectiveness of distraction has also been noted in research on delay of gratification (Mischel, 1974; Rodriguez, Mischel, & Shoda, 1989). Children who succeeded in waiting for a delayed larger reward commonly employed some technique of self-distraction. They found some way—whether playing games with their feet, singing, covering their eyes, or trying to sleep—to occupy their attention with something (anything!) other than the tempting smaller prize that was immediately available (Mischel, 1974).

Religion can supply people with multiple avenues for distraction from temptation.

Religious conversion is often accompanied by new goals and motives (Paloutzian, Richardson, & Rambo, 1999). Although the person's old, inappropriate desires still exist, they may be overpowered by the force of the newly acquired goals. This is, essentially, the concept of transcendence again. The person focuses on the new high-order religious goal, ignoring desires to engage in activities that are incompatible with his or her religious goals. For example, someone who used to go to wild parties on the weekend may, after a religious conversion, suddenly prefer to attend a religious meeting. To the extent that people can immerse themselves in the pursuit of religious or virtuous goals, they will become too preoccupied and distracted to feel very strongly the temptation to sin. Dealing with an inappropriate desire may be relatively easier for a person who has managed to get him- or herself caught up in something else even more engrossing, such as an activity that produces a state of "flow" (Csikszentmihalyi, 1990). Furthermore, people may learn to "develop a taste for" virtuous or spiritual satisfactions, such that their zeal in pursuing religious goals and rewards continues to increase. The more strongly people desire their moral or religious goals, the more likely are those goals to outweigh sinful desires. Simultaneously, we could speculate that people's cravings for sinful pleasures may fade slightly with disuse; after not indulging in a sin for a period of time, people may gradually begin to forget slightly how much they had once enjoyed that sinful activity. This may be especially likely if the person is motivated to forget, or, put differently, if the person is motivated to remember their past in a negative light.

Regulating Affect

Although latent motivations are often activated by external stimuli, sometimes the cue comes not from the environment so much as from the person him- or herself. Emotional distress may function like a cue for people to engage in vices. Baumeister (2005) has proposed that behavior pursues emotion. According to this theory, people do what they think will make them feel positive emotions and avoid what they think will make them feel negative emotions. Consistent with that view, Tice, Bratslavsky, and Baumeister (2001) found that when people are emotionally distressed, they indulge their immediate impulses in an attempt to make themselves feel better. In short, they sacrifice their self-regulatory goals in order to boost their mood. However, when participants believed their bad mood was frozen (unchangeable), their tendencies to eat fattening foods, seek immediate gratification, and engage in frivolous procrastination disappeared. Thus it seems that people believe that indulging will improve their mood. When people are distressed, the goal of affect regulation sometimes conflicts with other self-control goals. Prioritizing the goal of affect regulation over other self-control goals is a common cause of self-control failures. For example, if a woman who is in a bad mood believes that buying new clothes will make her feel better, she may choose to go shopping, even if that causes her to fail in her goal of saving money (Baumeister, 2002). In summary, emotional distress can prompt failures of self-control because in general people behave in a way that they think will make them feel good. When distressed, many people believe that indulging themselves will improve their mood. People's emotion regulation goals often take precedence over their self-control goals.

Emotional distress is an internal cue, not as easily controlled as stimuli in the external environment. In general, people don't have direct control over whether they are going to be in a bad mood. However, some beliefs commonly associated with religion tend to reduce people's emotional distress during experiences of misfortune, discomfort, or suffering. Many religious people believe that God is sovereign—in other words, that God has ultimate control over everything that happens. Another common religious belief is that God is benevolent, that God's intentions toward humankind are good and trustworthy. Those two beliefs together comprise a tremendous resource for people who are coping with distressing events. People who hold those kinds of beliefs can derive comfort from the assumption that what they are undergoing is not meaningless, but rather has some good purpose—regardless of whether they know exactly what that purpose is. Belief in ultimate religious salvation or fulfillment can also enable people to endure far more tribulation than they otherwise would. Because they have not yet sampled this ideal future, people are free to assume that the coming happiness will more than compensate them for their present troubles. This principle is mentioned often in the Bible—for example, "I consider that our present sufferings are not worth comparing with the glory that will be revealed in us" (Romans 8:18).

Thus, religious beliefs may supply people with motivation, hope, and comfort that can allow them to maintain virtuous behavior, even when to do so is painful or difficult. Furthermore, since the religious beliefs themselves may reduce people's emotional distress during difficult or unpleasant experiences, religious people may feel less tempted to regulate their mood by indulging in some vice. In other words, religion may prevent or weaken the activating cue of emotional distress; consequently, the impulse to indulge in some sin may be less likely to arise.

There is another way in which religion may help prevent people's affect regulation goals from interfering with their self-control goals. We suggested that behavior pursues emotion, in that people will tend to do what they believe will produce positive emotion or alleviate negative emotion. Religion sometimes entails beliefs about what will and what will not make people happy, satisfied, or fulfilled. A person's religion may teach that engaging in a certain sin will not truly produce the satisfaction or positive emotion that he or she is seeking. To the extent that the person is convinced that this is true, he or she should be less likely to turn to sinful indulgences in order to regulate his or her affect. If the person does not expect sinning to bring positive emotion, the link between emotional distress and the impulse to indulge in that sin may be weakened or severed. It is possible that altering people's beliefs about what will make them happy might alter what they desire. So perhaps this could affect the latent motivation itself, although it is more likely that the motivation would be weakened than eliminated altogether. In addition, latent motivations that are biologically programmed are not likely to be greatly affected, no matter how fervent a person's beliefs might be.

In summary, religion can help people to regulate their affect because comforting beliefs in high-level meaning and in salvation can alleviate emotional distress. As a result, people may not feel as strong an urge to indulge in vices in an attempt to regulate their affect. Furthermore, when people are emotionally distressed, religion may discourage them from turning to vices to make themselves feel better, if their religion teaches them that indulging in sinful activities will not bring them the positive emotions and satisfaction that they are craving. If religious beliefs can interfere with a person's association between sin and pleasure, they may lessen that person's desire or motivation to sin.

Beliefs and Expectations about Failure and Success

Both religion and the broader culture can promote beliefs that affect people's self-control. Particular beliefs can influence the degree of success people experience in their self-control endeavors, as well as the way they react to lapses and setbacks.

Whether people think it is possible to control themselves affects whether and how hard they are going to try to maintain control. Baumeister, Heatherton, and Tice (1994) argued that, although the evidence suggests that people generally acquiesce in their own loss of control, cultural trends may be leading people to believe that impulses such as aggression or violence are impossible to resist. This belief may be problematic in that people's beliefs that they are helpless to resist may lead them to reduce their efforts. Furthermore, if people are indeed helpless, then they cannot be held morally accountable for their actions. Consequently, these beliefs are likely to contribute to an increase in actual violent behavior. Similarly, if people believe they are powerless to resist their addiction to alcohol or drugs, they may be more likely not to attempt to control themselves. They may not consciously intend to not control themselves; nevertheless, they may unconsciously more easily acquiesce with the loss of self-control. Thus, cultural trends that support the belief that people cannot control, and therefore cannot be held accountable for, their actions may actually detract from people's success at self-control.

Some religious beliefs may counteract those cultural trends. For example, some religious beliefs include an emphasis on personal responsibility. Furthermore, as noted earlier, religion gives directives for moral behavior. Some religious people may take the divine command about what to do as implying that obedience is possible. If obedience is possible, then there is no excuse for disobedience. Perceiving that their behavior is under their own control may spur people to acknowledge their own complicity in their loss of self-control. It is harder for them to deceive themselves; they have to admit to acquiescence. While this understanding is likely to be uncomfortable for the individual, it is likely to be beneficial for the rest of society.

However, a limit must be acknowledged: It may be counterproductive for people to believe that they have control over things they cannot actually control, such as impulses. Baumeister, Heatherton, and Tice (1994) concluded that most impulses cannot themselves be controlled (rather, at best, one can only control the behavior that might stem from the impulse). Some religious authorities have voiced similar opinions. The Jewish sages taught that the "evil inclination" was created by God, and thus it was not in man's power to completely uproot, although it was in man's power to rule (Urbach, 1979). Christian ascetics of the fourth century concurred. In fact, in the stories of the desert fathers, when a hermit claimed to have succeeded in "killing" sinful passion—even one who had "fasted valiantly for fifty years"—that person was corrected or warned by the others. They viewed such claims as an indication of self-deception or lack of insight, and even considered that the person's seemingly passionless state could be spiritually harmful. Likewise, when a younger member of the monastic community was upset about his failure to eradicate sinful impulses, he was reassured that eradicating the impulses was both impossible and unnecessary, and that all that mattered was how he responded to the sinful impulses when they did arise (Merton, 1960). Most people today likely would consider eradicating the passions or controlling the occurrence of impulses to be impossible. However, a significant number of religious groups have held that type of view. For example, Christians in the "Holiness Movement" believed in a doctrine called "entire sanctification," which meant that a person can be sinless in this life, or perfected in holiness. This doctrine seems to have proved problematic, both for interpersonal relationships and for the psychological health of individuals (Henry, 1984). Overall, unrealistic beliefs about the degree to which people can control themselves seem to be a problem to which religious people, more than nonreligious people, might be prone.

One reason that religious people may be more likely to entertain unrealistic expectations about their own perfectability is that religious beliefs can increase people's sense of self-efficacy. For example, religious persons may believe that God is helping them, or that their methods are endorsed by God and thus more likely to be effective. Religious persons may also pray for success and expect that their requests will be granted. Many Christians believe that God's Holy Spirit dwells within them and works to change and sanctify their hearts. The Bible specifies self-control as one of the "fruits," or products, of the presence of God's Spirit. Irrespective of whether the beliefs themselves are accurate, the ensuing heightened sense of self-efficacy may affect the degree of success at self-control that people experience. These beliefs may bolster people's self-control efforts.

In some cases, though, religious beliefs could negatively affect self-control attempts. Religious beliefs may give people false confidence or lead them to believe that they don't have to put forth any effort—this might be termed the "let go and let God" mentality. Such persons might focus on God's power so much that they underemphasize the active role of the person. Persons whose religious beliefs hinder their self-control in this way might be described as having low spiritual intelligence, as defined by Emmons (2000). The problem is not that they are religious, but that they have failed to adaptively balance the components of their spirituality (Emmons, 2000). Unrealistic self-assessments can also lead to other forms of misregulation such as overcommitment or persisting too long at a doomed project (Baumeister, Heatherton, & Tice, 1994).

Religious beliefs can also affect how people respond to failure and setbacks. The way people deal with lapses in self-control has the potential to sabotage their efforts. Religion can contribute either to constructive or to maladaptive responses to lapses, depending on the person's specific beliefs. For example, for some people, religious beliefs may cause them to base their sense of self-worth on their success at being virtuous. Therefore, when they fail, they may be especially prone to fall prey to discouragement. By contrast, other people's religious beliefs may cause them to base their sense of self-worth on God's unconditional grace. When these people fail, they may feel free simply to try again, without being overly burdened by guilt.

Guilt

Failures of self-control—such as not studying, overeating, or not exercising—are one of the most common sources of guilt feelings. The other major topic of guilt, according to Baumeister, Stillwell, and Heatherton (1995), is interpersonal transgressions. Arising when people fail to behave in a virtuous way or when people hurt one another, guilt is widely considered to be a moral emotion or moral affect (e.g., Tangney, 1991, 1992).

The generally prosocial, relationship-enhancing effects of guilt were documented in a literature review by Baumeister, Stillwell, and Heatherton (1994). Guilt motivates people to try to restore or maintain relationships, such as by making amends for wrongs they have committed, apologizing to people they have hurt, and trying not to commit the same offense again in the future. This last effect indicates the function of guilt to teach lessons: Guilt teaches people the lesson that they should not do again what they had done to arouse the guilt they feel (Baumeister et al., 1995). Guilt focuses attention on what the person did that caused the guilt. The feeling of guilt is experienced as aversive, but guilt is not subject to volitional control. If people could get over their guilt just by snapping their fingers or wishing it away, guilt's power to teach lessons and to enforce relationship-enhancing behaviors would be greatly reduced. Thus, guilt functions to promote relationships. The desire to avoid guilt may be one of the most powerful motivators for moral behavior.

Cultural changes may have slightly weakened guilt's efficacy at spurring people to be virtuous (Baumeister & Exline, 1999). The emotional roots of guilt may lie partly in anxiety over possibly losing a relationship, which is why people generally feel more guilt about wronging a loved one than wronging a stranger (see Baumeister et al., 1994, for a review). However, over time, social relationships have become less stable. People are more mobile. They can easily move to a different geographic location. In addition, they can easily move from one level of society to another, and from one economic class to another. As a result, people have fewer long-term, stable relationships. Because people are most likely to feel guilty about harm done to someone with whom they have a stable long-term relationship, a reduction in long-term relationships diminishes guilt's power to enforce morality. Friedman's (2002) history of U.S. law makes the important point that laws and morals often use similar rules to promote similar behaviors, but insofar as morality depends on reputation and long-term relationship contexts to provide its force, it loses effectiveness in promoting prosocial behavior between strangers. Therefore, as society changes to increase the amount of dealings people have with relative strangers, they rely steadily more on law than on morality to ensure fair treatment.

Religion, on the other hand, may reinforce the power of guilt for promoting prosocial behavior. As mentioned earlier, some religious beliefs include an emphasis on the moral accountability of the individual. Religious persons may be less likely to think that their failures were outside of their control and therefore not something for which they could be blamed. Religion also puts forth clear moral standards, which enables people to know clearly when they have failed to meet those standards.

In addition, people who join a religion do not simply acquire a set of beliefs; they also become part of a group. Some people may stay with the same religious group over a long period of time and develop intimate relationships with other group members. However, the extreme mobility of people in contemporary society surely also affects the quality of people's affiliation with religious groups. Perhaps many religious people do not become deeply personally invested in one particular group of people, but rather may move from group to group. Nevertheless, people who belong to the same religious group are likely to share similar self-control goals. Membership in the group often entails a certain degree of moral accountability. Sometimes members of a religious group feel entitled or obligated to inform on or to confront each other when they perceive each other as falling short of virtue. Thus, they help to monitor each others' behavior. They may, in addition, reward virtuous behavior with acceptance or status, while punishing sinful behavior with ostracism or public shame. Despite cultural changes, religious groups still retain a unique position in terms of being able to enforce moral codes.

Another way in which guilt is connected to religion for some people is that religion supplies an additional relationship about which to feel guilty. Many Christians, for example, consider themselves to have a relationship with God on the basis of God's sacrificial love for them. They believe that in return they owe God gratitude and love. Some Christians also hold the belief that sin, in a sense, offends or hurts God; they may even speak in (metaphorical) terms about God's heart or God's feelings of sorrow. This conception of God as being like a person with whom they have a relationship endows them with an additional source of guilt upon sinning: Not only do they feel guilty because they have failed to self-regulate or to uphold a moral rule, they also feel guilty because they believe that their sin negatively affects God and possibly also may threaten their relationship with God.

The principle that behavior pursues emotion applies to guilt too. People try to behave in such a way that they will not have to feel guilty. The two most common sources of guilt are failures of self-control and interpersonal transgressions. The function of guilt is to make people less likely to commit the same failures of self-control or the same interpersonal transgressions again in the future. Thus, although the experience of guilt is unpleasant for the individual, guilt is a prosocial emotion in that it facilitates relationships and benefits society.

Summary: Religion and Virtue

Religiosity can affect self-control efforts in multiple ways, most of them positive. The evolution of a capitalist economy and the elevation of the self into a value base have complicated the moral landscape. Nevertheless, religion remains an important source of moral standards to guide people's self-control endeavors. As a source of motivation for moral behavior, religion is unparalleled. Religious organizations also have in place helpful traditions and practices that facilitate people's self-monitoring.

People may try to use a variety of strategies to deal with inappropriate or immoral desires. Preventing tempting stimuli from coming to one's attention is often the place one begins and is possibly the most effective way to stay on the path of virtue. This can often be accomplished most effectively by controlling one's environment. When a tempting stimulus does catch a person's eye, merely trying to suppress thoughts about the temptation is unlikely to be particularly productive. Distraction has been shown to be very helpful, both in the white bear thought suppression experiments and in the delay of gratification research. People who are religious may want not only to distract themselves from sinful desires, but to replace those sinful desires with virtuous or spiritual ones.

People's bad moods and emotional distress can lead them to try to remedy their mood by indulging in some vice or allowing their other self-control goals to fail. Religion is a helpful resource for those who are experiencing some sort of trouble or suffering. Because religion helps people to cope with negative situations, religious people may escape some of the self-control failures that occur as a result of immediate affect regulation goals taking precedence over normal self-control goals. Another possibility is that religious beliefs about what will or will not bring happiness and fulfillment can reduce people's inclination to indulge in vices for affect-regulating purposes.

A recurring theme in this chapter has been that the specific content of a religious belief often matters. This is also true of beliefs that the culture in general promotes. There is a disturbing trend for U.S. culture to support people's belief that they are sometimes incapable of controlling their actions. We are generally skeptical of people's efforts to abnegate personal responsibility for losses of self-control and ensuing misdeeds. However, there are some responses that are not directly controllable, including many impulses and emotions. Even so, people can control their behavior. In other words, people may be mostly unable to prevent themselves from having sinful thoughts, feelings, or impulses, but they can prevent themselves from acting on them.

Religious beliefs can directly affect people's expectations of success in their self-control projects. It seems likely that Christians, for example, would have higher expectations of success if they believe that God is blessing their efforts. However, it would be hard to predict what the overall effect would be on people's level of success. Similarly, religious beliefs seem likely to influence the way people cope with setbacks and lapses in their efforts at self-control. However, any research on this topic would have to be willing to undertake a fairly fine-grained analysis, because merely assessing "religiosity" in general might yield results that would be ambiguous.

Guilt is the all-purpose moral emotion. Guilt teaches a lesson to the person experiencing it, and is one of the most important motivators for moral behavior. Some motivations for morality are specific to religion, but guilt is available to all—religious or secular. The great mobility of people in contemporary society may slightly undermine the process by which guilt enforces morality. But religion continues to make good use of guilt. The religious groups to which people belong are often excellent at prompting guilt feelings in people who do not meet the group's moral standards. Christians also have an ever present guilt source, in that any time a Christian sins, he or she can interpret that sin as having hurt or offended God. In other words, according to some Christians' theology, there is no such thing as a victimless sin.

CONCLUSION

Religion offers many benefits, both to individual believers and to society as a whole. One large indirect means by which these benefits are obtained is probably self-control. By offering a framework that supports self-control, religion promotes a trait that enables people to do what is morally and pragmatically best for society and that also helps them do what best serves their own long-term, enlightened self-interest. We have characterized self-control as the master virtue because the capacity to override one's impulsive tendencies in order to do what is best or right is central to moral action. Most vices involve failures of self-control, and most virtues involve effective self-control.

At present, psychology has a better understanding of how self-control works than of how religiosity promotes self-control, and so our discussion of the latter has necessarily been somewhat speculative. Religion may promote self-control by upholding specific moral standards, by motivating people to want to be good, by exploiting the prosocial power of guilt, by linking the religious individual to a stable network of relationships with other believers and with God, by promoting character strength through regular exercise of the moral muscle, by fostering self-criticism, and by making people feel that their good and bad deeds are being observed and recorded. Possibly there are other ways as well. As knowledge continues to accumulate, it seems likely that self-control will continue to loom large in accounting for the earthly benefits of religiosity.

REFERENCES

Bargh, J. (1982). Attention and automaticity in the processing of self-relevant information. *Journal of Personality and Social Psychology, 43,* 425–436.

Baumeister, R. F. (1991). *Meanings of life.* New York: Guilford Press.

Baumeister, R. F. (1997). *Evil: Inside human violence and cruelty.* New York: Freeman.

Baumeister, R. F. (2002). Yielding to temptation: Self-control failure, impulsive purchasing, and consumer behavior. *Journal of Consumer Research, 28,* 670–676.

Baumeister, R. F. (2005). *The cultural animal: Human nature, meaning, and social life.* New York: Oxford University Press.

Baumeister, R. F., & Boden, J. M. (1998). Aggression and the self: High self-esteem, low self-control, and ego threat. In R. G. Geen & E. Donnerstein (Eds.), *Human aggression: Theories, research, and implications for social policy* (pp. 111–137). San Diego: Academic Press.

Baumeister, R. F., Bratslavsky, E., Muraven, M., & Tice, D. M. (1998). Ego depletion: Is the active self a limited resource? *Journal of Personality and Social Psychology, 74,* 1252–1265.

Baumeister, R. F., & Exline, J. J. (1999). Virtue, personality, and social relations: Self-control as the moral muscle. *Journal of Personality, 67,* 1165–1194.

Baumeister, R. F., & Exline, J. J. (2000). Self-control, morality, and human strength. *Journal of Social and Clinical Psychology, 19,* 29–42.

Baumeister, R. F., & Heatherton, T. F. (1996). Self-regulation failure: An overview. *Psychological Inquiry, 7,* 1–15.

Baumeister, R. F., Heatherton, T. F., & Tice, D. M. (1994). *Losing control: How and why people fail at self-regulation.* San Diego: Academic Press.

Baumeister, R. F., Muraven, M., & Tice, D. M. (2000). Ego depletion: A resource model of volition, self-regulation, and controlled processing. *Social Cognition, 18,* 130–150.

Baumeister, R. F., Stillwell, A. M., & Heatherton, T. F. (1994). Guilt: An interpersonal approach. *Psychological Bulletin, 115,* 243–267.

Baumeister, R. F., Stillwell, A. M., & Heatherton, T. F. (1995). Personal narratives about guilt: Role in action control and interpersonal relationships. *Basic and Applied Social Psychology, 17,* 173–198.

Berg, M. B., Janoff-Bulman, R., & Cotter, J. (2001). Perceiving value in obligations and goals: Wanting to do what should be done. *Personality and Social Psychology Bulletin, 27,* 982–995.

Carver, C. S., & Scheier, M. F. (1981). *Attention and self-regulation: A control theory approach to human behavior.* New York: Springer-Verlag.

Csikszentmihalyi, M. (1990). *Flow: The psychology of optimal experience.* New York: Harper & Row.

Diener, E., Fraser, S. C., Beaman, A. L., & Kelem, R. T. (1976). Effects of deindividuation variables on stealing among Halloween trick-or-treaters. *Journal of Personality and Social Psychology, 33,* 178–183.

Diener, E., & Wallbom, M. (1976). Effects of self-awareness on antinormative behavior. *Journal of Research in Personality, 10,* 107–111.

Emmons, R. A. (1999). *The psychology of ultimate concerns: Motivation and spirituality in personality.* New York: Guilford Press.

Emmons, R. A. (2000). Is spirituality an intelligence?: Motivation, cognition, and the psychology of ultimate concern. *The International Journal for the Psychology of Religion, 10,* 3–26.

Emmons, R. A., & King, L. A. (1988). Conflict among personal strivings: Immediate and long-term implications for psychological and physical well-being. *Journal of Personality and Social Psychology, 54,* 1040–1048.

Friedman, L. M. (2002). *Law in America: A short history.* New York: Random House.

Glass, D. C., Singer, J. E., & Friedman, L. N. (1969). Psychic cost of adaptation to an environmental stressor. *Journal of Personality and Social Psychology, 12,* 200–210.

Gottfredson, M. R., & Hirschi, T. (1990). *A general theory of crime.* Stanford, CA: Stanford University Press.

Habermas, J. (1973). *Legitimation crisis* (T. McCarthy, Trans.). Boston: Beacon Press.

Haidt, J., Rosenberg, E., & Hom, H. (2003). Differentiating diversities: Moral diversity is not like other kinds. *Journal of Applied Social Psychology, 33,* 1–36.

Henry, M. (1984). *Hannah Whitall Smith.* Minneapolis, MN: Bethany House.

Hirsch, S. R. (Trans.) (1989). *Chapters of the Fathers.* Jerusalem: Feldheim.

Hogan, R. (1973). Moral conduct and moral character: A psychological perspective. *Psychological Bulletin, 79,* 217–232.

Hull, J. G. (1981). A self-awareness model of the causes and effects of alcohol consumption. *Journal of Abnormal Psychology, 90,* 586–600.

James, W. (1950). *The principles of psychology* (Vol. 2). New York: Dover. (Original work published 1890)

Lyman, S. (1978). *The seven deadly sins: Society and evil.* New York: St. Martin's Press.

MacIntyre, A. (1981). *After virtue.* South Bend, IN: University of Notre Dame Press.

Merton, T. (1960). *The wisdom of the desert.* New York: New Directions.

Mischel, W. (1974). Processes in delay of gratification. In L. Berkowitz (Ed.), *Advances in experimental social psychology* (Vol. 7, pp. 249–292). New York: Academic Press.

Mischel, W., Shoda, Y., & Peake, P. K. (1988). Delay of gratification in children. *Science, 244,* 933–938.

Muraven, M., & Baumeister, R. F. (2000). Self-regulation and depletion of limited resources: Does self-control resemble a muscle? *Psychological Bulletin, 126,* 247–259.

Muraven, M., Baumeister, R. F., & Tice, D. M. (1999). Longitudinal improvement of self-regulation through practice: Building self-control through repeated exercise. *Journal of Social Psychology, 139,* 446–457.

Muraven, M., & Slessareva, E. (2003). Mechanism of self-control failure: Motivation and limited resources. *Personality and Social Psychology Bulletin, 29,* 894–906.

Muraven, M., Tice, D. M., & Baumeister, R. F. (1998). Self-control as limited resource: Regulatory depletion patterns. *Journal of Personality and Social Psychology, 74,* 774–789.

Paloutzian, R. F., Richardson, J. T., & Rambo, L. R. (1999). Religious conversion and personality change. *Journal of Personality, 67,* 1047–1079.

Rickaby, J. (1896). *Aquinas ethicus: The moral teaching of St. Thomas.* London: Burns & Oates.

Rodriguez, M. L., Mischel, W., & Shoda, Y. (1989). Cognitive person variables in the delay of gratification of older children at risk. *Journal of Personality and Social Psychology, 57,* 358–367.

Sansone, C., Weir, C., Harpster, L., & Morgan, C. (1992). Once a boring task, always a boring task?: Interest as a self-regulatory mechanism. *Journal of Personality and Social Psychology, 63,* 379–390.

Schmeichel, B. J., Vohs, K. D., & Baumeister, R. F. (2003). Intellectual performance and ego depletion: Role of the self in logical reasoning and other information processing. *Journal of Personality and Social Psychology, 85,* 33–46.

Tangney, J. P. (1991). Moral affect: The good, the bad, and the ugly. *Journal of Personality and Social Psychology, 61,* 598–607.

Tangney, J. P. (1992). Situational determinants of shame and guilt in young adulthood. *Personality and Social Psychology Bulletin, 18,* 199–206.

Tice, D. M., Bratslavsky, E., & Baumeister, R. F. (2001). Emotional distress regulation takes precedence over impulse control: If you feel bad, do it! *Journal of Personality and Social Psychology, 80,* 53–67.

Urbach, E. E. (1994). *The sages: Their concepts and beliefs* (Israel Abrahams, Trans.). Cambridge, MA: Harvard University Press.

Wegner, D. M., Schneider, D. J., Carter, S. R., & White, T. L. (1987). Paradoxical effects of thought suppression. *Journal of Personality and Social Psychology, 53,* 5–13.

Zube, M. J. (1972). Changing concepts of morality: 1948–1969. *Social Forces, 50,* 385–393.

PART V

PSYCHOLOGY OF RELIGION AND APPLIED AREAS

24

Do Religion and Spirituality Influence Health?

DOUG OMAN
CARL E. THORESEN

An important development in the scientific study of religion over the past decade has been an increasing number of studies that have persuasively documented positive relationships between religious involvement and physical and mental health outcomes (Miller & Thoresen, 2003). For example, a recent meta-analysis of over 40 independent samples has reported that religious involvement is significantly and positively associated with longevity (McCullough, Hoyt, Larson, Koenig, & Thoresen, 2000). One of the most thorough recent studies, an 8-year follow-up of more than 20,000 adults representative of the U.S. population, found a life expectancy gap of over 7 years between persons never attending services and those attending more than once weekly, "similar to the female–male and white–black gaps in U.S. life expectancy" (Hummer, Rogers, Nam, & Ellison, 1999, p. 277). Among African Americans, the life expectancy gap associated with religious attendance was nearly 14 years. After adjusting for demographics, socioeconomic status, health status, health behaviors, and social ties, mortality risk continued to be associated with nonattendance (50% elevation, i.e., relative hazard [RH] = 1.50), nearly as strongly as with heavy smoking (63% elevation, RH = 1.63). A critical review by a National Institutes of Health expert panel concluded that the evidence of frequent religious attendance (i.e., once a week or more) predicting longevity, independent of other well-established risk factors, is now "persuasive" (Powell, Shahabi, & Thoresen, 2003).

In this chapter, we explore relationships between religion and health, with primary emphasis on physical rather than mental health outcomes (see Miller & Kelley, Chapter 25, this volume, for a focus on mental health). However, mental and physical health outcomes are often interrelated, and therefore should not be rigidly dichotomized. For example, empirical evidence suggests that physical health benefits from religion are often mediated by gains in mental health correlates, such as improved social relationships, coping ability, and health behaviors. Physical health status, in turn, influences efforts to maintain mental health. Thus, ongoing reciprocal influence operates between physical and mental health. The boundary between them may sometimes be ambiguous, as in, for example, some forms of chronic pain that cannot be easily characterized as solely physical or solely mental. Although often not reflected in practice or in published research, more integrated, expanded views of the interrelationships between physical and mental health have long been available (e.g., see Antonovsky, 1980; Ryff & Singer, 1998).

Limited space prohibits detailed discussion of several phenomena that are affected by religion and that influence physical health. Such topics are discussed elsewhere in this volume, and include crime and delinquency (Donahue & Nielsen, Chapter 15, this volume), as well as war and other forms of intergroup violence (Silberman, Chapter 29, this volume).

In this chapter we begin by briefly tracing the historical emergence of empirical evidence for religion–health associations, and discussing certain definitional issues. Next we examine possible mechanisms by which religious and spiritual involvement may affect physical health, along with currently available empirical evidence. We close by discussing overarching issues viewed as relevant to deepening our understanding of the psychology of religion–health relationships. To save space, throughout the chapter, we use the term "RS" to signify "religious and/or spiritual." Spirituality and religion are often used interchangeably, yet actually represent somewhat distinct if not independent constructs for many persons (see Zinnbauer & Pargament, Chapter 2, this volume). We discuss these topics more fully later in this chapter.

HISTORICAL DEVELOPMENT

Scientific investigation of RS–health relationships extends more than a century. Indeed, the value for physical health of faith-induced positive expectancies was recognized by the founders of modern biomedicine (e.g., Osler, 1910). More than 75 years ago, the *Journal of the American Medical Association* reviewed psychological factors in faith healing, concluding that "the medical problem is to . . . recognize the true function of the mental and the spiritual as well as the material in the alleviation of human ills" (Paulsen, 1926, p. 1696). The *Journal* also gave suggestions for enhancing positive expectancies, noting that "the religious appeal . . . is calculated to affect the largest number of persons [and] may afford the soundest basis for the expectation of lasting results" (p. 1696). Three-quarters of a century later, more than 1,000 published studies of religion–health relationships are available. Reports of positive associations vastly outnumber reports of negative associations (Koenig, McCullough, & Larson, 2001). Why, then, has religion so often been ignored or deprecated as a health-related variable through much of the 20th century? Why do many biomedical and social-scientific researchers still lack awareness of scientific findings about religion, spirituality, and health?

Psychology has played a role, both in overlooking religion and in rediscovering it as a health-related variable. With systematic empirical evidence about religion–health relationships largely unavailable to them, influential founders of modern psychology were free to adopt a variety of disparate approaches to religion. In his *Varieties of Religious Experience* (1902/1961), William James followed a pluralistic approach to religion, viewing positive or "healthy-minded" forms of religion as capable of producing, in some persons, genuine physical cures through expectancy effects. Drawing on case studies and a range of reasoned arguments, James wrote that healthy-minded religion "prevents certain forms of disease as well as science does, or even better in a certain class of persons" (p. 110).

In stark contrast to James, Sigmund Freud relentlessly deprecated religion throughout much of his career, characterizing it as a "universal obsessional neurosis" (Freud, quoted in Koenig et al., 2001, p. 61). Despite Freud's failure to marshal any systematic empirical evidence to support his negative views, they remained highly influential through much of the middle of the 20th century, when religion–health relationships, and religion itself, received little scientific scrutiny (see also Paloutzian & Park, Chapter 1, this volume).

After World War II, the expansion of empirical science of all kinds led to a gradual increase in the number of studies relating religion and health. Some of these studies were conducted by psychologists, some by sociologists or other social scientists, and some by physicians, epidemiologists, or related health professionals. While psychologists sometimes employed multidimensional measures that distinguished internal and external forms of religious involvement (e.g., Allport & Ross, 1967), most confined themselves to single, more institutionally focused measures, such as denominational affiliation and frequency of attendance at religious services. These single-dimension measures were often conceptualized as substitutes or proxies for health behaviors or social connections (e.g., Seventh-Day Adventist affiliation used as an indicator of likely vegetarian diet; see also Oman & Thoresen, 2002). Relatively few studies providing evidence about religion–health relationships focused upon religion itself. More often, religion was seen as an incidental covariate or adjustment variable (e.g., necessary to disentangle and remove religion's unwanted "confounding" effects from estimates of relationships between other higher interest variables). In this period, few scientists studying religion were aware that considerable evidence for religion–health relationships was accumulating, or that it tended to show a positive overall pattern of relationships between religious involvement and health.

The post-World War II period was characterized by a steady increase in both the quality and the quantity of studies. More were published in the 1950s and 1960s than before the war, but efforts still remained relatively sporadic (Koenig et al., 2001). Meanwhile, capitalizing upon cultural changes that swept the Western world in the 1960s, the 1970s saw the initiation of scientific research on secularized or religious forms of meditation, a practice indigenous to both Eastern and Western religious traditions (Keating, 1986/1997; Murphy, Donovan, & Taylor, 1999). Even as they broke new ground, however, many major meditation studies from this period excluded or radically deemphasized meditation's religious and cognitive components, often focusing purely on physiological correlates (Seeman, Dubin, & Seeman, 2003; Shapiro, 1994).

In the 1980s and 1990s, religion qua religion began to draw sustained and more systematic scientific attention as a health-related factor. In the beginning of this period, Bergin (1983) challenged psychological orthodoxy with evidence and arguments that religion was not always associated with psychopathology, initiating a decade of intensified study of religion and mental health. Psychiatrist David Larson also began publishing systematic reviews documenting the neglect of religious factors in medical journals (e.g., Larson, Pattison, Blazer, Omran, & Kaplan, 1986). Levin (1996b), who is a sociologist and epidemiologist, began publishing reviews and theoretical discussions on questions of validity, causal direction, and mediating factors between religion and physical health. These articles alerted scientific readers to the existence of a large but neglected body of research on religion and physical health. During this time, Pargament (1997), a psychologist, initiated an extensive research program on religious forms of coping with stress. Finally, beginning in the late 1990s, several large-scale population-based studies drew much public and scientific attention to the field, showing that frequent attendance at religious services was associated with greater longevity, independent of other well-established risk factors (see McCullough, Hoyt, et al., 2000; Powell et al., 2003). To explain these effects, several authors suggested that greater longevity among religiously involved persons might be due to unmeasured psychological factors, such as religious methods of coping with stress.

Most studies recently linking religious factors to physical health have been conducted by sociologists, epidemiologists, and physicians, rather than by psychologists. While psychologists have studied potential mediating variables, such as mental health and religious coping, the psychological variables used in most studies have been relatively simplistic and few in number, if not essentially absent. This state of affairs has led some to assert that contemporary psychology has been too often "missing in action" in research on religion, spirituality, and health (Thoresen & Harris, 2002).

Still, signs of growing and more sophisticated interest regarding religion and health, mental as well as physical, have become highly evident within psychology. Recently in the United States, the *American Psychologist* published a special section on religion, spirituality, and health that included several papers prepared by an expert panel appointed by the National Institutes of Health (NIH). Several of these papers are cited or discussed in the present chapter (Miller & Thoresen, 2003; Powell et al., 2003; Seeman et al., 2003). Other international or United States-based psychology journals have also published special issues on religion that have included or focused upon health (e.g., Thoresen, 1999). In the last decade, the American Psychological Association has published a series of books on the implications of spirituality or religion for health and clinical practice (e.g., Richards & Bergin, 1997). The widely used fourth edition of the *Diagnostic and Statistical Manual of Mental Disorders* (DSM-IV; American Psychiatric Association, 1994) has for a decade acknowledged religious and spiritual issues to be normal and important rather than pathogenic factors in diagnosis and treatment as in previous editions.

Clearly psychology has not been alone in its interest. Parallel books and journals have been published in medical and other social scientific fields (Koenig et al., 2001; Oman & Thoresen, 2002; Thoresen & Harris, 2002), and the NIH have requested funding applications for studies of spirituality and alcohol abuse. Interest is also abundantly evident in popular media (e.g., a *Newsweek* cover story [Kalb, 2003]).

DEFINITIONAL ISSUES

Many challenges confront the researcher who seeks to formulate a broadly generalizable definition of religion or spirituality (Miller & Thoresen, 2003). Religion and spirituality each may be viewed as multidimensional and latent constructs (i.e., possessing some features that are not directly observable). Often, religion is seen as more institutionally oriented, and spirituality as more personally oriented, although some warn that this approach risks polarization (see Zinnbauer & Pargament, Chapter 2, this volume). Many earlier studies of health largely avoided definitional issues by relying on secondary analyses of data sets containing primarily institutionally based measures of religiosity (e.g., denomination or attendance at worship services in epidemiological studies), or by focusing upon decontextualized mediating factors, such as clinical forms of meditation. Increasingly, data collection is now designed more specifically for understanding the relationships of religion and spirituality to physical health. Thus, clarity about definitions is becoming more important (on measurement issues, see Hill, Chapter 3, this volume).

Influential recent definitions of religion and spirituality have used the concept of the "sacred" as a pivotal point of reference. In major variants of this approach, spirituality is defined as a "search for the sacred." Religion is also defined as a search related in some way to the sacred (for details on two variants of this approach, see Zinnbauer & Pargament, Chapter 2, this volume). Such approaches go beyond a static understanding of religion as centered on group membership, beliefs, and rituals. Instead, they highlight the more dynamic, experiential, emotional, and goal-directed features of religion and spirituality (Allport & Ross, 1967). Doing so offers rich potential linkages to mainstream psychological theory, stress and coping theory, and health psychology (Emmons, Chapter 13, this volume; McCullough & Snyder, 2000; Pargament, 1997; Park, Chapter 16, this volume).

Definitions of spirituality and religion can be most useful if they are not only conceptually grounded, but resonate well with popular usage. Resonance with common speech facilitates validity of the self-report questionnaire measures frequently used in health research (e.g., "To what extent are you spiritual?"). Furthermore, psychoeducational interventions that target spiritual and religious factors need to confront evolving popular as well as scientific meanings of these terms. Dissonance between popular and scientific definitions risks fostering superficial understanding of a growing number of persons who identify themselves as "spiritual but not religious." This group constitutes approximately 20% of the U.S. population (Fuller, 2001). Some within this group engage in nontraditional but *committed* forms of spiritual practice that clearly possess a moral dimension and a "binding quality" (Wuthnow, 1998, p. 184).

Finding cross-cultural definitions of religion and spirituality that are generalizable seems crucial for accumulating cross-cultural corroboration that religious involvement provides health benefits, as well as health hazards. Some initial efforts at cross-cultural generalizability for an RS outcome measure can be seen in the World Health Organization Quality of Life questionnaire, developed and validated in 14 countries, with 24 dimensions, one of which is "spiritual" (The WHOQOL Group, 1998). Similar efforts are needed on RS involvement measures.

MEDIATING FACTORS

It is seldom evident to untrained academics or others how religion or spirituality could "get into the body." For example, why should a worship practice that media stereotypes associate with choir singing and formal Sunday clothing lead to improved health? To explain observed health benefits, researchers on religion–health relationships have typically identified at least five broad pathways or causal mechanisms by which religious or spiritual involvement might lead to better health (Levin, 1996b; Oman & Thoresen, 2002). Some mechanisms are conceptualized as buffering against stressful life events, while others are viewed as direct main effects (see Chatters, 2000, on alternative analytic approaches). Most of these mechanisms may operate simultaneously, partially overlapping, rather than separately. Of five broad classes of mechanisms commonly cited, four are widely recognized by psychologists as well as many other scientists:

- *Health behaviors.* Religious or spiritual groups may discourage smoking and heavy drinking, or encourage exercise, appropriate health service utilization, or other positive health practices out of respect for the body as an instrument of God's service (see sections below on lifestyle health behaviors, health service utilization, and meditation).
- *Psychological states.* RS involvement may foster improved mental health and more positive psychological states such as joy, hope, and compassion, bringing enhanced physical health through reduced burden on physical organ systems, often now termed reduced "allostatic load" (McEwen, 1998).
- *Coping.* RS involvement may foster more effective ways of dealing with stressful events and conditions. Healthier, more effective coping orientations can lead to improved physical health through reductions in maladaptive health behaviors (e.g., less substance abuse) and improvements in psychological states (e.g., reduced chronic anger).
- *Social support.* RS involvement may foster larger and stronger social networks and a greater availability of social support, a well-established salutary factor that may protect health in part by fostering effective coping with stressors.

Many researchers suggest that RS involvements may lead to physical health through a fifth mode of influence, what have been termed "superempirical" or "psi" mechanisms. For example, certain religious practices, such as intercessory prayer (Targ, 1997), may act partially through natural laws—laws perhaps governing "subtle energies" (Levin, 1996a)—that are beyond current modern scientific understanding. Such laws and the phenomena they seek to explain, commonly called "psi" phenomena in psychology, may be amenable in time to being understood scientifically (see Levin, 1996a, for fuller discussion).

As noted above, these five mechanisms are not seen as acting in isolation. For example, a person who becomes active in a faith community may obtain increased social support, which causes enhanced positive psychological states and improved mental health, which in turn brings the person even greater social support, resulting in a beneficial upward spiral of positive effects (Ryff & Singer, 1998). Evidence suggests such ascending positive psychological states and perceived social support from others could engender better immune competence and less cardiovascular reactivity that, in turn, could strengthen physical health. Improved positive psychological states and social support might also result in enhanced health behaviors, also leading to better health.

But a basic question emerges here. What if, for example, religious involvement were shown to foster reduced smoking, and reduced smoking, in turn, were shown (as it has been) to foster improved physical health (e.g., lower rates of numerous diseases, including lung cancer). Would such evidence logically suggest that religious involvement *causally* benefits physical health in this "indirect" way? In the language we use in this chapter, it clearly does. However, readers of the published debates about the strength of the evidence should be aware that differing interpretations have been advanced (e.g., Sloan, Bagiella, & Powell, 1999). In fact, Oman and Thoresen (2002) point out that in scientific research literature as well as in popular culture, confusion arises from *several* different interpretations of claims that religious involvement causes better health outcomes.

Observers sometimes focus selectively on hypothesized mechanisms, on ones that pique their interest, their fear, or their annoyance (e.g., alleged superempirical effects). In doing so they may dismiss or ignore evidence for other mechanisms as irrelevant or uninteresting. Apparently they prefer to view the phrase "religion causally influences health" as applying solely or primarily to their favored or feared mechanism. For example, one can be committed to demonstrating that any religious factor that seems to enhance health can be readily explained simply as the product in some way of greater social support. Therefore, if a form of religious coping is identified as helping to explain the observed health benefit, that evidence may be ignored, dismissed, or reinterpreted without evidence as simply due to the generic features of social support. On the other hand, medically oriented studies that claim evidence for health effects from religion, but fail to measure or even acknowledge potential mediating factors such as social support and health behaviors, can also promote confusion. Such studies risk being seen as overly tendentious, or as "cheerleading" (Thoresen & Harris, 2004). To avoid such confusion, we urge readers to bear in mind the diverse relevant pathways through which RS factors are hypothesized to causally influence health. We should also be aware of present constraints in our abilities to draw clear-cut causal inferences (Levin, 1994; Thoresen, Oman, & Harris, 2005).

Denominational differences appear secondary in their influence, although they clearly exist (Krause, 2004). That is, evidence to date suggests that major classes of protective mechanisms operate in most or perhaps all faiths and denominations, although specific manifestations and magnitudes of protection may vary. For example, Latter-Day Saints, Seventh-Day Adventists, Jews, or other religious groups may benefit by promoting specific protective health behaviors, such as vegetarian diets, not smoking, or not using alcohol. Such health effects from denominational affiliation have been confirmed (e.g., Phillips, Kuzma, Beeson, & Lotz, 1980; see appendices in Koenig et al., 2001). Few if any studies, however, have examined possible psychological mechanisms involved in denominational transmission of such behaviors, or the relative contributions of motives (e.g., for refraining from smoking). For example, is the motive that leads to nonsmoking primarily social conformity or stewardship of the body as a sacred instrument of service? We deemphasize in this chapter denominational differences and instead focus on processes that are shared to a greater or lesser extent by most if not all denominations.

EVIDENCE LINKING RS FACTORS DIRECTLY TO THE BODY

We may conceive of RS factors as affecting bodily conditions, such as blood pressure or immune competence, through mediating factors described above, such as health behaviors and stress-related psychological states. Changed bodily conditions in turn can affect physical health and disease outcomes. This chain of causal influence may be represented as follows:

RS → Mediators → Physiological Measures → Physical Health/Disease Outcomes

In this section, we examine empirical evidence that links RS factors directly with measures of what is "in the body," that is, with physiological measures and physical health and disease outcomes.

Physical Health and Disease Outcomes

Empirical studies have explored direct relationships between several RS dimensions and a wide range of physical health outcomes. Here, we summarize major patterns of interest rather than examining each pairwise combination of an RS dimension with a health outcome. We review findings relating RS factors to three relatively well-studied health outcomes: mortality, morbidity, and disability.

Mortality

In one of the few well-studied pairings between an individual health outcome and an individual dimension of religiosity, Powell and colleagues (2003) found a large and "persuasive" quantity of evidence that attendance at religious services was associated with lower mortality in large population samples. Evidence rated as high-quality from seven studies indicated that the direct association persisted after adjustment for potential confounders (i.e., background variables that if unadjusted might obscure true relationships). Six studies indicated that the association was also independent of established risk factors. More specifically, "the strength of the relationship was, on average, approximately a 30% reduction in mortality after adjustment for demographic, socioeconomic, and health-related confounders and approximately a 25% reduction in mortality after adjustment for established risk factors" (p. 40). This review used very conservative a priori criteria and "levels of evidence" methods modeled on Cochrane Library techniques that have been influential in medical research (see Miller & Thoresen, 2003).

Powell and colleagues' (2003) findings of persuasive religious service attendance–mortality associations were consistent with a meta-analysis by McCullough and colleagues (McCullough, Hoyt, et al., 2000) that weighted evidence among more than 125,000 study participants according to sample size and controlled for over 10 other factors (covariates). The meta-analysis found an average mortality reduction of about 25% associated with religious involvement (primarily religious attendance) across 42 independent samples. Three other findings of the meta-analysis seem notable: when only private religious involvement was used (e.g., reading Scripture), results failed to predict changes in mortality; women showed a much greater benefit than men (59% vs. 33% less mortality); and considerable variability was found in mortality outcomes between the studies used in the analyses.

Regarding specific causes of death, two large community-based epidemiological studies have examined multiple causes of death within a single cohort, and have produced remarkably similar findings (Hummer et al., 1999; Oman, Kurata, Strawbridge, & Cohen, 2002). Compared to nonattendance, both studies found that weekly attendance at religious services predicted an approximately 40% reduction in circulatory disease mortality, even after adjusting for demographics and prior health status. Both studies also found a relatively strong and independent protective effect against respiratory disease mortality, but a lack of significant protective effect against cancer mortality, consistent with review findings by Powell and colleagues (2003).

Morbidity

RS factors and morbidity outcomes were reviewed by Koenig and colleagues (2001), who devoted separate chapters to physical health outcomes that included heart disease, hypertension, stroke, immune disease, cancer, and pain. While religious involvement is generally associated with lower morbidity, most religion–morbidity studies to date have been cross-sectional rather than prospective, and very few have adequately controlled for possible confounding factors. For example, of 16 studies of cancer risk that were identified by Koenig and colleagues (2001, pp. 560–561), only three included multivariate controls such as age, previous health, or health behaviors. Increased physical pain has been associated with more frequent praying in several cross-sectional studies, but a longitudinal study reported that more frequent prayer predicted later decreases in pain (McCullough & Larson, 1999).

Disability and Recovery

Other findings from the methodologically conservative review by Powell and colleagues (2003) included generally stronger effects from religious involvement in protecting healthy persons against disease than in promoting patient recovery, which may actually be impeded by certain factors such as "religious struggle" (Exline & Rose, Chapter 17, this volume). Powell and colleagues (2003) also noted insufficient evidence to draw firm conclusions regarding protection against disability, as reported by some studies, as well as consistent failures of evidence to support hypotheses that religious involvement slows the progression of cancer or improves recovery from acute illness.

Physiological Measures

High blood pressure, termed "hypertension" when it surpasses a designated threshold, is regarded as a risk factor for serious forms of heart disease as well as for cerebrovascular diseases, such as stroke. Empirical evidence links religious involvement with lower blood pressure and reduced hypertension. The critical review by Seeman and colleagues (2003), mentioned above, found "reasonable" levels of evidence linking religion and spirituality with lower blood pressure. For example, Steffan, Hinderliter, Blumenthal, and Sherwood (2001) studied 24-hour ambulatory blood pressure among 77 blacks and 78 whites. Higher levels of religious coping were associated with lower blood pressure among blacks, both when awake and when asleep. The review by Seeman and colleagues also reported finding reasonable evidence for an association with better immune function (e.g., Woods, Antoni, Ironson, & Kling, 1999).

EVIDENCE ON MEDIATING FACTORS

In this section, we examine empirical evidence regarding *how* RS factors might get into the body. That is, we examine possible mediators between RS factors and bodily conditions, such as measures of physiological states and physical health outcomes.

Compelling demonstration that a factor operates as a mediator must include evidence that (1) RS involvement gives rise to the proposed mediating factor, and (2) The mediating factor gives rise to physical health. The first few mediators discussed below are relatively well established, and hence the second type of evidence (mediator causing health) is well known and readily available (see Koenig et al., 2001). For these relatively well-established health factors, the discussion below emphasizes evidence that the mediator correlates with RS factors.

Several less established (more novel) potential mediating factors are also discussed below: meditation, forgiveness, service to others, virtues, and distant intentionality. These factors are often seen as accompanying religious or spiritual involvement, but mainstream research does not typically consider them to be established predictors of health. For these proposed mediators, we discuss both forms of evidence listed above. The importance that religious traditions have placed on some of these practices has led many authors to classify them as RS factors. However, unlike purely theistic prayer or attendance at religious worship services, these factors as conceptualized here exist not only in their religious forms, but also in secular forms devoid of reference to the sacred. Historically, research on secular forms of these practices has helped to clarify their effects and their underlying modes of operation. Yet these practices might be altered or enhanced in their effects if embedded in a spiritual or religious context, and full understanding requires that their effects be investigated in spiritual as well as secular settings (Shapiro, 1994; Thoresen et al., 2005).

Lifestyle Health Behaviors

Several dimensions of religious involvement have been associated with well-established behavioral risk factors. For example, behaviorally strict denominations may discourage smoking and drinking of alcohol or encourage good diets (Troyer, 1988). More broadly, many denominations may encourage good health behaviors out of respect for the body as an instrument of God's service. In cross-sectional community-based studies, persons attending religious services more frequently have been found to engage in more exercise and less smoking and heavy drinking (Oman & Reed, 1998; Strawbridge, Shema, Cohen, & Kaplan, 2001) (see Koenig et al., 2001, for extensive discussion). Other studies, primarily cross-sectional, also report that higher levels of religious involvement are associated with less risky sexual behavior (Koenig et al., 2001). These patterns extend to more religiously involved adolescents, who engage in less smoking, less drinking of alcohol, and more frequent use of seat belts (Oman & Thoresen, 2005; Wallace & Forman, 1998; see also Levenson & Aldwin, Chapter 8, this volume). One study of twins suggests that RS factors may mitigate the impact of genotype on measures of disinhibition, a correlate of substance abuse and other risky health behaviors (Boomsma, de Geus, van Baal, & Koopmans, 1999). But in an exception to the generally very positive patterns of RS correlates, several studies report higher prevalence of excessive body weight among more religious persons (Koenig et al., 2001, pp. 569–572; Oman & Reed, 1998).

Does religious involvement encourage better health behaviors, or do these associations arise because people with better health behaviors are more likely to become religious or spiritual? In a rare if not unique longitudinal investigation, Strawbridge and colleagues (2001) followed a representative sample of more than 2,500 community-dwelling adults over three decades. Persons who frequently attended religious services were more likely to adopt and maintain positive health behaviors, such as exercising and refraining from smoking and heavy drinking. Overall, beneficial effects on health behaviors from religious attendance were stronger for women than for men.

Research also suggests that spiritual factors, for example, as provided through 12-step programs, may be implicated in the recovery from addictions (Gorsuch, 1995). A recent study speaks to this point. Tonigan (2003) found that RS practices did not directly predict abstinence from alcohol. However, RS factors predicted continuing participation in Alcoholics Anonymous (AA) meetings, which predicted abstinence. More specifically, AA participation at 3 years follow-up had no direct effect on AA participation at 10 years. Instead, AA participation at 3 years predicted RS practices at 10 years, which predicted AA participation at 10 years (beta = .24 and .71, $p < .05$). This AA participation at 10 years predicted abstinence at 10 years (beta = .40, $p < .05$). Thus, the mediating effect of RS experiences and practices emerged gradually over time, and did not exercise a direct main effect on a health outcome.

Improved Coping

Relationships between physical health and personal styles of appraising and coping with stress have been extensively studied (Pargament, 1997). Effective coping fosters adaptive health behaviors and may lead to stress-related personal growth (Park, Chapter 16, this volume). More effective coping styles are also thought to reduce physiological wear and tear on the organism (i.e., reduce allostatic load), thereby improving physical health (McEwen, 1998). Recently, Pargament (1997) synthesized a large body of research on distinctively religious methods of coping (see also Pargament, Ano, & Wacholtz, Chapter 26, this volume). Findings suggest that religious coping measures help predict adjustment to stressful life events beyond purely secular measures of coping. Religious coping "complements nonreligious coping . . . by offering responses to the limits of personal powers" (Pargament, 1997, p. 310). For example, persons adopting a "collaborative" coping orientation with the divine, viewing God as a partner, experienced better outcomes than persons using either a primarily "deferring" coping style (involving a passive attitude toward problems) or a primarily "self-directive" coping style (p. 294). Viewing religious coping as a distinctive RS dimension, Powell et al. (2003) found evidence to date inadequate for predicting longevity.

Social Support

Social support is another established health factor that may partly mediate RS–health associations. Like religion and spirituality, social support is multidimensional (Cohen, Underwood, & Gottlieb, 2000), with social support sometimes construed to include largely psychological concepts, such as perceived emotional support. Several dimensions, including social networks and perceived social support, have been found to predict lower risk of morbidity and mortality, but the mechanisms remain unclear. Difficulties in the research include differences in how social support is viewed (e.g., size of support network or perceived level of social/emotional support) and the lack of well-controlled randomized trials showing that changes in support influence health (Cohen et al., 2000). Some have suggested that social support may be conceived as a kind of coping assistance, which might explain why different dimensions of social support are sometimes most protective among different populations that possess different resources and experience different stressors (Thoits, 1986).

Several studies have linked various dimensions of religious and spiritual involvement with larger or more stable social networks and/or with more perceived social and emotional support (e.g., Oman & Reed, 1998; Strawbridge et al., 2001). (Koenig et al., 2001, p. 215, mentioned 19 studies showing statistically significant relationships, but failed to cite them.) Evidence, however, that social support explains more than a small portion of any RS–health relationship is lacking (George, Ellison, & Larson, 2002).

To our knowledge, the only longitudinal studies of RS factors and social support are by Strawbridge and colleagues (2001), who reported that frequent service attenders were less likely over 28 years to become or to remain socially isolated, and were more likely to become or to remain married. Considerable evidence also suggests that religious families offer more stable social support through lower divorce rates and improved marital functioning, with some findings suggesting more positive parenting and better child adjustment (Mahoney, Pargament, Tarakeshwar, & Swank, 2001; see also Mahoney & Tarakeshwar, Chapter 10, this volume).

Positive Psychological States

Religiously or spiritually involved persons may experience better mental health and more positive psychological states, such as joy, hope, and compassion, perhaps from using religious coping methods to buffer stress. Also they may gain from adhering to spiritually related goals and "personal strivings" learned in part from family, community, or historical spiritual exemplars (Emmons, Chapter 13, this volume; Oman & Thoresen, 2003b). Such states may include reduced negative emotional states (e.g., fear, sadness, anger), as well as expectancy-related positive states such as optimism and faith (Osler, 1910). Also involved may be other well-studied or potentially health-relevant states such as meaning, conscientiousness, or perceptions of primary or secondary control (Cole & Pargament, 1999; Park, Chapter 16, this volume). Positive emotional states could lead to improved physical health by reducing overall chronic burden on organ systems from adapting to environmental challenges (reduced "allostatic load"). Benefits of less allostatic load may include reduced cardiovascular reactivity and enhanced immune competence (McEwen, 1998). Positive psychological states derived from spiritual or religious coping might also help people to overcome internal barriers in adopting positive health behaviors, to obtain appropriate health services, and/or to form supportive social connections.

Much evidence links religious and spiritual involvement to measures of improved mental health. A recent meta-analysis demonstrated a negative correlation between religious involvement and measures of depression (Smith, McCullough, & Poll, 2003). Many studies have examined relationships between nonmeditative prayer and mental health, with mixed findings (McCullough & Larson, 1999; Spilka, Chapter 20, this volume; Thoresen et al., 2005). Most studies of RS factors and mental health factors have been cross-sectional, and prospective evidence about mediating effects from well-controlled studies is lacking (George et al., 2002; see also Miller & Kelley, Chapter 25, this volume).

Health Services Utilization

Some evidence demonstrates relationships between spirituality, religion, and health services utilization. These studies tend to report patterns of greater use of preventive care and compliance with medical regimens among individuals with higher levels of religion or spirituality (Koenig et al., 2001, p. 408). For example, a recent study found that both men and women who reported religion as more important in their lives were more likely to use a variety of preventive services, including flu shots, cholesterol screening, breast self-exams, mammograms, Pap smears, and prostate screening (Reindl Benjamins & Brown, 2004).

Meditation

Meditation, as noted earlier, has been the focus of much research. Unfortunately, many meditation studies have suffered from design flaws, including inadequate assessments, lack of a comparison group, or failure to control for other factors that could explain health effects (Murphy et al., 1999; Seeman et al., 2003). However, some well-designed studies have linked meditation with physical and mental health benefits. These include improved stress management skills as well as reduced somatic and mental arousal, lower blood pressure, and lower cholesterol (e.g., Patel, Marmot, Terry, Carruthers, Hunt, & Patel, 1985). The critical review by Seeman and colleagues (2003) reported that evidence is now "persuasive" that meditation is associated with better outcomes among clinical populations. Furthermore, one randomized study of 73 older persons found that two forms of meditation produced much higher rates of survival over 3 years (100% and 88%) than did relaxation training (65%) or merely assessing participants over time (63%) (Alexander, Langer, Newman, Chandler, & Davies, 1989).

Research in the affective neurosciences is beginning to show that meditation may be a crucial factor in altering prefrontal brain processes, thus changing physiological processes influencing major organ systems, such as immune, neuroendocrine, and cardiovascular functioning. Davidson and colleagues (2003) reported that meditation increased activity in the left prefrontal cortex area and reduced activity in the right prefrontal cortex area. The left area is often associated with positive emotions, such as compassion, and the right area with negative emotions, such as fear. Also found were increased immune competence in dealing with an influenza vaccine, as well as less cortisol and more positive emotions. Neurological studies of meditation have now advanced to the point where general models of neural correlates and functioning of meditation have been offered (Newberg & Newberg, Chapter 11, this volume).

Forgiveness

Forgiving attitudes and behaviors are commonly endorsed in most religious and spiritual traditions (McCullough, Bono, & Root, Chapter 22, this volume; McCullough, Pargament, & Thoresen, 2000). Emerging evidence indicates that forgiveness may lead to better physical and mental health by reducing rumination and enhancing positive emotions. For example, unforgiving thoughts have been linked with aversive emotions and significantly higher facial tension (corrugator electromyogram), skin conductance, heart rate, and blood pressure. In contrast, forgiving thoughts have been linked with greater perceived control and comparatively lower physiological stress responses (Witvliet, Ludwig, & Vander Laan, 2001). Health benefits of forgiveness may arise from reductions in excessive self-focus and angry rumination, more adaptive coping, and overall enhancements of mental and social health. A few experimental studies demonstrate that interventions can promote forgiveness, thereby also fostering health-related outcomes such as reduced chronic stress and anger (see Thoresen et al., 2005). However, with rare exception, studies have not yet compared the effectiveness of spiritually versus secularly presented forgiveness interventions.

Service to Others

Altruism is also strongly endorsed by religious traditions, in theory and often in practice. Emerging research has linked altruistic attitudes and behaviors to health. Protective effects may occur through mechanisms such as reduction in excessive self-focus, reduced stress reactivity, and increased social support (Oman, Thoresen, & McMahon, 1999; Post, Underwood, Schloss, & Hurlbut, 2002). Formal volunteer work, which may be undertaken for a variety of altruistic and nonaltruistic motives, has been linked to greater longevity as well as improved self-rated health and mental health (Oman et al., 1999; Schwartz, Meisenhelder, Ma, & Reed, 2003). Informal helping has also been studied, and peer helping among patients has been related to reduced depression and increased confidence, self-awareness, self-esteem, and role functioning (Schwartz & Sendor, 1999). Two studies have found that the protectiveness of volunteering was significantly larger in fostering longevity among frequent attenders at religious services (Harris & Thoresen, in press; Oman et al., 1999).

Virtues

Virtues such as compassion, self-control, hope, wisdom, and love have been suggested as "classical human strengths" that may promote health by a variety of mechanisms (Levin, 1996b; McCullough & Snyder, 2000). Along with other positive qualities such as focused attention and mindfulness, each of these virtues seems likely to have its own profile of specific properties and correlates (Brown & Ryan, 2003; McCullough, Bono, & Root, Chapter 22, this volume; Oman, Hedberg, Downs, & Parsons, 2003). Yet these religiously related virtues may still be mutually reinforcing features of character strength, and may promote health through similar processes, such as enhancing wise judgment and fostering self-control (Geyer & Baumeister, Chapter 23, this volume).

Distant Healing

Finally, much research has explored the effects of distant healing, that is, mentally based efforts to heal or influence from a distance (shielded from all ordinary social or material influences). Guidelines for future research have recently been offered (Jonas & Chez, 2003). Most research on distant healing has been purely secular, investigating effects on humans, animals, or other biological systems (e.g., Kiang, Marotta, Wirkus, & Jonas, 2002). Research on intercessory prayers offered by religious persons can also be understood as research on distant healing (e.g., Levin, 1996a; Targ, 1997).

This is a very controversial area of research, in part because conventional scientific paradigms do not readily allow explanations for such phenomena. The theological assumptions supposed to underlie such studies have also been criticized (Chibnall, Jeral, & Cerullo, 2001). At present, reviews suggest that reasonable, but not persuasive, evidence exists for healing benefits from being the recipient of prayers by others (Powell et al., 2003). A much larger body of evidence suggests the existence of some type of distant mental influence (Levin, 1996a). However, it is unclear to what extent such phenomena may mediate the religious benefits of spiritual and religious involvement. This is because it is not yet known whether religiously or spiritually involved persons, when compared to others in the general population, are the targets of a larger quantity of distant healing intentionality, or more fervent prayers for healing (Oman & Thoresen, 2002). Indeed, "it is conceivable that distant healing largely functions unconsciously, subtly integrated into each procedure. . . . It may be that our challenge is . . . to find doctors or other healthcare providers who are *not* using some form of psychic healing" (Targ, 1997, p. 77).

STRENGTH OF THE EVIDENCE

The currently available empirical evidence, reviewed above, provides powerful refutation of claims that, across the board, religious and spiritual involvement are physically and mentally unhealthy if not dangerous. Persuasive evidence now demonstrates the existence of positive associations between health and practices such as attendance at worship services and meditation. However, from a scientific standpoint, underlying issues of causal direction are still very much open to debate. Some longitudinal data *do* strongly suggest that RS factors operate over time to produce the conditions for better health (e.g., Strawbridge et al., 2001). Still, additional replication in other populations using a much wider variety of designs and measures of RS factors, along with plausible mediators, could provide a more comprehensive and persuasive picture (Levin, 1994; Thoresen, 1999). A fully persuasive picture will require much more attention to contextual factors, treated not as static constructs, but as variables that in themselves often change over time.

RESEARCH NEEDS

The empirical findings described above, while encouraging in linking RS factors to health, fall short of offering a solid understanding of how religious and spiritual involvement promote or hinder physical health. Most areas clearly require additional research, as reflected by previously cited NIH panel review papers. Clarification of effects from a wider range of specifically religious and spiritual factors is needed, along with a broader variety of assessment strategies. Questionnaires are very useful yet cannot be the only method used if we are to understand relationships more fully (see Hill, Chapter 3, this volume). More qualitative studies, longitudinal studies, and multiwave panel studies can help reveal which findings are robustly supported across diverse designs.

Another key limitation is that existing research has been conducted largely in North America, with fewer studies conducted in Europe or Israel, and very small numbers conducted elsewhere. Religion, spirituality, and health are all in many ways multicultural issues. We need to move forward in acknowledging the multicultural reality of RS factors (American Psychological Association, 2003). The contexts in which religious and spiritual practices typically occur are not homogeneous entities, but are dynamic, multicultural, and heterogeneous (Chatters, 2000). A tremendous variety of unexplored person factors, such as specific beliefs, experiences, and behaviors, may help explain why some RS factors appear more protective than others against specific risks in specific populations. Contextual features may also clarify why detrimental health associations have sometimes been observed for specific RS factors in some populations.

Psychologists can make important contributions to future studies in this area by developing and using multidimensional measures of religion and spirituality that capture the most health-relevant dimensions of religion in various cultural settings. The importance of cultural variability is demonstrated by Krause and colleagues, who offer evidence and theoretical arguments that service attendance may be less relevant to health in Japanese culture than in U.S. culture (Krause, Ingersoll-Dayton, Liang, & Sugisawa, 1999). Of course, many findings regarding religion may generalize across cultures. Hood and colleagues, for example, offer evidence of similar factorial patterns underlying mystical experience in Islamic and Christian cultures (Hood et al., 2001). But without *many* more high-quality studies in non-Western populations, it will be impossible to know which findings will reliably generalize to a majority of the world's population.

We now discuss several areas where research is needed, some of them involving themes and concepts from religion (e.g., higher consciousness), and some from mainstream psychology (e.g., self-regulation, self-efficacy, and attachment). We believe these areas share a common potential for advancing understanding of spirituality, religion, and physical health.

Higher Consciousness and Primal Energies

Most major religious traditions affirm the existence of qualitatively higher states of consciousness that can persist over long periods of time within privileged individuals, such as saints or advanced meditators (Goleman, 1988; Underhill, 1911). Empirical study of these states of consciousness to date has been limited, but evidence suggests that correlates of advanced states may include atypical, high-theta brain wave patterns (Hood, Spilka, Hunsberger, & Gorsuch, 1996), as well as changes in prefrontal cortical areas of the brain (Davidson et al., 2003). Other research suggests that meditators may gain a degree of conscious control over biological processes such as bodily temperature (Murphy et al., 1999).

Scientific study of the psychological and biological homeostatic processes that permit higher states to be maintained is constrained by difficulties in identifying, recruiting, and validating the eligibility of persons with higher states of consciousness. Still, such studies are feasible in principle and constitute basic research that could yield fundamental insights relevant to health, the nature of the human being, and the capacities of the human organism.

One question meriting study is similarities and differences between high spiritual states and experiences of "flow" described by psychologists (e.g., Csikszentmihalyi, 1990). Does maintaining higher states require the convergence of specific measurable physiological processes involving energy flows (e.g., Shang, 2001) with specific mental schemas that structure experience into a flow-like activity (e.g., schemas regulating devotion to God or beliefs about higher being as described in Smith, 1976)? To date, "relatively little research has addressed the experience of flow when attention is trained on internal sources of information (e.g., . . . spiritual experience)," although more "culturally defined domains (e.g., prayer) . . . may be understandable in terms of existing flow theory" (Nakamura & Csikszentmihalyi, 2002, p. 102).

A deeper understanding of homeostatic processes underlying higher states of spiritual consciousness might also help clarify the complex relationship between adult sexual energies, risky sexual behaviors, and physical and mental health. Most professionally administered public health efforts to prevent the spread of AIDS have focused almost exclusively on disseminating condoms and promoting safe rather than unprotected sex. Such efforts have met with only limited success in reducing HIV infection rates in many parts of the developing world. Recently, campaigns by faith-based organizations for sexual restraint, as a more "primary" form of behavioral change, have brought unprecedented reductions in HIV infection rates in Uganda and some other developing countries (Green, 2003). These efforts may have succeeded partly because persons who maintain celibacy or abstain from extramarital sex have functioned as behavioral models who contribute to what epidemiologists term "herd immunity," a social condition in which low case retransmission rates of a disease lead to its elimination from a population (Levin, 1996b; Oman & Thoresen, 2003b).

But can sexual restraint that could reduce disease risk be a viable long-term pattern for entire societies as well as for individuals? Freud saw dangers in both excessive repression and excessive expression of primal human energies that he characterized as fundamentally sexual. His psychodynamic perspective allowed for the possibility of a third route for these energies, a redirection into nonsexual activities, a process he called "sublimation." Similarly, all major religious faiths have affirmed, especially in their mystical traditions, that a higher being (such as God or a true Self) can function as an absorbing and fulfilling focus of a human being's love, to be given "with all thine heart, and with all thy soul, and with all thy might" (Deuteronomy 6:5).

In contrast to the common perception of "sublimation" as involving a derivative and probably diluted and second-rate experience, worldwide mystical traditions affirm that divine love can be *fulfilling*—that as Protestant Christian mystic Jacob Boehme affirms, union with the divine is "is brighter than the sun, it is sweeter than anything called sweet; it is stronger than all strength; it is more nutrimental than food, more cheering to the heart than wine, and more pleasant than all the joy and pleasantness of the world" (quoted in Perry, 1991, p. 614). Long-term faith/health dialogue and collaboration to address the AIDS pandemic might benefit from improved scientific understanding of persons who function as stable exemplars of the rewards and processes underlying the intense spiritual transformation of primal human energies (Oman & Thoresen, 2003b).

Spiritual Self-Efficacy

Within social-cognitive theory, the self-efficacy (domain-specific self-confidence) construct has been widely applied to understanding and promoting many types of health behavior change (Bandura, 1997). Similarly, the self-efficacy construct might be used to study effective ways of transmitting practices of interest to religion and spirituality, such as meditation, prayer, forgiveness, and service to others (Thoresen et al., 2005). However, such measures need to be interpreted in view of changes in the conceptions of self that may accompany spiritual growth. Tendencies to attribute achievements to God, as in St. Paul's statement that "not I, but Christ liveth in me" (Galatians 2:20), illustrate this concern (Oman & Thoresen, 2003a). Would, for example, measures of individual self-efficacy be less relevant than measures of dyadic (the individual with God) self-efficacy for persons with a "collaborative" religious coping orientation (Pargament, 1997)? Does the collective spiritual self-efficacy of a religious group predict more success in engaging in spiritual practices than each person's individual self-efficacy?

Spiritual Self-Regulation

Self-regulation has benefited from decades of study in mainstream psychology and health psychology. Domain-specific forms of self-regulation have been studied in organizational, health, counseling/clinical, and educational psychology, but application to religion has only received explicit attention recently (Boekaerts, Pintrich, & Zeidner, 2000; Geyer & Baumeister, Chapter 23, this volume). Still unarticulated and unstudied to our knowledge is the construct of spiritual self-regulation, that is, the regulation of one's conduct in order to attain spiritual goals. The construct of spiritual self-regulation has a strong commonsensical appeal for explaining daily choices that many religious people actually make (e.g., "I avoid taverns because I experience them as a temptation to sin"). Tools for developing and operationalizing the construct of spiritual self-regulation have recently become more available through goal-oriented definitions and research programs on spirituality and religion (Emmons, Chapter 13, and Zinnbauer & Pargament, Chapter 2, this volume). Such regulation is also closely related to spiritual modeling (Oman & Thoresen, 2003b). Social-cognitive theory recognizes that the self-evaluative processes underlying self-regulation are shaped in part by standards acquired from models (Bandura, 2003). "Modeling is an excellent vehicle for transmitting knowledge and skills, but it is infrequently studied as a maintainer of standards" (Bandura, 1986, p. 371). We believe that the concept of spiritual self-regulation could be useful for understanding nontraditional but committed forms of spirituality (Wuthnow, 1998), as well as for clarifying the operation of spiritual interventions (e.g., 12-step programs), refining the concept of spiritual health, and developing new spiritual interventions.

Attachment Styles

Attachment styles are a plausible but unstudied potential mediator between RS factors and physical health. Attachment theory has expanded from its initial focus on infant–parent relationships to examination of adult attachments, and has recently been extended to attachments to personified higher or sacred powers. Similarities to human attachment relationships offer "more than an interesting analogy: Perceived relationships with God meet all of the defining criteria of attachment relationships and function psychologically as true attachments" (Kirkpatrick, 1999, p. 804). God as an attachment figure appears to function analogously to childhood attachment figures as a safe haven in crisis and a secure base for exploration. More secure attachment to God has been associated with greater life satisfaction, agreeableness, religious symbolic immortality, positive affect, as well as with less negative affect, neuroticism, loneliness, anxiety, depression, and physical illness (Rowatt & Kirkpatrick, 2002). Considerable evidence, often indirect, supports the plausibility that secure attachment relationships promote physical health (Maunder & Hunter, 2001).

Does a secure attachment relationship with a divinity, or with a human figure understood as a channel of grace, provide a causal source of personal growth and mental and physical health? To our knowledge, relationships between secure *spiritual* attachments and physical health remain unstudied.

Negative Effects from Religion

We have focused on positive effects on physical health, partially because empirical evidence suggests primarily positive effects on physical and mental health. However, negative effects on health have also been documented. For example, "religious struggle" has been associated with elevated mortality (see Exline & Rose, Chapter 17, this volume). Also, some religious groups discourage certain forms of medical care, such as vaccinations or blood transfusions (Koenig et al., 2001). Recently, the highly publicized controversies surrounding physical and sexual abuse by members of religious orders also speak to egregiously harmful effects (Plante, 2004). These effects should be viewed in context: as a major social institution that provides professionally based care and service, institutionalized religion, like institutionalized education, law, and medicine, will undoubtedly contribute at times to certain negative health effects for some people. Such damage should be detected and corrected. Empirical research can contribute to needed institutional improvements as well as to understanding and perhaps alleviating negative consequences of phenomena such as religious struggle. The possibility should not be excluded that some short-term negative effects may precede longer term positive effects, perhaps mediated by stress-related growth (e.g., Richards, Acree, & Folkman, 1999).

Spiritual and Religious Interventions

Understanding how interventions might be used to alter religious and spiritual factors is a topic of both practical and theoretical importance. If RS factors do indeed foster improved mental and physical health, then respectful, ethically grounded interventions to alter these practices may be warranted (Post, Puchalski, & Larson, 2000; see also Shafranske, Chapter 27, this volume). Furthermore, experimental intervention studies are an important complement to observational studies in providing underlying evidence about causal mechanisms, and may provide crucial information for drawing well-founded causal inferences about effects from religion and spirituality (Thoresen et al., 2005).

Unfortunately, only a small number of studies to date have examined the extent to which RS factors can be experimentally altered (Thoresen et al., 2005). For example, some studies of meditation interventions have examined self-reported measures of spiritual experiences or self-rated spirituality (Astin, 1997; Oman, Hedberg, & Thoresen, 2005). Few if any studies, however, have examined longer term outcomes on a broader range of spiritual or religious dimensions—for example, beliefs, participation in spiritual/religious fellowship or worship, spiritual/religious coping, spiritual attachment, or various forms of prayer. Also largely unstudied is the ability of interventions to affect a person's confidence (self-efficacy) that he or she can properly or effectively engage in practices promoted by religion and spirituality—for example, worship, prayer, meditation, and forgiveness (Oman & Thoresen, 2003a; Oman, Thoresen, Flinders, & Flinders, 2003). Self-confidence (self-efficacy), as noted above, is one of the strongest predictors of behavior in many domains of human functioning. We know of no evidence suggesting that RS practices are an exception to this pattern (Bandura, 1997).

Interventions that merit study for their ability to alter RS factors could be as simple as a clinician performing a brief "spiritual history" with a patient, perhaps thereby motivating the patient through increased ability to believe that medical and spiritual goals are aligned (Koenig, 2000). Other viable clinical interventions include brief 5- to 7-minute interviews using a very structured yet unintrusive pattern of inquiry into patients' overall and spiritual coping strategies and needs for assistance (Rhodes & Kristeller, 2000). Some medical patients or counseling clients may benefit from interventions aimed at reducing maladaptive rumination by teaching repetition of a holy name or mantram (Easwaran, 1977/1998; Oman & Driskill, 2003). Spiritual and religious values can also be integrated into longer term counseling in a variety of ways (Richards & Bergin, 1997). Evidence suggests that even largely secularized forms of meditation may promote spiritual experiences, perhaps through processes such as the training of attention that are intrinsic to most forms of meditation (Goleman, 1988; Kass, Friedman, Leserman, Zuttermeister, & Benson, 1991). Interventions can also offer tools to enhance processes, such as attention and retention, that underlie learning from spiritual exemplars (Bandura, 2003; Oman & Thoresen, 2003b). For example, recent nonsectarian interventions have taught participants how to meditate on memorized passages from personally selected Scriptures such as the Psalms and Gospels, or spiritual figures such as St. Francis, the Buddha, and Rumi (Oman et al., 2005). Doing so produced substantial reductions maintained over several months in several health-related factors, such as perceived stress and burnout, and increases in caregiving self-efficacy.

Spiritual Health

Further study is also needed of the theological bases and implications for modern healthcare systems of various ways to operationalize the notion of "spiritual health." Historical and cross-cultural studies confirm that modern Western medicine, "shorn of every vestige of mystery, faith, or moral portent, is actually an aberration in the world scene" (Barnard, Dayringer, & Cassel, 1995, p. 807). The construct of spiritual health holds promise as a pivot around which modern healthcare systems might reintegrate spiritual sensitivity into their daily operations (see also Hathaway, 2003). However, it is unclear to what extent multiple and sometimes competing definitions of spiritual health may function as a constraint. For example, although most systems of complementary and alternative medicine address spirituality, it is unclear to what extent these meanings agree with each other, with spirituality defined as a search for the sacred (Zinnbauer & Pargament, Chapter 2, this volume), or with spirituality as operationalized in recently constructed measures (e.g., WHOQOL Group, 1998). Research is needed to identify and operationalize common ground among various approaches to spirituality and spiritual health, and to document their relationships with physical health.

CONCLUSION

The empirical evidence available from a variety of disciplines now clearly shows that robust relationships exist between some physical health outcomes and some dimensions of religious and spiritual involvement, especially attendance at religious services. The evidence is suggestive, but clearly not yet persuasive, that many other relationships may exist. However, the causal nature of the observed relationships is still scientifically a very open question. Results linking religious and spiritual involvement with better health contradict the belief that religion in general is hazardous to health. But we do not yet understand what processes occurring over time might best describe how religious or spiritual beliefs and practices lead to better health (or to diminished health).

We offer the following as additional conclusions for consideration:

• Conceptions of spirituality continue to evolve, reflecting its multidimensional nature. Its relationship to religion remains fluid in that some see it as central to if not the core of religion, while others view it as essentially independent of religion. Relatedly, applications of the concept of the sacred appear to be evolving as well, with some believing it to be the centerpiece of religion and of spirituality.

• Psychology is very well positioned in terms of contemporary theories, research methods, and practices to advance our understanding of the role in health of religion and spirituality. However psychologists need to collaborate in this work with other scientists and professionals, including religious professionals.

• Research on the relationship of religion with health needs to embrace more diversified and pluralistic methods. This includes recognizing that some phenomena may be very difficult to assess through existing approaches. A variety of qualitative and quantitative methods (not just survey questions) is required, with assessment spanning more than one or two occasions, since most variables themselves are variable, often changing over time.

• The search for possible mediators of relationships between religious and spiritual factors and health indicators deserves top priority at this time. Other studies are important, but identifying mediators holds special promise to accelerate and advance our understanding.

• Several research topics have been suggested. These include ones that we believe have often not received any attention or inadequate attention: studies of higher consciousness linking physiological, cognitive, and emotional/mood factors; spiritual self-regulation, including spiritual modeling and spiritual self-efficacy and dyadic efficacy; attachment style over the lifespan, including quality of attachment to God and other sacred persons or spiritual exemplars; spiritual interventions focusing on a variety of spiritual and religious practices, and in secular compared to religious or spiritual formats; spiritual health as a concept and as assessed; and negative effects on health of specific religious or spiritual beliefs, behaviors, or practices.

The present is a very exciting time for the emerging transdisciplinary field of religion, spirituality, and health. Research findings are slowly coalescing into a coherent picture of how the human body and human health is affected by the perennial human quest in various forms for spiritual and religious truth. Many psychologists and religionists, but perhaps not enough, are moving beyond earlier mutual stereotypes and learning to collaborate. Only through such collaboration, we believe, can we apply the fullest range of knowledge and wisdom to fostering human health and well-being in the context of today's dire global needs.

REFERENCES

Alexander, C. N., Langer, E. J., Newman, R. I., Chandler, H. M., & Davies, J. L. (1989). Transcendental meditation, mindfulness, and longevity: An experimental study with the elderly. *Journal of Personality and Social Psychology, 57,* 950–964.

Allport, G. W., & Ross, M. J. (1967). Personal religious orientation and prejudice. *Journal of Personality and Social Psychology, 5,* 432–443.

American Psychiatric Association. (1994). *Diagnostic and statistical manual of mental disorders* (4th ed.). Washington, DC: Author.

American Psychological Association. (2003). Guidelines on multicultural education, training, research, practice, and organizational change for psychologists. *American Psychologist, 58,* 377–402.

Antonovsky, A. (1980). *Health, stress and coping.* San Francisco: Jossey-Bass.

Astin, J. A. (1997). Stress reduction through mindfulness meditation: Effects on psychological symptomatology, sense of control, and spiritual experiences. *Psychotherapy and Psychosomatics, 66,* 97–106.

Bandura, A. (1986). *Social foundations of thought and action.* Englewood Cliffs, NJ: Prentice Hall.

Bandura, A. (1997). *Self-efficacy: The exercise of control.* New York: Freeman.

Bandura, A. (2003). On the psychosocial impact and mechanisms of spiritual modeling. *The International Journal for the Psychology of Religion, 13,* 167–174.

Barnard, D., Dayringer, R., & Cassel, C. K. (1995). Toward a person-centered medicine: Religious studies in the medical curriculum. *Academic Medicine, 70,* 806–813.

Bergin, A. E. (1983). Religiosity and mental health: A critical reevaluation and meta-analysis. *Professional Psychology: Research and Practice, 14,* 170–184.

Boekaerts, M., Pintrich, P. R., & Zeidner, M. (Eds.). (2000). *Handbook of self-regulation.* New York: Academic Press.

Boomsma, D. I., de Geus, E. J., van Baal, G. C., & Koopmans, J. R. (1999). A religious upbringing reduces the influence of genetic factors on disinhibition: Evidence for interaction between genotype and environment on personality. *Twin Research, 2,* 115–125.

All biblical quotations are from the King James Bible translation.

Brown, K. W., & Ryan, R. M. (2003). The benefits of being present: Mindfulness and its role in psychological well-being. *Journal of Personality and Social Psychology, 84,* 822–848.

Chatters, L. M. (2000). Religion and health: Public health research and practice. *Annual Review of Public Health, 21,* 335–367.

Chibnall, J. T., Jeral, J. M., & Cerullo, M. A. (2001). Experiments on distant intercessory prayer: God, science, and the lesson of Massah. *Archives of Internal Medicine, 161,* 2529–2536.

Cohen, S., Underwood, L., & Gottlieb, B. H. (2000). *Social support measurement and intervention: A guide for health and social scientists.* New York: Oxford University Press.

Cole, B. S., & Pargament, K. I. (1999). Spiritual surrender: A paradoxical path to control. In W. R. Miller (Ed.), *Integrating spirituality into treatment* (pp. 179–198). Washington, DC: American Psychological Association.

Csikszentmihalyi, M. (1990). *Flow: The psychology of optimal experience.* New York: Harper & Row.

Davidson, R. J., Kabat-Zinn, J., Schumacher, J., Rosenkrantz, M., Muller, D., Santorelli, S. F., Urbanowski, F., Harrington, A., Bonus, K., & Sheridan, J. F. (2003). Alterations in brain and immune function produced by mindfulness meditation. *Psychosomatic Medicine, 65,* 564–570.

Easwaran, E. (1998). *Mantram handbook* (4th ed.). Tomales, CA: Nilgiri Press. (Original work published 1977)

Fuller, R. C. (2001). *Spiritual, but not religious: Understanding unchurched America.* New York: Oxford University Press.

George, L. K., Ellison, C. G., & Larson, D. B. (2002). Explaining the relationships between religious involvement and health. *Psychological Inquiry, 13,* 190–200.

Goleman, D. (1988). *The meditative mind: The varieties of meditative experience.* New York: Tarcher.

Gorsuch, R. L. (1995). Religious aspects of substance abuse and recovery. *Journal of Social Issues, 51,* 65–83.

Green, E. C. (2003). *Rethinking AIDS prevention.* Westport, CT: Praeger.

Harris, A. H. S., & Thoresen, C. E. (in press). Volunteering is associated with delayed mortality in older people: Analysis of the Longitudinal Study of Aging. *Journal of Health Psychology.*

Hathaway, W. L. (2003). Clinically significant religious impairment. *Mental Health, Religion and Culture, 6,* 113–129.

Hood, R. W., Jr., Ghorbani, N., Watson, P. J., Ghramaleki, A. F., Bing, M. N., Davison, H. K., Morris, R. J., & Williamson, W. P. (2001). Dimensions of the Mysticism Scale: Confirming the three-factor structure in the United States and Iran. *Journal for the Scientific Study of Religion, 40,* 691–705.

Hood, R. W., Spilka, B., Hunsberger, B., & Gorsuch, R. (1996). *The psychology of religion: An empirical approach.* New York: Guilford Press.

Hummer, R. A., Rogers, R. G., Nam, C. B., & Ellison, C. G. (1999). Religious involvement and U.S. adult mortality. *Demography, 36,* 273–285.

James, W. (1961). *The varieties of religious experience: A study in human nature.* New York: Collier. (Original work published 1902)

Jonas, W. B., & Chez, R. A. (2003). The role and importance of definitions and standards in healing research. *Alternative Therapies in Health and Medicine, 9,* A5–A9.

Kalb, C. (2003, November 10). Faith and healing. *Newsweek,* pp. 40–44, 53–54, 56.

Kass, J. D., Friedman, R., Leserman, J., Zuttermeister, P. C., & Benson, H. (1991). Health outcomes and a new index of spiritual experience. *Journal for the Scientific Study of Religion, 30,* 203–211.

Keating, T. (1997). *Open mind, open heart.* New York: Continuum. (Original work published 1986)

Kiang, J. G., Marotta, D., Wirkus, M., & Jonas, W. B. (2002). External bioenergy increases intracellular free calcium concentration and reduces cellular response to heat stress. *Journal of Investigative Medicine, 50,* 38–45.

Kirkpatrick, L. A. (1999). Attachment and religious representations and behavior. In J. Cassidy & P.

R. Shaver (Eds.), *Handbook of attachment: Theory, research, and clinical applications* (pp. 803–822). New York: Guilford Press.

Koenig, H. G. (2000). Religion, spirituality, and medicine: Application to clinical practice. *Journal of the American Medical Association, 284*, 1708.

Koenig, H. G., McCullough, M. E., & Larson, D. B. (2001). *Handbook of religion and health*. New York: Oxford University Press.

Krause, N. (2004). Common facets of religion, unique facets of religion, and life satisfaction among older African Americans. *Journals of Gerontology: Series B, Psychological Sciences and Social Sciences, 59*, S109–S117.

Krause, N., Ingersoll-Dayton, B., Liang, J., & Sugisawa, H. (1999). Religion, social support, and health among the Japanese elderly. *Journal of Health and Social Behavior, 40*, 405–421.

Larson, D. B., Pattison, E. M., Blazer, D. G., Omran, A. R., & Kaplan, B. H. (1986). Systematic analysis of research on religious variables in four major psychiatric journals, 1978–1982. *American Journal of Psychiatry, 143*, 329–334.

Levin, J. S. (1994). Religion and health: Is there an association, is it valid, and is it causal? *Social Science and Medicine, 38*, 1475–1482.

Levin, J. S. (1996a). How prayer heals: A theoretical model. *Alternative Therapies in Health and Medicine, 2*, 66–73.

Levin, J. S. (1996b). How religion influences morbidity and health: Reflections on natural history, salutogenesis and host resistance. *Social Science and Medicine, 43*, 849–864.

Mahoney, A., Pargament, K. I., Tarakeshwar, N., & Swank, A. B. (2001). Religion in the home in the 1980s and 1990s: A meta-analytic review and conceptual analysis of links between religion, marriage, and parenting. *Journal of Family Psychology, 15*, 559–596.

Maunder, R. G., & Hunter, J. J. (2001). Attachment and psychosomatic medicine: Developmental contributions to stress and disease. *Psychosomatic Medicine, 63*, 556–567.

McCullough, M. E., Hoyt, W. T., Larson, D. B., Koenig, H. G., & Thoresen, C. (2000). Religious involvement and mortality: A meta-analytic review. *Health Psychology, 19*, 211–222.

McCullough, M. E., & Larson, D. B. (1999). Prayer. In W. R. Miller (Ed.), *Integrating spirituality into treatment: Resources for practitioners* (pp. 85–110). Washington, DC: American Psychological Association.

McCullough, M. E., Pargament, K. I., & Thoresen, C. E. (Eds.). (2000). *Forgiveness: Theory, research, and practice*. New York: Guilford Press.

McCullough, M. E., & Snyder, C. R. (2000). Classical sources of human strength: Revisiting an old home and building a new one. *Journal of Social and Clinical Psychology, 19*, 1–10.

McEwen, B. S. (1998). Protective and damaging effects of stress mediators. *New England Journal of Medicine, 338*, 171–179.

Miller, W. R., & Thoresen, C. E. (2003). Spirituality, religion, and health: An emerging research field. *American Psychologist, 58*, 24–35.

Murphy, M., Donovan, S., & Taylor, E. (1999). *The physical and psychological effects of meditation: A review of contemporary research with a comprehensive bibliography 1931–1996* (2nd ed.). Sausalito, CA: Institute of Noetic Sciences.

Nakamura, J., & Csikszentmihalyi, M. (2002). The concept of flow. In C. R. Snyder & S. J. Lopez (Eds.), *Handbook of positive psychology* (pp. 89–105). New York: Oxford University Press.

Oman, D., & Driskill, J. D. (2003). Holy name repetition as a spiritual exercise and therapeutic technique. *Journal of Psychology and Christianity, 22*, 5–19.

Oman, D., Hedberg, J., Downs, D., & Parsons, D. (2003). A transcultural spiritually-based program to enhance caregiving self-efficacy: A pilot study. *Complementary Health Practice Review, 8*, 201–224.

Oman, D., Hedberg, J., & Thoresen, C. E. (2005). *Passage meditation reduces stress among health professionals*. Manuscript under review.

Oman, D., Kurata, J. H., Strawbridge, W. J., & Cohen, R. D. (2002). Religious attendance and cause of death over 31 years. *International Journal for Psychiatry in Medicine, 32*, 69–89.

Oman, D., & Reed, D. (1998). Religion and mortality among the community-dwelling elderly. *American Journal of Public Health*, *88*, 1469–1475.

Oman, D., & Thoresen, C. E. (2002). "Does religion cause health?": Differing interpretations and diverse meanings. *Journal of Health Psychology*, *7*, 365–380.

Oman, D., & Thoresen, C. E. (2003a). The many frontiers of spiritual modeling. *The International Journal for the Psychology of Religion*, *13*, 197–213.

Oman, D., & Thoresen, C. E. (2003b). Spiritual modeling: A key to spiritual and religious growth? *The International Journal for the Psychology of Religion*, *13*, 149–165.

Oman, D., & Thoresen, C. E. (2005). Religion, spirituality, and children's physical health. In E. C. Roehlkepartain, P. E. King, L. Wagener, & P. L. Benson (Eds.), *The handbook of spiritual development in childhood and adolescence* (pp. 399–415). Thousand Oaks, CA: Sage.

Oman, D., Thoresen, C. E., Flinders, T., & Flinders, C. (2003, June 9). *Reduced stress and improved spiritual practice self-efficacy from an integrated meditation program*. Paper presented at 5th Meeting on Spiritual Modeling, Santa Clara University, Santa Clara, CA.

Oman, D., Thoresen, C., & McMahon, K. (1999). Volunteerism and mortality among the community-dwelling elderly. *Journal of Health Psychology*, *4*, 301–316.

Osler, W. (1910). The faith that heals. *British Medical Journal*, *2*, 1470–1472.

Pargament, K. I. (1997). *The psychology of religion and coping: Theory, research, practice*. New York: Guilford Press.

Patel, C., Marmot, M. G., Terry, D. J., Carruthers, M., Hunt, B., & Patel, M. (1985). Trial of relaxation in reducing coronary risk: Four year follow up. *British Medical Journal*, *290*, 1103–1106.

Paulsen, A. E. (1926). Religious healing: Preliminary report [series]. *Journal of the American Medical Association*, *86*, 1519–1524, 1617–1623, 1692–1697.

Perry, W. (1991). *A treasury of traditional wisdom*. Cambridge, UK: Quinta Essentia.

Phillips, R. L., Kuzma, J. W., Beeson, W. L., & Lotz, T. (1980). Influence of selection versus lifestyle on risk of fatal cancer and cardiovascular disease among Seventh-Day Adventists. *American Journal of Epidemiology*, *112*, 296–314.

Plante, T. G. (Ed.). (2004). *Sin against the innocents: Sexual abuse by priests and the role of the Catholic Church*. Westport, CO: Praeger.

Post, S. G., Puchalski, C. M., & Larson, D. B. (2000). Physicians and patient spirituality: Professional boundaries, competency, and ethics. *Annals of Internal Medicine*, *132*, 578–583.

Post, S. G., Underwood, L. G., Schloss, J. P., & Hurlbut, W. B. (2002). *Altruism and altruistic love: Science, philosophy, and religion in dialogue*. New York: Oxford University Press.

Powell, L. H., Shahabi, L., & Thoresen, C. E. (2003). Religion and spirituality: Linkages to physical health. *American Psychologist*, *58*, 36–52.

Reindl Benjamins, M., & Brown, C. (2004). Religion and preventative health care utilization among the elderly. *Social Science and Medicine*, *58*, 109–118.

Rhodes, M., & Kristeller, J. L. (2000, August 8). *The OASIS project: Oncologist-assisted spirituality intervention study*. Paper presented at the annual meeting of the American Psychological Association, Washington, DC.

Richards, P. S., & Bergin, A. E. (1997). *A spiritual strategy for counseling and psychotherapy*. Washington, DC: American Psychological Association.

Richards, T. A., Acree, M., & Folkman, S. (1999). Spiritual aspects of loss among partners of men with AIDS: Postbereavement follow-up. *Death Studies*, *23*, 105–127.

Rowatt, W. C., & Kirkpatrick, L. A. (2002). Two dimensions of attachment to God and their relation to affect, religiosity, and personality constructs. *Journal for the Scientific Study of Religion*, *41*, 637–651.

Ryff, C. D., & Singer, B. (1998). The contours of positive human health. *Psychological Inquiry*, *9*, 1–28.

Schwartz, C., Meisenhelder, J. B., Ma, Y., & Reed, G. (2003). Altruistic social interest behaviors are associated with better mental health. *Psychosomatic Medicine*, *65*, 778–785.

Schwartz, C. E., & Sendor, M. (1999). Helping others helps oneself: Response shift effects in peer support. *Social Science and Medicine*, *48*, 1563–1575.

Seeman, T. E., Dubin, L. F., & Seeman, M. (2003). Religiosity/spirituality and health: A critical review of the evidence for biological pathways. *American Psychologist, 58*, 53–63.

Shang, C. (2001). Emerging paradigms in mind–body medicine. *Journal of Alternative and Complementary Medicine, 7*, 83–91.

Shapiro, D. H. (1994). Examining the content and context of meditation: A challenge for psychology in the areas of stress management, psychotherapy, and religion/values. *Journal of Humanistic Psychology, 34*, 101–135.

Sloan, R. P., Bagiella, E., & Powell, T. (1999). Religion, spirituality, and medicine. *The Lancet, 353*, 664–667.

Smith, H. (1976). *Forgotten truth: The primordial tradition*. New York: Harper & Row.

Smith, T. B., McCullough, M. E., & Poll, J. (2003). Religiousness and depression: Evidence for a main effect and the moderating influence of stressful life events. *Psychological Bulletin, 129*, 614–636.

Steffen, P. R., Hinderliter, A. L., Blumenthal, J. A., & Sherwood, A. (2001). Religious coping, ethnicity, and ambulatory blood pressure. *Psychosomatic Medicine, 63*, 523–530.

Strawbridge, W. J., Shema, S. J., Cohen, R. D., & Kaplan, G. A. (2001). Religious attendance increases survival by improving and maintaining good health practices, mental health, and stable marriages. *Annals of Behavioral Medicine, 23*, 68–74.

Targ, E. (1997). Evaluating distant healing: A research review. *Alternative Therapies in Health and Medicine, 3*, 74–78.

Thoits, P. A. (1986). Social support as coping assistance. *Journal of Consulting and Clinical Psychology, 54*, 416–423.

Thoresen, C. E. (1999). Spirituality and health: Is there a relationship? [Special issue on spirituality and health]. *Journal of Health Psychology, 4*, 293–300.

Thoresen, C. E., & Harris, A. H. (2002). Spirituality and health: What's the evidence and what's needed? *Annals of Behavioral Medicine, 24*, 3–13.

Thoresen, C. E., & Harris, A. H. S. (2004). Spirituality, religion, and health: A scientific perspective. In J. M. Raczynski & L. C. Leviton (Eds.), *Handbook of clinical health psychology* (pp. 269–298). Washington, DC: American Psychological Association.

Thoresen, C. E., Oman, D., & Harris, A. H. S. (2005). The effects of religious practices: A focus on health. In W. R. Miller & H. D. Delaney (Eds.), *Human nature, motivation, and change: Judeo-Christian perspectives on psychology* (pp. 205–226). Washington, DC: American Psychological Association.

Tonigan, J. S. (2003, March 21). *Spirituality and AA practices: 10-year Project MATCH follow-up*. Paper presented at the annual meeting of the Society for Behavioral Medicine, Salt Lake City, UT.

Troyer, H. (1988). Review of cancer among 4 religious sects: Evidence that life-styles are distinctive sets of risk factors. *Social Science and Medicine, 26*, 1007–1017.

Underhill, E. (1911). *Mysticism: A study in the nature and development of man's spiritual consciousness* (3rd ed.). New York: Dutton.

Wallace, J. M., Jr., & Forman, T. A. (1998). Religion's role in promoting health and reducing risk among American youth. *Health Education and Behavior, 25*, 721–741.

WHOQOL Group. (1998). The World Health Organization Quality of Life assessment (WHOQOL): Development and general psychometric properties. *Social Science and Medicine, 46*, 1569–1585.

Witvliet, C.v., Ludwig, T. E., & Vander Laan, K. L. (2001). Granting forgiveness or harboring grudges: Implications for emotion, physiology, and health. *Psychological Science, 12*, 117–123.

Woods, T. E., Antoni, M. H., Ironson, G. H., & Kling, D. W. (1999). Religiosity is associated with affective and immune status in symptomatic HIV-infected gay men. *Journal of Psychosomatic Research, 46*, 165–176.

Wuthnow, R. (1998). *After heaven: Spirituality in America since the 1950s*. Berkeley, CA: University of California Press.

25

Relationships of Religiosity and Spirituality with Mental Health and Psychopathology

LISA MILLER
BRIEN S. KELLEY

This chapter's purpose is to delineate the ways in which religiosity and spirituality interact with psychological functioning and buffer against, or exacerbate, mental illness. In addressing religion and mental health, it is important to realize that the absence of pathology does not necessarily imply "mental health," nor does it guarantee happiness or an optimistic worldview, two factors that a spiritual life often imbues in its adherents. Also, the beliefs and practices that characterize a spiritual life fluctuate over the lifespan, waxing and waning in response to life circumstances and developmental progress. For this reason, it is useful to think of religiosity's relationship to psychological health as a developmental process throughout ontogeny. From this perspective, we must consider questions such as:

1. How is religiousness defined and measured in people of different ages, faiths, and cultures?
2. What are the salient features of the beliefs and practices interacting with mental health or pathology?
3. What are the effects of religious and spiritual activity at different ages, and how do these activities affect the protection against, or the expression of, different mental disorders?

In seeking the answers to these questions, we present the relevant literature regarding religiosity, mental health, and psychopathology in a manner that, while not as comprehensive as several recently published literature review articles and books (e.g., Koenig, 1998; Regnerus, Smith, & Fritsch, 2003; Spilka, Hood, Hunsberger, & Gorsuch, 2003), raises questions and suggests refinements of the experimental psychology of religion in two directions, both inexorably connected to issues of mental health and pathology: a more complex developmental theory of life-course religiosity, and a broader perspective that draws from, and is mindful of, cultural differences and the diversity of the world's religious believers.

METHODOLOGICAL AND CONCEPTUAL POINTS OF CONTENTION

Before examining the positive or negative effects of religiosity or spirituality on mental health, it is necessary to briefly address methodological and conceptual issues that have been noted repeatedly throughout the literature. First, results of studies exploring religiosity and spirituality are highly dependent upon the definitions of the constructs being used, and a consensus on the essential features of both (and their differences) is far from achieved (see Hackney & Sanders, 2003; Zinnbauer & Pargament, Chapter 2, this volume). Similarly, researchers' a priori assumptions about what constitutes the religious or spiritual life affect the scales they choose for their investigations, with researchers having hundreds of possibilities to choose from and little in the way of specific theoretical models for guidance (Hill & Hood, 1999; Tsang & McCullough, 2003). Most now agree that these constructs are multidimensional and include a variety of motivational and behavioral elements, and therefore researchers are increasingly using more sensitive and specific measures to address the salient issues in question. Furthermore, there is no clear consensus on what constitutes "mental health," either within the psychology of religion or clinical psychology as a whole; it is accepted as a largely relative construct, though many researchers have wisely explicated their operating assumptions as part of the conceptual foundation supporting their research (e.g., Ventis, 1995).

Second, culture is often extremely important in influencing how people interpret mental illness, characterize the relationship between spirituality and mental health, and determine how that spirituality is organized and practiced in the service of mental health (Al-Issa, 1995). Although primarily discussed in investigations of cultural influence in the psychology of religion, the issue of generalizability is pertinent to all interpretations of empirical results. Borrowing terms from anthropology, the *etic* versus *emic* demarcation is a useful heuristic in attempting to make, or cautioning against, sweeping statements about the potency of religiosity or spirituality in mental health. *Etic* refers to human universals, and is applied to studies that use objective methods that are presumed to be consistent across cultural differences. In contrast, *emic* is an "experience-close" frame of reference, in which pure objectivity and universality are seen as unattainable and unrealistic upon detailed inquiry, and therefore the subjective impressions of those studied *and* those studying receive paramount attention. These latter studies are more idiographic or qualitative, and deal with particulars, such as examining the role of African American religious folk-healing strategies (Parks, 2003), or evaluating the influence of specific religious activities, like *dhikr* in the Muslim faith (Al-Issa, 2000b). As noted by Al-Issa (2000a), it is nearly impossible to conduct a study that takes either position in its pure form. Any question and all answers are contextual and thus relative, and derive meaning from comparison and specificity; the best that can be asked of researchers at this stage in the burgeoning field of psychology of religion is an explicit awareness of these issues to safeguard against misinterpretation of results or an overly narrow focus that contributes little to the goals of empirical science.

Related to this issue, scholars are divided over the primary mechanisms of religious and spiritual influence on mental health. Some postulate a sui generis quality of religious belief and practice, something above and beyond the secular variables that inform any belief system or behavior pattern (e.g., Smith, 2003). Others find religious variables reducible to factors that have been previously hypothesized to buttress mental health, such as explanatory style, positive emotions, or most commonly, socialization (e.g., Fredrickson, 2002; Wallace & Williams, 1997). This often involves the search for secular mediator and moderator variables that may influence or determine the relationship between religiosity and mental health. Which operating mechanisms are studied is an issue that dovetails with the discussions of measurement and of methodology presented by Hill (Chapter 3, this volume) and by Hood and Belzen (Chapter 4, this volume). Results presented in this chapter should be viewed through the prism of the conceptual and practical choices made by the researchers in order to best understand each author's specific contribution to the field.

DIRECTIONALITY OF THE RELATIONSHIP

In teasing apart the multiplicity of influences on mental health, it quickly becomes clear that a consistent, robust, and unidirectional relationship between mental health and religiosity or spirituality is an illusion—the reality is far more subtle and complex. Researchers are often forced to pin down a narrow spectrum of religious variables and compare those with ranges of clinical symptomatology or health indicators. In this way, correlations can be found that point statistically to either a positive or a negative relationship. However, a moment of introspection (for the religious) or creative imagination (for those less sure) is all that is necessary to realize that "religion" works in mysterious and dynamic ways–over one person's lifespan, religion might be magical in childhood, a social network in adolescence, a factor in choosing a life-mate and childrearing in adulthood, and a solace in old age. Therefore, a one-time measure of church attendance or a Likert-scale rating of belief cannot capture the essence of religion's fluid and reciprocal influence.

A more sophisticated analysis of correlational data can indicate a curvilinear relationship between religious variables and mental health outcomes over the life course (Ingersoll-Dayton, Krause, & Morgan, 2002), on depressive expression (Schnittker, 2001), death anxiety (Pressman, Lyons, Larson, & Gartner, 1992), general anxiety disorders (Koenig, Ford, George, Blazer, & Meador, 1993), and overall distress (Ross, 1990). In some of these studies, nonbelievers, and, on the opposite end of the spectrum, those in whom religion is an extremely potent and orienting factor in their lives show the most favorable association with mental health outcomes. In others, those at the far ends of the religious continuum are the most susceptible to suffering, and those that adhere to a more moderate practice or belief system show better functioning. The linearity of association between mental health and religiosity has not been established, though this makes intuitive sense when interpreting the interaction from a developmental perspective throughout the lifespan.

Furthermore, while the direction of association is far from clear, so too is the direction of causality. It might be that happier and healthier people gravitate to worship, communal activity, or divine appreciation, as opposed to religion or spirituality in itself causing well-being. Determining temporal and causal precedence is all but impossible in correlational research, but longitudinal and large, epidemiological survey studies do suggest the latter (e.g., Kendler, Gardner, & Prescott, 1997; Levin & Taylor, 1998).

SALIENT DIMENSIONS OF RELIGIOSITY FOR MENTAL HEALTH

Although it is now accepted that religiosity and spirituality are multidimensional constructs, it is difficult, yet very necessary, to specify exactly which dimensions are assessed by any one study, and to have theoretical justification for expecting that dimension (or dimensions) to interact with specific symptoms or mental health outcomes. Leading researchers acknowledge this necessity, and most suggest dimensional paradigms that overlap with those posed by others in the field (e.g., Kendler et al., 2003). These commonly include factors such as identity constituents, motivation, prayer or ritual practice, social support, some type of personal devotion or feeling of closeness to the divine, explanatory style, and intensity of belief (Hodges, 2002; Levin & Chatters, 1998). Each of these components can influence mental health, and their variety requires researchers to clearly define and assess the constructs being investigated. For instance, Kendler and colleagues (2003) found that dimensions such as social religiosity and thankfulness, as well as unvengefulness, protected against internalizing disorders, while general religiosity, conceptions of an involved and judging God, and forgiveness protected against externalizing disorders (e.g., substance abuse), illustrating the differential effect of distinct components of religiosity on psychopathological symptoms.

One well-investigated heuristic in the psychology of religion is the extrinsic, intrinsic, quest formulation of religious orientation (Allport & Ross, 1967; Ventis, 1995; Donahue & Nielsen, Chapter 15, this volume). "Extrinsic religiosity" refers to a "means" approach, in which a person uses religion as the means to some secular end, like ego reinforcement or social approval, and is generally found to correlate with higher levels of psychological distress, less effective coping abilities, and a higher likelihood of prejudice, intolerance, and socially inappropriate behavior (see Batson, Schoenrade, & Ventis, 1993, for a meta-analysis of the literature, and Ventis, 1995, for a discussion of consequences; also see Smith, McCullough, & Poll, 2003). In contrast, "intrinsic religiosity" refers to an "ends" orientation, in which the belief and practice of the religious life *is* the goal; this style of worship is related to greater well-being, more realistic and effective coping, and more appropriate social behavior (Batson et al., 1993; Ventis, 1995). "Quest," on the other hand, a relative newcomer to the literature, refers to those adherents that continually question and challenge their beliefs in an effort to make sense of the world they are confronted with (Batson et al., 1993). The elements of skepticism and doubt that can accompany the quest orientation can account for the mixed findings regarding this outlook's relation to mental health: such uncertainty could lead to anxiety and such doubts to depression, while the questing search can also be experienced as a rewarding spiritual path in which beliefs are refined in response to the world, and not merely to Scripture or other forms of dogmatic certainty (which could account for the positive association between the quest orientation and open-mindedness) (Batson et al., 1993). These three religious orientations have been studied extensively with a diverse set of samples, personality variables, and individual differences. However, scholars have expressed doubts about these constructs, noting their simplicity, their failure to account for combinations of orientations, and the Judeo-Christian context of the orientations to which they refer (e.g., Kirkpatrick & Hood, 1990).

RELIGIOSITY/SPIRITUALITY, POSITIVE PSYCHOLOGY, AND WELL-BEING RESEARCH

This chapter considers the different ways that religion and spirituality interact with and influence mental health, well-being, and psychopathology. These broad constructs cover the full spectrum of human psychological functioning, from the happiest of exalted states to the most pervasive and dysfunctional of psychoses. The science of well-being, or "hedonic psychology" seeks to elucidate "what makes experiences and life pleasant or unpleasant," and takes a strength-based approach to framing the discussion of mental health (Kahneman, Diener, & Schwarz, 1999, p. ix). Although this positive stance is a relatively recent zeitgeist in academic psychology, William James pondered and elucidated the association between religious faith and "healthy-mindedness" at the turn of the 20th century (James, 1902/1985).

Overall, the preponderance of empirical research and clinical wisdom suggests that religion has a positive influence on mental health and functioning (e.g., Levin & Chatters, 1998). This goes beyond the mere absence of psychopathology or suffering to include such positive traits as general happiness, satisfaction with life, constructing meaning and life goals, and other, more objective outcomes such as longevity, education, and income (Chamberlain & Zika, 1992; Ferriss, 2002). Kim (2003) summarizes the relevant research and theoretical writings by proposing five distinct yet interrelated models of influence that often guide understanding of the relationship between religiosity and well-being. Most of these models are considered by Park in her discussion of meaning issues (Chapter 16, this volume), and by Oman and Thoresen in their examination of religiosity's impact on physical health (Chapter 24, this volume).

Kahneman et al.'s (1999) landmark edited volume, Well-Being: The Foundations of Hedonic Psychology, devotes only two pages (of 572) to religion or spirituality, although Argyle's (1999) review concisely sums up the prevailing conclusions of relevant investigations: "happiness is greater for those who are more religious, however this is assessed, though the effect is often small" (p. 365). Argyle concludes that social support accounts for most of the impact of religiosity on well-being, and hypothesizes that the atmosphere of love and the ideology of brotherhood, along with the interpretive power of religion to frame rites of passage in a communal way, accounts for that social potency. Furthermore, a subjective feeling of closeness to God is pointed to (what the present authors and other researchers conceptualize as *personal devotion*) as a primary mechanism, as is "existential certainty."

NEGATIVE EFFECTS OF RELIGION OR SPIRITUALITY ON MENTAL HEALTH

Although most studies indicate a protective effect of religiosity or spirituality on mental health, there is evidence that some religious configurations can inflame psychopathological expression or even contribute to its etiology (e.g., see Exline & Rose, Chapter 17, and Paloutzian, Chapter 18, this volume). Indeed, for every diagnostic disorder we consider there are at least a few studies that display a positive correlation between religious belief or activity and pathological symptoms. Some examples of these exceptions include the possibility of reinforcing deluded beliefs and exacerbating guilt and worry, actually constituting psychopathological expression (through excessive ritual, glossolalia, delusions of persecution or reference, etc.), or perpetuating mental illness by providing a structured framework from which to interpret the pathological symptoms in ways that preclude seeking treatment for the disorder (e.g., Askin, Paultre, White, & Van Ornum, 1993; Prince, 1992). Furthermore, mystical states or religious experiences are often difficult to distinguish from psychotic behavior or hallucinations, with the final conclusion likely to reflect the effect of the experience, such that if it was pleasurable or meaningful, then it was a mystical experience, while if it was distressing or uncultivated, it is thought to be pathological in nature (Eeles, Lowe, & Wellman, 2003; Hood, Chapter 19, this volume). Additionally, many elements of sudden religious conversion can be related to a weakened sense of ego or identity, psychopathological symptomatology, or existential anxiety (Hunter, 1998; James, 1902/1985; Zinnbauer & Pargament, 1998). Finally, while some evidence points to increased optimism and subjective well-being among very religious (fundamentalist Christians, Orthodox Jews, etc.) adherents, there is a body of research that suggests that overly rigid orientations can have negative ramifications, such as bigotry, homophobia, and general intolerance of others' beliefs (e.g., Altemeyer & Hunsberger, Chapter 21, this volume; Ferriss, 2002; Sethi & Seligman, 1991).

RELIGION AND SPIRITUALITY IN CHILDREN: EFFECTS ON MENTAL HEALTH

While research on the effects of religion and spirituality on mental health is increasing and becoming more refined, there is a lack of empirical study of those effects on children (Spilka et al., 2003). Benson, Roehlkepartain, and Rude (2003) surveyed the social sciences databases and found that less than 1% of articles on children or adolescents examined spirituality or spiritual development. Studies have found a negative relationship between religiosity and psychotic symptoms in children (Francis, 1994), as well as symptoms of depression (Miller, Warner, Wickramatne, & Weissman, 1997) and anxiety (Schapman & Inderbitzen-Nolan, 2002), although here again there are a few exceptions to these generalizations. In these circumstances, authors often point to a restrictive and rigid authoritarian religious parenting style, in which guilt and excessively proscribed behavior influence a still-malleable worldview (e.g., Josephson, 1993). However, even if religiously conservative families are more likely to use threats or physical punishment, they are also more likely to hug and praise their children (Wilcox, 1998). Moreover, the similarly conservative congregation that commonly accompanies such strong personal beliefs likely produces a positive sense of community and social support (Mahoney & Tarakeshwar, Chapter 10, this volume). There is evidence that depression suffered in childhood can lead to decreased or distorted forms of religiosity in adulthood, which may suggest that a foundation of psychological well-being is necessary in childhood to engender strong and protective spiritual or religious adherence as adults (Miller, Weissman, Gur, & Adams, 2002).

Several theoretically derived, developmental stage models exist, in which the transitions of childhood and young adulthood, along with social and intellectual integration, are examined through the prism of religious involvement or complexity of belief (see Sperry, 2001, for a review of these models, as well as Boyatzis, Chapter 7, this volume). This developmental paradigm, then, is the exact opposite of what is found in the psychology of religion overall: for children and adolescents, much is viewed developmentally but lacks empirical investigation, while the body of the adult research is too often seen in snapshot, cross-sectional focus, with little developmental activity accounted for (Gorsuch, 1988).

Viewed from the perspective of the family, children have been found to be closer to mothers who report attending church more often (Pearce & Axinn, 1998), a factor that also contributes to higher satisfaction with life in the child (Varon & Riley, 1999). Religious families in general have been found to exert influence through the types of discipline and religious interpretation they use (see Spilka et al., 2003, for a review). However, since children whose mothers suffer from depression have been shown to display lower levels of religiosity, and since specifically depressogenic forms of spirituality have been found in the adult offspring of depressed mothers, it may be that growing up in an environment deficient in hope and happiness distorts the child's sense of the spiritual (Gur, Miller, & Weissman, 2004). Kirkpatrick and Shaver (1990) postulate a "compensation hypothesis," in which children who are reared with insecure attachment styles with their parents find solace in the notion of a loving and personal God; this seems to be especially relevant to children from nonreligious homes, and has received some empirical support.

Conversely, Glass, Bengtson, and Dunham (1986) showed that the spirituality of children from nonreligious homes was often higher than that of their parents, and that the child's spirituality may impact adults as readily as the reverse, implying that the origin of childhood spirituality is not entirely a socialization process, but could be either innate or an extension of other types of supernatural thinking. With respect to possible innateness, there is empirical support for the notion of inherent spirituality or religiosity, especially concerning the construct of personal devotion. Kendler and colleagues' (1997) study found that the dimension of a personal sense of connection to God correlated moderately ($r = .33$) with close adherence to a religious creed and weakly ($r = .18$) with religious denomination, suggesting that a strong spiritual connection to God exists both within and outside communal religious observance. Furthermore, in this study, an analysis of the heritable versus the environmental contribution to between-person variance showed that 29% of the difference between women endorsing items reflecting personal devotion can be explained by broad heritability. To the extent that differences among us are explained by heredity, the very entity itself appears to be part of our fundamental nature, providing some genetic evidence for the existence of inherent spirituality. D'Onofrio, Eaves, Murrelle, Maes, and Spilka (1999) expanded on this study with 14,781 twins from the "Virginia 30,000" epidemiological data set, and found that though affiliation is a culturally transmitted process, religious attitudes and practices are moderately influenced by genetic factors (accounting for 40–50% of the variance in religiosity), above and beyond personality trait variables. Miller, Weissman, Gur, and Adams's (2001) study of the spirituality of children of opiate addicts showed that the children were eight times more likely to endorse spirituality as personally important than were their mothers, suggesting that the children either held independent and possibly innate connections to a spiritual reality, or that they had "cast a wide net" across religious and spiritual experiences with abusing and nonabusing adults, essentially using selective religious socialization, and had ultimately assimilated healthy understandings of spirituality.

Regarding the later interpretation of the Glass et al.'s (1986) finding presented above, children have been found to exhibit an extensive range of magical thinking, and these supernatural ideas or assumptions are often religious in nature, or co-opt religious formulations from the adult milieu surrounding the child (Rosengren & Johnson, 2000). Whether these often literal beliefs are soothing to the child's psyche or a source of anxiety is likely determined by the support and interpretation they are given by the parental and community dynamic. So, while the empirical data is at times contradictory or ambiguous regarding the protective effects of religiosity or spirituality in children, the majority of the few studies that examine this relationship suggest that a religious family or belief system is an effective buffer against many types of childhood psychopathology, which is consistent with clinical, anecdotal reports of childhood spiritual and religious coping.

RELIGION AND SPIRITUALITY IN ADOLESCENCE: EFFECTS ON MENTAL HEALTH

Adolescence is a "stage" of life in which a sense of self and identity begins to crystallize and the social/peer group usurps influence from the family dynamic. Also, unfortunately, it is a time in which many psychiatric disorders have their root and the first indications of disturbance appear—creating a window of risk for concurrent and future psychopathology or deviance. Adolescence is therefore a fertile period for the study of religion, spirituality, and mental health, as recent review reports (Regnerus et al., 2003) and issues of peer-reviewed journals (King & Boyatzis, 2004) can attest. Adding to the complications of studying religiosity and spirituality in children, empirical research with adolescents must be interpreted within a larger contextual framework, as teens are far more susceptible to peer and cultural influence than are children.

In general, religious belief and involvement have been found to exert salutary effects on the psychological functioning of teens in domains as diverse as academic performance, subjective well-being, self-esteem, and motivation toward civic involvement, as well as in fostering healthy lifestyles (Batson et al., 1993; Cochran, 1992; Wallace & Forman, 1998). Religious adolescents also suffer from fewer depressive or anxious symptoms, are at lesser risk for suicide, and overwhelmingly reject promiscuous or premarital sex and delinquent behaviors such as drug or alcohol abuse (Regnerus et al., 2003; Smith & Faris, 2003; Wallace & Williams, 1997). In terms of psychological well-being, Smith and Faris (2003) report that 12th graders who attend church once a week or to whom religion is very important are more likely than nonbelievers or nonattenders to "have positive attitudes towards themselves . . . feel hopeful about the future . . . feel like life is meaningful, and enjoy being in school" (p. 5). Reasons for these effects can often reduce to the dual function of religion and spirituality as a major constituent and foundation of identity formation, and the related self-selection of a peer group that mutually reinforces prosocial and healthy lifestyles (see Levenson & Aldwin, Chapter 8, this volume). Regnerus et al. (2003) reiterate a focus on adolescent religiosity that includes development and culture in order to understand the individual's own developmental processes and changing worldview, while situating that ontogeny within a broader, culturally sensitive frame of reference.

Among the myriad variables studied with respect to resilience in adolescence, the most consistently protective appear to be the previously described combination of personal devotion and spiritual or religious social support. Religious social support has been understood as unique for its level of acceptance of the individual, a quality that must be reassuring during the transitions and individuation that characterize the adolescent years (Oman & Reed, 1998). Religious social support also may derive potency from interpersonal religious experience, a collective experience of the divine, or simply from the spiritually mindful treatment of one another (Miller et al., 2002). These two factors have been shown to be far more protective than other, more secular variables. For instance, a strong sense of personal devotion is 80% protective against depression among adolescents at high risk and 65% protective against onset of heavy substance use in adolescence (Miller, Davies, & Greenwald, 2000), far exceeding the magnitude of 10–30% found for social functioning and cognitive style (Hammen, 1992; Reivich & Gillham, 2003).

RELIGION AND SPIRITUALITY AND ADULT PSYCHOPATHOLOGY

The DSM-IV-TR now includes a catch-all category of a "condition that may be a focus of clinical attention" that addresses religious or spiritual problems (V62.89) (American Psychiatric Association, 2000). These problems include "distressing experiences that involve loss or questioning of faith, problems associated with conversion to a new faith, or questioning of spiritual values." Although these crises can stand alone as a pathological condition, religion and spirituality can also influence the expression of the more prevalent Axis I mental disorders. A brief and selective review of the literature, broken down by clinical disorder, constitutes the next section of our discussion.

Mood Disorders

Depression is by far the most studied clinical disorder in relation to religiosity and spirituality, with good reason, as most religions seek fundamentally to impart hope, happiness, and a fulfilling worldview in their adherents in ways antithetical to depressive symptomatology. Smith and colleagues (2003) found a statistically reliable and highly robust inverse association of modest effect size (similar to the association between gender and depressive symptoms) between religious involvement and depressive symptoms in a meta-analysis covering 147 studies that used close to 99,000 subjects, confirming the conclusions drawn by other researchers who have reviewed the literature (e.g., McCullough & Larson, 1999). This association was not moderated by age, gender, or ethnicity, but was affected by measure of religiousness used (church attendance, frequency of prayer, etc.). It seems that religiosity is generally protective against suicidality among adolescents and adults, across many world religions (e.g., Al-Issa, 1995; Regnerus et al., 2003). Factors that have been suggested to affect the protective influence of religiosity on depression include genetic influence, developmental and familial dynamics, social support, event appraisal, stress coping, and others (e.g., Smith et al., 2003). Both Smith and colleagues (2003) and Kendler, Gardner, and Prescott (1999) found support for both a main effect of religiosity on depressive symptoms and a buffering effect, which suggests that religious factors gain protective or ameliorative potency as life stress increases.

In contrast to the many studies that found a positive association between religious social support (or church attendance) and treatment outcomes (i.e., reduction of symptoms), Loewenthal, Cinnirella, Evdoka, and Murphy (2001) found that private beliefs and activities that indicate high personal devotion, such as faith and prayer, were *perceived* as the most helpful in coping with depression compared with more social religious mechanisms, although some denominational differences were found (between Christians, Jews, Hindus, and Muslims). Interestingly, although personal devotion was viewed as effective, subjects perceived religious coping as less effective than counseling or medication, and those who had been depressed at some point considered it to be less effective than those who had never been depressed, suggesting either a preventative effect for religious activity or the destructive power of learned skepticism on religious coping.

Much more investigation of religiosity and spirituality's relation to affective disorders *other* than major depression needs to occur before any generalizations can be made. Clinical experience and inpatient treatment have long associated religious delusions of grandeur and persecution with the affective and verbal overflow typical of manic patients. Wilson (1998) notes that religious experiences can "precipitate an attack of mania," and that common manic symptoms such as delusions and hurried, anxious speech can often include religious elements. Mitchell and Romans (2002) investigated 147 outpatient subjects with bipolar affective disorder in remission. They found that 78% of patients held strong religious or spiritual beliefs, and 81.5% practiced their religion frequently. Furthermore, most perceived a direct link between their religiosity and religious coping techniques and the management of their symptoms, even when those beliefs and practices contradicted medical models of etiology or treatment. It seems that, like religion's relation to other mental disorders, religiosity is generally protective against psychopathology, and helpful in facing symptoms, but when that pathology does occur, the religious often incorporate religious elements into their symptomatic presentation.

Anxiety Disorders

Reviews of the literature on religiosity and psychopathology reveal a smaller relationship between anxiety and religiosity, and in the opposite direction from depression—people who are more anxious may also be more religious, although this does not necessarily mean that those who are religious are more susceptible to anxiety. It is likely that strong religious beliefs impart a confidence surrounding existential issues, but those less sure of their beliefs or who actively question those beliefs may be more likely to be anxious about them (Harris, Schoneman, & Carrera, 2002). There is some evidence that studies that find a positive association between religiosity and anxiety disorders are too general and fail to account for other salient variables. In two studies conducted by Koenig and colleagues in 1993 (Koenig, Ford, et al., 1993; Koenig, George, Blazer, Pritchett, & Meador, 1993), the relationship between the two variables disappeared when social support, chronic illness, low socioeconomic status, and greater disability were accounted for. For the most reliable investigation of religiosity's relation to anxiety it is recommended that measures that gauge intrinsic orientation be used. Research has exposed sex differences in the ability of religiosity to moderate anxiety among teenagers (Davis, Kerr, & Kurpius, 2003). In a controlled clinical study, healthy subjects were more likely to report that religion could make a person sick than subjects with mood or anxiety disorders (Pfeifer & Waelty, 1999). The clinically diagnosed anxious or depressed subjects experienced religion as a support, but perceived their symptoms as interfering with the expression of their faith.

Death anxiety seems a pertinent and viable area of concern in the study of religion and mental distress. Research done in the United States and abroad points to denominational differences, as well as to differences between religiosity versus spirituality's effects on anxiety surrounding death (e.g., Abdel-Khalek, 2003; Al-Issa, 2000b; Thorson, 1998). Although this kind of research is commonly conducted among elderly samples, and less frequently with college students, anxiety surrounding what happens after death can occur at any point during the life course. Researchers studying death anxiety often conclude that culture and cultural norms have just as strong an impact as religious belief or religious involvement on existential anxiety, raising questions about cultural confounds in other areas of empirical research with religion.

Schizophrenia-Spectrum Disorders

Wilson (1998) proposed that since schizophrenia is predominantly biologically determined, religion and spirituality exert influence more in the expression of symptomatology (delusions and hallucinations, and subsequent behaviors) and in coping with the disorder than in actual etiology. One often-cited study found no difference in rates of delusions in German and Japanese schizophrenics, but did find that Germans had significantly more religious delusions (21.3%) than did the Japanese (6.8%), mostly as the result of cultural factors mediating between religious variables and psychopathology (Tateyama et al., 1993).

In a study from the United Kingdom, religious delusions or hallucinations were relatively common among patients admitted to the hospital for schizophrenia (24%); those evidencing religious delusions had higher symptom scores, functioned less well, and were prescribed more medication than those without religious symptoms (Siddle, Haddock, Tarrier, & Faragher, 2002). Other researchers have found that religious delusions can precipitate self-harm, are held more strongly than secular delusions, and are associated with poorer outcomes from treatment (see Siddle et al., 2002, for a review). Atallah, El-Dosoky, Coker, Nabil, and El-Islam (2001) analyzed decades of Egyptian medical and impatient records and discovered that the prevalence of religious symptoms closely paralleled the fluctuating religious fundamentalism in Egypt, such that in more religious periods more schizophrenics presented with religious symptoms, and in more liberal periods those rates decreased. These findings suggest that the content of delusions and hallucinations is sensitive to the cultural, political, and religious climate the sufferer is embedded within. Future research should take these dimensions into account when exploring the association between religiosity and psychotic disorders.

Obsessive–Compulsive Disorder

Most studies find ambiguous results for the influence of religiosity in obsessive–compulsive disorder (OCD) symptomatology, often concluding that religious rituals *can* constitute the obsessions and compulsions of patients with OCD, but there is little evidence that religious adherents are universally *more* susceptible to the disorder (e.g., Raphael, Rani, Bale, & Drummund, 1996). Greenberg and Witztum (1994) found that religious symptoms are quite common in ultra-Orthodox Jews. They explained this finding by noting that religion provides the setting for the disorder in highly religious outpatients, who are more likely to subscribe to the emphasis on ritual-based purity found in Jewish dietary law and daily practice. This manifestation of OCD is often investigated as "religious scrupulosity." Greenberg and Shefler (2002) have argued that pathological religious obsessions are distinguishable from religious rites or rituals by the distress they cause to individuals and those individuals' resistance to change. Research has shown that adherents of a particular faith are more likely to see a religious leader or counselor for religious compulsion problems and a secular therapist for more general obsessions and compulsions, indicating that the two types, religious and secular, are experienced differently and consciously by sufferers (Hermesh, Masser-Kavitzky, & Gross-Isseroff, 2003). Islam and Orthodox Judaism are both very ritualistic traditions, and the frequency of religious obsessions and compulsions has been found to be greater among Muslim and Jewish adherents in Middle Eastern countries than their European and American, Catholic and Protestant counterparts (Greenberg & Witztum, 1994; Mahgoub & Abdel-Hafeiz, 1991).

CULTURAL INFLUENCES IN THE RELATIONSHIP
BETWEEN RELIGION/SPIRITUALITY AND MENTAL HEALTH

The cultural component of the interaction between religiosity or spirituality and mental health is implicit in many theoretical discussions of the topic, and is not to be underestimated, even though it is one of the newer topics in the field to receive empirical attention. Culture can be examined in a number of ways, including focusing similar types of correlational studies on specific cultural groups, using large epidemiological studies to compare demographic data, and conducting more ideographic or qualitative investigations. There are also studies that seek to apply U.S. academic paradigms of religious–psychological interaction to international populations or diverse religious systems (see Al-Issa, 2000a for a review of such studies and a discussion of their merits and shortcomings). Findings from these very different types of investigation are ambiguous and often run counter to what is typically found among U.S. Judeo-Christian, white subjects, and hence serve as a caution against interpreting empirical results as human universals from which to assert the pros and cons of different lifestyles and worldviews.

Researchers point to cultural differences in rates of religious delusions, hallucinations, or "visions," and the preponderance of certain types of rituals that resemble OCD, as evidence that culture plays a large role in the interaction between religiosity or spirituality and mental health and disorder. The particular modes of expression and praxis encouraged by each of the world's religions highly influence the daily lives of their adherents, and therefore the manifestation of the adherents' symptoms—so, it becomes a challenge for researchers to tease apart the influence of culture from the doctrinally based differences of each respective religion practiced within those cultures (Tarakeshwar, Stanton, & Pargament, 2003). Furthermore, Western psychotherapy is predominantly a European and American phenomenon, and there are broad swaths of the world in which religion is the primary etiological framework from which to think about mental illness, as well as the primary mechanism for symptom alleviation. This raises questions, too, about culturally sensitive definitions of "mental health"; in some African communities a person would be considered insane *not* to believe that the spirits of the dead actively influence an individual's life (Boyer, 2001), whereas that same conviction would be a sign of a major thought disorder in the United States.

Ritual is an important facet of religious life, and yet when unchecked or overly emphasized can metastasize into OCD-like presentation. As noted, Muslims and Orthodox Jews have been found to more rigidly and excessively practice certain rituals, which are emphasized from birth and which are invested with religious importance, but can border on psychopathology in certain predisposed people. The idea of *waswaas*, or the whispering of the devil, can disrupt a devout Muslim's prayer ritual and force numerous repetitions of cleaning and absolution (Pfeiffer, 1982); in India, purity mania (or *suci bhay*) can arise out of Hinduism's focus on ritual purity, and can severely delimit what a person can touch and can require holy water blessings that interfere with daily life (Chakraborty & Banerji, 1975). Again, the ritual cleaning necessary to prepare for *salat* (five times a day) prayer in Islam can be taken too far; this phenomena has been encountered in Saudi Arabia, Egypt, and Qatar, suggesting that religious prescription is exerting more influence than cultural variables, as the cultural environment is quite different in those countries (Mahgoub & Abdel-Hafeiz, 1991; Okasha, Saad, Khalil, El-Dawla, & Yahia, 1994). Similarly, beliefs in spirit possession, ghosts, and anthropomorphized ritual objects are common throughout many parts of the world, leading some theorists to posit cognitive and/

or neural underpinnings to certain types of religious belief (e.g., Boyer, 2001). These are but a few examples of the ways "psychopathology" can manifest through the religious convictions and behaviors of adherents of diverse world religions.

Furthermore, the less accepting a culture or faith is of Western notions of empirical, medical science, the less likely it is that its people or adherents will seek out psychotherapy or psychopharmacological treatment. In one study, Muslims in the United Kingdom endorsed all types of religious activity as more efficacious in coping with depression, above and beyond other, more Western treatments, and far surpassing the depressed of other faiths investigated (Loewenthal et al., 2001). Al-Issa's (2000b) description of indigenous therapeutic methods in the Arab-Muslim world confirm this—folk remedies and religious prescriptions administered by the local *imam*, or religious leader, are far more likely to be used by a Muslim practitioner, even as psychology in Muslim communities often takes the form of religious therapy (e.g., El-Islam & Ahmed, 1971).

Ways that religion might be used in the process of therapy are beyond the scope of this chapter (see Shafranske, Chapter 27, this volume), but suffice it to say that different types of psychotherapeutic discourse and techniques are needed within different cultures or when treating patients of different religious and spiritual beliefs. Pargament, Poloma, and Tarakeshwar (2001) outlined the psychological potency of several religious practices and beliefs, such as *karma*, spiritual healing, and rituals like the bar/bat mitzvah. A familiarity with the effective uses of these and other religious beliefs and practices is critical for a therapist seeking to utilize religion in a clinical setting. This partial review of the cultural influence between religiosity and mental health was meant to impart the realization that the relationship between the two broad constructs is particular to person, place, denomination, and time, meaning that much more cross-cultural research must take place in order to understand the role of specific theologies, practices, and ethnicities in impacting mental health.

CONCLUSION

Research in the psychology of religion indicates that religiosity and spirituality contribute to mental health, can be subverted or distorted to influence psychopathology, and are expressed and related to psychological functioning differently depending on the culture and specific religion studied. This chapter has sought to caution against the overgeneralization of results across religious group or culture. Though researchers consider themselves to be studying "religion" or "spirituality," the actual studies they have conducted tend to elucidate the nature of a very narrow spectrum of the whole of human religiousness. If conclusions are to be made regarding this possibly universal human impulse to believe in the unverifiable, and the psychological consequences of these beliefs and the practices they engender, research must be conducted outside the United States with populations from non-Abrahamic religions.

A corollary to this call for the broadening of the field is the need for the theoretical to catch up with the empirical—associations and mechanisms receive replication after replication without proper theoretical justification or exposition of exactly why or how these factors relate. This requires methodological diversification, including increases in longitudinal and qualitative investigations. If each person's mental health, and his or her degree and manifestation of religiosity, vary throughout the life course, it only makes sense to unpack that fluctuating association from a developmental perspective, and in ways that give full credence to the individual's personal narrative. A careful consideration of the results of such studies would exponentially increase our ability to accurately theorize, and hence uncover the causal mechanisms and relationships that underlie the interdependence between mental health and religious or spiritual belief. An example of this confluence of the qualitative and the theoretical is the topic of religious scrupulosity and anxiety. Several case studies of Orthodox Jews have been published, exploring in depth their worries and compulsions and the relationship between those symptoms and their religious beliefs (e.g., Hoffnung, Aizenberg, Hermesh, & Munitz, 1989). This has in turn driven theory to postulate a more complex interaction between praxis and pathology, such that well-designed and controlled clinical studies have since been performed to quantify and replicate that proposed relationship (e.g., Greenberg & Shefler, 2002; Hermesh et al., 2003).

Although scholars in the psychology of religion have bemoaned the lack of attention to religious and spiritual variables (e.g., Larson & Larson, 1994) in the broader field of academic psychology, there is actually a large body of research and writings on the subject, one that has expanded exponentially within the last 15–20 years. Clinical work is growing more accepting of the religious dimension of life, and researchers have begun to consider distorted or atrophied spirituality or religious belief as a component in the etiological constellation of many psychiatric disorders (specifically depression and substance abuse). For the field to better consider the function and range of religious belief, more attention must be paid to the nonbelievers, those who are happy and healthy *without* reference to the divine or the spiritual. Clinically, conceptualizations such as Richards and Bergin's (1997) "Spirit of Truth" may help spiritually minded therapists surmount denominational differences by acknowledging the suppositions at the root of many world religions: people exist in a living, dynamic universe, and their behavior is best rewarded by adhering to social principles such as honoring commitments and kinship, showing compassion to those in need, and caring for the well-being of the planet and its inhabitants, as well as by embracing existential principles such as believing in a meaning and purpose to life (these correspond to the personal devotion and social support dimensions so often exposed as being the most beneficial from the empirical literature). Both atheists and the full spectrum of believers can often agree on such formulations, indicating the degree to which the study of spirituality and religion is often, at its most elemental *and* expansive, the study of what makes humankind most happy and healthy, loving and just. While this chapter has proffered many distinctions, and coupled each theme with its caveats, this fundamental core of belief, behavior, and community underlies inquiries of both mental health and the spiritual life, rendering their reflexive influence difficult to articulate, but ultimately the most natural thing in the world.

REFERENCES

Abdel-Khalek, A. M. (2003). Death anxiety in Spain and five Arab countries. *Psychological Reports*, *93*(2), 527–528.

Al-Issa, I. (1995). Culture and mental illness in an international perspective. In I. Al-Issa (Ed.), *Culture and mental illness: An international perspective* (pp. 3–49). Madison, CT: International Universities Press.

Al-Issa, I. (Ed.). (2000a). *Al-Junuun: Mental illness in the Islamic world*. Madison, CT: International Universities Press.

Al-Issa, I. (2000b). Does the Muslim religion make a difference in psychopathology? In I. Al-Issa (Ed.), *Al-Junuun: Mental illness in the Islamic world* (pp. 315–353). Madison, CT: International Universities Press.

Allport, G. W., & Ross, J. M. (1967). Personal religious orientation and prejudice. *Journal of Personality and Social Psychology, 5,* 432–433.

American Psychiatric Association. (2000). *Diagnostic and statistical manual of mental disorders* (4th ed., text rev.). Washington, DC: Author.

Argyle, M. (1999). Causes and correlates of happiness. In D. Kahneman, E. Diener, & N. Schwarz (Eds.), *Well-being: The foundations of hedonic psychology* (pp. 353–373). New York: Russell Sage Foundation.

Askin, H., Paultre, Y., White, R., & Van Ornum, W. (1993, August). *The quantitative and qualitative aspects of scrupulosity.* Paper presented at the annual convention of the American Psychological Association, Toronto, Canada.

Atallah, S. F., El-Dosoky, A. R., Coker, E. M., Nabil, K. M., & El-Islam, M. F. (2001). A 22-year retrospective analysis of the changing frequency and patterns of religious symptoms among inpatients with psychotic illness in Egypt. *Social Psychiatry and Psychiatric Epidemiology, 36,* 407–415.

Batson, C. D., Schoenrade, P., & Ventis, W. L. (1993). *Religion and the individual: A social psychological perspective.* London: Oxford University Press.

Benson, P. L., Roehlkepartain, E. C., & Rude, S. P. (2003). Spiritual development in childhood and adolescence: Toward a field of inquiry. *Applied Developmental Science, 7,* 204–212.

Boyer, P. (2001). *Religion explained: The evolutionary origins of religious thought.* New York: Basic Books.

Chakraborty, A., & Banerji, G. (1975). Ritual: A culture-specific neurosis, and obsessional states in Bengali culture. *Indian Journal of Psychiatry, 17,* 211–216.

Chamberlain, K., & Zika, S. (1992). Religiosity, meaning in life, and psychological well-being. In J. F. Shumaker (Ed.), *Religion and mental health* (pp. 138–148). New York: Oxford University Press.

Cochran, J. K. (1992). The effects of religiosity on adolescent self-reported frequency of drug and alcohol use. *Journal of Drug Issues, 22,* 91–104.

Davis, T. L., Kerr, B. A., & Kurpius, S. E. (2003). Meaning, purpose, and religiosity in at-risk youth: The relationship between anxiety and spirituality. *Journal of Psychology and Theology, 31*(4), 356–365.

D'Onofrio, B. M., Eaves, L. J., Murrelle, L., Maes, H. H., & Spilka, B. (1999). Understanding biological and social influences on religious affiliation, attitudes, and behaviors: A behavior genetic perspective. *Journal of Personality, 67*(6), 953–984.

Eeles, J., Lowe, T., & Wellman, N. (2003). Spirituality or psychosis?: An exploration of the criteria that nurses use to evaluate spiritual-type experiences reported by patients. *International Journal of Nursing Studies, 40*(2), 197–206.

El-Islam, M. F., & Ahmed, S. A. (1971). Traditional interpretation and treatment of mental illness in an Arab psychiatric clinic. *Journal of Cross-Cultural Psychology, 2*(3), 301–307.

Ferriss, A. L. (2002). Religion and the quality of life. *Journal of Happiness Studies, 3,* 199–215.

Francis, L. J. (1994). Personality and religious development during childhood and adolescence. In L. B. Brown (Ed.), *Religion, personality, and mental health* (pp. 94–118). New York: Springer-Verlag.

Fredrickson, B. L. (2002). How does religion benefit health and well-being?: Are positive emotions active ingredients? *Psychological Inquiry, 13*(3), 209–213.

Glass, J., Bengtson, V. L., & Dunham, C. C. (1986). Attitude similarity in three-generation families: Socialization, status inheritance, or reciprocal influence? *American Sociological Review, 51,* 685–695.

Gorsuch, R. L. (1988). Psychology of religion. *Annual Review of Psychology, 39,* 201–221.

Greenberg, D., & Shefler, G. (2002). Obsessive compulsive disorder in ultra-orthodox Jewish patients: A comparison of religious and non-religious symptoms. *Psychology and Psychotherapy: Theory, Research and Practice, 75*(2), 123–130.

Greenberg, D., & Witztum, E. (1994). The influence of cultural factors on obsessive compulsive disorder: Religious symptoms in a religious society. *Israel Journal of Psychiatry and Related Sciences*, *31*(3), 170–182.

Gur, M., Miller, L., & Weissman, M. M. (2004). *Maternal depression and offspring religiousness*. Manuscript submitted for publication.

Hackney, C. H., & Sanders, G. S. (2003). Religiosity and mental health: A meta-analysis of recent studies. *Journal for the Scientific Study of Religion*, *42*(1), 43–55.

Hammen, C. (1992). The family–environmental context of depression: A perspective on children's risk. In D. Cicchetti & S. Toth (Eds.), *Developmental perspectives on depression* (pp. 251–281). Rochester, NY: University of Rochester Press.

Harris, J. I., Schoneman, S. W., & Carrera, S. R. (2002). Approaches to religiosity related to anxiety among college students. *Mental Health, Religion and Culture*, *5*(3), 253–265.

Hermesh, H., Masser-Kavitzky, R., & Gross-Isseroff, R. (2003). Obsessive–compulsive disorder and Jewish religiosity. *Journal of Nervous and Mental Disease*, *191*(3), 201–203.

Hill, P. C., & Hood, R. W., Jr. (Eds.). (1999). *Measures of religiosity*. Birmingham, AL: Religious Education Press.

Hodges, S. (2002). Mental health, depression, and dimensions of spirituality and religion. *Journal of Adult Development*, *9*(2), 109–115.

Hoffnung, R. A., Aizenberg, D. V., Hermesh, H., & Munitz, H. (1989). Religious compulsions and the spectrum concept of psychopathology. *Psychopathology*, *22*(2–3), 141–144.

Hunter, E. (1998). Adolescent attraction to cults. *Adolescence*, *33*, 709–714.

Ingersoll-Dayton, B., Krause, N., & Morgan, D. (2002). Religious trajectories and transitions over the life course. *International Journal of Aging and Human Development*, *55*(1), 51–70.

James, W. (1985). *The varieties of religious experience*. Cambridge, MA: Harvard University Press. (Original work published 1902)

Josephson, A. M. (1993). The interactional problems of Christian families and their relationship to developmental psychopathology: Implications for treatment. *Journal of Psychology and Christianity*, *12*(4), 312–328.

Kahneman, D., Diener, E., & Schwarz, N. (Eds.). (1999). *Well-being: The foundations of hedonic psychology*. New York: Russell Sage Foundation.

Kendler, K. S., Gardner, C. O., & Prescott, C. A. (1997). Religion, psychopathology, and substance use and abuse: A multimeasure, genetic-epidemiological study. *American Journal of Psychiatry*, *154*, 322–329.

Kendler, K. S., Gardner, C. O., & Prescott, C. A. (1999). Clarifying the relationship between religiosity and psychiatric illness: The impact of covariates and the specificity of buffering effects. *Twin Research*, *2*, 137–144.

Kendler, K. S., Liu, X., Gardner, C. O., McCullough, M. E., Larson, D., & Prescott, C. A. (2003). Dimensions of religiosity and their relationship to lifetime psychiatric and substance use disorders. *American Journal of Psychiatry*, *160*(3), 496–503.

Kim, A. E. (2003). Religious influences on personal and societal well-being. *Social Indicators Research*, *62–63*(1–3), 149–170.

King, P. E., & Boyatzis, C. J. (Eds.). (2004). Exploring adolescent spiritual and religious development: Current and future theoretical and empirical perspectives [Special issue]. *Applied Developmental Science*, *8*(1).

Kirkpatrick, L. A., & Hood, R. W., Jr. (1990). Intrinsic–extrinsic religious orientation: The boon or bane of contemporary psychology of religion? *Journal for the Scientific Study of Religion*, *29*, 442–462.

Kirkpatrick, L. A., & Shaver, P. R. (1990). Attachment theory and religion: Childhood attachments, religious beliefs, and conversion. *Journal for the Scientific Study of Religion*, *29*, 315–334.

Koenig, H. G. (Ed.). (1998). *Handbook of religion and mental health*. New York: Academic Press.

Koenig, H. G., Ford, S. M., George, L. K., Blazer, D. G., & Meador, K. G. (1993). Religion and anxiety disorder: An examination and comparison of associations in young, middle-aged, and elderly adults. *Journal of Anxiety Disorders, 7,* 321–342.

Koenig, H. G., George, L. K., Blazer, D. G., Pritchett, J. T., & Meador, K. G. (1993). The relationship between religion and anxiety in a sample of community-dwelling older adults. *Journal of Geriatric Psychiatry, 26,* 65–93.

Larson, D. B., & Larson, S. S. (1994). *The forgotten factor.* Rockville, MD: National Institute for Healthcare Research.

Levin, J. S., & Chatters, L. M. (1998). Research on religion and mental health: An overview of empirical findings and theoretical issues. In H. G. Koenig (Ed.), *Handbook of religion and mental health* (pp. 34–47). New York: Academic Press.

Levin, J. S., & Taylor, R. J. (1998). Panel analyses of religious involvement and well-being in African Americans: Contemporaneous vs. longitudinal. *Journal for the Scientific Study of Religion, 37*(4), 695–709.

Loewenthal, K. M., Cinnirella, M., Evdoka, G., & Murphy, P. (2001). Faith conquers all?: Beliefs about the role of religious factors in coping with depression among different cultural-religious groups in the UK. *British Journal of Medical Psychology, 74,* 293–303.

Mahgoub, O. M., & Abdel-Hafeiz, H. B. (1991). Pattern of obsessive–compulsive disorder in eastern Saudi Arabia. *British Journal of Psychiatry, 158,* 840–842.

McCullough, M. E., & Larson, D. B. (1999). Religion and depression: A review of the literature. *Twin Research, 2,* 126–136.

Miller, L., Davies, M., & Greenwald, S. (2000). Religiosity and substance use and abuse among adolescents in the National Comorbidity Survey. *Journal of the American Academy of Child and Adolescent Psychiatry, 39*(9), 1190–1197.

Miller, L., Warner, V., Wickramaratne, P., & Weissman, M. M. (1997). Religiosity and depression: Ten-year follow-up of depressed mothers and offspring. *Journal of the American Academy of Child and Adolescent Psychiatry, 36,* 1416–1425.

Miller, L., Weissman, M. M., Gur, M., & Adams, P. (2001). Religiousness and substance use in children of opiate addicts. *Journal of Substance Abuse, 13,* 323–336.

Miller, L., Weissman, M., Gur, M., & Greenwald, S. (2002). Adult religiousness and history of childhood depression: Eleven-year follow-up study. *Journal of Nervous and Mental Disease, 190*(2), 86–93.

Mitchell, L., & Romans, S. (2002). Spiritual beliefs in bipolar affective disorder: Their relevance for illness management. *Journal of Affective Disorders, 75*(3), 247–257.

Okasha, A., Saad, A., Khalil, A. H., El-Dawla, A. S., & Yahia, N. (1994). Phenomenology of obsessive–compulsive disorder: A transcultural study. *Comprehensive Psychiatry, 35,* 191–197.

Oman, D., & Reed, D. (1998). Religion and mortality among community dwelling elderly. *American Journal of Public Health, 88,* 1469–1475.

Pargament, K. I., Poloma, M. M., & Tarakeshwar, N. (2001). Methods of coping from the religions of the world: The bar mitzvah, karma, and spiritual healing. In C. R. Snyder (Ed.), *Coping with stress: Effective people and processes* (pp. 259–284). New York: Oxford University Press.

Parks, F. M. (2003). The role of African-American folk beliefs in the modern therapeutic process. *Clinical Psychology: Science and Practice, 10*(4), 456–475.

Pearce, L. D., & Axinn, W. G. (1998). The impact of family religious life on the quality of mother-child relations. *American Sociological Review, 63,* 810–828.

Pfeifer, S., & Waelty, U. (2000). Anxiety, depression, and religiosity: A controlled clinical study. *Mental Health, Religion, and Culture, 2*(1), 35–45.

Pfeiffer, W. (1982). Culture-bound syndromes. In I. Al-Issa (Ed.), *Culture and psychopathology* (pp. 201–218). Baltimore: University Park Press.

Pressman, P., Lyons, J. S., Larson, D. B., & Gartner, J. (1992). Religion, anxiety, and fear of death. In J. F. Schumaker (Ed.), *Religion and mental health* (pp. 98–109). New York: Oxford University Press.

Prince, R. H. (1992). Religious experience and psychopathology. In J. F. Schumaker (Ed.), *Religion and mental health* (pp. 281–290). New York: Oxford University Press.

Raphael, F. J., Rani, S., Bale, R., & Drummund, L. M. (1996). Religion, ethnicity and obsessive–compulsive disorder. *International Journal of Social Psychiatry, 42,* 38–44.

Regnerus, M., Smith, C., & Fritsch, M. (2003). *Religion in the lives of American adolescents: A review of the literature.* Chapel Hill, NC: National Study of Youth and Religion.

Reivich, K., & Gillham, J. (2003). Learned optimism: The measurement of explanatory style. In S. J. Lopez, & C. R. Snyder (Eds.), *Positive psychological assessment: A handbook of models and measures* (pp. 57–74). Washington, DC: American Psychological Association.

Richards, P. S., & Bergin, A. E. (1997). *A spiritual strategy for counseling and psychotherapy.* Washington, DC: American Psychological Association.

Rosengren, K. S., & Johnson, C. N. (2000). *Imagining the impossible: Magical, scientific, and religious thinking in children.* New York: Cambridge University Press.

Ross, C. E. (1990). Religion and psychological distress. *Journal for the Scientific Study of Religion, 29*(2), 236–245.

Schapman, A. M., & Inderbitzen-Nolan, H. M. (2002). The role of religious behavior in adolescent depressive and anxious symptomatology. *Journal of Adolescence, 25*(6), 631–643.

Schnittker, J. (2001). When is faith enough?: The effects of religious involvement on depression. *Journal for the Scientific Study of Religion, 40*(3), 393–411.

Sethi, S., & Seligman, M. E. P. (1991). Optimism and fundamentalism. *Psychological Science, 4*(4), 256–259.

Siddle, R., Haddock, G., Tarrier, N., & Faragher, E. B. (2002). Religious delusions in patients admitted to hospital with schizophrenia. *Social Psychiatry and Psychiatric Epidemiology, 37*(3), 130–138.

Smith, C. (2003). Theorizing religious effects among American adolescents. *Journal for the Scientific Study of Religion, 42*(1), 17–30.

Smith, C., & Faris, R. (2003). *Religion and American adolescent delinquency, risk behaviors and constructive social activities.* Chapel Hill, NC: National Study of Youth and Religion.

Smith, T. B., McCullough, M. E., & Poll, J. (2003). Religiousness and depression: Evidence for a main effect and the moderating influence of stressful life events. *Psychological Bulletin, 129*(4), 614–636.

Sperry, L. (2001). *Spirituality in clinical practice: Incorporating the spiritual dimension in psychotherapy and counseling.* New York: Brunner/Routledge.

Spilka, B., Hood, R. W., Jr., Hunsberger, B., & Gorsuch, R. (2003). *The psychology of religion: An empirical approach* (3rd ed.). New York: Guilford Press.

Tarakeshwar, N., Stanton, J., & Pargament, K. I. (2003). Religion: An overlooked dimension in cross-cultural psychology. *Journal of Cross-Cultural Psychology, 34*(4), 377–394.

Tateyama, M., Asai, M., Kamisada, M., Hashimoto, M., Bartels, M., & Heimann, H. (1993). Comparison of schizophrenic delusions between Japan and Germany. *Psychopathology, 26,* 151–158.

Thorson, J. A. (1998). Religion and anxiety: Which anxiety? Which religion? In H. G. Koenig (Ed.), *Handbook of religion and mental health* (pp. 147–160). New York: Academic Press.

Tsang, J., & McCullough, M. E. (2003). Measuring religious constructs: A hierarchical approach to construct organization and scale selection. In S. J. Lopez & C. R. Snyder (Eds.), *Positive psychological assessment: A handbook of models and measures* (pp. 345–360). Washington, DC: American Psychological Association.

Varon, S. R., & Riley, A. W. (1999). Relationship between maternal church attendance and adolescent mental health and social functioning. *Psychiatric Services, 50,* 799–805.

Ventis, W. L. (1995). The relationships between religion and mental health. *Journal of Social Issues, 51*(2), 33–48.

Wallace, J. M., Jr., & Forman, T. A. (1998). Religion's role in promoting health and reducing risk among American youth. *Health Education and Behavior, 25,* 721–741.

Wallace, J. M., Jr., & Williams, D. R. (1997). Religion and adolescent health-compromising behavior. In J. Schulenberg & J. L. Maggs (Eds.), *Health risks and developmental transitions during adolescence* (pp. 444–468). New York: Cambridge University Press.

Wilcox, W. B. (1998). Conservative Protestant childrearing: Authoritarian or authoritative? *American Sociological Review, 63,* 796–809.

Wilson, W. P. (1998). Religion and psychoses. In H. G. Koenig (Ed.), *Handbook of religion and mental health* (pp. 161–174). New York: Academic Press.

Zinnbauer, B., & Pargament, K. I. (1998). Spiritual conversion: A study of religious change among college students. *Journal for the Scientific Study of Religion, 37,* 161–180.

The Religious Dimension of Coping

Advances in Theory, Research, and Practice

KENNETH I. PARGAMENT
GENE G. ANO
AMY B. WACHHOLTZ

Each time I knew everything would be all right because I asked
God to carry me through—I know that He's got his arms around
me.
—KIDNEY DIALYSIS PATIENT following several cardiac
arrests and surgeries (in O'Brien, 1982, p. 76)

A year ago this week, Satan drove up 5th Street in a Ryder truck.
He blew my babies up. He may have looked like a normal man,
but he was Satan.
—GRANDFATHER OF TWO CHILDREN killed in the Oklahoma
City bombing (in *Newsweek*, 1996, p. 19)

I am told God lives in me—and yet the reality of darkness and
coldness and emptiness is so great that nothing touches my soul.
—MOTHER TERESA (in *Newsweek*, 2001, p. 23)

Major life events touch people spiritually as well as emotionally, socially, and physically. Crises can be viewed through a spiritual lens as threats, challenges, losses, or opportunities for the growth of whatever the individual may hold sacred. In coming to terms with trauma and tragedy, people can draw on a number of resources that have been prescribed by the religions of the world for thousands of years. Yet it is also true that religion can be a burden and a source of struggle for people facing difficult life situations, adding another dimension to the pain and hardship of coping.

Perhaps, then, it should come as no surprise that where we find crisis and tragedy, we often find religion. "In times of crisis," psychologist Paul Johnson (1959, p. 82) wrote, "religion usually comes to the foreground." For example, in a survey of a national sample of Americans shortly after the 9/11 attacks, Schuster et al. (2001) found that 90% reportedly turned to their religion for solace and support. As singular an event as 9/11 was, it was not unusual in a religious sense. Other groups experiencing traumatic life events also frequently draw upon their religion to cope. Segall and Wykle (1988–1989) asked black primary caregivers of family members with dementia to identify the one special way they dealt with caring for their relative. Prayer or faith in God were, by far, the most common responses. Among hospitalized and long-term care patients, 86% reported using religious activities to cope with their problems (Ayele, Mulligan, Gheorghui, & Reyes-Ortiz, 1999). Bulman and Wortman (1977) asked a group of people paralyzed in severe accidents how they explained their misfortune. The most common response to the question "Why me?" was that God had a reason.

Historically, researchers and theorists have neglected the role of religion in coping or have viewed it from a critical perspective. More recently, however, this picture has begun to change. Over the past two decades, there has been a sharp increase in the number of studies of religion and coping by researchers in the social sciences and health (see Harrison, Koenig, Hays, Eme-Akwari, & Pargament, 2001; Pargament, 1997). Health practitioners have also begun to draw upon religious coping resources in their efforts to ameliorate a variety of problems and conditions. In this chapter, we review the current theoretical and empirical status of the psychology of religion and coping, the practical interventions that have grown out of this body of work, and future directions for research and practice to advance this exciting area of study further.

WHAT WE KNOW ABOUT RELIGION AND COPING

Freud (1927/1961) argued that religion is rooted in the child's sense of helplessness in the face of a world filled with dangerous and uncontrollable forces. By transforming the natural into the supernatural, he maintained, the child is able to defend him- or herself against the threats posed by the external environment. He wrote: "If the elements have passions that rage as they do in our own souls, if death itself is not something spontaneous but the violent act of an evil Will, if everywhere in nature there are Beings around us of a kind that we know in our own society, then we can breathe freely, can feel at home in the uncanny and can deal by psychical means with our senseless anxiety" (p. 20). For Freud, religion was defensive in nature, designed to allay anxiety and avoid the confrontation with reality. This perspective is still widely held within psychology. It is, however, a stereotype, one that oversimplifies religious life and one that is inconsistent with an emerging literature on religion and coping (see Pargament & Park, 1995, for an extensive review).

Religion Is More Than a Defense

Like most stereotypes, there is a grain of truth to the "religion as defense" view. As noted above, many people do, in fact, turn to their faith to reduce their anxiety and to gain solace and support in times of stress. Shrimali and Broota (1987) captured this defensive process at work in their comparative study of Indian patients undergoing major surgery, patients receiving minor surgery, and a control group. Before surgery, the patients facing major surgery reported higher levels of anxiety, superstitious beliefs, and beliefs in God than the other two groups. After surgery, however, the levels of anxiety

and religious beliefs declined significantly among those experiencing the serious procedures, while the levels of anxiety and belief remained constant in the other two groups.
It is also the case that religion can help people avoid a direct confrontation with painful situations. The responsibility for problem solving can be deferred passively to God
(Pargament, Kennell, Hathaway, Grevengoed, Newan, & Jones, 1988), religious systems of belief can provide justifications for a status quo that perpetuates injustice and
inequality, and faith can serve as a cloak for the denial of problems, as we hear in the
words of the prison inmate who said: "Since I got Jesus, I don't have no memories of
the past" (quoted in Peck, 1988). Nevertheless, while there may be a grain of truth to
the notion that religion can serve as a defense, there is little foundation to the idea that
religion is *merely* a defense.

In fact, several lines of study suggest that religion is more than defensive in nature.
First, religion has been linked theoretically and empirically to a variety of functions in
coping that go beyond anxiety reduction, including meaning making (Paloutzian, 1981;
Park & Folkman, 1997); intimacy (Johnson & Mullins, 1989); personal mastery, growth,
and actualization (Park & Cohen, 1993); and the search for the sacred itself (Pargament,
Magyar, & Murray-Swank, 2005). These motivations are not necessarily mutually exclusive; in fact, part of the power of religion lies in its ability to serve a wide variety of needs
among its adherents.

Second, empirical studies indicate that religion is not generally linked with the blanket denial of the situation. Most religious traditions provide their members with rites of
passage that encourage them to acknowledge and mark difficult life transitions (e.g., funerals) rather than deny their reality. For example, Acklin, Brown, and Mauger (1983)
found no relationships between measures of religiousness and denial among patients with
cancer. Rather than encouraging denial, religion promotes reinterpretations of negative
events through the sacred lens. Thus, a major life crisis can be viewed as an opportunity
for spiritual growth, a crisis can be attributed to a loving God who is trying to teach the
individual a valuable lesson, and a tragedy can be perceived as part of a larger, mysterious, but ultimately benevolent plan. Certainly, these benevolent views may make the pain
of the situation more bearable, but people do not necessarily "shut down" emotionally to
reach this point. In this vein, McIntosh, Silver, and Wortman (1993) studied parents of infants who died of sudden infant death syndrome (SIDS). Parents who were more religious
found greater meaning in their child's death over time and, in turn, experienced less distress. Interestingly, religious parents engaged in *more* rather than less cognitive processing
of the event, suggesting that they were actively working through the experience rather
than denying it. Similar results have been reported by people coping with war trauma (Ai,
Peterson, & Huang, 2003) and breast cancer (Gall & Cornblat, 2002).

Third, although religion has been accused of passivity in response to critical life
events, empirical studies suggest otherwise. For example, various studies have shown that
measures of religiousness have been linked more consistently to active coping than to passive coping (see Pargament & Park, 1995, for a review). Furthermore, it is possible to
identify active as well as passive forms of religious coping. Pargament et al. (1988) distinguished among three ways in which religion can be involved in the search for control in
the problem-solving process: a deferring approach in which the individual relinquishes
the responsibility for problem solving to God; a self-directing approach in which the individual perceives God giving him or her the skills and resources to solve problems independently; and a collaborative approach in which the individual perceives God to be a
partner who shares in the responsibility for problem solving. This and subsequent studies

revealed that the collaborative problem-solving style was more common than the deferring or self-directing styles.

The idea that religion is merely a defense oversimplifies and stereotypes religious life. Empirical studies of people grappling with life crises reveal a much richer, multidimensional picture of religious coping.

Religion Expresses Itself in Many Ways in Coping

When religion has been examined within the general coping literature, it has usually been assessed by only one or two items. For example, in the widely used Ways of Coping Scale by Lazarus and Folkman (1984), religiousness is measured by two items: "found new faith" and "I prayed." This approach can offer only the smallest window into religious life. Religiousness is neither simple nor uniform. It is instead a complex process consisting of cognitive, behavioral, emotional, interpersonal, and physiological dimensions. Empirical investigations have repeatedly revealed multidimensionality in religious life. For example, in their extensive review of the literature, Hill and Hood (1999) identified 125 measures of religiousness representing 17 different categories (e.g., beliefs, congregational involvement, attitudes, religious orientations).

Religious coping represents a rich phenomenon in and of itself. Although religious coping could be defined and measured in terms of the degree to which religion is a part of the process of understanding and dealing with critical life events, it is important to consider not only *how much* religion is involved in coping, but also *how* religion is involved in coping: specifically, the *who*'s (e.g., clergy, congregation members, God), *what*'s (e.g., prayer, Bible reading, ritual), *when*'s (e.g., acute stressors, chronic stressors), *where*'s (e.g., within a congregation, privately), and *why*'s (e.g., to find meaning, to gain control) of coping.

In perhaps the most comprehensive effort to identify various religious coping methods, Pargament, Koenig, and Perez (2000) developed a measure of 21 types of religious coping activities through interviews and a literature review. The coping methods encompass active, passive, and interactive strategies; emotion-focused and problem-focused approaches; and cognitive, behavioral, interpersonal, and spiritual domains. As can be seen in Table 26.1, the religious coping activities represent five key religious functions: the search for meaning, the search for mastery and control, the search for comfort and closeness to God, the search for intimacy and closeness to God, and the search for a life transformation. As comprehensive as this measure is, though, it still does not capture many of the religious coping methods specific to various religious traditions among Western and non-Western cultures (e.g., karma, spiritual healing, pilgrimage). Clearly, religion can express itself in a variety of ways in the coping process.

To digress for a moment, the transformational role of religion in coping is particularly noteworthy (see Pargament, 1997, for discussion; also see Park, Chapter 16, this volume). Generally, religion has been viewed as a conservational force in coping: an attempt to hold on to or sustain the sense of meaning, control, comfort, intimacy, or spiritual connection in the midst of life crisis. At times, however, conservation is no longer possible. Internal changes, developmental transitions, or external life events may result in the loss of those goals and strivings that have given direction to the individual's life. During these times religious coping methods (e.g., religious conversion, seeking religious direction, religious forgiving) are also available to assist the individual in the process of acknowledgment of the loss, letting go of old goals and values, and moving toward new purpose and meaning (see Park & Folkman, 1997).

TABLE 26.1. The Many Methods of Religious Coping

Religious methods of coping to find meaning

Benevolent religious reappraisal—redefining the stressor through religion as potentially beneficial
Punishing God reappraisal—redefining the stressor as a punishment from God for the individual's sins
Demonic reappraisal—redefining the stressor as an act of the devil
Reappraisal of God's powers—redefining God's power to influence the stressful situation

Religious methods of coping to gain mastery and control

Collaborative religious coping—seeking control through a partnership with God in problem solving
Passive religious deferral—passive waiting for God to control the situation
Active religious surrender—active giving up of control to God in coping
Pleading for direct intercession—seeking control indirectly by pleading to God for a miracle or divine intervention
Self-directing religious coping—seeking control through individual initiative rather than help from God

Religious methods of coping to gain comfort and closeness to God

Seeking spiritual support—searching for comfort and reassurance through God's love and care
Religious focus—engaging in religious activities to shift focus from the stressor
Religious purification—searching for spiritual cleansing through religious actions
Spiritual connection—seeking a sense of connectedness with forces that transcend the self
Spiritual discontent—expressing confusion and dissatisfaction with God' relationship to the individual in the stressful situation
Marking religious boundaries—clearly demarcating acceptable from unacceptable religious behavior and remaining within religious boundaries

Religious methods of coping to gain intimacy with others and closeness to God

Seeking support from clergy or members—searching for intimacy and reassurance through the life and care of congregation members and clergy
Religious helping—attempting to provide spiritual support and comfort to others
Interpersonal religious discontent—expressing confusion and dissatisfaction with the relationship of clergy or members to the individual in the stressful situation

Religious methods of coping to achieve a life transformation

Seeking religious direction—looking to religion for assistance in finding a new direction for living
Religious conversion—looking to religion for a radical change in life
Religious forgiving—looking to religion for help in shifting from anger, hurt, and fear associated with an offense to peace

Religious Coping Methods Can Be Helpful or Harmful

In the past, macroanalytic studies that investigated religiousness as a global, dispositional variable yielded mixed results. Consequently, the efficacy of religious coping for people undergoing stressful life events remained unclear. However, advances in the measurement of religious coping have led to microanalytic studies that clarify the efficacy of religious coping by focusing on the relationships of specific religious coping strategies to the outcomes of stressful situations. The results of these studies show that religious coping can be helpful or harmful, depending upon the particular type of religious coping strategy employed.

While some studies have examined specific types of religious coping in fine detail, higher order factor analyses have revealed that particular religious coping methods can also be grouped into two broad overarching categories: positive and negative religious coping (Pargament, Smith, Koenig, & Perez, 1998). In general, positive religious coping strategies, those that reflect a secure relationship with God and a sense of spiritual connectedness with others, tend to be more beneficial for people undergoing stressful life events. For example, in a recent meta-analytic review of research on religious coping and psychological adjustment to stress, positive religious coping strategies, such as spiritual connectedness, benevolent religious reappraisals, collaborative religious coping, seeking spiritual support, and seeking support from clergy or members, were positively associated with positive outcomes, such as stress-related growth, spiritual growth, and greater life satisfaction, and negatively associated with negative outcomes, such as depression, anxiety, distress, hopelessness, and guilt, among various samples dealing with a variety of life stressors (Ano & Vasconcelles, 2005). Positive religious coping methods have also been associated with indices of better physical health in a few studies (see Koenig, McCullough, & Larson, 2001, for a review)

In contrast, negative religious coping methods, those that reflect an insecure relationship with God and tension between congregation members, are generally more maladaptive (see Exline & Rose, Chapter 17, this volume). For example, in their meta-analysis of the literature on religious coping and psychological adjustment to stress, Ano and Vasconcelles (2005) found that negative religious coping strategies, such as spiritual discontent, punishing God reappraisals, reappraisals of God's powers, demonic reappraisals, and interpersonal religious discontent, were positively associated with negative psychological outcomes, such as depression, anxiety, callousness, posttraumatic stress disorder (PTSD) symptoms, and spiritual injury, among different samples coping with a variety of negative life events. Such negative religious coping strategies also have harmful implications for physical functioning, as evidenced by findings from longitudinal studies with medical samples. For example, in a longitudinal study of religious coping among medically ill, elderly patients, Cox's regression analysis revealed that spiritual discontent and demonic reappraisals at baseline were associated with a 19–28% increased risk of mortality 2 years later, even after controlling for other important demographic and predictor variables, such as baseline illness severity and mental health status (Pargament, Koenig, Tarakeshwar, & Hahn, 2001). Additional analyses suggested that it was the group of patients who displayed consistently high levels of spiritual struggle over 2 years that was at greatest risk for declines in physical and mental health. In a sample of medical rehabilitation patients, Fitchett, Rybarczyk, DeMarco, and Nicholas (1999) found that spiritual struggles during hospital admission were significantly related to poorer recovery of somatic autonomy at follow-up 4 months postadmission, even after controlling for activities of daily living at admission, depression, social support, and relevant demographic variables. Thus, religious coping is not automatically beneficial; some types are more harmful than others.

Three additional points are important here. First, although much of the existing literature has demonstrated relationships between measures of religious coping and psychological indicators of adjustment, several studies have also linked religious coping to measures of social, spiritual, and physical well-being (e.g., Koenig, Pargament, & Nielsen, 1998; Pargament, Koenig, Tarakeshwar, & Hahn, 2004). Second, the relationships between religious coping and adjustment have remained significant after adjusting for the effects of demographic variables and nonreligious coping measures. For example, in their study of patients undergoing kidney transplants, Tix and Frazier (1998) found that religious coping predicted life satisfaction 12 months after transplantation, after controlling for measures of cognitive restructuring, internal control, and social support. Findings such as these suggest that religious coping represents a distinctive resource, one that cannot be "explained away" in terms of presumably more basic phenomena (Pargament, 2002). Finally, some studies of religious coping have reported nonsignificant or contradictory findings (e.g., Culver, Arena, Antoni, & Carver, 2002; VanNess & Larson, 2002). Differences in samples, stressors, and measures may partly account for these discrepancies. It is also possible that some forms of religious coping have mixed rather than exclusively positive or negative implications for health and well-being. For example, religious groups that respond to threats by marking boundaries (i.e., sharply distinguishing between insiders and outsiders) may preserve the integrity of the group and the psychological well-being of its members (e.g., Seth & Seligman, 1993), but at the cost of prejudice toward outsiders (Altemeyer & Hunsberger, 1992).

People Draw on a General Orienting System in Religious Coping

Research examining the nature of religious coping has shown that people do not come to coping empty-handed. They enter the coping process with a general orienting system of resources and burdens that influences the particular ways they interpret and handle stressful situations. The *orienting system* is a general disposition to the world that involves beliefs, feelings, practices, and relationships from religious, personality, and social domains (Pargament, 1997). In specific situations, people draw on religious coping methods that are a part of their general orienting system. For example, in studies employing hierarchical multiple regression analyses, dispositional variables (e.g., neuroticism, attachment to God, religious orientation), significantly predicted different types of religious coping strategies above and beyond the effects of other potentially relevant demographic and predictor variables (Ano, 2003; Pargament et al., 1992).

Furthermore, path analytic studies have shown that elements of the general orienting system, such as religious orientation (Roesch & Ano, 2003), church attendance and prayer (Nooney & Woodrum, 2002), and attachment to God (Belavich & Pargament, 2002) differentially shape the specific religious coping strategies that are employed in stressful life events. In these studies, religious coping mediated the relationship between dispositional variables (e.g., religious orientation and attachment to God) and the outcomes to stressful events. Thus, as a general disposition, the orienting system appears to influence the types of religious coping strategies that are employed in specific situations, with general resources (e.g., intrinsic religious orientation, secure attachment to God, church attendance) leading to more positive religious coping strategies and general burdens (e.g., insecure attachment to God, neuroticism) leading to more negative religious coping methods. However, it is the specific religious coping methods that are related more directly to the resolution of critical situations.

Effects of Religious Coping Are Moderated by Different Factors

Religious coping does not occur in a vacuum. It is employed by particular people, in particular contexts, in response to particular stressful situations. As such, different factors have been identified that moderate the links between religious coping and outcomes to stressful events. First, religious coping appears to be more helpful for those who are more religious. In two studies of religious coping among a national sample of Presbyterian members, elders, and clergy in the United States, religious coping was more strongly associated with psychological adjustment for those who were more religious (i.e., for clergy than for elders, and for elders than for members) (Krause, Ellison, & Wulff, 1998; Pargament, Tarakeshwar, Ellison, & Wulff, 2001). More specifically, among those who were more religious, positive religious coping and church-based emotional support were more strongly related to positive affect and less depression, whereas negative religious coping and interpersonal conflicts in the church were associated with less positive affect and greater depression.

Second, religious coping appears to be more helpful during more taxing situations that push people to the bounds of their human limitations, when immediate personal and social resources are depleted. For example, in a study of religious coping among parents dealing with the loss of a child, spiritual support was more strongly associated with lower levels of depression among those who were more distressed (i.e., recently bereaved parents) than for those who were less distressed (i.e., parents who lost a child more than 2 years ago) (Maton, 1989).

Third, religious coping has differential effects for people from different religious affiliations. In two different studies, religious coping was more helpful for Protestants than for Catholics. For example, in a sample of hospital patients and their loved ones dealing with the stress of a kidney transplant surgery, Tix and Frazier (1998) found that religious coping was associated with greater life satisfaction and less distress for Protestants, but not for Catholics. In another study involving a sample of Hispanic women coping with breast cancer, higher levels of religious coping were associated with less distress among Evangelicals, but greater distress among Catholics (Alferi, Culver, Carver, Arena, & Antoni, 1999). However, these findings do not necessarily mean that Protestants are "better off" than Catholics. In a study of religious doubting among parochial school adolescents, religious doubts were more strongly associated with distress among Dutch Reformed Protestants than Catholics (Kooistra & Pargament, 2002). Thus, religious affiliation clearly moderates the effects of religious coping, but it does so in complex ways (see Park, Cohen, & Herb, 1990).

FROM RESEARCH TO PRACTICE

Building on the growing body of research that has demonstrated empirical links between religious coping and adjustment, researchers and practitioners have begun to develop and evaluate therapeutic methods that draw upon religious coping resources or address religious struggles in the counseling process. Spiritually integrated psychotherapeutic approaches are still in their infancy. However, promising models of treatment that build on religious coping methods are in the process of development (e.g., Avants & Margolin, 2004). Although empirical evidence of efficacy is only just beginning to emerge (see Harris, Thoresen, McCullough, & Larson, 1999; McCullough, 1999; Worthington, Kurusu, McCullough, & Sandage, 1996), the results are encouraging.

A number of studies have demonstrated the positive effects of meditation on various aspects of health and well-being (e.g., Shapiro, Schwartz, & Bonner, 1998). Wachholtz and Pargament (in press) conducted a study that underscores the potential value of a more explicitly spiritual form of meditation. They compared the effects of spiritual meditation with secular meditation. Participants in the two groups meditated either to a sacred mantra (e.g., God loves me) or a secular mantra (e.g., I am loved) over a 2-week period. Spiritual meditation was associated with significantly greater anxiety reduction, greater spiritual well-being, and greater ability to withstand pain than the secular meditation or a relaxation group. These findings suggest that spiritual meditation may be a distinctive therapeutic resource, one that could potentially improve patients' quality of life and activity level without some of the financial expense and negative side effects of pain medications.

Researchers have also evaluated the effects of prayer as a form of intervention. However, prayer is a global resource that can encompass many types of religious coping. For example, Rajagopal, Mackenzie, Bailey, and Lavizzo-Mourey (2002) studied the effects of using a prayer wheel on anxiety and depression among an elderly population. The prayer wheel actually embodied several types of prayer and coping, such as requests for spiritual protection and guidance, forgiveness of oneself and others, and offering spiritual support to others. Participants who made use of the prayer wheel reported significant decreases in anxiety and, to a lesser degree, depression.

Confession represents another potentially important, yet understudied, religious coping resource that could be integrated into treatment. Working with a sample of college students, Murray-Swank (2003) compared the effects of spiritual confession to secular confession and a control condition. Participants in the spiritual confession condition wrote a letter to God asking for forgiveness for something they had done wrong. Participants in the nonspiritual confession condition simply wrote a letter about something they had done wrong. The results were interesting and complex. In comparison to the other two conditions, spiritual confession was associated with greater reports of spiritual growth immediately after writing the letter to God and 2 weeks later. However, spiritual confession was also linked with higher levels of guilt in comparison to the nonspiritual confession condition. Finally, the participants' images of God moderated the impact of spiritual confession on positive affect, such that those who perceived God in loving terms experienced increases in positive affect from baseline to the 2-week follow-up, and those with less loving images of God showed a decrease in positive affect. In another study with implications for confession, Exline, Smith, Gregory, Hockemeyer, and Tulloch (2005) found that people with PTSD who wrote about their trauma in positive religious terms experienced more positive mood by the third session of writing.

Several researchers have developed and tested psychospiritual interventions that use mixed religious and spiritual resources to facilitate the health and well-being of women with cancer (Cole, 1999; Targ & Levine, 2002). For example, Targ and Levine (2002) compared the effects of a mind–body–spirit group intervention for women with breast cancer with a support group. The spiritual group was taught to use meditation, imagery, ritual, and affirmation. Participants in both groups demonstrated positive changes in quality of life, depression, anxiety, and spiritual well-being. In comparison to the support group, the spiritual group also showed greater increases in spiritual integration and less avoidance. However, the support group showed more declines in confusion and helplessness/hopelessness.

A number of studies have been conducted that evaluate the effects of religious coping resources that are specific to particular religious traditions. For instance, religious support, encouragement, and guidance have been shown to be helpful to Muslim religious patients from Malaysia coping with bereavement (Azhar & Varma, 1995) and with generalized anxiety disorder (Azhar, Varma, & Dharap, 1994). In these studies, patients who were encouraged to pray, discuss religious issues, and read verses from the Qur'an reported more significant and more rapid improvement than patients in support groups. Similarly, McCullough (1999) conducted a meta-analysis of five studies that compared the effectiveness of a Christian-accommodative form of cognitive-behavioral therapy with standard cognitive-behavioral therapy. The Christian treatments emphasized the use of religious imagery, prayer, and biblical perspectives. While both forms of treatment produced positive results, the Christian-accommodative and standard treatments did not differ from each other in their efficacy.

One program examined the impact of an intervention that encouraged religious transformation. Gruner (1984) evaluated a residential drug rehabilitation program for adolescents administered through the Assemblies of God church. The program was designed to help participants challenge feelings of meaninglessness, hopelessness, and alienation, and overcome their addiction through a reprioritization of their values and new dedication of their lives to God. The retention and rehabilitation rates in this program were higher than those reported by other comparable, secular programs.

Finally, a few researchers have begun to examine the impact of spiritually oriented interventions on people encountering spiritual struggles. Murray-Swank and Pargament (2003) developed and evaluated an 8-week manualized individual intervention that drew on spiritual resources to help women who had experienced childhood sexual abuse. The treatment draws on a variety of spiritual coping resources and modalities (e.g., visualizations of a loving God, letter writing to God, benevolent spiritual appraisals, prayer/meditation, rituals) to address spiritual struggles (e.g., feelings of abandonment by God, anger at God, and feelings of shame). Following the intervention and at 1 month follow-up, 80% of the women reported reductions in psychological and spiritual distress. Similarly, Phillips, Lakin, and Pargament (2002) implemented a psychospiritual intervention specifically designed for individuals experiencing serious mental illness. This 7-week intervention provided group members with an opportunity to share their religious journeys and discuss topics such as spiritual resources, spiritual strivings, spiritual struggles, forgiveness of others, and hope. In contrast to concerns that have been raised about raising spiritual matters among people with serious mental illness, the intervention did not trigger any serious psychological disturbances in group members. In fact, the participants asked the leaders to continue the group over the next year.

As a whole, this body of research suggests that religious coping resources may offer valuable adjuncts to the treatment process. As yet, however, we do not know which religious coping methods may be particularly helpful in the therapeutic process. Additional studies are needed to pinpoint and evaluate the efficacy of specific religious coping methods in treatment.

FUTURE DIRECTIONS FOR RESEARCH AND PRACTICE

In the past quarter century, the psychology of religion has reemerged as a significant area of scientific inquiry (see Emmons & Paloutzian, 2003). Within this context, there has also been a dramatic rise in studies of religion and coping. Nevertheless, the study of religion and coping remains in its infancy. We conclude this chapter by pointing to several important directions for future research and practice.

First, studies of religion and coping remain somewhat parochial, designed, implemented, and interpreted by researchers within the scientific study of religion. Given its significance for the physical, psychological, social, and spiritual well-being of people, research in the domain of religion and coping should be more fully integrated into mainstream research and practice within the applied health professions and the social and health sciences. Toward this end, researchers in the area of religion and coping should draw more fully upon theory and research from other disciplines and, in turn, make more concerted efforts to disseminate their findings to the wider applied and scientific community.

Second, although empirical advances in the psychology of religion and coping have yielded a reasonable base of established findings, the majority of research has been conducted with Caucasian/European-American samples. Future research should investigate religious coping in ethnically and religiously diverse samples. A few studies have examined religious coping among particular ethnic groups, such as African Americans (Woods, Antoni, Ironson, & Kling, 1999), Hispanics (Alferi et al., 1999), and Koreans (Kim & Seidlitz, 2002), but very few studies have compared religious coping across ethnicities, with the exception of one study that examined appraisals, coping, and distress among Korean American, Filipino American, and Caucasian American Protestants (Bjorck, Cuthbertson, Thurman, & Lee, 2001). Drawing from research on multicultural psychology, it would be interesting to examine the nature and prevalence of specific religious coping strategies, such as interpersonal religious discontent and seeking support from clergy and members in such ethnic groups as Asian Americans, given the greater value such groups place upon collectivism compared to Caucasian/European Americans. In terms of religious diversity, the majority of research on religious coping has been conducted with Christian samples, with the exception of a few studies that have examined religious coping among Hindus (Tarakeshwar, Pargament, & Mahoney, 2003), Jews (Dubow, Pargament, Boxer, & Tarakeshwar, 2000), and Muslims (Ai et al., 2003). Future studies should examine religious coping in Eastern and nontheocentric religious traditions to identify other forms of religious coping and to understand how other religious beliefs and practices might contribute to the coping process.

Third, there is a need for more longitudinal studies of religious coping. Cross-sectional findings could either reflect the impact of religious coping on adjustment, or the stress mobilization effects of distress on religious coping. Fortunately, a few longitudinal studies of religious coping have begun to clarify the temporal relationships between stressors, religious coping, and adjustment as well as the longer-term impact of religious coping (e.g., Fitchett et al., 1999; Pargament, Koenig, Tarakeshwar, & Hahn, 2001; Pargament et al., 1994; Tix & Frazier, 1998). Longitudinal studies are also needed to examine fluctuations in religious coping over time and their implications for adjustment. In this vein, Keefe et al. (2001) conducted a diary study of religious coping with rheumatoid arthritis patients and found significant variation in religious coping scores from day to day over the course of 30 consecutive days, indicating that religious coping was a dynamic phenomenon sensitive to changing times and circumstances. Diary studies represent one promising and creative way to study religious coping "up close," as it unfolds over time.

Fourth, future studies should investigate religious coping among relatively neglected groups, such as people with serious mental illness. Tepper, Rogers, Coleman, and Malony (2001) examined religious coping among a sample of 406 participants with persistent mental illness and found that more than 80% of the sample used religion to cope with daily frustrations. Given the prevalence of religious coping among this sample, future research should examine the unique implications that religious coping might have for those with serious mental illness. Another neglected group in the literature on religious coping is children (Mahoney, Pendleton, & Ihrke, 2005; Pendleton, Cavalli, Pargament, & Nasr, 2002). Researchers should examine religious coping from a developmental perspective and investigate how religious coping evolves throughout the lifespan or between developmental stages. For example, it would be interesting to explore how cognitive development influences religious coping. Are children in the concrete operational stage of cognitive development capable of more meaning-based religious coping strategies? How does religious coping evolve from childhood and adolescence, when cognitions might be more fantasy-laden and egocentric, to adulthood, when cognitions may be more rational and reality-based? Such research would draw upon cognitive-developmental theory and could, in turn, inform cognitive-developmental psychology. For example, could spending more time in contemplative prayer (a particular type of religious coping strategy) improve abstract cognitive reasoning? Ideas such as these illustrate how the psychology of religion might be influenced by and simultaneously impact mainstream general psychology.

Fifth, there is a need for studies of specific religious coping methods. For example, while a number of studies have examined forgiveness (for reviews, see McCullough, Pargament, & Thoresen, 2000; McCullough, Bono, & Root, Chapter 22, this volume), particularly from the perspective of the victim, few studies have examined its flip side, confession, which may have unique and important implications for social psychology, since most transgressions are interpersonal in nature. Religious rites of passage (e.g., confirmations, bar/bat mitzvahs, and funerals) are another type of specific religious coping activity that involve ceremonial rituals to signify the passing from one stage of spiritual identity to the next (see Pargament, Poloma, & Tarakeshwar, 2001). These rites of passage are often imbued with deep emotions and significance, and thus represent rich targets for studies of the affective basis of spirituality. These studies, in turn, may hold important implications for more general psychological theories of emotion. Finally, researchers should pay closer attention to situations that could be perceived as a threat or violation to whatever people may hold sacred. This type of primary appraisal may be particularly powerful. Magyar, Pargament, and Mahoney (2000) examined the degree to which college students perceived an offense in a romantic relationship as a sacred violation (i.e., desecration) and its impact on health and well-being. People who perceived the romantic offense as a desecration were more likely to report negative affect, more physical health symptoms, and more intrusive and avoidant thoughts and behaviors related to the event, even after controlling for the negativity of the offense. These results were largely replicated in a community sample faced with a wider range of stressful life events (Pargament, Magyar, Benore, & Mahoney, 2005).

Sixth, future research should incorporate both quantitative and qualitative methods of studying religious coping. In this vein, Ganzevoort (1998) conducted a qualitative study of religious coping by examining people's life narratives and weaving the storylines of religion together with other prominent life themes. Ganzevoort (2001) then integrated quantitative methods with this qualitative narrative reformulation of religious coping by conducting cluster analyses of story themes and examining their intercorrelations. This innovative methodology allows for an even more fine-grained analysis of this complex construct, providing a richer picture of religious coping that could lead to unique insights.

Seventh, because religious coping has implications for people across a variety of domains, there is a need for studies that include multiple criteria of well-being. Most of the research on religious coping has been conducted by psychologists who are predominantly interested in mental health. However, there is a need for studies that consider the implications of religious coping for other social, spiritual, and physical dimensions to expand knowledge on religious coping and make the psychology of religion more relevant to other academic and applied disciplines. For example, with respect to the social dimension, Mahoney et al. (2002) found that college students who perceived the 9/11 terrorist attacks as desecrations of something sacred adopted more severe retaliatory attitudes toward the terrorists responsible for these acts. From a sociological perspective, these findings could explain the perpetuation and exacerbation of tensions between societies, cultures, and nations that simultaneously perceive the other as desecrating their own sacred objects, lands, values, and ideals.

Finally, although researchers and practitioners have begun to develop and evaluate religiously oriented treatments, additional studies are needed to compare the efficacy of these treatments with other traditional secular interventions through experimental designs. For example, Rye and Pargament (2002) developed a group-based, religiously oriented forgiveness intervention for college women who were hurt in a romantic relationship and compared its efficacy with a secular forgiveness treatment group and a no-treatment control condition. Results of the study showed that, although both treatment groups were more effective than the control group, as evidenced by improvements on measures of forgiveness and existential well-being, there was no difference between the religious and secular interventions. However, post hoc content analyses revealed that participants in the secular treatment group reported that they drew upon religious resources, even though psychospiritual techniques were not explicitly integrated in the intervention. Thus, more controlled experimental studies that successfully distinguish between religious and secular interventions are needed to examine the unique contributions that particular psychospiritual techniques might make toward well-being. Furthermore, most psychospiritual interventions augment traditional approaches to the treatment of psychological problems. Additional studies are needed to develop and evaluate spiritually based interventions that specifically address religious problems, such as spiritual struggles.

There is no shortage of basic or applied questions about the roles of religion in coping. A rapidly growing body of research, however, suggests that this is a promising area of study, one that holds significant implications for our efforts to understand and help people come to terms with the most significant problems of their lives.

REFERENCES

Acklin, M. W., Brown, E. C., & Mauger, P. A. (1983). The role of religious values in coping with cancer. *Journal of Religion and Health*, 22, 322–333.

Ai, A. L., Peterson, C., & Huang, B. (2003). The effect of religious spiritual coping on positive attitudes of adult Muslim refugees from Kosovo and Bosnia. *The International Journal for the Psychology of Religion*, 12, 29–47.

Alferi, S. M., Culver, J. L., Carver, C. S., Arena, P. L., & Antoni, M. H. (1999). Religiosity, religious coping, and distress: A prospective study of Catholic and Evangelical Hispanic women in treatment for early-stage breast cancer. *Journal of Health Psychology*, 4, 343–356.

Altemeyer, B., & Hunsberger, B. (1992). Authoritarianism, religious fundamentalism, quest, and prejudice. *The International Journal for the Psychology of Religion*, 2, 113–133.

Ano, G. G. (2003). *Correlates of religious struggles: An exploratory study*. Unpublished master's thesis, Bowling Green State University, Bowling Green, OH.

Ano, G. G., & Vasconcelles, E. B. (2005). Religious coping and psychological adjustment to stress: A meta-analysis. *Journal of Clinical Psychology*, 61, 1–20.

Avants, S. K., & Margolin, A. (2004). Development of spiritual self-schema therapy for the treatment of addictive and HIV risk behavior: A convergence of cognitive and Buddhist psychology. *Journal of Psychotherapy Integration*, 14, 253–289.

Ayele, H., Mulligan, T., Gheorghiu, S., & Reyes-Ortiz, S. (1999). Religious activity improves life satisfaction for some physicians and older patients. *Journal of the American Geriatrics Society, 47,* 453–455.

Azhar, M. Z., & Varma, S. L. (1995). Religious psychotherapy as management of bereavement. *Acta Psychiatric Scandinavica, 91,* 233–235.

Azhar, M. Z., Varma, S. L., & Dharap, A. S. (1994). Religious psychotherapy in anxiety disorder patients. *Acta Psychiatrica Scandinavica, 90,* 1–3.

Belavich, T. G., & Pargament, K. I. (2002). The role of attachment in predicting spiritual coping with a loved one in surgery. *Journal of Adult Development, 9,* 13–29.

Bjorck, J. P., Cuthbertson, W., Thurman, J. W., & Lee, Y. S. (2001). Ethnicity, coping, and distress among Korean Americans, Filipino Americans, and Caucasian Americans. *Journal of Social Psychology, 141,* 421–442.

Bulman, R. J., & Wortman, C. B. (1977). Attributions of blame and coping in the "real world": Severe accident victims react to their lot. *Journal of Personality and Social Psychology, 35,* 351–363.

Cole, B. S. (1999). *The integration of spirituality and psychotherapy for people who have confronted cancer: An outcome study.* Unpublished doctoral dissertation, Bowling Green State University, Bowling Green, OH.

Culver, J. L., Arena, P. L., Antoni, M. H., & Carver, C. S. (2002). Coping and distress among women under treatment for early stage breast cancer: Comparing African Americans, Hispanics, and non-Hispanic whites. *Psycho-Oncology, 11,* 495–504.

Dubow, E. F., Pargament, K. I., Boxer, P., & Tarakeshwar, N. (2000). Religion as a source of stress, coping, and identity among Jewish adolescents. *Journal of Adolescent Research, 20,* 418–441.

Emmons, R. A., & Paloutzian, R. F. (2003). The psychology of religion. *Annual Review of Psychology, 54,* 377–402.

Exline, J. J., Smyth, J., Gregory, J., Hockemeyer, J., & Tulloch, H. (2005). Religious framing by individuals with PTSD when writing about traumatic experiences. *The International Journal for the Psychology of Religion, 15,* 17–34.

Fitchett, G., Rybarczyk, B. D., DeMarco, G. A., & Nicholas, J. J. (1999). The role of religion in rehabilitation outcomes: A longitudinal study. *Rehabilitation Psychology, 44,* 1–22.

Freud, S. (1961). *The future of an illusion.* In J. Strachey (Ed. and Trans.), *The standard edition of the complete psychological works of Sigmund Freud* (Vol. 11, pp. 5–56). London: Hogarth. (Original work published 1927)

Gall, T. L., & Cornblat, M. W. (2002). Breast cancer survivors give voice: A qualitative analysis of spiritual factors in long-term adjustment. *Psycho-Oncology, 11,* 524–535.

Ganzevoort, R. R. (1998). Religious coping reconsidered, part two: A narrative reformulation. *Journal of Psychology and Theology, 26,* 276–286.

Ganzevoort, R. R. (2001). Religion in rewriting the story: Case study of a sexually abused man. *The International Journal for the Psychology of Religion, 11,* 45–62.

Gruner, L. (1984). Heroin, hashish, and hallelujah: The search for meaning. *Review of Religious Research, 26,* 176–186.

Harris, A. H. S., Thoresen, C. E., McCullough, M. E., & Larson, D. B. (1999). Spiritually and religiously oriented health interventions. *Journal of Health Psychology, 4,* 413–433.

Harrison, M. O., Koenig, H. G., Hays, J. C., Eme-Akwari, A. G., & Pargament, K. I. (2001). The epidemiology of religious coping: A review of recent literature. *International Review of Psychiatry, 13,* 86–93.

Hill, P. C., & Hood, R. W., Jr. (Eds.). (1999). *Measures of religiosity.* Birmingham, AL: Religious Education Press.

Johnson, D. P., & Mullins, L. C. (1989). Religiosity and loneliness among the elderly. *Journal of Applied Gerontology, 9,* 110–131.

Johnson, P. E. (1959). *Psychology of religion.* Nashville, TN: Abingdon Press.

Keefe, F. J., Afflect, G., Lefebvre, J., Underwood, L., Caldwell, D. S., Drew, J., Egert, J., Gibson, J., &

Pargament, K. I. (2001). Living with rheumatoid arthritis: The role of daily spirituality and daily religious and spiritual coping. *Journal of Pain, 2,* 101–110.

Kim, Y., & Seidlitz, L. (2002). Spirituality moderates the effect of stress on emotional and physical adjustment. *Personality and Individual Differences, 32,* 1377–1390.

Koenig, H. G., McCullough, M. E., & Larson, D. B. (2001). *Handbook of religion and health.* New York: Oxford University Press.

Koenig, H. G., Pargament, K. I., & Nielsen, J. (1998). Religious coping and health status in medically ill hospitalized older adults. *Journal of Nervous and Mental Disease, 186,* 513–521.

Kooistra, W. P., & Pargament, K. I. (1999). Religious doubting in parochial school adolescents. *Journal of Psychology and Theology, 27,* 33–42.

Krause, N., Ellison, C. G., & Wulff, K. M. (1998). Church-based emotional support, negative interaction, and psychological well-being: Findings from a national sample of Presbyterians. *Journal for the Scientific Study of Religion, 37,* 725–741.

Lazarus, R. S., & Folkman, S. (1984). *Stress, appraisal, and coping.* New York: Springer.

Magyar, G. M., Pargament, K. I., & Mahoney, A. (2000, August). *Violating the sacred: A study of desecration among college students.* Paper presented at the annual meeting of the American Psychological Association, Washington, DC.

Mahoney, A. M., Pargament, K. I., Ano, G. G., Lynn, Q., Magyar, G. M., McCarthy, S., Pristas, E., & Wachholtz, A. (2002, August). *The devil made them do it: Demonization and desecration of the 9/11 terrorist attacks.* Paper presented at the annual meeting of the American Psychological Association, Chicago, IL.

Mahoney, A. M., Pendleton, S., & Ihrke, H. (2005). Religious coping by children and adolescents: Unexplored territory in the realm of spiritual development. In E. C. Roehlkepartain, P. E. King, L. Wagner, & P. E. Benson (Eds.), *The handbook of spiritual development in childhood and adolescence.* Thousand Oaks, CA: Sage.

Maton, K. I. (1989). The stress-buffering role of spiritual support: Cross-sectional and prospective investigations. *Journal for the Scientific Study of Religion, 28,* 310–323.

McCullough, M. E. (1999). Research on religion-accommodative counseling: Review and meta-analysis. *Journal of Counseling Psychology, 46,* 92–98.

McCullough, M. E., Pargament, K. I., & Thoresen, C. E. (Eds.). (2000). *Forgiveness: Theory, research, and practice.* New York: Guilford Press.

McIntosh, D. N., Silver, R. C., & Wortman, C. B. (1993). Religion's role in adjustment to a negative life event: Coping with the loss of a child. *Journal of Personality and Social Psychology, 65,* 812–823.

Murray-Swank, A. (2003). *Exploring spiritual confession: A theoretical synthesis and experimental study.* Unpublished doctoral dissertation, Bowling Green State University, Bowling Green, OH.

Murray-Swank, N., & Pargament, K. (2003, April). *Solace for the soul: A psycho-spiritual intervention for female survivors of sexual abuse.* Paper presented at the meeting for the International Center for the Integration of Health and Spirituality, Bethesda, MD.

Newsweek. (1996, April 29). Perspectives. p. 19.

Newsweek. (2001, September 17). Perspectives. p. 23.

Nooney, J., & Woodrum, E. (2002). Religious coping and church-based social support as predictors of mental health outcomes: Testing a conceptual model. *Journal for the Scientific Study of Religion, 4,* 359–368.

O'Brien, M. E. (1982). Religious faith and adjustment to long-term hemodialysis. *Journal of Religion and Health, 21,* 68–80.

Paloutzian, R. F. (1981). Purpose in life and value changes following conversion. *Journal of Personality and Social Psychology, 41,* 1153–1160.

Pargament, K. I. (1997). *The psychology of religion and coping: Theory, research, practice.* New York: Guilford Press.

Pargament, K. I. (2002). Is religion nothing but . . . ?: Explaining religion versus explaining religion away. *Psychological Inquiry, 13,* 239–244.

Pargament, K. I., Ishler, K., Dubow, E. G., Stanik, P., Rouiller, R., Crowe, P., Cullman, E. P., Albert, M., & Royster, B. J. (1994). Methods of religious coping with the Gulf War: Cross-sectional and longitudinal analyses. *Journal for the Scientific Study of Religion, 33*, 347–361.

Pargament, K. I., Kennell, J., Hathaway, W., Grevengoed, N., Newman, J., & Jones, W. (1988). Religion and the problem-solving process: Three styles of coping. *Journal for the Scientific Study of Religion, 27*, 90–104.

Pargament, K. I., Koenig, H. G., & Perez, L. (2000). The many methods of religious coping: Development and initial validation of the RCOPE. *Journal of Clinical Psychology, 56*, 519–543.

Pargament, K. I., Koenig, H. G., Tarakeshwar, N., & Hahn, J. (2001). Religious struggle as a predictor of mortality among medically ill elderly patients: A two year-longitudinal study. *Archives of Internal Medicine, 161*, 1881–1885.

Pargament, K. I., Koenig, H. G., Tarakeshwar, N., & Hahn, J. (2004). Religious coping methods as predictors of psychological, physical, and spiritual outcomes among medically ill elderly patients: A two-year longitudinal study. *Journal of Health Psychology, 9*, 713–730.

Pargament, K. I., Magyar, G. M., Benore, E., & Mahoney, A. M. (2005). Sacrilege: A study of sacred loss and desecration and their implications for health and well-being in a community sample. *Journal for the Scientific Study of Religion, 44*, 59–78.

Pargament, K. I., Magyar, G. M., & Murray-Swank, N. (2005). The sacred and the search for significance: Religion as a unique process. *Journal of Social Issues, 61*(4).

Pargament, K. I., Olson, H., Reilly, B., Falgout, K., Ensing, D., & Van Haitsma, K. (1992). God help me (II): The relationship of religious orientation to religious coping with negative life events. *Journal for the Scientific Study of Religion, 22*, 393–404.

Pargament, K. I., & Park, C. L. (1995). Merely a defense?: The variety of religious means and ends. *Journal of Social Issues, 51*, 13–32.

Pargament, K. I., Poloma, M., & Tarakeshwar, N. (2001). Spiritual healing, karma, and the bar mitzvah: Methods of coping from the religions of the world. In C. R. Snyder (Ed.), *Coping and copers: Adaptive processes and people* (pp. 259–284). New York: Oxford University Press.

Pargament, K. I., Smith, B. W., Koenig, H. G., & Perez, L. (1998). Patterns of positive and negative religious coping with major life stressors. *Journal for the Scientific Study of Religion, 37*, 710–724.

Pargament, K. I., Tarakeshwar, N., Ellison, C. G., & Wulff, K. M. (2001). Religious coping among the religious: The relationship between religious coping and well-being in a national sample of Presbyterian clergy, elders, and members. *Journal for the Scientific Study of Religion, 40*, 497–513.

Park, C. L., & Cohen, L. H. (1993). Religious and nonreligious coping with the death of a friend. *Cognitive Therapy and Research, 17*, 561–577.

Park, C. L., Cohen, L. H., & Herb, L. (1990). Intrinsic religiousness and religious coping as life stress moderators for Catholics vs. Protestants. *Journal of Personality and Social Psychology, 59*, 562–574.

Park, C. L., & Folkman, S. (1997). Meaning in the context of stress and coping. *Review of General Psychology, 1*, 115–144.

Peck, D. L. (1988). Religious conviction, coping, and hope: The relation between a functional corrector and a future prospect among life-without-parole inmates. *Case Analyses, 2*, 201–219.

Pendleton, S. M., Cavalli, K. S., Pargament, K. I., & Nasr, S. Z. (2002). Spirituality in children with cystic fibrosis: A qualitative analysis. *Pediatrics, 109*, 1–11.

Phillips, R. E., III, Lakin, R., & Pargament, K. I. (2002). The development of a psychospiritual intervention for people with serious mental illness. *Community Mental Health Journal, 38*, 487–495.

Rajagopoal, D., Mackenzie, E., Bailey, C., & Lavizzo-Mourey, R. (2002). The effectiveness of a spiritually-based intervention to alleviate subsyndromal anxiety and minor depression among older adults. *Journal of Religion and Health, 41*, 153–166.

Roesch, S. C., & Ano, G. (2003). Testing an attribution and coping model of stress: Religion as an orienting system. *Journal of Psychology and Christianity, 22*(3), 197–209.

Rye, M. S., & Pargament, K. I. (2002). Forgiveness and romantic relationships in college: Can it heal the wounded heart? *Journal of Clinical Psychology, 58*, 419–441.

Schuster, M. A., Stein, B. D., Jaycox, L. H., Collins, R. L., Marshall, G. N., Elliott, M. N., Zhou, A. J., Kanouse, D. E., Morrison, J. L., & Berry, S. H. (2001). A national survey of stress reactions after the September 11, 2001, terrorist attacks. *New England Journal of Medicine, 345*, 1507–1512.

Segall, M., & Wykle, M. (1988–1989). The black family's experience with dementia. *Journal of Applied Social Sciences, 13*, 170–191.

Seth, S., & Seligman, M. E. P. (1993). Optimism and fundamentalism. *Psychological Science, 4*, 256–259.

Shapiro, S. L., Schwartz, G. E., & Bonner, G. (1998). Effects of mindfulness-based stress reduction on medical and premedical students. *Journal of Behavioral Medicine, 21*, 581–599.

Shrimali, S., & Broota, K. D. (1987). Effect of surgical stress on beliefs in God and superstition: An in situ investigation. *Journal of Personality and Clinical Studies, 3*, 135–138.

Tarakeshwar, N., Pargament, K. I., & Mahoney, A. (2003). Initial development of a measure of religious coping among Hindus. *Journal of Community Psychology, 31*, 607–628.

Targ, E. F., & Levine, E. G. (2002). The efficacy of a mind–body–spirit group for women with breast cancer: A randomized controlled trial. *General Hospital Psychiatry, 24*, 238–248.

Tepper, L., Rogers, S. A., Coleman, E. M., & Malony, H. N. (2001). The prevalence of religious coping among persons with persistent mental illness. *Psychiatric Services, 52*, 660–665.

Tix, A. P., & Frazier, P. A. (1998). The use of religious coping during stressful life events: Main effects, moderation, and mediation. *Journal of Consulting and Clinical Psychology, 66*, 411–422.

VanNess, P. H., & Larson, D. B. (2002). Religion, senescence, and mental health: The end of life is not the end of hope. *American Journal of Geriatric Psychiatry, 10*, 386–397.

Wachholtz, A. B., & Pargament, K. I. (in press). Is spirituality a critical ingredient of meditation?: Comparing the effects of spiritual meditation, secular meditation and relaxation on pain sensitivity and endurance. *Journal of Behavioral Medicine.*

Woods, T. E., Antoni, M. H., Ironson, G. H., & Kling, D. W. (1999). Religiosity is associated with affective status in symptomatic HIV-infected African American women. *Journal of Health Psychology, 4*, 317–326.

Worthington, E. L., Jr., Kurusu, T. A., McCullough, M. E., & Sandage, S. J. (1996). Empirical research on religion and psychotherapeutic processes and outcomes: A 10-year review and research and prospectus. *Psychological Bulletin, 119*, 448–487.

27

The Psychology of Religion in Clinical and Counseling Psychology

EDWARD P. SHAFRANSKE

A confluence of developments is leading to the emergence of an applied psychology of religion in which knowledge gained through theoretical and empirical scholarship contributes to the practice of clinical and counseling psychology. Foremost among the factors contributing to this convergence of science and practice is a burgeoning literature in the psychology of religion reflecting "a full-force, leading edge research area that contributes new knowledge, data, and professional activity to the rest of psychology" (Emmons & Paloutzian, 2003, p. 379). Of particular relevance to clinical practice are the results of empirical investigations in which correlations between religious involvement and mental and physical health have been found (Mills, 2002; Pargament, Koenig, Tarakeshwar, & Hahn, 2001; Powell, Shahabi, & Thoresen, 2003; also see Oman & Thoresen, Chapter 24, and Miller & Kelley, Chapter 25, this volume). Although the findings are subject to debate and further inquiry (Miller & Thoresen, 2003; Sloan, Bagiella, & Powell, 1999) and not all forms of religious involvement enhance psychological adjustment (Pargament, 2002a, 2002b), meta-analyses have generally found religious commitment to be associated with reduced risk factors important to mental health (Koenig & Larson, 2001) and may contribute to the enhancement of positive emotions, which "can transform individuals for the better, helping them to be more resilient, more creative, and wise, more virtuous, more socially integrated, and on top of all this physically healthier" (Fredrickson, 2002, p. 211).

In addition to these developments, religion and spirituality have been recognized to play integral roles in the transmission of beliefs, values, and practices, which coalesce into a worldview (American Psychological Association, 2002b, p. 8), and constitute essential features of diversity that must be considered when conducting research or providing clinical services (American Counseling Association, 1996; American Psychological Association, 2002a). For many clients, religion or spirituality serves as "the overarching framework for living, applicable to the widest range of human experience" (Pargament, 1997, p. 132); it is the "ultimate value base" (Baumeister, 1992, p. 196) upon which personal goals are established and resources for well-being and psychological coping are found. This is the case in many cultures in which spirituality not only concerns faith in transcendent realities but is central to physical, mental, and/or health issues (Fukuyama & Sevig, 1999; Tarakeshwar, Stanton, & Pargament, 2003).

Consistent with such an appreciation of diversity is the acknowledgment that the provision of psychological treatment is a values-based enterprise and that clinical understanding is obtained within socially constructed, culturally embedded spheres of meaning in which religious forms contribute to "making sense" of the other's conflicts and suffering. Psychological theory implicitly contains values perspectives concerning what constitutes the good life, human nature, and morality. Clinical practice necessarily involves beliefs and values (Bergin, 1980) in which the division between personal and professional beliefs is poorly demarcated or, in fact, nonexistent (cf. O' Donohue, 1989). Psychotherapy may be considered a form of "moral engagement" (Miller, 2004; Richardson, Fowers, & Guignon, 1999) and its outcomes have been found to be influenced by the internalization of the professional and personal values of the therapist (Beutler, Machado, & Neufeldt, 1994). These findings, taken together with the recognition of the high importance most Americans place on religion (Newport, 2004; Roof, 1999), requires clinicians to become aware of their present *practice orientation* to religion as a clinical variable as well as to develop increased competence in bringing spiritual factors into assessment and treatment.

APPROACHES TO RELIGION AND SPIRITUALITY WITHIN THE CLINICAL SETTING

Clinical competence is enhanced through the performance of an *intentional orientation* in which religion and spirituality are addressed as variables relevant to assessment and intervention. Such an approach proactively considers the role that religion plays in a client's worldview and brings into focus the unique contributions of religion to the conception of psychological difficulties as well as its ability to provide resources for coping. Such an approach does not minimize appreciation for the psychological, behavioral, or biological contributions to mental health but rather aims for a more comprehensive and holistic approach. Richards and Bergin (2005, pp. 16–17) called for a viable spiritual strategy that would be empirical in nature, and Shafranske (2002a) asserted that the necessary and sufficient conditions for an applied psychology of religion would include the development of empirically supported approaches (see also Shafranske & Malony, 1996). Although these requirements remain for the most part aspirational, a body of literature exists from which practice recommendations can be derived.

ASSESSING RELIGION AND SPIRITUALITY AS CLINICAL VARIABLES

The overarching goal of assessing religion and spirituality within the clinical setting is to obtain an accurate understanding of the salience and expression of these dimensions to the client's orienting system. Attention is directed to the contributions of both religion and spirituality as distinct yet interrelated constructs (Hill & Pargament, 2003; Zinn-bauer, Pargament, & Scott, 1999). Clinicians need to be aware of any personal biases (e.g., the simplistic view of spirituality as good and religion as bad) that may affect their clinical inquiry. Richards and Bergin (2005) suggest that conducting a religious–spiritual assessment can help therapists:

1) understand their clients' worldviews and thus increasing the capacity to empathically understand and sensitively work with each client;

2) determine whether clients' religious–spiritual orientation is healthy or unhealthy and what impact it has on presenting problems;

3) determine whether clients' religious and spiritual beliefs and community could be used as a resource to help them better cope, heal, and grow;

4) determine which spiritual interventions could be used in therapy to help clients; and

5) determine whether clients have unresolved spiritual doubts, concerns, or needs that should be addressed in therapy (cf. pp. 220–223).

Such an assessment can also be useful diagnostically in providing a cultural context to understand the normative status of client beliefs, experiences, and practices. For example, communication with the dead, apparitions, and ritual devotions are relatively common features of the *religiosidad popular* of Latinos (Romero, 1991) but rare among many other groups. Situating such phenomena within a cultural framework aids in differentiating between religious experiences and manifestations of psychopathology, although such discriminations are complicated by the fact that "psychiatric difficulties can coexist with ecstatic spiritual experiences and normative religious affiliation and practice" (Galanter, 1996, p. 289). Clinical inquiry also signifies openness on the part of the clinician to consider religion and spirituality to be personally relevant to the mental health of the client.

Preliminary Religious–Spiritual Assessment

The procedures for conducting a clinical assessment must be tailored to the salience of the spiritual dimension in the client's mental health and psychological coping. A two-tiered approach in interviewing is useful in which religion and spirituality are considered within a multimodal or multisystemic assessment (see Table 27.1). At the first level of inquiry, broad-based questions, for example, "How important is religion or spirituality in your daily life?," are asked to assess the importance the client places on spirituality. Prompts may be offered to encourage self-reflection and to make explicit the nature of the client's spiritual involvement. Clients may be asked to discuss previous hardships, the meaning these circumstances had for them, and the means by which they coped with these challenges. These self-reports provide historical snapshots of the client's use of religious beliefs, attributions, and resources and their effects on coping. Assessment is conducted with the understanding that religiosity and spirituality are embedded within family and cultural contexts and assessment is specific to the life of an individual, at a specific time, facing a given psychological challenge. The outcome of the initial phase of assessment should include an understanding of salience, which will determine the extent to which the therapist will focus further inquiry into religion and spirituality as clinical variables.

TABLE 27.1. Assessment and Integration of Religious and
Spiritual Interventions

Stage 4: Implementation of integration

Integration, consultation, collaboration
Explicit intervention approach/informed consent
Mode of process and outcome evaluations

Stage 3: Mode of integration

Salience
Informed consent
Alliance
Client–therapist faith/values congruence
Tasks and goals of treatment
Psychotherapy orientation
Therapist competence
Resources and barriers to treatment
Nature of integration: implicit–explicit continuum

Stage 2: Level-II assessment
In-depth assessment

Beliefs
God image, God representations
Compensatory or complementary religious attachment figures
Religious/spiritual affiliation(s)
Practices and rituals
Moral prescriptions/proscriptions
Participation in faith community
Family and community contexts
Religious training/developmental milestones
Use and form of religious coping
Degree of integration in orienting system

Stage 1: Level-I assessment
Screening for salience

Salience
Degree of integration in orienting system
Use of religious coping
Presenting complaints associated with religion/spirituality
Impairments in religious and spiritual functioning

In-Depth Religious–Spiritual Assessment[1]

A second level of assessment is recommended when religion or spirituality figures promi-
nently in the client's worldview, presents the potential to serve as a resource or obstacle to
the therapeutic progress, religious or spiritual problems are themselves the focus of clinical attention (Code V62.89; American Psychiatric Association, 1994, p. 685), or when
impairment in religious or spiritual functioning exists (Hathaway, 2003). Further assessment is warranted when psychological crisis has led to a sudden loss or change in spiritual orientation, particularly for those whom religious faith had previously played a
significant role or in situations in which religion or spirituality appears to be producing a
detrimental effect. Similarly, if spirituality had served in the past as protective, it is important to assess the risk factors that overwhelmed the resources that religious faith had
provided (Gorsuch & Miller, 1999).

The contents and processes constituting a complete religious–spiritual assessment have not been standardized. Richards and Bergin (2005), for example, consider meta-physical worldview, religious affiliation, religious orthodoxy, religious problem-solving style, spiritual identify, God image, value–lifestyle congruence, doctrinal knowledge, and religious and spiritual health and maturity (pp. 224–234). Sperry (2001) includes a spiritual history, involvement in a spiritual community, God representation, the role of prayer, other spiritual practices, and basic values and beliefs (pp. 112–114). Chirban (2001, pp. 284–287) presents a comprehensive Religion and Spiritual History Inventory that delineates multiple lines of inquiry (See also Gorsuch & Miller, 1999).

Assessment may also incorporate procedures derived from specific treatment orientations. For example, within cognitive-behavioral therapy, focus may be placed on assessing cognitive distortions, dysfunctional schemas, and the client's *style* of thinking about his or her relationship with God (cf. Nielson, Johnson, & Ellis, 2001, p. 113) that may contribute to the development or alleviation of symptoms (Nielson, 2004; Tan & Johnson, 2004) . . . Within psychoanalysis a religious history may be discerned in which beliefs, practices, rituals, religious training, and other experiences are considered in light of their reciprocal impacts on the formation of God representations and in intrapsychic conflict (Rizzuto, 1979, 1996; Shafranske, 2004a, 2004b). The client's apparent relationship with God may provide a window into the client's relational capacities and attachment style (Kirkpatrick, 1992, 1998) and reflects a correspondence or compensation in object relations (cf. Sorenson, 2004). Further, culturally derived religious narrative may be understood to articulate self-experience (Shafranske, 2002b) and in the Jungian tradition is seen to reflect the religious function of the psyche (Corbett, 1996).

Assessment of Religious Coping

Pargament (1997, 2002a, 2002b, and Chapter 26, this volume) has demonstrated the importance of religion and spirituality in coping. An assessment should consider that some forms of religious involvement are more helpful than others (e.g., internalized, intrinsically motivated, secure relationship with God) and appreciate that even more controversial ones (e.g., fundamentalism) offer advantages and disadvantages, particularly when religious beliefs and practices are well integrated into life. Religion plays a particularly valuable role as an available resource for coping for socially marginalized groups and when people are pushed to the limits of their resources (cf. Pargament, 2002a, p. 168). Pargament (2002a) further suggested that "those who benefit most from their religion are more likely to (a) be part of a larger social context that supports their faith; (b) apply means that are appropriate to their religious ends; (c) select religious appraisals and solutions that are tailored to the problem at hand; and (d) blend their religious beliefs, practices, and motivations harmoniously with each other" (p. 178). These conclusions direct clinical inquiry to the nature of personal integration and to the flow of religious coping and its end effects on the problem at hand (Butter & Pargament, 2003). Attention should also be placed on the style of religious coping (self-directing, deferring, or collaborative) in respect to the degree of autonomous control the client may have in responding to the immediate crisis (Pargament, 1997, p. 181) and how the client is utilizing his or her existing sources of significance.

The use of religious coping may provide important benefits to the client; however, there are forms of religious–spiritual involvement that may produce negative effects and actually exacerbate psychiatric symptoms. Specific "red flags" (Pargament, 1997, p. 375) such as religious beliefs, experiences of disappointment, anger and distrust of God, interpersonal strains associated with affiliation within a faith community, and problems faced in attempting to exercise the values or moral standards of religious faith may produce distress (Exline, 2002, 2003; Exline, Yali, & Sanderson, 2000; Pargament, 2002b; Pargament, Smith, Koenig, & Perez, 1998; see Exline & Rose, Chapter 17, this volume).

Taking into consideration Snyder, Sigmon, and Feldman's (2002) perspective "that every religion offers a prepackaged matrix of goals, pathways for accomplishing those goals, and agency thoughts for applying those pathways," an assessment of "how these three elements work together to the benefit or detriment of the individual" (p. 235) is important. For example, it may be relevant to consider such questions as: "Has the client lost faith in the goals or in the means or self-agency to attain the goals?" or "Does the client participate in a community or in relationships that sustain and support spiritual goals and the means to attain those goals?"

This body of literature points to the necessity to consider the *function* religious or spiritual participation serves in the life of the individual, particularly in times of loss, hardship, or ennui, when spiritual crises may parallel or contribute to psychological distress or religious faith may provide an ontological footing for psychological coping. In addition, consideration of the direction that religious participation encourages—openness versus closedness, broadness versus narrowness in perspective, and degrees of rigidity versus degrees of flexibility—may point to the relative adaptive or pathological consequences in the way in which individuals hold their beliefs (Meissner, 1996). Evaluation is not aimed at the specific religion or spiritual group per se but rather assesses the dynamic nature of the functions—for example, adaptive or defensive, well integrated or brittle. Hathaway (2003) has suggested that assessment should also consider "clinically significant religious/spiritual impairment (CSRI)," in which the ability "to perform religious/spiritual activities, achieve religious/spiritual goals, or experience religious/spiritual states" (Hathaway, Scott, & Garver, 2004, p. 97) is reduced because of a psychological disorder. This is important to assess for clients for whom religious involvement had served constructive, life-enhancing, and stress-buffering functions. Hathaway et al. (2004) reported the findings of a national survey of clinical psychologists in which 91% stated that their "clients spontaneously report changes in their religious/spiritual functioning associated with their disorders" and 92% of the respondents reported "changes in clients' religious/spiritual functioning during the course of psychotherapy" (p. 100).

Techniques and Resources in Religious–Spiritual Assessment

Assessment of the spiritual dimension within the clinical setting is accomplished primarily through the use of interview procedures, which draw upon interpersonal competencies and skills in obtaining specific information while simultaneously encouraging open-ended exploration. The task is particularly challenging given the varieties and multidimensionality of religious experience (Wulff, 1997) and the lack of an empirically supported interview protocol. Familiarity with the major religious traditions readies the clinician to assess dimensions of religious involvement that are clinically salient. For example, knowledge of beliefs, practices, moral prescriptions and proscriptions, rituals, and milestones assists in understanding the normative status of the client's religious involvement, the context out of which psychological conflict may develop, or circumstances in which a client's behavior is at variance with his or her religious values or those of his or her faith community (Richards & Bergin, 2000).

Other techniques may be incorporated to obtain qualitatively rich descriptions, to engage the client in self-refection, or to arrive at valid and reliable assessments of specific dimensions of religiosity or spirituality. Clients may be asked to write a spiritual autobiography; to construct a spiritual map depicting on a timeline the significant milestones, events, and challenges within their spiritual journeys (Sperry, 2001, pp. 115–116); or to develop a spiritual genogram in which the role and functions of religion and spirituality as well as divergences and problems can be explored from intergenerational and systems perspectives (Frame, 2000, 2003).

Instruments developed within the psychology of religion may also be used to supplement interview data, although few have been systematically evaluated for their application in clinical practice (Hill & Hood, 1999; Sherman & Simonton, 2001). Instruments that may have particular utility in the clinical setting include the Age Universal I–E Scale (Gorsuch & Venable, 1983), the Spiritual Well-Being Scale (Ellison, 1994), the Index of Core Spiritual Experience (INSPIRIT) (Kass, Friedman, & Lesserman, 1991), and the recently developed Multidimensional Measurement of Religiousness/Spirituality (John E. Fetzer Institute, 1999), Spiritual Assessment Inventory (Hall & Edwards, 2002), and Clients' Attitudes Towards Spirituality in Therapy survey (Rose, Westefeld, & Ansley, 2001). The following instruments offer valid and reliable means to assess religious coping: Religious Coping Scale (RCOPE) (Pargament, Koenig, & Perez, 2000); Brief RCOPE (Pargament, Smith, et al., & Perez, 1998), Negative Religious Coping Scale (Pargament, Zinnbauer, et al., 1998) and, with further development, the measure of religious coping and strain (Exline et al., 2000).

Through the exercise of an *intentional orientation*, the nature, salience, and integration of religion and spirituality in the client's orienting system can be assessed. A two-stage or tier approach has been proposed in which the initial screening of salience delimits the scope of further assessment and sets the stage for the degree to which attention will be focused on the spiritual dimension, religious or spiritual interventions will be employed, and religious coping, including the use of religious and spiritual resources, will be incorporated into treatment.

ADDRESSING RELIGIOUS AND SPIRITUAL DIMENSIONS IN PSYCHOLOGICAL INTERVENTION

The use of an *intentional orientation* promotes congruence between the salience of the religious dimension for the client and the degree of attention and integration undertaken in the treatment. The incorporation of religious or spiritual interventions or resources should not be determined by the psychotherapist's personal faith orientation; rather, it should correspond to the salience and function of religion in the client's life, with informed consent, and within the scope of the clinician's competence, established through appropriate training and supervision. The degree of integration should be tailored to the mutually defined goals and tasks of the treatment and in respect to an established therapeutic alliance (Shafranske & Sperry, 2004; Sperry, 2004).

A Conceptual Framework for Integration

Tan (1996) proposed a model that presents two distinct forms of integration, which exist on a continuum. *Implicit integration* refers to a more covert approach that does not initiate the discussion of religious or spiritual issues and does not openly, directly, or systematically use spiritual resources like prayer and Scripture or other sacred texts in therapy . . . [and] *Explicit integration*, [which refers to] a more overt approach that directly and systematically deals with spiritual or religious issues in therapy, and uses spiritual resources like prayer, Scripture or sacred texts, referrals to church or other religious groups or lay counselors, and other religious practices. (p. 368)

In addition to salience, the psychotherapy approach also prescribes the nature of integration and delimits the kinds of religious or spiritual interventions to be employed. In cognitive-behavioral psychotherapy, for example, explicit forms of integration may readily be assimilated such as addressing selective abstraction and misinterpretations of Scripture similar to working with other forms of dysfunctional thinking. Psychodynamic and other insight-oriented approaches usually employ implicit integration, in which religious content is addressed through exploration and interpretation consistent with the clinician's usual mode of activity. A comprehensive discussion of the ways in which each therapeutic modality may approach integration is beyond the scope of this chapter; however, there are a number of clinical texts that contain exemplar clinical illustrations of integration (Richards & Bergin, 2000, 2004; Shafranske, 1996a; Sperry & Shafranske, 2004; see also Frame, 2003; Fukuyama & Sevig, 1999; Griffifth & Griffifth, 2001; Kelly, 1995; Lovinger, 1984; Miller, 1999, 2003; Nielson et al., 2001; Randour, 1993; Sperry, 2001; Steere, 1997; Stern, 1985; West, 2000).

These approaches emphasize integrating religion and spirituality as clinically relevant dimensions into preexisting therapeutic frameworks and do not challenge the implicit epistemic, values-based foundations of the therapeutic modalities or require accommodation to a spiritual worldview. Such integration might be metaphorically expressed as taking place on the "home turf" of psychology, with its assumptions and rules in effect, rather than playing on a neutral field, let alone within the heavens. Models have also been developed that draw more equally from an integration of psychological and religious–spiritual worldviews. A rich and identifiable literature, professional academies, and training programs exist that contribute to such efforts, particularly in respect to the dialogue between Christianity and psychology (Vande Kemp, 1996). Clinical models have been developed (although rarely have they been scientifically evaluated or presented within the mainstream of clinical training) that integrate secular and religious (e.g., Buddhist, Christian, Jewish, and Muslim) viewpoints, beliefs, traditions, and healing practices (Richards & Bergin, 2000). There are also approaches, such as Alcoholics Anonymous programs, that offer a spiritual perspective and incorporate spiritual beliefs, values, and practices without being located within specific religious traditions. Although many questions remain concerning the functional contributions of spirituality (Tonigan, Toscova, & Connors, 1999), 12-step programs illustrate the potential benefits of integrating a spiritual dimension.

There are also clinical models that involve integration at the most fundamental level and assert not only a posture of "theistic realism" (Bergin, 1980), in which respect for the client's objects and practices of faith are afforded the legitimacy of reality, but go further to *affirm* an empirically based theistic, spiritual view of human nature and of the world (Richards & Bergin, 2005). Such approaches bring directly into the therapeutic relationship the faith commitments of both the client and the clinician, belief in the healing power of God, consideration of a theistic moral framework, and the explicit use of spiritual inventions, such as prayer, Scripture, spiritual direction, or meditation practices (Richards, 2004). In such approaches psychological and spiritual dimensions may be viewed as distinct, parallel, and complementary trajectories; as interwoven; or as an amalgam in which the psychological is subsumed into the spiritual (Sperry & Shafranske, 2004).

The Integration of Religious and Spiritual Interventions and Resources

Central to the consideration of integration is whether the client has expressed an explicit desire (and given informed consent) for religion and spirituality to be included as areas of focus within the course of treatment. Survey research suggests that many patients believe that the spiritual dimension should be considered in consultation; however, as with clinicians, patients have not demonstrated a clear consensus as to how such integration is to be accomplished. MacLean et al. (2003), for example, reported that one-third of the medical patients wanted to be asked about their religious beliefs and two-thirds felt that physicians should be aware of their beliefs (p. 38). Rose et al. (2001) surveyed 75 clients from nine different counseling settings and found that 55% of the respondents wanted to discuss religious or spiritual issues in psychological treatment. Surveys of psychologists, psychiatrists, and rehabilitation physicians have also found that religious and spiritual issues often are involved in treatment (Shafranske, 2000, 2001). Recently, respondents to an online survey of over 200 psychologists, employing a real-time behavior sampling (RTBS) methodology, reported that spirituality contributed to the solution in 37% of the cases and in 26% of cases were involved in both problem and solution (American Psychological Association Practice Directorate, 2003).

A range of interventions, reflecting varying degrees of explicit integration of religious and spiritual perspectives and practices, are available. Richards and Bergin (2005, pp. 287–288) identified 19 examples of religious and spiritual interventions that could be applied within explicit integration, including therapist prayer, teaching scriptural concepts, reference to Scripture, spiritual self-disclosure, spiritual confrontation, spiritual assessment, religious relaxation or imagery, therapist and client prayer, blessing by the therapist, encouragement for forgiveness, use of religious community, client prayer, encouragement of client confession, referral for blessing, religious journal writing, spiritual meditation, religious bibliotherapy, Scripture memorization, and dream interpretation. Although the majority of clinicians consider religion and spirituality to be relevant to treatment, reviews of the literature (Worthington, Kurusu, McCullough, & Sandage, 1996; see also McCullough, 1999; Worthington & Sandage, 2001, 2002) suggest the use of religious and spiritual interventions (1) does not appear to be consistent or systematic across clinicians; (2) is influenced by the personal commitments of the clinicians; and (3) varies according to the degree of involvement of the clinician in the performance of explicit religious–spiritual behavior (Shafranske, 1996b, 2000). Little is known about the decision-making processes that inform a clinician's introduction of religious or spiritual interventions or resources.

In a recent national survey of clinical psychologists, Hathaway et al. (2004) reported that over 80% of the clinicians believe that "religious/spiritual functioning is a significant and important domain in human adjustment," yet "over half reported asking about client religiousness or spirituality 50% of the time or less" and 12% and 18% reported that they never asked "about client religiousness or spirituality, respectively, during assessment" (p. 100). This inconsistency within and between clinicians may reflect differences in personal religious–spiritual commitment as well as education and training. Survey research has indicated that the greater the extent to which clinicians self-identify as religious, the more likely it is that they will perform religious interventions (Shafranske, 1996b, 2000, 2001; see also Worthington et al., 1996). Also, it has been found that as the intervention becomes more active and requires direct clinician participation, the endorsement and performance of the intervention decreases (Shafranske, 1996b, 2000, 2001); Figure 27.1 presents an example of this trend in a survey of rehabilitation psychologists. Although clinicians almost universally endorse gaining knowledge about the religious backgrounds of their clients and the majority of clinicians do so, almost no one reports praying with a client. This is of interest in light of the importance many individuals place on prayer (McCaffrey, Eisenberg, Legedza, Davis, & Philips, 2004) and the results of a 1999 CBS News Poll in which 63% of adults stated that they believed that physicians should join their patients in prayer if requested and 34% believed that prayer should be a standard part of the practice of medicine. Similar to clinicians, MacLean et al. (2003) found that "patient interest in religious or spiritual interaction decreased when the intensity of the interaction moved from a simple discussion of spiritual issues (33% agree) to physician silent prayer (28% agree) to physician prayer with a patient (19% agree; $p < .001$)" (p. 38).

The use of clinical interventions is best established on a foundation of clinical investigation, education, training, and supervision. In the first respect, few empirical studies of religious and spiritual interventions in psychotherapy have been conducted. Worthington and Sandage (2001, 2002) reported that only nine outcome studies of religion-accommodative psychotherapy had been conducted in which cognitive or cognitive-

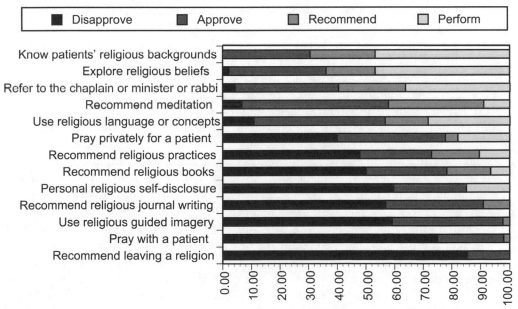

FIGURE 27.1. Attitudes and performance of religious and spiritual interventions by psychologists specializing in rehabilitation. From Shafranske (2000). Copyright 2000 by Slack, Inc. Reprinted by permission.

behavioral psychotherapy had been accommodated to religious clients through the introduction of religious interventions. They concluded that in all cases "religious CBT [cognitive-behavioral therapy] has been at least as effective as secular CBT for religious clients; in several cases, it has been better" (Worthington & Sandage, 2001, p. 476; see also Propst, Ostrom, Watkins, Dean, & Mashburn, 1992). Such findings are promising; however, further studies are required to establish empirical support.

Education and Training

Historically, most clinicians receive little or no training in assessing religiousness or spirituality as clinical variables or in the use of religious and spiritual interventions (Shafranske, 1996b, 2000, 2001), and up until recently, religion as a feature of diversity has been underrepresented in the scientific literature (Nilsson et al., 2003). However, Hathaway et al. (2004) in a more recent survey found that over one-third of the clinicians surveyed indicated that they had received prior training, although the extent of the exposure was not defined. Shafranske (2002a) and Weaver, Flannelly, and Oppenheimer (2003) report significant increases in the coverage of religion and spirituality as clinical issues within scholarly journals. Surveys of doctoral programs provide additional information regarding the present state of preparation. Schulte, Skinner, and Claiborn (2002), Brawer, Handal, Fabricatore, Roberts, and Wajda-Johnson (2002), and Young, Cashwell, Wiggins-Frame, and Belaire (2002), in their respective studies of counseling, clinical, and Council for Accreditation of Counseling and Related Educational Programs (CACREP)-accredited psychology and counseling programs, found that specific courses are rarely or never offered; this content area is most often subsumed into more broad areas, such as the diversity or cultural component(s) of the curriculum or in supervision; considerable variability exists in respect to the nature and extent of coverage; and it is unclear how considerations of religion and spirituality are addressed. Although the groundswell of research as well as continued efforts to ensure diversity competence may prompt increased attention to religion and spirituality as relevant to clinical practice, at present there is no evidence to suggest significant curricular investment to ensure systematic and comprehensive education and training in this area. Doctoral programs, which have as their mission the explicit integration of a faith dimension, will continue to train psychologists with unique competencies in this area. Moreover, clinical supervision provides important opportunities to assist novice clinicians to become sensitive and effective in addressing religious and spiritual variables (Miller, Korinek, & Ivey, 2004; Polanski, 2003; Shafranske & Falender, 2005). The development of competence in understanding the contributions of religion and spirituality to mental health as well as in the applied psychology of religion, in the near term, is likely to rest on unique training experiences rather than on systematic attention throughout all levels of graduate education and clinical training. To a great extent the personal faith commitment of the clinician will continue to serve as a salient feature of motivation and determine the extent to which a psychologist obtains expertise in this area. Survey research has shown that personal faith, intrinsic religious orientation, and religious involvement play significant roles in the use of religious interventions (Shafranske & Gorsuch, 1985; Shafranske & Malony, 1990a, 1990b) and, given the current state of training, this is likely to continue.

The role of personal faith in influencing the manner in which the spiritual dimension is addressed in psychological consultation is important in light of the differences in religious and spiritual beliefs, preference, and involvement between mental health practitioners and the general public (Bergin & Jensen, 1990; Shafranske, 1996b, 2000, 2001; Shafranske & Malony, 1990a, 1990b, 1996). Psychologists, as a group, appear to be less institutionally religious compared with the general population, and within the academy the majority of psychology professors report "None" when asked about religious preference (Roper Center for Public Opinion Research, 1991, pp. 86–87). When salience is measured in terms of spirituality, psychologists (and psychiatrists) appear to be more similar than previously assumed to the general population. This may suggest that the majority of psychologists appreciate the religious–spiritual dimension; however, they are less likely to participate in organized religion, which may influence their perspective when working with clients for whom participation in denominational religion is central (see Table 27.2).

Consultation and Collaboration

The integration of religious and spiritual resources can be accomplished through collaboration with religious professionals, and yet it appears that psychologists rarely consider clergy as potential collaborators (Weaver et al., 1997). Consultation can enhance psychologists' understanding of religious worldviews and practices and can facilitate familiarity with the faith communities in which their clients are involved. Collaboration can provide a means for clients to receive consultation directly from clergy, which may support the treatment process and in many instances is the ethically appropriate response to a client's needs. Referral to a religious professional, who by virtue of education and training offers competence in matters of religion, is often, if not always, the ethically appropriate intervention when clients are addressing explicitly religious issues. Consultation and collaboration are competencies that can be developed (McMinn, Aikins, & Lish, 2003; McMinn, Chaddock, Edwards, Lim, & Campbell, 1998; McMinn, Meek, Can-

TABLE 27.2. Salience of Religion and Spirituality to Psychologists and Public at Large (Percentages)

	Very important	Fairly important	Not very important	No opinion
National sample[a]	58	30	11	1
National sample[b]	59	29	12	<1
Education[b]				
Postgraduate	50	35	15	<1
College graduate	51	35	15	<1
College incomplete	56	33	11	<1
No college	64	29	7	<1
Clinical and counseling psychologists[c]				
Salience of religion	26	22	51	0
Salience of spirituality	48	25	26	0
Rehabilitation psychologists[d]				
Salience of religion	27	28	43	2
Salience of spirituality	50	30	19	1

Note. From Shafranske (2000). Copyright 2000 by Slack, Inc. Reprinted by permission.
[a] Gallup Poll (April 30–May 2, 1999).
[b] 1993 Gallup Poll (Gallup, 1994).
[c] Random sample of American Psychological Association members listing degrees in clinical psychology or counseling psychology (N = 253) (Shafranske, 1995).
[d] Random sample of American Psychological Association Division 22 members (N = 242) (Shafranske, 1998).

ning, & Pozzi, 2001), and offer an advantageous approach to integrating the full complement of religious and spiritual resources in cases when appropriate.

Ethics

Clear guidelines exist regarding the requirement of taking religion (and spirituality) into consideration as a feature of diversity (American Psychological Association, 2002a, 2002b). However, psychologists face a number of ethical challenges when addressing client beliefs and values and integrating religious–spiritual interventions and resources into psychological treatment. Richards and Bergin (2005) cite the following ethical pitfalls: "dual relationships (religious and professional), displacing or usurping religious authority, imposing religious values on clients, violating work setting (church–state) boundaries, and practicing outside the boundaries of professional competence" (p. 183). They also present general process suggestions to inform ethical practice (see Table 27.3). Among their suggestions, Yarhouse and VanOrman (1999) recommend including "perspectives on religion in informed consent . . . offering treatment that has been adapted to the language and experience of religious clients . . . [and] incorporating interventions that are congruent with the values, priorities, and concerns of religious clients" (p. 561; see also Richards, Rector, & Tjeltveit, 1999; Tan, 1994, 2003; Tjeltveit, 1986; Younggren, 1993). Therapists must also consider that explicit integration, in particular, leads into a territory in which statutory authority for such practices and empirical support for the use of such interventions have not been established and client informed consent is a reasonable but may not be a sufficient safeguard. A firm foundation for practice will be established through advances in the empirical standing of these procedures within the clinical setting; systematic and comprehensive attention

TABLE 27.3. General Process Suggestions for Therapists Who Are Using Religious and Spiritual Interventions

1. Tell clients during informed consent procedures that they approach therapy with a theistic spiritual perspective. When appropriate, use religious and spiritual interventions.

2. Assess clients' religious and spiritual background and current status before using religious and spiritual interventions.

3. Establish a relationship of trust and rapport with clients.

4. Consider carefully whether religious and spiritual interventions are indicated (or contraindicated) before using them.

5. Describe the interventions they wish to use and obtain clients' permission to do so before implementing them.

6. Use interventions in a respectful manner, remembering that many of the interventions are regarded as sacred religious practices by religious believers.

7. Work within clients' value framework and be careful not to push spiritual beliefs and values on clients; it is appropriate, however, to challenge and help clients examine beliefs that are irrational, self-defeating, and linked to the presenting problem.

8. Do not apply interventions rigidly or uniformly with all clients but use them in a flexible, treatment-tailoring manner.

9. Seek spiritual enlightenment and inspiration to guide them in what interventions to use and when to use them.

Note. From Richards and Bergin (2005). Copyright 2005 by the American Psychological Association. Reprinted by permission.

in education, training, and supervision; and initiatives to identify and evaluate levels of competence and to credential expertise and specialized competence (Hathaway, 2003; Yarhouse & Fisher, 2002).

CONCLUSION

Advances in clinical practice, drawing on the scholarship within the psychology of religion, offer the possibility of addressing and incorporating religious and spiritual dimensions, which are salient in the lives of most individuals, into clinical practice, and encourages a more comprehensive approach to human suffering and healing. Although science is firmly establishing the connection between religion and spirituality and health, much work lies ahead in developing empirically supported intervention protocols and guidelines to ensure ethical conduct; to enhance education, training, and supervision; and to institute processes to evaluate levels of competence in the provision of religious and spiritual interventions.

NOTE

1. "In-depth" rather than "comprehensive" has been selected to describe the nature of the second level of assessment. The scope of the assessment is limited to the requirements of the clinical evaluation and as such usually does not include a comprehensive, all-encompassing examination of each facet of an individual's religious–spiritual life.

REFERENCES

American Counseling Association. (1996). Spirituality Competencies. Summit on Spirituality. Retrieved December 10, 2003, from www.counseling.org/site/PageServer pagename=aservic_Spirituality_Competencies.

American Psychiatric Association. (1994). *Diagnostic and statistical manual of mental disorders* (4th ed.). Washington, DC: Author.

American Psychological Association. (2002a). Ethical principles of psychologists and code of conduct 2002. Retrieved May 1, 2003, from www.apa.org/ethics/code2002.html.

American Psychological Association. (2002b). *Guidelines for multicultural education, training, research, practice, and organizational change for psychologists.* Washington, DC: Author.

American Psychological Association Practice Directorate. (2003). *PracticeNet* survey: Clinical practice patterns. Retrieved December 1, 2004, from www.apapracticenet.net/results/Summer2003/2.asp.

Baumeister, R. F. (1992). *Meanings of life.* New York: Guilford Press.

Bergin, A. E. (1980). Psychotherapy and religious values. *Journal of Consulting and Clinical Psychology, 48,* 95–105.

Bergin, A. E., & Jensen, J. P. (1990). Religiosity of psychotherapists: A national study. *Psychotherapy, 27,* 3–7.

Beutler, L. E., Machado, P. P. P., & Neufeldt, S. A. (1994). Therapist variables. In A. E. Bergin & S. L. Garfield (Eds.), *Handbook of psychotherapy and behavior change* (4th ed., pp. 229–269). New York: Wiley.

Brawer, P. A., Handal, P. J., Fabricatore, A. N., Roberts, R., & Wajda-Johnston, V. A. (2002). Training and education in religion/spirituality within APA-accredited clinical psychology programs. *Professional Psychology: Research and Practice, 33*, 203–206.

Butter, E. M., & Pargament, K. I. (2003). Development of a model for clinical assessment of religious coping: Initial validation of the process evaluation model. *Mental Health, Religion and Culture, 6*(2), 175–194.

CBS News. (1999). Should doctors pray with their patients? National Institute for Healthcare Research. Retrieved August 4, 1999, from www.nihr.org/media/poll.html.

Chirban, J. T. (2001). Assessing religious and spiritual concerns in psychotherapy. In T. G. Plante & A. C. Sherman (Eds.), *Faith and health: Psychological perspectives* (pp. 265–290). New York: Guilford Press.

Corbett, L. (1996). *The religious function of the psyche.* New York: Routledge.

Ellison, C. (1994). *The spiritual well-being scale.* Nyack, NY: Life Advance.

Emmons, R. A., & Paloutzian, R. F. (2003). The psychology of religion. *Annual Review of Psychology, 54*, 377–402.

Exline, J. J. (2002). Stumbling blocks on the religious road: Fractured relationships, nagging vices, and the inner struggle to believe. *Psychological Inquiry, 13*(3), 182–189.

Exline, J. J. (2003). Anger toward God: A brief overview of existing research. *Psychology of Religion Newsletter, 29*(1), 1–8.

Exline, J. J., Yali, A. M., & Sanderson, W. C. (2000). Guilt, discord, and alienation: The role of religious strain in depression and suicidality. *Journal of Clinical Psychology, 56*, 1481–1496.

Frame, M. W. (2000). The spiritual genogram in family therapy. *Journal of Marital and Family Therapy, 26*, 211–216.

Frame, M. W. (2003). *Integrating religion and spirituality into counseling.* Pacific Grove, CA: Brooks/Cole.

Fredrickson, B. L. (2002). How does religion benefit health and well-being?: Are positive emotions active ingredients? *Psychological Inquiry, 13*(3), 209–213.

Fukuyama, M. A., & Sevig, T. D. (1999). *Integrating spirituality into multicultural counseling.* Thousand Oaks, CA: Sage.

Galanter, M. (1996). Cults and charismatic group psychology. In E. P. Shafranske (Ed.), *Religion and the clinical practice of psychology* (pp. 269–296). Washington, DC: American Psychological Association.

Gallup, G., Jr. (1994). *The Gallup poll: Public opinion 1993.* Wilmington, DE: Scholarly Resources.

Gallup. (1999). CNN/USA Today Poll. Retrieved June 1, 1999, from brain.gallup.com/documents/questionnaire. ASPX?/STUDY-92990425

Gorsuch, R. L., & Miller, W. R. (1999). Assessing spirituality. In W. R. Miller (Ed.), *Integrating spirituality into treatment* (pp. 47–64). Washington, DC: American Psychological Association.

Gorsuch, R. L., & Venable, G. D. (1983). Development of an "age universal" I–E scale. *Journal for the Scientific Study of Religion, 22*, 181–187.

Griffith, J. L., & Griffith, M. L. (2001). *Encountering the sacred in psychotherapy: How to talk with people about their spiritual lives.* New York: Guilford Press.

Hall, T. W., & Edwards, K. J. (2002). The Spiritual Assessment Inventory: A theistic model and measure for assessing spiritual development. *Journal for the Scientific Study of Religion, 41*, 341–357.

Hathaway, W. L. (2003). Clinically significant religious impairment. *Mental Health, Religion and Culture, 6*, 39–55.

Hathaway, W. L., Scott, S. Y., & Garver, S. A. (2004). Assessing religious/spiritual functioning: A neglected domain in clinical practice. *Professional Psychology: Research and Practice, 35*(1), 97–104.

Hill, P. C., & Hood, R. W., Jr. (1999). *Measures of religiosity.* Birmingham, AL: Religious Education Press.

Hill, P. C., & Pargament, K. I. (2003). Advances in the conceptualization and measurement of religion and spirituality. *American Psychologist, 58*(1), 64–74.

John E. Fetzer Institute. (1999). *Multidimensional measurement of religiousness/spirituality for use in health research*. Kalamazoo, MI: Author.

Kass, J. D., Friedman, R., & Lesserman, J. (1991). Health outcomes and a new index of spiritual experience. *Journal for the Scientific Study of Religion, 30*, 203–211.

Kelly, E. W., Jr. (1995). *Spirituality and religion in counseling and psychotherapy: Diversity theory and practice*. Alexandria, VA: American Counseling Association.

Kirkpatrick, L. A. (1992). An attachment-theory approach to the psychology of religion. *The International Journal for the Psychology of Religion, 2*, 3–28.

Kirkpatrick, L. A. (1998). God as a substitute attachment figure: A longitudinal study of adult attachment style and religious change in college students. *Personality and Social Psychology Bulletin, 24*(9), 961–973.

Koenig, H. G., & Larson, D. B. (2001). Religion and mental health: Evidence for an association. *International Review of Psychiatry, 13*(2), 67–78.

Lovinger, R. J. (1984). *Working with religious issues in therapy*. Northvale, NJ: Aronson.

MacLean, C. D., Susa, B., Phifer, N., Bynum, D., Franco, M., Klioze, A., Monroe, M., Garrett, J., & Cykert, S. (2003). Patient preference for physician discussion and practice of spirituality: Results from a multicenter patient survey. *Journal of General Internal Medicine, 18*(1), 38–43.

McCaffrey, A. M., Eisenberg, D. M., Legedza, A. T. R., Davis, R. B., & Philips, R. S. (2004). Prayer for health concerns. *Archives of Internal Medicine, 164*(8), 858–861.

McCullough, M. E. (1999). Research on religion-accomodative counseling: Review and meta-analysis. *Journal of Counseling Psychology, 46*, 92–98.

McMinn, M. R., Aikins, D. C., & Lish, R. A. (2003). Basic and advanced competence in collaborating with clergy. *Professional Psychology: Research and Practice, 34*(2), 197–202.

McMinn, M. R., Chaddock, T. P., Edwards, L. C., Lim, R. K. B., & Campbell, C. D. (1998). Psychologists collaborating with clergy: Survey findings and implications. *Professional Psychology: Research and Practice, 29*, 564–570.

McMinn, M. R., Meek, K. R., Canning, S. S., & Pozzi, C. F. (2001). Training psychologists to work with religious organizations: The center for church–psychology collaboration. *Professional Psychology: Research and Practice, 32*(3), 324–328.

Meissner, W. W. (1996). The pathology of beliefs and the beliefs of pathology. In E. P. Shafranske (Ed.), *Religion and the clinical practice of psychology* (pp. 241–267). Washington, DC: American Psychological Association.

Miller, G. (2003). *Incorporating spirituality into counseling and psychotherapy*. New York: Wiley.

Miller, M. M., Korinek, A., & Ivey, D. C. (2004). Spirituality in MFT training: Development of the Spiritual Issues in Supervision Scale. *Contemporary Family Therapy: An International Journal, 26*(1), 71–81.

Miller, R. B. (2004). *Facing human suffering: Psychology and psychotherapy as moral engagement*. Washington, DC: American Psychological Association.

Miller, W. R. (1999). *Integrating spirituality into treatment: Resources for practitioners*. Washington, DC: American Psychological Association.

Miller, W. R., & Thoresen, C. E. (2003). Spirituality, religion, and health: An emerging research field. *American Psychologist, 58*(1), 24–35.

Mills, P. J. (Ed.). (2002). Spirituality, religiousness, and health [Special issue]. *Annals of Behavioral Medicine, 24*(1).

Newport, F. (2004, March 23). A look at Americans and religion today. The Gallup Organization. Retrieved on March 24, 2004, from http://gallup.com/content/default.aspx?ci=11089.

Nielson, S. L. (2004). A Mormon rational emotive behavior therapist attempts Qur'anic rational emotive therapy. In P. S. Richards & A. E. Bergin (Eds.), *Casebook for a spiritual strategy in counseling and psychotherapy* (pp. 213–230). Washington, DC: American Psychological Association.

Nielson, S. L., Johnson, W. B., & Ellis, A. (2001). *Counseling and psychotherapy with religious persons: A rational emotive behavior therapy approach*. Mahwah, NJ: Erlbaum.

Nilsson, J. E., Berkel, L.-V. A., Flores, L. Y., Love, K. M., Wendler, A. M., & Mecklenburg, E. C. (2003). An 11-year review of *Professional Psychology: Research and Practice*: Content and sample analysis with an emphasis on diversity. *Professional Psychology: Research and Practice*, *34*, 611–616.

O'Donohue, W. (1989). The (even) bolder model: The clinical psychologist as metaphysician-scientist-practitioner. *American Psychologist*, *44*(12), 1460–1468.

Pargament, K. I. (1997). *The psychology of religion and coping*. New York: Guilford Press.

Pargament, K. I. (2002a). The bitter and the sweet: An evaluation of the costs and benefits of religiousness. *Psychological Inquiry*, *13*(3), 168–181.

Pargament, K. I. (2002b). Is religion nothing but . . . ?: Explaining religion versus explaining religion away. *Psychological Inquiry*, *13*(3), 239–244.

Pargament, K. I., Koenig, H. G., & Perez, L. M. (2000). The many methods of religious coping: Development and initial validation of the RCOPE. *Journal of Clinical Psychology*, *56*, 519–543.

Pargament, K. I., Koenig, H. G., Tarakeshwar, N., & Hahn, J. (2001). Religious struggle as a predictor of mortality among medically ill elderly patients. *Archives of Internal Medicine*, *161*, 1881–1886.

Pargament, K. I., Smith, B. W., Koenig, H. G., & Perez, L. (1998). Patterns of positive and negative religious coping with major life stressors. *Journal for the Scientific Study of Religion*, *37*, 710–724.

Pargament, K. I., Zinnbauer, B. J., Scott, A., Butter, E. M., Zerowin, J., & Stanik, P. (1998). Red flags and religious coping: Identifying some religious warning signs among people in crisis. *Journal of Clinical Psychology*, *54*, 77–89.

Polanski, P. J. (2003). Spirituality in supervision. *Counseling and Values*, *47*(2), 131–141.

Powell, L. H., Shahabi, L., & Thoresen, C. E. (2003). Religion and spirituality: Linkages to physical health. *American Psychologist*, *58*(1), 36–52.

Propst, L. R. (1988). *Psychotherapy in a religious framework: Spirituality in the emotional healing process*. New York: Human Sciences.

Propst, L. R., Ostrom, R., Watkins, P., Dean, T., & Mashburn, D. (1992). Comparative efficacy of religious and nonreligious cognitive-behavioral therapy for the treatment of clinical depression in religious individuals. *Journal of Consulting and Clinical Psychology*, *60*, 94–103.

Randour, M. L. (Ed.). (1993). *Exploring sacred landscapes*. New York: Columbia University Press.

Richards, P. S. (2004). Theistic psychotherapy approach. In L. Sperry & E. P. Shafranske (Eds.), *Spiritually oriented psychotherapy*. Washington, DC: American Psychological Association.

Richards P. S., & Bergin, A. E. (Eds.). (2000). *Handbook of psychotherapy and religious diversity*. Washington, DC: American Psychological Association.

Richards, P. S., & Bergin, A. E. (Eds.). (2004). *Religion and psychotherapy: A casebook*. Washington, DC: American Psychological Association.

Richards, P. S., & Bergin, A. E. (2005). *A spiritual strategy for counseling and psychotherapy* (2nd ed.). Washington, DC: American Psychological Association.

Richards, P. S., Rector, J. M., & Tjeltveit, A. C. (1999). Values, spirituality, and psychotherapy. In W. R. Miller (Ed.), *Integrating spirituality in treatment: Resources for practitioners* (pp. 133–160). Washington, DC: American Psychological Association.

Richardson, F., Fowers, B., & Guignon, C. (1999). *Re-envisioning psychology: Moral dimensions of theory and practice*. San Francisco: Jossey-Bass.

Rizzuto, A.-M. (1979). *The birth of the living God*. Chicago: University of Chicago Press.

Rizzuto, A.-M. (1996). Psychoanalytic treatment and the religious person. In E. P. Shafranske (Ed.), *Religion and the clinical practice of psychology* (pp. 409–431). Washington, DC: American Psychological Association.

Romero, C. G. (1991). *Hispanic devotional piety*. Maryknoll, NY: Orbis.

Roof, C. W. (1999). *Spiritual marketplace*. Princeton, NJ: Princeton University Press.

Roper Center for Public Opinion Research. (1991, April–May). Politics of the professorate. *The Public Perspective*, pp. 86–87.

Rose, E. M., Westefeld, J. S., & Ansley, T. N. (2001). Spiritual issues in counseling: Clients' beliefs and preferences. *Journal of Counseling Psychology*, *48*, 61–71.

Schulte, D. L., Skinner, T. A., & Claiborn, C. D. (2002). Religious and spiritual issues in counseling psychology training. *The Counseling Psychologist*, *30*, 118–134.

Shafranske, E. P. (1995). *Religiosity of clinical and counseling psychologists.* Unpublished manuscript.

Shafranske, E. P. (1998). *Religiosity of APA Division 22 members.* Unpublished manuscript.

Shafranske, E. P. (Ed.). (1996a). *Religion and the clinical practice of psychology.* Washington, DC: American Psychological Association.

Shafranske, E. P. (1996b). Religious beliefs, affiliations, and practices of clinical psychologists. In E. P. Shafranske (Ed.), *Religion and the clinical practice of psychology* (pp. 149–162). Washington, DC: American Psychological Association.

Shafranske, E. P. (2000). Religious involvement and professional practices of psychiatrists and other mental health professionals. *Psychiatric Annals, 30,* 1–8.

Shafranske, E. P. (2001). The religious dimension of patient care within rehabilitation medicine: The role of religious beliefs, attitudes, and personal and professional practices. In T. G. Plante & A. C. Sherman (Eds.), *Faith and health: Psychological perspectives* (pp. 311–335). New York: Guilford Press.

Shafranske, E. P. (2002a). The necessary and sufficient conditions for an applied psychology of religion. *Psychology of Religion Newsletter, 27*(4), 1–11.

Shafranske, E. P. (2002b). The psychoanalytic meaning of religious experience [Il significanto dell'esperienza religiosa]. In M. Arieti & F. De Nardi (Eds.), *Psychoanalisi e religione* (pp. 227–257). Turin, Italy: Centro Scientifico Editore.

Shafranske, E. P. (2004a). A psychodynamic case study. In P. S. Richards & A. E. Bergin (Eds.), *Casebook for a spiritual strategy in counseling and psychotherapy* (pp. 153–170). Washington, DC: American Psychological Association.

Shafranske, E. P. (2004b). Psychoanalytic approach. In L. Sperry & E. P. Shafranske (Eds.), *Spiritually oriented psychotherapy* (pp. 105–130). Washington, DC: American Psychological Association.

Shafranske, E. P., & Falender, C. A. (2005). *Addressing religious and spiritual issues in clinical supervision.* Manuscript in preparation.

Shafranske, E., & Gorsuch, R. (1985). Factors associated with the perception of spirituality in psychotherapy. *Journal of Transpersonal Psychology, 16,* 231–241.

Shafranske, E., & Malony, H. N. (1990a). Clinical psychologists' religious and spiritual orientations and their practice of psychotherapy. *Psychotherapy, 27*(1), 72–78.

Shafranske, E. P., & Malony, H. N. (1990b). California psychologists' religiosity and psychotherapy. *Journal of Religion and Health, 29*(3), 219–231.

Shafranske, E. P., & Malony, H. N. (1996). Religion and the clinical practice of psychology: A case for inclusion. In E. P. Shafranske (Ed.), *Religion and the clinical practice of psychology* (pp. 561–586). Washington, DC: American Psychological Association.

Shafranske, E. P., & Sperry, L. (2004). Addressing the spiritual dimension in psychotherapy: Introduction and overview. In L. Sperry & E. P. Shafranske (Eds.), *Spiritually oriented psychotherapy* (pp. 11–29). Washington, DC: American Psychological Association.

Sherman, A. C., & Simonton, S. (2001). Assessment of religiousness and spirituality in health research. In T. G. Plante & A. C. Sherman (Eds.), *Faith and health: Psychological perspectives* (pp. 139–163). New York: Guilford Press.

Sloan, R., Bagiella, E., & Powell, T. (1999). Religion, spirituality, and medicine. *The Lancet, 353,* 664–667.

Snyder, C. R., Sigmon, D. R., & Feldman, D. B. (2002). Hope for the sacred and vice versa: Positive goal-directed thinking and religion. *Psychological Inquiry, 13*(3), 234–238.

Sorenson, R. L. (2004). *Minding spirituality.* Hillsdale, NJ: Analytic Press.

Sperry, L. (2001). *Spirituality in clinical practice.* Philadelphia: Brunner-Routledge.

Sperry, L. (2004). Integrative spiritually oriented psychotherapy. In L. Sperry & E. P. Shafranske (Eds.), *Spiritually oriented psychotherapy* (pp. 307–329). Washington, DC: American Psychological Association.

Sperry, L., & Shafranske, E. P. (2004). *Spiritually oriented psychotherapy.* Washington, DC: American Psychological Association.

Steere, D. (1997). *Spiritual presence in psychotherapy: A guide for caregivers.* New York: Brunner/Mazel.

Stern, E. M. (Ed.). (1985). *Psychotherapy and the religiously committed patient.* New York: Haworth Press.

Tan, S.-Y. (1994). Ethical considerations in religious psychotherapy: Potential pitfalls and unique resources. *Journal of Psychology and Theology, 22,* 389–394.

Tan, S.-Y. (1996). Religion in clinical practice: Implicit and explicit integration. In E. P. Shafranske (Ed.), *Religion and the clinical practice of psychology* (pp. 365–387). Washington, DC: American Psychological Association.

Tan, S.-Y. (2003). Integrating spiritual direction into psychotherapy: Ethical issues and guidelines. *Journal of Psychology and Theology, 31,* 14–23.

Tan, S.-Y., & Johnson, W. B. (2004). Spiritually-oriented cognitive-behavioral approach. In L. Sperry & E. P. Shafranske (Eds.), *Spiritually oriented psychotherapy* (pp. 77–103). Washington, DC: American Psychological Association.

Tarakeshwar, N., Stanton, J., & Pargament, K. I. (2003). Religion: An overlooked dimension in cross-cultural psychology. *Journal of Cross-Cultural Psychology, 34*(4), 377–394.

Tjeltveit, A. C. (1986). The ethics of values conversion in psychotherapy: Appropriate and inappropriate therapist influence on client values. *Clinical Psychology Review, 6,* 515–537.

Tonigan, J. S., Toscova, R. T., & Connors, G. J. (1999). Spirituality and the 12-step programs: A guide for clinicians. In W. R. Miller (Ed.), *Integrating spirituality into treatment* (pp. 111–131). Washington, DC: American Psychological Association.

Vande Kemp, H. (1996). Historical perspective: Religion and clinical psychology in America. In E. P. Shafranske (Ed.), *Religion and the clinical practice of psychology* (pp. 71–112). Washington, DC: American Psychological Association.

Weaver, A. J., Flannelly, K. J., & Oppenheimer, J. E. (2003). Religion, spirituality and chaplains in the biomedical literature: 1965–2000. *International Journal of Psychiatry in Medicine, 33,* 155–161.

Weaver, A. J., Samford, J. A., Kline, A. E., Lucas, L. A., Larson, D. B., & Koenig, H. G. (1997). What do psychologists know about working with clergy?: An analysis of eight APA journals: 1991–1994. *Professional Psychology: Research and Practice, 28,* 471–474.

West, W. (2000). *Psychotherapy and spirituality: Crossing the line between therapy and religion.* London: Sage.

Worthington, E. L., Jr., Kurusu, T. A., McCullough, M. E., & Sandage, S. J. (1996). Empirical research on religion and counseling: A ten-year update and prospectus. *Psychological Bulletin, 119,* 448–487.

Worthington, E. L., Jr., & Sandage, S. J. (2001). Religion and spirituality. *Psychotherapy, 38*(4), 473–478.

Worthington, E. L., Jr., & Sandage, S. J. (2002). Religion and spirituality. In J. C. Norcross (Ed.), *Psychotherapy relationships that work: Therapist contributions and responsiveness to patients* (pp. 383–399). New York: Oxford University Press.

Wulff, D. M. (1997). *Psychology of religion* (2nd ed.). New York: Wiley.

Yarhouse, M. A., & Fisher, W. (2002). Level of training to address religion in clinical practice. *Psychotherapy, 39,* 171–176.

Yarhouse, M. A., & VanOrman, B. T. (1999). When psychologists work with religious clients: Applications of the general principles of ethical conduct. *Professional Psychology: Research and Practice, 30,* 557–562.

Young, J. S., Cashwell, C., Wiggins-Frame, M., & Belaire, C. (2002). Spiritual and religious competencies: A national survey of CACREP-accredited programs. *Counseling and Values, 47,* 22–33.

Younggren, J. N. (1993). Ethical issues in religious psychotherapy. *Register Report, 19,* 7–8.

Zinnbauer, B. J., Pargament, K. I., & Scott, A. B. (1999). The emerging meanings of religiousness and spirituality: Problems and prospects. *Journal of Personality, 67,* 889–919.

28

From Advocacy to Science

The Next Steps in Workplace Spirituality Research

ROBERT A. GIACALONE
CAROLE L. JURKIEWICZ
LOUIS W. FRY

WORKPLACE SPIRITUALITY: AN OVERVIEW

A burgeoning interest in issues regarding religion and spirituality can found in nearly every academic discipline as well as in the popular media. These issues have received increased attention in the organizational sciences, where the topic of workplace spirituality is one of the fastest growing areas of new research and inquiry by scholars (see Cavanaugh, 1999; Sass, 2000) and practitioners alike (Laabs, 1996). Why this is occurring is a matter of some debate (see Giacalone & Jurkiewicz, 2003, for a full review). The most viable arguments are that society seeks spiritual solutions to ease tumultuous social and business changes (e.g., Cash, Gray, & Rood, 2000; Mitroff & Denton, 2000); that profound change in values globally has brought a growing social consciousness and spiritual renaissance (e.g., Inglehart, 1997; Neal, 1998); and that growing interest in Eastern philosophies (Brandt, 1996) has prompted a general increase in spiritual yearnings. Whatever the reasons, the increased attention directed toward spiritual issues in the workplace is undeniable.

Interest in workplace spirituality has spurred curiosity beyond the capacity of scholars to keep pace with it either theoretically or methodologically. Elementary attempts at a noetic understanding of workplace spirituality began in the early 1990s as evidenced in books, articles, and special journal issues or sections (e.g., *Journal of Managerial Psychology*, *Journal of Management Inquiry*, *Journal of Management Education*, *Organization*, and the *Journal of Organizational Change Management*). Organizational consultants have also embraced the value of workplace spirituality for their clients, with some

(Barrett, 1998) taking a more pragmatic, data-based approach, and others providing training seminars and coaching on the topic. In the Academy of Management, the professional organization for scholars in business management, a formal interest group has emerged whose primary focus is the intersection of management, spirituality, and religion. Most recently, a 32-chapter volume, *The Handbook of Workplace Spirituality and Organizational Performance* (Giacalone & Jurkiewicz, 2003) established a new paradigm for this field of inquiry in the social sciences.

The emergence of workplace spirituality in the organizational sciences emerged from a very different mind-set than one would expect from a subarea in an organizational science. Organizational behavior, for example, borrowed heavily from psychology and sociology in its early development. Similarly conjoined, the field of human resource management developed a symbiotic relationship with industrial psychology. While many may have expected workplace spirituality to emerge from research on the psychology of religion, given the connotations suggested by the title of this book, that is not at all the case. While the research may sometimes parallel or intersect now, the field of workplace spirituality was born of organizational and social psychology, ethics, and management. It was one of the goals of the *Handbook* to establish these linkages and draw upon their strengths in developing this new science.

It is a point worthy of further elaboration and discussion. The disconnection between these fields can be best understood if we consider that the psychology of religion, particularly over the past 30 years, has been characterized by data gathering, while the study of workplace spirituality emerged through theoretical advocacy and organizational case study rather than by data sets compiled from individual respondents. Thus, the concept of workplace spirituality emerged from recognition and documentation of the phenomenon, and an articulated need for formalized study to address this salient aspect of organizational life. The stream of research that has arisen from this ontological tradition (see Biberman & Whitty, 2000) has led to important and groundbreaking forays into complex and emerging issues in the social sciences (Fairholm, 1997; Mirvis, 1997; Mitroff & Denton, 1999; Neal, 2001).

But in a nascent field that has undergone enormous change, where theoretical advocacy and organizational case study is increasingly being supplanted by scientific data, the question of direction looms large. What are the variables of interest? What conceptual distinctions are appropriate? What should the focus of measurement be? It is to these questions that we now turn.

WHERE DO WE GO FROM HERE?: THE NEXT ITERATION IN WORKPLACE SPIRITUALITY RESEARCH

The charge in *The Handbook of Workplace Spirituality and Organizational Performance* was clear: a scientific, data-based approach to workplace spirituality was warranted and necessary. But while theory development was important, what Giacalone and Jurkiewicz (2003) argued was that the study of workplace spirituality needs to demonstrate *effects* in order for it to be seen as a legitimate discipline in the field of organizational science. While the potentially constructive benefits of spiritual pursuits have been lauded effectively in psychological (Koenig, 1998), and medical (Koenig, McCullough, & Larson, 2001) writing, the organizational treatises prior to the *Handbook* focused on the normative, humanistic necessity of workplace spirituality. Indeed, if for no other reason, these scholars served an important function in introducing the concept to organizational leaders. But organizations, by their very nature, are far less interested in ideologies concerned with normative necessities and ultimately more entrenched in outcomes. Legitimizing workplace spirituality therefore requires a demonstrable positive impact of spiritual variables on workplace-related functioning. Without this demonstration, the topic of workplace spirituality would be marginalized as a philosophical and impractical pursuit. Thus, this chapter establishes a research framework by which one can assess the impact of spirituality on work-related functioning, with an emphasis on methodologies to demonstrate the predictive validity of the spirituality concept.

Assumptions of Our Approach

First, the study of workplace spirituality has, to date, been relatively free of denominational politics and the faith blanket in which such polemics are frequently cloaked. In fact, religious ideology itself has been virtually disregarded. Under the rubric of spirituality, the issues that have surfaced have avoided any mention of a comparatively right and wrong ideology. The approach set forth here follows that of Fry (2003), who distinguishes religion from spirituality and differentiates spiritual concerns from the search for God and the sharing of beliefs of any particular religious group (Veach & Chappel, 1991). The Dalai Lama (1999, p. 22) makes the distinction between spirituality and religion by noting that religion is concerned with faith in the claims of one faith tradition or another and is connected with systems of belief, ritual prayer, and related formalized practices and ideas. In contrast, spirituality is concerned with qualities of the human spirit including positive psychological concepts such as love and compassion, patience, tolerance, forgiveness, contentment, personal responsibility, and a sense of harmony with one's environment.

From this perspective, spirituality is necessary for religion but religion is not necessary for spirituality. Workplace spirituality can therefore be inclusive or exclusive of religious theory and practice. Institutionalists or traditionalists focus on time-honored beliefs and practices of their church; rationalists study prodigiously and engage in reflective thought; mystics use silent, intuitive contemplation; and moralists devote themselves to active obedience to duty. Spirituality is found in pursuit of a vision of service to others; through humility as having the capacity to regard oneself as an individual equal in value to other individuals; through charity, or altruistic love; and through veracity beyond basic truth telling to engage the capacity to see things exactly as they are, freed from subjective distortions.

Second, in trying to establish the parameters of a relationship between spirituality and work, it is essential that we entertain both the positive and the negative potential that spirituality brings. It is necessary to assume that spirituality can have both desirable and undesirable effects on organizational performance and that these could occur simultaneously. For example, negative spiritual traits such as judgmentalism and authoritarianism are grounded in selfish egoistic values and pride. One would expect negative personal and organizational outcomes to the extent that the attitudes and behaviors from these values create frustration, resentment, anger, worry, and fear within and across individuals and workgroups. An example would be a judgmental and authoritarian professional manager who mistrusted his or her people, and who therefore took on the most challenging projects him- or herself while micromanaging the routine work he or she delegated to similarly competent professional subordinates.

Furthermore, there may be unforeseen costs as well as benefits of employing a spiritual employee. For example, if we found that a spiritual employee held higher ethical standards than other employees held, those higher standards could also lead the employee to have higher expectations for what constitutes appropriate ethical behavior. Such standards could prove costly, in terms of both time (trying to reach a consensus on what is appropriate) and price (implementation), and could lead to whistleblowing behaviors if the concerns of the highly spiritual employee are not effectively addressed within the organizational structure. Conversely, if we extrapolate from a growing body of research that demonstrates a positive relationship between spirituality and health (see Koenig, 1998; Koenig, McCullough, & Larson, 2001; Oman & Thoresen, Chapter 24, this volume), understanding such a relationship could prove fruitful in allaying the costs of healthcare to the organization, an increasingly worrisome concern in the United States.

It is important, then, in moving the paradigm of workplace spirituality forward that we seek first to establish a foundation of theoretical and empirical knowledge, building upon the basic elements contributed to the field thus far, and keeping an open mind toward the questions that must be asked as well as how they are asked.

THE FUTURE OF WORKPLACE SPIRITUALITY RESEARCH

In calling for a scientific inquiry into workplace spirituality, Giacalone and Jurkiewicz, (2003) identify four major weaknesses that must be addressed if this newly emerging paradigm is to achieve acceptance within the scientific community: (1) the lack of an accepted conceptual definition, (2) inadequate measurement tools, (3) limited theoretical development, and (4) legal concerns. To address these weaknesses and to advance as a workplace spirituality paradigm rooted in science, three critical issues will need to be addressed: levels of conceptual analysis, conceptual distinctions and measurement foci, and clarification of the relationship between criterion variables. These issues lie at the heart of scientific inquiry and the theory building and testing process central to it (Dubin, 1978).

Level of Conceptual Analysis

There are many possible levels of analysis for workplace spirituality. The work of Giacalone and Jurkiewicz (2003; also see Jurkiewicz & Giacalone, 2004) has conceptualized it at both the individual and the organizational levels of analysis. Workplace spirituality at the individual level refers to a personal set of values that promote the experience of transcendence through the work process, facilitating a sense of connectedness to others in a way that provides feelings of completeness and joy (Giacalone & Jurkiewicz, 2003). Research has not determined whether employees necessarily bring spiritual values into the workplace or adopt them as an organizational ethic (Jurkiewicz, 2003). In much the same way that some employees may feel that it is best to leave personal ethics at home, some employees may sense that personal spirituality does not fit the work environment either. When employees bring their spirituality and related values to work, such spirituality might be considered an *integrative spirituality* in which personal spirituality is woven into various facets of the job. Conversely, when employees fail to bring their spirituality into work, it would be defined as a *segmented spirituality*. Segmented spirituality may be the result of the individual's unwillingness to bring spiritual beliefs to work (they don't want to share this part of their lives, they fear reprisal), or it may be a function of the individual's inability to enact it (they don't know how to integrate these beliefs into their work). Thus, in understanding workplace spirituality at the individual level, we must determine not only the level of spirituality, but also the level or integration of that spirituality into the organizational environment.

At the organizational or strategic level, workplace spirituality is a descriptor of the organization as an entity. Giacalone and Jurkiewicz (2003) defined it as a framework of organizational values evidenced in the culture that promote employees' experience of organizational transcendence through the work process, facilitating their sense of being connected to others in a way that provides feelings of completeness and joy. As such, workplace spirituality at this level can be considered both in terms of vision and cultural values.

Strategic leaders are ultimately responsible for creating vision and value congruence across the individual, group or team, and organizational levels, as well as for developing effective relationships between the organization and environmental stakeholders (Fry, 2003; Maghroori & Rolland, 1997). Of utmost importance is a clear and compelling vision. This vision should vividly portray a journey which, when undertaken, will give one a sense of calling, of one's life having meaning (see Park, Chapter 16, this volume) and making a difference. The vision, coupled with the organization's purpose (i.e., its reason for existence) and mission (i.e., what the organization does and who it serves), work in concert to define the organization's core values. This visioning process then forms the basis for the social construction of the organization's culture and the ethical system and core values underlying it, which will in turn form the foundation for relating to and meeting or exceeding the expectations of high-power and/or high-importance stakeholders (e.g., customers, employees, chain of command, regulatory agencies).

At the group or team level, organizations must establish a culture with values that reflect the organization's culture and values. Especially important for workplace spirituality is empowerment. Empowerment is power sharing, the delegation of both power and authority and all but symbolic responsibility to organizational followers (Bowen & Lawler, 1995; Spreitzer, 1996). Strategic leaders, in addition to delegating power, should provide followers with knowledge of how their jobs are relevant to the organization's performance. It is this linkage that creates the cross-level connection between individual and group jobs and the organization's vision and values, thereby giving followers a sense of direction by which to act. In addition to empowerment, this process of providing directed autonomy, competence, and relatedness is also the foundation for intrinsic motivation and workplace spirituality (Deci & Ryan, 2000; Ford & Fotler, 1995; Fry, 2003).

Conceptual Distinctions and Measurement Focus

An indisputable difficulty that must be addressed in workplace spirituality research is the conceptual overlap between spirituality and related concepts (see Zinnbauer & Pargament, Chapter 2, this volume). Conceptually, there are aspects of workplace spirituality, particularly at the individual level, that are theoretically and empirically connected to other areas—notably those behaviors and dispositional traits identified in the areas of positive psychology (Snyder & Lopez, 2001) and character ethics (Lickona, 1991). While the work of Fry (2004), Emmons (2003), Emmons and Paloutzian (2003), Giacalone and Jurkiewicz (2003), and Jurkiewicz and Giacalone (2004) have identified the core values, attitudes, and behavior of ethical and spiritual well-being, their approach integrates and envelopes other frameworks, theories, and concepts. Both Fry (2004) and Giacalone and

Jurkiewicz (2003) use conceptualizations that are mainstays in social psychology and political science.

Among other issues, such conceptual overlaps raise concerns over measurement (see Hill, Chapter 3, this volume). With many good treatises written on spiritual and religious measurement (Hill & Hood, 1999; MacDonald, Friedman, & Kuentzel, 1999; MacDonald, Kuentzel, & Friedman,1999), none has confronted the complexity of firmly distinguishing among these conceptual overlaps, nor have they addressed whether such conceptualizations can be aggregated at a macro (organizational) level. Getting to the root of this complexity is critical if workplace spirituality is to develop as a scientific area of inquiry. We know from related research on postmaterialist values (Inglehart, 1990) that conceptual ambiguities, when coupled with measurement problems, create a voluminous research output that focuses on conceptual problems rather than theoretical advances. In the case of postmaterialist values, for example, the assessment problems have embroiled researchers in trying to determine the number of dimensions involved, the level at which responses can be aggregated, and the theoretically appropriate way to determine how a hypothesis might be tested (e.g., Davis & Davenport, 1999).

Workplace spirituality research is now in a similarly difficult stage of development. The lack of conceptual clarity related to level of analysis makes measurement questionable. Whether one assesses at the individual or at the organizational level depends on one's conceptualization, but since there is no agreement on the level of analysis, researchers must decide for themselves. Such decisions are pivotal in developing foundations for further research. This lack of clarity is an example of unrationalized categorization at the theoretical level (Fry & Smith, 1987; Stanfield, 1976), and, like the research on postmaterialist values, could result in a hodgepodge of empirical studies that, even though reliable and valid, will serve to muddy rather than clarify theory building on workplace spirituality.

But even when such a pivotal decision is made, an equally important issue remains: What should be measured? The literature on spirituality is replete with measures of spirituality predicated on different conceptualizations (e.g., Hill & Hood, 1999). Inasmuch as a large body of published work has already focused attention upon two different types of measures (those of religiosity and those of spirituality separate from religiosity), the specifics and consequences of these measurement differences are not explored in this chapter (see Zinnbauer & Pargament, Chapter 2, this volume). It is pragmatic to assume that varying conceptualizations will have significantly different impacts upon the relationship outcomes between workplace spirituality and criterion variables.

Measures of religiosity are designed to assess individual adherence to theistic connection, or membership affiliation, though not necessarily an experience of transcendence. A measure in the study of religiosity and health outcomes, the DUREL (Duke University Religion Index) scale, has been used extensively in Koenig's ongoing research on the health–religion relationship. The DUREL scale measures organizational religiosity (e.g., How often do you attend church or other religious meetings?), nonorganizational religiosity (e.g., How often do you spend time in private religious activities, such as prayer, meditation, or Bible study?), and intrinsic religiosity (e.g., My religious beliefs are what really lie behind my whole approach to life). From a different conceptualization, the Human Spirituality Scale (HSS; Wheat, 1991) assesses substantive individual attributes constituting nondenominational personal spirituality (e.g., beliefs and attitudes) apart from religious affiliation. The HSS is a 20-item instrument with Likert-type scaling, and includes such statements as "I experience a sense of the sacred in living things" and "I set aside time for personal reflection and growth." Previous work (Belaire & Young, 2000) has shown this measure to be effective in assessing spirituality.

For the workplace spirituality researcher, what differentiates these measures from spiritual measures is not simply a matter of denominational affiliation or context. Rather, it is a matter of the more complex interactive relationship of the organizational and personal beliefs and their impact on criterion variables. For example, in an organization affiliated with a religious ideology, the individual's spirituality may be less important than her denominational affiliation. Similarly, in an organization that has a more generic, spiritual orientation, doctrinal employees may find themselves at odds over specific theological tenets.

A further complexity arises when trying to establish a relationship between individual spirituality and religiosity, group spirituality and religiosity, and organizational spirituality and religiosity: Is it appropriate to aggregate individual-level responses to the organizational level to determine the organizational level of these variables? Indeed, in the postmaterialism literature, this problem of aggregation has been a source of continual debate (e.g., Grendstad, & Selle, 1997). If workplace spirituality is conceptualized at the group and/or organizational level much work is needed to determine if and how current measures can be developed that do not suffer from aggregation bias (Fry, 1982; James, Demaree, & Wolf, 1993).

Despite the more traditional measures of religiosity and spirituality, recent scientific approaches to workplace spirituality have turned to conceptualizations focusing on the experience of transcendence apart from an individual's theistic connection, or membership affiliation. Unlike the previous conceptualizations and measures that were explicitly spiritual (such as the HSS), these other conceptualizations and measures of spirituality are not so explicit but instead represent characteristics long associated with spiritual and religious pursuits (Emmons, 2000; Giacalone & Jurkiewicz, 2003). Conceptualizations of leadership (Malone & Fry, 2003), hope (Snyder et al., 1996), forgiveness (Worthington, 1998), gratitude (Emmons & McCullough, 2003), generativity (McAdams & de St. Aubin, 1992), and agency/communion (Helgeson, 1994) all provide measures that can be used to ascertain how particular aspects of spirituality may impact organizationally related outcomes. Again, the complexity of aggregation from individual-level to organizational-level responses is problematic and must be considered in future work.

Establishing Clear Relationships with Criterion Variables

Inasmuch as workplace spirituality work was to a large extent driven by advocacy, workplace spirituality has been associated with a normative sense of goodness. Spiritual organizations were organizations with a higher purpose and calling characterized by cultures that incorporate humanitarian concerns and outcomes. Who can, after all, argue against such transcendent goals and love-based cultures, where completeness and joy are an integral part of the organizational purpose? But organizations, with their bottom-line mentality, while not opposed to these outcomes, are understandably interested in whether there is a relationship between spirituality and specific organizationally desirable outcomes. Political correctness aside, there is the "so what" question: If people are happy, if humanitarian purposes are achieved, and if completeness and joy abound, does that improve my profit/productivity picture? If workplace spirituality is associated with these positive outcomes, but fails to increase profitability/productivity (or decreases it), it will not have achieved the venerated value of wealth creation (or, in the public and nonprofit sectors, taxpayer return on investment). Albeit positive from a normative sense, organizations are likely to remain disinterested in creating spiritual workplaces without a demonstrable practical outcome (e.g., profits) associated with it, or other pressures (e.g., social responsibility, hiring) that demand that such environments be developed. Even if an association between spiritual workplaces and humanitarian outcomes could be demonstrated, it might not interest the power elite in organizations. Therefore, even if one accepts that spirituality is associated with a normative sense of goodness, creating spiritual workplaces will require demonstrating that workplace spirituality is aligned to organizational goals.

The legitimacy of this association has been discussed by Fry (2003), who notes that by understanding the vision of the organization and being empowered with the autonomy to act as they see fit, participants have an experience of competence in that, through their work, they are making a positive difference in other peoples' lives, which in turn enriches their own. It is such outcomes, ultimately based in the satisfactions that result from work performed as if it were a calling, that will result in higher levels of organizational commitment and productivity, and reduced stress—the same organizational goals most often reported as affective outcomes of organizational research. Conceptually, organizations would be interested in workplace spirituality if it demonstrated either a positive relationship with desirable outcomes or an inverse relationship with undesirable outcomes. These relationships need not be directly tied to a financial outcome (such as increased individual productivity or decreased theft), but could be tied indirectly to financially related outcomes such as associations with positive employee attitudes (yielding lower turnover), lowered rates of illness (reducing healthcare costs and absenteeism), or improved public image (yielding more interest in the company).

One such conceptualization, tied to leadership, has been proposed by Fry (2003). His causal theory of spiritual leadership is developed within an intrinsic motivation model that incorporates vision, hope/faith, and altruistic love, theories of workplace spirituality, and spiritual survival through calling and membership. The purpose of spiritual leadership is to tap into the fundamental needs of both leader and follower to create vision and value congruence across the strategic, empowered team, and individual levels and, ultimately, to foster higher levels of organizational commitment and productivity. Fry (2004) further extended spiritual leadership theory as a predictor of ethical well-being and spiritual well-being, positive human health, and corporate social responsibility.

Spiritual leadership is defined as comprising the values, attitudes, and behaviors that are necessary to intrinsically motivate one's self and others so that they have a sense of spiritual survival through calling and membership (see Figure 28.1). This entails:

1. Creating a vision wherein organization members experience a sense of calling in that their life has meaning and makes a difference;
2. Establishing a social/organizational culture based on altruistic love whereby leaders and followers have genuine care, concern, and appreciation for *both* self and others, thereby producing a sense of membership and feeling understood and appreciated.

To summarize the hypothesized relationships among the variables of the causal model of spiritual leadership (see Figure 28.1), "doing what it takes" through hope and faith in the organization's vision keeps followers looking forward to the future and provides the desire and positive expectation that fuels effort through intrinsic motivation. In

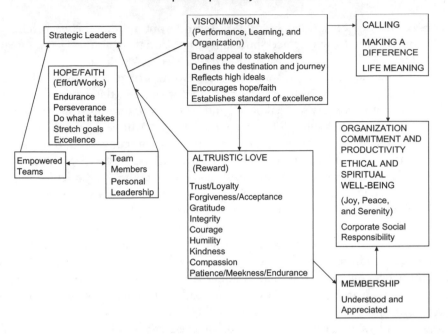

FIGURE 28.1. Spiritual leadership as a source of ethical and spiritual well-being and corporate social responsibility.

pursuing its vision, an organizational culture based in the values of altruistic love is also received by followers. This drives out and removes fears associated with worry, anger, jealousy, selfishness, failure, and guilt and gives one a sense of membership—that part of spiritual survival that gives one an awareness of being understood and appreciated. This is, of course, one of the most fundamentally motivating factors in the workplace overall.

Ultimately, this intrinsic motivation cycle based on vision (performance), altruistic love (reward), and hope/faith (effort) results in an increase in one's sense of spiritual survival (e.g., calling and membership) and ultimately positive personal, group, and organizational outcomes such as increased ethical and spiritual well-being, positive human health, organizational commitment and productivity, and corporate social responsibility.

Spirituality versus Religion Hypothesis

A central hypothesis to be tested relates to the distinction between spirituality and religious approaches to workplace spirituality across the individual, group, and organizational levels (see Zinnbauer & Pargament, Chapter 2, this volume). Many feel that viewing workplace spirituality through the lens of religious traditions and practice is divisive in that, to the extent that a specific religion views itself as the only path to God and salvation, it excludes those who do not share in the denominational tradition (Cavanaugh, 1999). Furthermore, religious practices often conflict with the social, legal, and ethical foundations of business, law, and public and nonprofit administration (Nadesan, 1999). Thus, religion can lead to the arrogant attitude that a particular company, faith, or society is better, morally superior, or more worthy than another (Nash, 1994). Promoting religion and pushing it into workplace spirituality can foster zealotry at the expense of organizational goals, offend constituents and customers, and decrease morale and employee well-being (Giacalone & Jurkiewicz, 2003). Accentuating the line between religion and spirituality in regards to workplace spirituality is essential to honoring the integrity of both disciplines.

There is even the potential, if spirituality is viewed through the lens of religion, for it to be divisive in that it may exclude those who do not share in the denominational tradition or conflict with a society's social, legal, and ethical foundations of business and public administration (Cavanaugh, 1999; Nadesan, 1999). "Adherence to a religious workplace orientation can lead to arrogance that a particular company, faith, or even nation is somehow 'better' or worthier than another" (Giacalone & Jurkiewicz, 2003, p. 13).

Indeed, if one looks at church organizations in general as the model for implementing religious ideology in secular organizations, one finds that while allowing some discretion at the church level, these organizations are mostly highly centralized. Pastors have minimum authority because of the manner in which leadership has been defined in constitutions, by-laws, and position descriptions. From the perspective of spiritual leadership theory, religious traditions and practices (as described above) would be seen as having a negative influence on organizational commitment and productivity. This is because exclusionary "our way is the one best way to lead and manage" values, attitudes, and behaviors tend to increase bureaucratic oversight. In the most extreme cases, a legacy of bureaucratic leadership steeped in hundreds or even thousands of years of creeds and practice can stifle creativity and intrinsic motivation for those excluded, while increasing stress, avoidance behaviors, and fear on the part of believers who demonstrate a mind-set focused on wrongdoing and punishment for deviance.

A major proposition of spiritual leadership theory is that spiritual leadership is necessary for the transformation to and continued success of learning organizations. Spiritual leadership can be viewed as an intrinsically motivating force that enables people to feel alive, energized, and connected with their work. It is this force that translates spiritual survival into feelings of attraction, fascination, and caring for work and people in the work environment into committed and productive organizational behavior (Covey, 1990). Spiritual leaders in these organizations must influence others through vision, values, and loving relationships rather than through fear, power, and control. Any workplace practices, whether under the guise of religion or some other spiritual tradition, that stifles this process would therefore lead to negative individual and organizational outcomes (e.g., in terms of commitment, productivity, ethical and spiritual well-being).

FUTURE DIRECTIONS FOR WORKPLACE SPIRITUALITY RESEARCH

Table 28.1 offers a tentative research agenda for workplace spirituality research that proposes differences between spiritual and religious approaches to workplace spirituality for common criterion variables across the individual, group, organizational, and societal levels.

Workplace spirituality research is undoubtedly in the initial concept/elaboration stage of development (Hunt, 1999; Reichers & Schneider, 1990). It therefore follows that the four components viewed as necessary and sufficient conditions for the development of any theoretical model (Dubin, 1978) are important to the study of workplace spirituality at this point in time: (1) identifiable units or variables of interest to the researcher; (2) congruence as defined by the laws of relationship among units of the model that specify how they are associated; (3) boundaries within which the laws of relationships are

TABLE 28.1. Proposed Research Agenda for Workplace Spirituality Research

Category	Purpose of measure	Individual variables	Group variables	Organizational variables	Society variables
Spiritual	To assess the experience of spiritual survival through transcendence (calling) and membership	Ethical and spiritual well-being (e.g., joy, peace, and serenity), commitment, productivity	Empowerment, effectiveness, productivity	Culture with values of altruistic love, profitability, competitive positions, reputation	Impact on stakeholders; corporate social responsibility
Religious	To assess the experience of spiritual survival through transcendence (calling), membership, and adherence to beliefs	Ethical and spiritual well-being (e.g., joy, peace, and serenity), attachment, productivity, decisions	Empowerment, effectiveness, and productivity	Culture with values of altruistic love, profitability, competitive positions, reputation	Impact on stakeholders; corporate social responsibility

expected to operate; and (4) contingency effects that specify system states within which the units of the theory take on characteristic values that are deterministic and have a persistence through time (see also Fry & Smith, 1987). It is toward fulfilling these components that scholarship in workplace spirituality must now focus.

In the context of Table 28.1 and spiritual leadership, the prospects for workplace spirituality are far more advanced. Research on several fronts is necessary to establish the validity of spiritual leadership theory before it should be widely applied as a model of organizational and professional development with the goal of fostering systemic change and transformation. Research suggests that increased organizational commitment strengthens motivation and reduces turnover (Mowday, Porter, & Steers, 1982), and that organizational productivity is at the heart of the total quality management (TQM) movement. Research is just beginning on the relationship between the qualities of spiritual leadership and organizational outcomes (Fry, Vitucci, & Cedillo, in press; Malone & Fry, 2003; Townsend, 1984). Still, outcomes across levels (e.g., ethical and spiritual well-being; joy, peace, and serenity; corporate social responsibility) hypothesized to be affected by spiritual leadership (Fry, 2004) also need to be validated for spiritual leadership theory to develop. Finally, the conceptual distinction between spiritual leadership theory variables and other workplace spirituality and workplace religion theories and constructs needs to be refined in order to further advance this key new paradigm in organizational studies.

REFERENCES

Barrett, R. (1998). *Liberating the corporate soul*. Boston: Butterworth-Heinemann.

Belaire, C., & Young, J. S. (2000). Influences of spirituality on counselor selection. *Counseling and Values, 44*, 189–197.

Biberman, J., & Whitty, M. (Eds.). (2000). *Work and spirit: A reader of new spiritual paradigms for organizations*. Scranton, PA: University of Scranton Press.

Bowen, D. E., & Lawler, E. E., III. (1995). Empowering service employees. *Sloan Management Review*, 70, 73–84.

Brandt, E. (1996, April). Corporate pioneers explore spirituality. *HRMagazine*, pp. 82–87.

Cash, K. C., Gray, G. R., & Rood, S. A. (2000). A framework for accommodating religion and spirituality in the workplace. *The Academy of Management Executive*, 14, 124–134.

Cavanagh, G. F. (1999). Spirituality for managers: Context and critique. *Journal of Organizational Change Management*, 12, 186–199.

Covey, S. (1990). *The seven habits of highly effective people.* New York: Simon and Schuster.

Dalai Lama XIV. (1999). *Ethics for the new millennium.* New York: Putnam Publishing Group.

Davis, D. W., & Davenport, C. (1999). Assessing the validity of the Postmaterialism Index. *American Political Science Review*, 93, 649–664.

Deci, E. L., & Ryan, R. M. (2000). The "what" and "why" of goal pursuits: Human needs and self-determination of behavior. *Psychological Inquiry*, 11, 227–268.

Dubin, R. (1978). *Theory building.* New York: Free Press.

Emmons, R. A. (2000). Is spirituality an intelligence?: Motivation, cognition, and the psychology of ultimate concern. *The International Journal for the Psychology of Religion*, 10, 3–26.

Emmons, R. A. (2003). Acts of gratitude in organizations. In K. S. Cameron, J. E. Dutton, & R. E. Quinn (Eds.), *Positive organizational scholarship: Foundations of a new discipline.* San Francisco: Berrett-Koehler.

Emmons, R. A., & McCullough, M. E. (2003). Counting blessings versus burdens: Experimental studies of gratitude and subjective well-being in daily life. *Journal of Personality and Social Psychology*, 84, 377–389.

Emmons, R. A., & Paloutzian, R. F. (2003). Psychology of religion. *Annual Review of Psychology*, 54, 377–402.

Fairholm, G. W. (1997). *Capturing the heart of leadership: Spirituality and community in the new American workplace.* Westport, CT: Praeger.

Ford, R. C., & Fottler, M. D. (1995). Empowerment: A matter of degree. *Academy of Management Executive*, 9, 21–31.

Fry, L. W. (1982). Technology-structure research: Three critical issues. *Academy of Management Journal*, 25, 532–552.

Fry, L. W. (2003). Toward a theory of spiritual leadership. *Leadership Quarterly*, 14, 693–727.

Fry, L. W. (2004). *Toward a theory of ethical and spiritual well-being and corporate social responsibility through spiritual leadership.* Paper presented at the meeting of the Academy of Management, New Orleans, LA.

Fry, L. W., & Smith, D. A. (1987). Congruence, contingency, and theory building. *Academy of Management Review*, 12, 117–132.

Fry, L. W., Vitucci, S., & Cedillo, M. (in press). Spiritual leadership and army transformation: Theory measurement and establishing a baseline. *Leadership Quarterly.*

Giacalone, R. A., & Jurkiewicz, C. L. (Eds.). (2003). *Handbook of workplace spirituality and organizational performance.* Armonk, NY: M.E. Sharpe.

Grendstad, G., & Selle, P. (1997). *Cultural theory, postmaterialism, and environmental attitudes.* Boulder, CO: Westview Press.

Helgeson, V. S. (1994). Relation of agency and communion to well-being: Evidence and potential explanations. *Psychological Bulletin*, 116, 412–428.

Hill, P. C., & Hood, R. W. (1999). *Measures of religiosity.* Birmingham, AL: Religious Education Press.

Hunt, J. G. (1999). Transformational/charismatic leadership's transformation of the field: An historical essay. *Leadership Quarterly*, 10, 129–143.

Inglehart, R. (1990). *Culture shift in advanced industrial society.* Princeton, NJ: Princeton University Press.

Inglehart, R. (1997). *Modernization and postmodernization: Cultural, economic and political change in 43 societies.* Princeton: Princeton University Press.

James, L. R., Demaree, R. G., & Wolf, G. (1993). An assessment of within-group interrater agreement. *Journal of Applied Psychology, 78,* 306–309.

Jurkiewicz, C. L., (2003). Strategic human resource management: Applying technology to function. In A. Farazmand (Ed.), *Strategic public personnel management.* New York: Marcel Dekker.

Jurkiewicz, C. L., & Giacalone, R. A. (2004). A values framework for measuring the impact of workplace spirituality on organizational performance. *Journal of Business Ethics, 49,* 129–142.

Koenig, H. (1998). *The handbook of religion and mental health.* San Diego: Academic Press.

Koenig, H. G., McCullough, M. E., & Larson, D. B. (2001). *Handbook on religion and health.* Oxford: Oxford University Press.

Laabs, J. (1996, March). Downshifters. *Personnel Journal,* 62–76.

Lickona, T. (1991). *Educating for character: How our schools can teach respect and responsibility.* New York: Bantam.

MacDonald, D. A., Friedman, H. L., & Kuentzel, J. G. (1999). A survey of measures of spiritual and transpersonal constructs: Part one—Research update. *Journal of Transpersonal Psychology, 31*(2), 137–154.

MacDonald, D. A., Kuentzel, J. G., & Friedman, H. L. (1999). A survey of measures of spiritual and transpersonal constructs: Part two—Additional instruments. *Journal of Transpersonal Psychology, 31*(2), 155–177.

Maghroori, R., & Rolland, E. (1997). Strategic leadership: The art of balancing organizational mission with policy, procedures, and external environment. *Journal of Leadership Studies, 2,* 62–81.

Malone, P., & Fry, L. *Transforming schools through spiritual leadership: A field experiment.* Unpublished manuscript.

McAdams, D. P., & de St. Aubin, E. (1992). A theory of generativity and its assessment through self-report, behavioral acts, and narrative themes in autobiography. *Journal of Personality and Social Psychology, 62,* 1003–1015.

Mirvis, P. (1997). "Soul work" in organizations. *Organization Science, 8*(2), 193–206.

Mitroff, I. I., & Denton, E. A. (1999). *A spiritual audit of corporate America: A hard look at spirituality, religion, and values in the workplace.* San Francisco: Jossey-Bass.

Mitroff, I. I., & Denton, E. A. (2000). *A spiritual audit of corporate America.* San Francisco: Jossey-Bass.

Mowday, R., Porter, L. W., & Steers, R. M. (1982). *Employee organization linkages.* New York: Academic Press.

Nadesan, M. H. (1999). The discourses of corporate spiritualism and evangelical capitalism. *Management Communication Quarterly, 13,* 3–42.

Nash, L. (1994). *Believers in business.* Nashville, TN: Thomas Nelson.

Neal, C. (1998). The conscious business culture. *Creative Nursing, 4,* 5–7.

Neal, J. A. (2001). Leadership and spirituality in the workplace. In R. N. Lusssier & C. F. Achua (Eds.), *Leadership theory, application, skill development* (pp. 464–473). New York: South-Western.

Reichers, A. E., & Schneider, B. (1990). Climate and culture: An evolution of constructs. In B. Schneider (Ed.), *Organizational climate and culture* (pp. 5–39). San Francisco: Jossey-Bass.

Sass, J. S. (2000). Characterizing organizational spirituality: An organizational communication culture approach. *Communication Studies, 51,* 195–207.

Snyder, C. R., & Lopez, S. J. (Eds.). (2001). *Handbook of positive psychology.* New York: Oxford University Press.

Snyder, C. R., Sympson, S. C., Ybasco, F. C., Borders, T. F., Babyak, M. A., & Higgins, R. L. (1996). Development and validation of the State Hope Scale. *Journal of Personality and Social Psychology, 2,* 321–335.

Spreitzer, G. (1996). Social structural characteristics of psychological empowerment. *Academy of Management Journal, 39*(2), 483–504.

Stanfield, G. (1976). Technology and structure as theoretical categories. *Administrative Science Quarterly, 21,* 489–493.

Townsend, J. S. (1984). The development of the spiritual leadership qualities inventory. *Journal of Psychology and Religion, 12,* 305–313.

Veach, T. L., & Chappel, J. N. (1991). Measuring spiritual health: A preliminary study. *Substance Abuse, 13,* 139–149.

Wheat, L. W. (1991). *Development of a scale for the measurement of human spirituality.* Unpublished doctoral dissertation, University of Maryland, College Park.

Worthington, E. (1998). *Dimensions of forgiveness.* Philadelphia, PA: Templeton.

29

Religious Violence, Terrorism, and Peace

A Meaning-System Analysis

ISRAELA SILBERMAN

> More wars have been waged, more people killed, and more evil
> perpetuated in the name of religion than by any other
> institutional force in human history. . . . At the center of
> authentic religions one always finds the promise of peace, both
> an inner peace for the adherent and the requirement to seek
> peaceful coexistence with the rest of creation.
> —KIMBALL (2002, p. 156)

The involvement of religion in national and international relations has been demonstrated in numerous historical and contemporary acts of violence and wars across the world (Hoffman, 1998; Juergensmeyer, 2003; Kimball, 2002; Silberman, 2002, 2003b) such as the Crusades and the Inquisition; the ongoing conflicts between Jews and Muslims in the Middle East, Hindus and Muslims in India, Catholics and Protestants in Ireland, and Christians and Muslims in the former Yugoslavia, East Timor, Lebanon, Russia, and many countries in Africa, such as Nigeria; and the killing of physicians and nurses by Christian antiabortion groups (Appleby, 2000; Carroll, 2001; Fox, 2001; Huntington, 2003; Silberman, 2005a). Special attention has been given in recent years to many acts of religious terrorism, which involve self-sacrifice and/or murder in the name of God. Some examples of such religious terrorism include the 1995 nerve gas attack on the Tokyo subway by Japanese followers of Shoko Asahara in the Aum Shinrikyo sect who were trying to hasten a new millennium, the September 11th, 2001, attacks on the United States in which thousands of civilians were killed by members of the Al-Qaeda organization, and a wave of bombings of civilian buses and public gathering places in Israel by the Islamic Hamas terrorists (Bergen, 2002; Hoffman, 1998; Silberman, 2003a; Silberman, Higgins, & Dweck, 2005).

Keeping this in mind, it is also important to realize that exemplary figures of faith, such as Martin Luther King, Jr., Abraham Joshua Heschel, Mohandas Gandhi, and Mother Theresa, and major organizations of faith have contributed significantly to social change that aims at the correction of injustice and that may be interpreted as a spiritual attempt to transform the world into a religiously ideal world, that is, to realize "God's kingdom" on earth. Religiously based social action to change society for the better is evidenced by numerous examples of religiously based charitable activities (e.g., Evans, 1979; Spilka & Bridges, 1992; Walzer, 1982), as well as by political activism. The latter is exemplified in the significant contribution of people of faith and organizations of faith to the mobilization of major movements such as the black civil rights movement, Poland's Solidarity movement, the South African antiapartheid movement, and the movement for Indian independence (Smith, 1996). It can also be seen in interfaith dialogues among religious leaders in both national and international arenas in order to facilitate the resolution of conflicts and bring about world peace (Appleby, 2000; Carroll, 2002; Gopin, 2000; Silberman et al., 2005).

The above description suggests that the role of religion in national and international relations is complicated. It raises the issue of how it is possible for religion to play the roles of both villain and hero in national and international relations. More specifically, it raises questions such as "What are the agents or the venues through which religion affects national and international relations?" and "What are the processes through which religion can facilitate violence, terrorism, and peace in these contexts?"

This chapter explores these questions by focusing on the role of religion as a unique system of meaning in national and international conflicts and their resolutions. It starts with a short introduction to the concept of religion as an individual or collective system of meaning and continues with an analysis of different agents and venues through which religion as a source of meaning can influence national and international relations. Next, it describes processes through which religion as a meaning system can influence either violence or peace. Finally, relevant implications for research and policy in the arena of religion are discussed.

RELIGION AS A UNIQUE MEANING SYSTEM

Within the psychological literature, *meaning systems* are usually defined as the idiosyncratic systems of beliefs that individuals construct about themselves, about others, about the world, and about their relations to the world. These beliefs or theories allow individuals to give meaning to the world around them and to their experiences, as well as to set goals, plan activities, and order their behavior (e.g., Eidelson & Eidelson, 2003; Epstein, 1985; Fox, 2001; Higgins, 2000; Park & Folkman, 1997; see Silberman, 1999, 2003a, 2005a for reviews).

The idiosyncratic religious meaning system of an individual, in similar ways to nonreligious meaning systems, functions as a lens through which reality is perceived and interpreted (McIntosh, 1995). It can influence the formation of goals for self-regulation, affect emotions, and influence behavior (e.g., Batson, Schoenrade, & Ventis, 1993; Emmons, 1999, 2005; Geertz, 1973; James, 1902/1982; Paloutzian & Silberman, 2003; Pargament, 1997; Park & Folkman, 1997; Park, 2005, Chapter 16, this volume; Silberman, Higgins, & Dweck, 2000, 2001; Silberman, 1999; see Silberman, 2003a, 2005a, for reviews). Yet religion as a meaning system is unique in that it centers on what is perceived to be the sacred (i.e., it centers on concepts of higher powers, such as the divine, God, or the transcendent, which are considered holy and worthy of special veneration and respect) (cf. Pargament's definition, 1997, p. 32; Pargament, Magyar, & Murray-Swank, 2005). Religion as a meaning system is also unique both in its comprehensiveness (i.e., the range of issues to which the system gives meaning) and in its quality (i.e., the type of meaning that it offers) (see Silberman, 2005a, 2005b, for reviews). In terms of comprehensiveness, religion offers meaning to history from the moment of creation until the end of time, as well as to every aspect of human life from birth to death and beyond (Emmons, 2005; Pargament et al., 2005). In terms of quality, religion has been described as unique in its ability to propose answers to life's deepest questions (Myers, 2000; Pargament et al., 2005; Park, 2005, Chapter 16, this volume). At times religion provides answers that offer hope and a sense of significance to people. However, at other times, it answers these questions in ways that can cause unique difficulties and distress (Kushner, 1989; Pargament et al., 2005). For additional discussion of the uniqueness of religion, see Emmons, 2005; Martin, 2005; Maton, Dodgen, Sto. Domingo & Larson, 2005; Pargament et al., 2005; Silberman, 2005a; and Silberman et al., 2005).

Religion, as a meaning system that centers on what is perceived as sacred, can give special content and value to any object (Pargament et al, 2005), as well as to each of the components of the meaning system, that is, to any belief, contingency, expectation, or goal, as well as to prescriptive postulates regarding any emotion or action (see Silberman, 2003a, 2005a, for reviews). For example, religious systems may include beliefs about humans as being sinful or pious, and of the world as being evil or holy. They can include the contingency that righteous people should be rewarded for their good deeds, while sinners should be punished for their bad actions, or contingencies that describe differential rules for treating ingroup versus outgroup members (Hunsberger & Jackson, 2005; Tsang, McCullough, & Hoyt, 2005). They can also give special sacred meaning to any positive or negative emotion (Silberman et al., 2001), as well as to any goal or action ranging from benevolent (Batson et al., 1993; Schwartz & Huismans, 1995; Tsang et al., 2005) to destructive ones (e.g., Hunsberger & Jackson, 2005; Martin, 2005; see Silberman et al., 2005 for a review).

Religion, like other meaning systems, can be viewed as a malleable system that can be learned, developed, and changed (e.g., see Dweck, 1999; Epstein, 1985; Higgins, 2000 on psychological meaning systems in general; see Firestone, 1999; Gopin, 2000; Lewis, 2003; Park, 2005; Park, Chapter 16, this volume; and Paloutzian, Chapter 18, this volume on religion; see Silberman, 2003a, 2004, 2005a for reviews). The basic postulates of religious meaning systems can be learned and modified in several ways that can be either conscious or nonconscious (see Silberman, 2004, for a review). For example, individuals can learn beliefs about God and about the nature of the world through the explicit oral or written teachings of religious leaders or through observation of persons serving as exemplars of how to live a spiritually meaningful life (Oman & Thoresen, 2003; Silberman, 2003a). Individuals can also change and develop their religious meaning systems in a way similar to that of scientific theories (Kuhn, 1962), by accommodating to observed phenomena that seem to disconfirm the basic, often subconscious, postulates of the system (Park, 2005; Park, Chapter 16, this volume). See Silberman (1999, 2005a, 2005c) for excellent discussions on the integrative power of the meaning system approach to religion, and Silberman (2005b) for a comprehensive demonstration of this power.

In the context of national and international relations, it is often important to consider not only the idiosyncratic meaning systems of individuals but also the religious and nonreligious collective worldviews of interacting religious groups (Beck, 1999; Eidelson & Eidelson, 2003; Kelman, 1990, 1997, 1999; Staub, 1989). These collective meaning systems compose the "shared reality" of each group (Hardin & Higgins, 1996) and can define the group's very essence (Bar-Tal, 1990, 2000). More specifically, these collective meaning systems allow groups and group members to interpret their shared experiences, including their historical and recent relations, with other groups. They can determine much of the goals, decision-making processes, and behaviors of groups on both national and international levels (Durkheim, 1933; Kearney, 1984; Moscovici, 1988; Thompson & Fine, 1999; Triandis, 1996; see Eidelson & Eidelson, 2003 and Silberman et al., 2005 for reviews).

In a parallel way to individual meaning systems, collective meaning systems can develop in both conscious and subconscious ways from culturally determined common experiences and through a variety of socialization processes (Bar-Tal, 1990, 2000; Ross, 1995, 1997; Volkan, 1997). However, like individual meaning systems, and perhaps even more than them, once they are constructed collective meaning systems are usually held with great conviction, as they tend to be viewed by a given group as basic unquestionable truths (Bar-Tal, 1990, 2000; Lustick, 1993; see Eidelson & Eidelson, 2003, for a review).

RELIGION AND NATIONAL AND INTERNATIONAL RELATIONS: AGENTS AND VENUES OF INFLUENCE

The above discussion of individual and collective meaning systems implies that religion as a meaning system may influence national and international relations through several venues and agents. One way in which religion can influence national and international relations involves influencing the worldviews that compose the meaning systems of political or religious leaders and of other policymakers, as well as their actions. For example, religion can encourage leaders to endorse either positive or negative perceptions of outgroups, and it can affect leaders' tendencies to approach other groups on both national and international levels in either peaceful or in violent ways (Silberman et al., 2005). In this context the religious views of Osama bin Laden or Ayatollah Khomeini could impact their hostile attitudes toward the West (Bergen, 2002), while the religious views of Mohandas Gandhi have made him, in the eyes of many, the catalyst if not the initiator of three of the major revolutions of the 20th century: against colonialism, against racism, and against violence. Beyond decisions to wage or end wars, the religious views of leaders may resonate in their attitudes toward other life-and-death issues such as abortion, capital punishment, euthanasia, and stem-cell research, as well as in issues regarding education, contraception, and same-sex marriages (e.g., Silberman, 2005a; Woodward, 2004).

In an interesting demonstration of this idea, religion seemed to echo in the following words of President George W. Bush and his rival, Senator John Kerry, as they were discussing their domestic and foreign policies during the final U.S. presidential debate on October 13, 2004:

> I believe we ought to love our neighbors like we love ourself, as manifested in public policy through the faith-based initiative where we've unleashed the armies of compassion to help heal people who hurt. I believe that God wants everybody to be free. . . . And that's been

part of my foreign policy. In Afghanistan, I believe that the freedom there is a gift from the Almighty. (Part of President George W. Bush's answer to the question "What part does your faith play in your policy decisions?") (Bush, Kerry Debate Domestic Policies, 2004a)

And I think that everything you do in public life has to be guided by your faith, affected by your faith, but without transferring it in any official way to other people. That's why I fight against poverty. That's why I fight to clean up the environment and protect this earth. That's why I fight for equality and justice. All of those things come out of that fundamental teaching and belief of faith. (Senator John Kerry) (Bush, Kerry Debate Domestic Policies, 2004b)

A second way in which religion as a source of meaning can influence national and international relations is by influencing the political and cultural milieus in which policymakers act (Fox, 2000). For example, states with Islamic populations have been found to be disproportionally autocratic (e.g., Fox, 2000, 2001; Midlarsky, 1998).

A third way involves the support of or the opposition to political leaders by religious institutions. It has been suggested that in modern times political movements tied to conservatism, tradition, family, nationalism, and militarism tend to be supported by conservative religious institutions (Beit-Hallahmi & Argyle, 1997). Another approach to the relations between religion and politics suggests that religions may differ in terms of their interactions with the dominant political parties. According to this approach (Lincoln, 1985), religions can be of the status quo (i.e., religions that support the dominant party and the sociopolitical status quo), of resistance (i.e., religions that define themselves in opposition to the religion of the status quo, defending themselves against the ideological domination of the latter), or of revolution (i.e., religions that define themselves in opposition to the dominant party itself, not its religious arm alone, promoting direct action against the dominant party's material control of society). Social, political, economic, and historical context variables that define circumstances under which religious groups tend to support the status quo or challenge it have been identified (see Silberman et al., 2005, for a review). In their efforts to support or oppose political leaders, religious institutions have often expressed positive or negative criticism of political leaders. For example, Senator John Kerry, the 2004 Democratic U.S. presidential candidate, was strongly criticized by some Catholic bishops who advocated taking a hard line with Catholic politicians-and—even voters—who stray from church teachings on issues such as abortion (Tumuly, 2004). In this context religious institutions have also provided organizational resources for political mobilization (Marty & Appleby, 1991; see Fox, 1999 and Silberman et al., 2005 for reviews). For example, during the 2004 presidential elections in the United States, religious groups from across the ideological spectrum intensified their level of political activity, getting involved in the distribution of campaign materials and in registering numerous voters ("Religious Groups Mobilize Voters," 2004) to an extent that was criticized at times as violating the U.S. constitutional separation between church and state (Kirkpatrick, 2004).

Fourth, religious (or nonreligious) meaning systems that individuals endorse can impact the general views of these individuals in terms of the desired role of religion in guiding the policy making of political leaders. According to a recent *Time* magazine poll (reported by Gibbs, 2004), 56% of U.S. voters agreed with the statement "We are a religious nation, and religious values should serve as a guide to what our political leaders do in office." Beyond that, the religious views of voters may influence the way in which they evaluate the religiosity of a specific political leader. For example, surveys reported that 85% of Bush voters said that President Bush's religious faith makes him a strong leader, while 65% of Kerry voters said that Bush's religious faith makes him too close-minded. In evaluating President George W. Bush's faith, some Democrats and Republicans criticized him for creating a faith-based presidency supported by his firm belief that he has a God-given mission, claiming that his faith may be a source of overconfidence for him, making questioning and analysis of facts unnecessary in his eyes (Suskind, 2004).

Fifth, as implied above, in countries where democratic elections are held, religion can influence not only the worldviews of laypeople and their evaluations of their leaders, but also their voting behavior (Beit-Hallahmi & Argyle, 1997; Religion and the 2004 Presidential Election, 2004). For example, Peres (1995) found a clear correlation between orthodoxy, militarism, and nationalism among Israeli Jews, and Nelson (1988) reported that disaffiliation from religious denominations was related to greater political liberalism among U.S. populations between 1973 and 1985. These findings are consistent with findings regarding the 2000 presidential elections in the United States where religious people voted at a rate of 62% for George W. Bush while only 31% of the least religious people voted for him (Election Analysis: The Religious Vote, 2000). They are also consistent with the analysis of the final voting results of the U.S. 2004 presidential elections, which suggests that President Bush's voters included a large group of more traditional religious people: 78% of white Evangelicals or born-again Christians and more than two thirds of Orthodox Jews voted for President Bush (Goodstein & Yardley, 2004).

A sixth way involves the influence of religion on the decisions of policymakers in national and international arenas via constraints placed on them by widely held beliefs within the population they represent (Fox, 2000). In other words, even in autocratic governments, policymakers might be reluctant to make decisions that are inconsistent with basic religious beliefs that are deeply held by their constituents. Thus, both Jewish and Arab leaders have had to take into account the religious meaning systems of their populations in making decisions regarding peace between Israel and its Arab neighbors, and Arab leaders sometimes take the religious values of their constituents into account in making decisions regarding their relations with the West (Fox, 2000). Leaders who make controversial decisions that are discrepant with strongly held religious values of the populations that they are supposed to represent may pay not only by losing political power but also by losing their lives, as in the cases of the former president of Egypt, Anwar Sadat, and the former prime minister of Israel, Yitzhak Rabin, who were both assassinated by religious extremists (Young, 1995). In a more recent example, the disengagement plan (a plan that would involve the evacuation of all Jewish settlers from the Gaza Strip and of additional settlers from the West Bank) of the prime minister of Israel, Ariel Sharon, has been attacked by some rabbis in the name of religion. Special attention was given to influential rabbis who, as part of their opposition to the plan, announced that soldiers in the Israeli army have an obligation to refuse to obey orders if they are asked to participate in this plan, which these rabbis perceive as an immoral plan that stands in direct contradiction to religious ruling. Their calls for disobedience in the name of religion have been viewed by some other rabbis and politicians as dangerous to the future of Israel (Ain, 2004).

Seventh, throughout history and in recent years, numerous acts of terrorism in the name of religion have been conducted with the aim of impacting national and international relations around the globe. While defining terrorism is challenging (Hoffman, 1998; Moghaddam, 2005), I follow those experts on terrorism who define *terrorism* as "an act or threat of violence against noncombatants with the objective of exacting revenge, intimidation, or otherwise influencing an audience" (Stern, 2003, p. xx). Terrorism in the name of religion, like any other act of terrorism, can be described as a war that is fundamentally psychological, a war that tries to create a crippling fear and psychological debilitation in the target community with the intention that this fear will be translated into pressure on governments to surrender to the terrorists' demands, helping them to achieve their ideological, religious, social, or economical goals (Ganor, 2002; Levant, Barbanel, & DeLeon, 2004).

THE PROCESSES THROUGH WHICH RELIGION CAN FACILITATE VIOLENCE, TERRORISM, AND PEACE

Religion, then, can influence national and international relations through several agents and venues by impacting the worldviews and behaviors of policymakers, their supporters, and their rivals, as well as the political culture within which they function. Beyond shedding light on the agents and the venues that religion can influence, viewing religion as a unique system of meaning that centers on the sacred (Park, 2005, Chapter 16, this volume; Pargament, 1997; Pargament et al., 2005; Silberman, 2005a, 2005b) can also illuminate the psychological-sociological processes through which religion can influence national and international conflicts and their resolutions. In other words, it can shed light on how religion can motivate people to conduct both violent and peaceful activism on both national and international levels.

In general, the meaning-making power of religion can encourage, at times, maintenance of the political and social status quo by providing a sacred basis for the existing order, and by enabling people to increase their satisfaction with it (Durkheim, 1912/1954; Glock, 1973; Marx, 1848/1964; see Schwartz & Huismans, 1995, for a review). At other times religion can facilitate intense activism by sanctifying acts of resistance or revolution (Lincoln, 1985; Marty & Appleby, 1991; Walzer, 1982), by offering both spiritual and nonspiritual rewards and punishments (Pargament, 1997; Silberman et al., 2001; Stern, 2003), and by encouraging a sense of self-efficacy to bring about both self-change and world change (Fox, 1999; Silberman, 1999, 2004; see Silberman et al., 2005, for a review). While the above processes can facilitate both peaceful and violent activism, the next section discusses processes that can facilitate *either* peaceful *or* violent activism.

Religion as a Facilitator of Violence and Terrorism

Religion when internalized as an individual or collective system of meaning can facilitate violent activism in a variety of ways. First, religions often contain values and ideas that may facilitate prejudice, hostility, and violence by encouraging the consciousness of belonging to a select and privileged community, and by emphasizing the "otherness" of those who are not following the tenets of the religion or those who belong to other religions (Appleby, 2000; Martin, 2005; Schwartz & Huismans, 1995; Wellman & Tokuno, 2004). According to Allport (1966), religion includes the following three basic invitations to bigotry: (1) the belief that one's religion teaches absolute and exclusive truth may lead to derogating views of the teachings of other religions and philosophical formulations as being wrong and a threat to human salvation (Hunsberger & Jackson, 2005; Kimball, 2002); (2) the doctrine of election (e.g., the concepts of God's chosen people or of God's country), which implies the inferiority of others because they have been rejected by God; and (3) theocracy (i.e., the view that a monarch rules by divine right, that the church is a legitimate guide for civil government, or that the legal code, being divinely ordained, is inviolable on the pain of punishment). In addition, religious teachings may explicitly or implicitly tolerate or even encourage prejudice against certain targets such as gay men and lesbians, Jews, or women (Altmeyer & Hunsberger, Chapter 21, this volume; see Hunsberger & Jackson, 2005 for a review).

An interesting example for a religious value that might facilitate violence would be "selflessness." This value means nullification in front of God and a focus on religious goals and objectives rather than on the self (Silberman, 2004). Under certain circumstances it can guide people to sacrifice other needs and even their lives in religious wars or in acts of homicide (suicide) bombings. Under other circumstances it can facilitate selfless acts of love and compassion. The same can be said about the value of "self-sacrifice."

Second, religion, because of its power to morally justify any goal or action through the process of sanctification, can provide an excellent source for the legitimization of the most violent acts within both individual and collective meaning systems (Fox, 1999). It can provide a particularly strong basis for processes of moral disengagement, such as moral justification, euphemistic labeling, and dehumanization. According to Bandura (2004), individuals adopt moral standards that serve as guides for positive conduct and as deterrents for negative conduct. When individuals wish to engage in behaviors that are seemingly inconsistent with their moral standards without experiencing a sense of self-condemnation, they endorse psychological mechanisms that disengage moral self-sanctions from the unethical behavior.

The moral disengagement process of moral justification involves the cognitive redefinition of a destructive conduct as servicing socially worthy or moral purposes, and, accordingly, as personally and socially acceptable (Bandura, 2004). One example of religious-based moral justification would be the attacks of the Al-Qaeda organization across the world, which have been described by Al-Qaeda members and supporters as part of a holy war, and as consistent with the teaching of spiritual leaders such as the Prophet Muhammad and Sheikh Omar Abdel Rahman, and as sanctified by ulema, or Muslim clergy (Bergen, 2002; Silberman, 2003a). This idea is expressed in the following description of the self-perception of religious terrorists: "They know they are right, not just politically but morally. They believe God is on their side" (Stern, 2003, p. 282).

Another way in which religious violence is presented as morally justified is by describing it as a response to pressing emergency situations (Appleby, 2000; Selengut, 2003; Stern, 2003). Whether these conditions involve difficult political or economic situations, a sense of threat to religious freedom, or threat from systems that promote values seen as danger to the religious system (e.g., pornography or sale of alcohol), they make it easier to define violence as morally legitimate. In the words of Appleby (2000, p. 88), "Fundamentalists believe themselves to be living in unusual extraordinary times of crisis, danger, or apocalyptic doom: the advent of the Messiah, the Second Coming of Christ, or the return of the Hidden Imam; and so on." The urgency of this special time requires true believers to make exceptions, to modify or ignore the general rules of the tradition (e.g., its adherence to peace), and to subordinate all other laws to the requirements of survival.

Beyond that, as implied above, religion can be very successful in the moral disengagement process of euphemistic labeling, which can be seen as based on the psychological idea that people behave much more cruelly when aggressive actions are given a sanitized label than when they are called aggression (Diener, Dineen, Endersen, Beaman, & Fraser, 1975). Religious violence and killing are often redefined through theological reinterpretation as holy wars, as sacred events, or as being fought for God and his honor.

These battles are not viewed within the religious meaning systems of those who participate in them as violence. On the contrary, they are viewed as religious battles for justice
aimed at making a more peaceful and just world. The battles are perceived as justified
means to educate those who are living in sin, to bring truth and redemption, and to inspire truth and faith for which even the fallen enemies will eventually be grateful
(Selengut, 2003, p. 20).

Finally, there are numerous historical and contemporary examples where basic beliefs that compose the religious meaning systems of individuals encourage the process of
dehumanization, which is defined as the stripping of individuals from their human qualities by redefining them as subhuman or even as satanic or evil (Bandura, 2004; Deutsch,
2000; Montville, 2001; Struch & Schwartz, 1989). Examples include the dehumanization
of the Jews in both Christian (Carroll, 2001) and Muslim (Bodansky, 2000) anti-
Semitism, and Muslim extremists' portrayals of Western nations as the "enemies of God"
and of the United States and Israel as the "great Satan" and the "small Satan," respectively (Lewis, 2003). Additional examples include Christian white supremacists' view of
Jews and nonwhites as "the literal children of the Satan" (Hoffman, 1993), and the dehumanization of Muslims by the Christian Crusaders (Bandura, 2004).

The third process through which religion can facilitate violence is desecration. Any
object, belief, goal, or action that is perceived as sacred can be desecrated by being lost,
destroyed, or violated. Since a perception of desecration has unique adverse effects, such
as intense negative affect (e.g., feeling distressed, nervous, scared, and upset; Pargament
et al., 2005), it may facilitate intensive political or violent activism against those who are
believed to have caused the desecration. For example, the Middle East conflict seems to
be fueled to a certain extent by a sense of desecration of both Jewish and Muslim holy
sites. A sense of desecration of Saudi Arabia (which is the Muslim Holy Land par excellence), especially of its two holy sites, Mecca and Medina, by a U.S. military presence has
been mentioned as one of the main sources of bin Laden's anger toward the United States
(Lewis, 2003).

Fourth, religion can facilitate violent activism by offering seemingly simple and powerful myths or stories that summarize very complicated situations in a cognitively man-
ageable way within individual or collective systems of meaning. "Such myths are critical
means of organizing the world and making sense of one's history, one's origins, and even
one's future" (Gopin, 2002, p. 7). Unfortunately, such myths often emphasize the "otherness" of the nonreligious or of those who hold different religious views in a derogating
way. "The facile invocation of religious symbols and stories can exacerbate ethnic tensions and foster a social climate conducive to riots, mob violence, or the random beatings
and killings known as hate crimes" (Appleby, 2000, p. 119).

A famous example of a powerful myth is the biblical story of the Abrahamic family—a
myth that is part of the lives of hundreds of millions of Jews, Christians, and Muslims.
The myth discusses the competition and rivalry between the two sons of Abraham—
Isaac, who is described as the key to the Jewish lineage, and Ishmael, the key to the Arab
Islamic lineage—and between their mothers. The sons compete over who is idolatrous
and who is authentic, and they also compete for the love of their father. "In this metaphor
of Abrahamic family, identities are established . . . old wounds are expressed . . . ancient
competitions and conflicts are given a quality of cosmic significance" (Gopin, 2002, p. 7).

Another famous myth is the portrayal of Jews and Judaism in early Christian writings. The Jews are portrayed there as the killers of Jesus, and the disagreements between
Jews and Christians are described dramatically as a cosmic struggle between evil and

good, with the Jews defined as the evil ones, as the offspring of Satan. By demonizing Jews as a symbol of "all evil," John's Gospel, for example, has aroused and legitimized hostility toward Jews throughout the course of Christian history (Carroll, 2001).

Fifth, several world religions have encouraged evangelism, which suggests that there is "either an obligation unfulfilled or spiritual reality unfulfilled as long as the whole world does not profess the tenets of a particular religion" (Gopin, 2000, p. 31). Evangelism, which requires the members of a particular religious group to make the effort to change the religious meaning systems of members of outgroups, does not inherently require violence, but, when imposed forcefully, it has brought about extreme violence throughout history (e.g., during the time of the Inquisition), and has the potential to do so in the future.

Beyond that, evangelism, which is restricted by law in many countries, can provoke a violent response against it. For example, the recent increase (particularly since September 11, 2001) in the activism of Christian missionaries in Islamic countries has been a source of tension. It has been interpreted by some individuals as a threat to the fragile peace among Muslims and Christians in countries like Lebanon, and even as a crusade against Islam on the part of the Bush Administration. This missionary activism has coincided with mounting restrictions on missionary efforts by the regimes of Islamic-majority countries and with increasing anti-Western militancy, which has involved the arrest and the imprisonment, or even the murder, of some Christian missionaries (Van Biema, 2003).

Religion as a Facilitator of Peace

Religions as meaning systems, then, can encourage hatred, discrimination, and violence. However, they seem to also have strong potential to facilitate conflict resolution and peace. For excellent discussions, see Appleby, 2000; Cox et al., 1994; Gopin, 2000, 2002; Helmick, 2001; Helmick & Petersen, 2001; Johnston & Sampson, 1994; Silberman et al., 2005. First, religious meaning systems (individual or collective) often include values that can facilitate peace (Gopin, 2000), such as (1) sanctity of life, which is sometimes supported by the religious idea that *all* humans are created in the image of God (Gopin, 2000; Montville, 2001); (2) selfless love and compassion (Poethig, 2002), including in some systems (e.g., Christianity) the idea that one must love or at least care for one's enemy (Gopin, 2000); (3) empathy (Gopin, 2000); (4) suspension of judgment of others; (5) forgiveness (Helmick & Petersen, 2001; Rye et al., 2000; Tsang et al., 2005); (6) humility (Gopin, 2000), self-examination and self-criticism (Carroll, 2002); (7) interiority, that is, the emphasis on the positive inner experience promoted by prayer, meditation, or feelings of divine love (Gopin, 2000); (8) religious discipline, that is, the religious idea that control of the senses may facilitate restraint in violent situations (Gopin, 2000); (9) the notion of interdependence, that is, the idea that the acts of one individual or nation can affect the whole world (Poethig, 2002); (10) the explicit encouragement of nonviolence, and the call for peace and pacifism (which is a critical concept of the inner life in the Eastern traditions of Jainism, Buddhism, and Hinduism) (Gopin, 2000; Poethig, 2002); and (11) messianism and imagination, that is, the vision of a more just social construction and new possibilities for the human social order (Gopin, 2000; Silberman et al., 2000).

Second, religion systems of meaning can include powerful myths in a way that may facilitate peaceful activism. For example, the powerful Abrahamic myth that was discussed above can be reframed as emphasizing the family relations between Jews and Muslims—a family that might have a somewhat disturbed history but that is still a family. Reports that religious Jewish and Muslim participants in conflict resolution efforts in the Middle East often refer to each other as "cousins" may reflect longings for this family unity (Gopin, 2000). When it comes to myths regarding the relations between Christianity and Judaism, there have been efforts by the Catholic Church since 1962 to change its history of hostility toward the Jews, which may eventually lead to a perception of Judaism within the meaning systems of many Catholics as the older sister of Christianity, rather than the rejected religion (Carroll, 2002).

Third, religions as systems of meaning can increase activism for peace by prescribing special rituals of forgiveness and reconciliation that can be applied in both interpersonal and intergroup contexts (Gopin, 2002).

CONCLUDING COMMENTS

This chapter explores the influence of religion on national and international relations by shedding light on agents, venues, and processes through which religion can impact national and international relations in both positive and negative ways. The chapter portrays religion as a complex (individual or collective) system of meaning that can be learned, developed, and changed in a variety of ways. The chapter suggests that religious (and nonreligious) policymakers and other agents have the ability to direct religious systems toward different goals by choosing to emphasize certain ends (e.g., forgiveness or conflict resolution) over other ends (e.g., revenge or victory over outgroups) (see Hunsberger & Jackson, 2005; Tsang et al., 2005; Martin, 2005; Silberman, 2005a; Silberman et al., 2005). These ideas have been demonstrated in a clear way in recent academic and nonacademic discussions about the continuous struggle between hardliners and moderates for the soul of Islam—that is, over the future of the faith and its relationship with the West (e.g., Benard, 2004; Lewis, 2003; Powell, 2004).

This chapter needs to be read with the following points in mind: First, the role of religion in national and international conflicts and their resolutions is very complicated and this chapter was not able to address all the relevant issues. Second, while this chapter focuses on the religious aspects of national and international relations, it is important to emphasize that most conflicts and other political events are motivated and influenced by complex combinations of factors (e.g., Fox, 2000; Silberman et al., 2005). Even when religion can be viewed as the main factor in certain national or international conflicts or in their resolutions, the role religion plays may be shaped by social, political, economic, and historical context variables, as well as by individual differences in personality variables that characterize the relevant leaders (see Silberman et al., 2005, for a review). Third, it is important to realize that, at times, religion can indeed serve as a causal factor of national and international conflicts and their resolutions. Yet at other times religion may be used just as an excuse or as an epiphenomenon for actions that are motivated by other factors. It would be important for future research to identify ways to distinguish between the two cases (Gopin, 2000).

Religion: The Missing Dimension in National and International Relations

Considering the historical and current significant positive and negative impacts of religion on national and international relations, and the predictions for its continuous future influence (e.g., Appleby, 2000; Huntington, 2003), the general neglect of the study of religion in academia and particularly in psychology is surprising and detrimental (Baumeister, 2002; Emmons, 1999; Emmons et al., 2003; Miller & Thoresen, 2003;

Wuthnow, 2003). This is clearly true in the context of national and international relations where religion has been described as the "missing dimension" because of the unfortunate tendency of scholars, policymakers, and diplomats to disregard the role of religion in facilitating both conflicts and their resolutions (Johnston, 2001; Johnston & Sampson, 1994; Rubin, 1994). This neglect is particularly surprising and disturbing considering the following facts: (1) religiously motivated national and international conflicts are very prevalent (Fox, 2004), and religious violence is described by experts on terrorism as being more intense and leading to more fatalities than the relatively more discriminating and less lethal incidents of violence committed by secular terrorist organizations (Appleby, 2000; Hoffman, 1998; Stern, 1999); (2) the number and impact of national and international intervention mediation and reconciliation efforts based on religious values is increasing (Silberman et al., 2005), and (3) religious leaders such as the Dalai Lama, Pope John Paul II, and Osama bin Laden are being viewed as some of the most influential people in the world today (*Time*, 2004).

Research and Policy Recommendations

First, it seems to me that the productivity of the meaning-system approach to the study of religion, as demonstrated in this chapter and in the *Journal of Social Issues* special interdisciplinary, multi-method issue on religion (Silberman, 2005b), suggests the use of this approach for future interdisciplinary theoretical and applied research on the role of religion in national and international relations and in many other contexts (Silberman, 2005a, 2005b, 2005c). Since there might be few, if any, important political events that are motivated purely by religion (Fox, 2001), it is important to continue to explore in a systematic way and from an interdisciplinary multimethod perspective the contextual factors (e.g., the social, political, economic, and historical factors, and the psychological variables) that influence the role of religion as a meaning system in national and international relations. For example, future research needs to further explore the context variables that facilitate religions' support of the status quo or their opposition to it (Martin, 2005; Roccas, 2005; Roccas & Schwartz, 1997; see Fox, 1999, and Silberman et al., 2005 for reviews). In a similar way it is necessary to shed more light on conditions that can influence whether religious systems develop in violent or peaceful ways (Appleby, 2000; Nepstad, 2004; Silberman et al., 2005 for a review). In this context Eidelson and Eidelson (2003) identified five belief domains, namely, superiority, injustice, vulnerability, distrust, and helplessness, as particularly important for further study of beliefs that propel groups toward conflicts. Some forms of religious meaning systems may be related positively to beliefs regarding superiority (e.g., Allport, 1966) and negatively to beliefs regarding hopelessness (Silberman et al., 2001; Silberman, 2004). It would be very interesting to explore the relations of religion to the other three beliefs and the extent to which the contribution of religion to conflicts is mediated by these beliefs.

Such research on contextual and psychological factors that influence the role of religion in national and international relations could contribute to a variety of fields within the psychology of religion and beyond. For example, it could contribute significantly to both research on religious violence and terrorism (e.g., Juergensmeyer, 2003; Kimball, 2002) and to general research on processes involved in violent group conflicts and their resolutions (e.g., Adams, 2000; Coleman, 2000; de Rivera, 2004; Gaertner, Dovidio, Nier, Ward, & Banker, 1999; Moghaddam, 2005; Moghaddam & Marsella, 2004; Staub, 2004; Sternberg, 2003; Volkan, Julius, & Montville, 1990; Zimbardo, 2001).

The second recommendation is for intensive national and international collaboration between researchers, policymakers, and religious leaders for the benefit of the larger society. For example, such collaboration could be productive in activism for those most in need in society (Maton et al., 2005; Pargament et al., 2005), as well as in national and international efforts to solve ethno-religious conflicts and to react to religious violence and terrorism. Several more specific recommendations are mentioned below. (See also Silberman, 2005a, 2005b; Silberman et al., 2005).

Conflict Resolution Efforts

Psychologists could contribute very significantly to the understanding and resolution of national and international conflicts where religion is a factor. First, they could combine existing knowledge of conflict and conflict resolution theories with knowledge about religion as a meaning system to develop conflict resolution theories and strategies that take into account the religious background of the participants (Gopin, 2000). For example, third-party mediators (Kressel, 2000) should be encouraged to learn about the religious systems of the involved parties so that the mediators can help the parties understand the role of their religions both in the facilitation of the conflicts and as one source for mutually acceptable solutions for their conflicts. More specifically, mediators could, on the one hand, increase the awareness of the parties to patterns within their religions that may facilitate the conflicts, such as the selection of targets for exclusion. On the other hand, they could encourage the parties to search their religious systems for values such as reciprocity, human equality, shared community, fallibility, and nonviolence that, according to Deutsch (2000), underline constructive conflict resolution. They could also help them find common ground (Bunker, 2000; Staub, 2004) for goals regarding desired world change or means to achieve them. Beyond that, psychologists as mediators of conflicts could be particularly helpful in developing creative ways to stop moral disengagement processes that are facilitated by religion. For example, by emphasizing to the parties the religious message that life is sacred and that *all* people are created in the image of God, they could overcome religious messages of prejudice and discrimination. Finally, they could further explore the psychological processes that are involved in religiously based rituals of reconciliation such as the Arab *sulh*, and incorporate variations of such rituals into the conflict resolution process (Gopin, 2002).

Second, psychologists could help evaluate existing national and international interfaith dialogue programs, which have become an increasingly popular response to religious conflicts, as was done recently by the Religion and Peacemaking Initiative of the U.S. Institute of Peace (Garfinkel, 2004).

Third, psychologists could contribute to the shaping of foreign policies by evaluating their effectiveness from a psychological point of view and by shedding light on the way these policies are perceived within different religious systems. They could also help the evaluation of different meaning systems (e.g., the four major ideological positions in the Muslim world today: fundamentalist, traditionalist, moderate, and secularist; Benard, 2004) in terms of their potential to communicate peacefully with the Western world.

Prevention of Religious Terrorism and Fighting against It

Psychologists, through their analyses of the conditions and the processes that facilitate religious terrorism, could contribute both to the prevention of religious terrorism and to the fight against religious terrorists. First, in addition to applying relevant conflict resolution strategies as mentioned above, psychologists could also suggest ways to remove some conditions that provide the contexts for religious violence and terrorism. For example, Moghaddam (2005) suggested that the best long-term policy against terrorism is prevention, which could be made possible by nourishing contextualized democracies. Time will test the validity of the idea, which has been promoted for years by leading scholars such as Lewis (2003), and supported by several influential journalists, some Arab intellectuals, and by President Bush (Zakaria, 2005).

Second, psychologists could help discourage religious (or nonreligious) ideas and prejudices that may facilitate terrorism. For example, in an effort to prevent additional acts of terrorism against Western civilians in the name of Islam, Muslim and non-Muslim psychologists together with peace-oriented religious leaders could help counter the anti-West, and particularly anti-United States, propaganda that seems to scapegoat the United States, blaming it for all of the difficulties of the Arab world, and portraying it inaccurately as heading a crusade against Islam (Lewis, 2003; Staub, 2004). Psychologists can help the development of public diplomacy programs aimed at providing more accurate images of the United States and the West in Muslim countries through cultural and educational exchange programs. This could include the creation of Arab-language television and radio networks (Powell, 2004) that would discuss Western culture and Western points of view on Muslim countries and their relations with the West, as well as provide factual information such as how the United States tried to save Muslims in Bosnia, Kosovo, and Albania (Lewis, 2003). Such public diplomacy could emphasize, for example, the responsibility of the leaders of repressive societies within the Muslim world for the difficult conditions of their citizens. It could also describe the corruption and the hypocrisy of certain political and religious leaders within the Muslim world, as well as their disregard for human life (including the life of Muslims). In certain cases, such public diplomacy could also highlight the vulnerabilities in the Islamic and ideological credentials of certain political and religious leaders who encourage violence and terrorism (Lewis, 2003).

Third, religious institutions, such as the Palestinian terrorist organization Hamas (see U.S. Department of State, 2004 for a list of designated foreign terrorist organizations), often provide critical social services and affordable educational opportunities. Unfortunately, the social welfare activists who run these welfare support organizations are often closely tied to the group's terrorist activities (Levitt, 2003), and their religious educational system tends to promote terrorism (Stern, 2003). Psychologists could help local and outside governments develop alternative affordable humanitarian systems that would provide the required social services, as well as educational systems that would educate youth in a more open-ended and tolerant way.

Further, psychologists could contribute significantly to the deterrence of religious terrorists by illuminating their decision-making processes, and by suggesting creative ways of influencing these process. More specifically, according to the *U.S. Army Field Manual*, as cited by the Terrorism Research Center (1997), a rationally motivated terrorist is a terrorist who makes decisions about terrorism through analyses of the presumed cost–benefit ratio of the intended actions. Ganor (2001) suggests that at least some of the religious terrorist organizations (e.g., Hamas, Islamic Jihad, and Hizbollah) are rational according to this definition, but emphasizes that both the variables that enter the ratio, the relative weight they are given, and what is considered to be an acceptable ratio may differ from what democratic liberal communities would conclude. Indeed, the meaning-system approach to the phenomenon of suicide bombing suggests that within certain religious meaning systems the act of suicide bombing can be perceived as a logical act, for which the perceived spiritual and material benefits outweigh the costs (i.e., losing one's life). Using the meaning-system approach, psychologists could suggest ways to deter potential suicide bombers by changing their perception of the cost–benefit ratio, as by convincing them that, according to their own religion, such homicide acts contradict the wish of God, thereby preventing them from reaching heaven (Lewis, 2003).

Coping with the Consequences of Religious Terrorism

Psychologists could significantly contribute to individual and communal efforts of coping with religious terrorism. First, psychologists could help individuals and communities cope in ways that would efficiently decrease the emotional, psychological, and political impacts of terrorism. They could promote resilience in response to terrorism, using existing knowledge of psychological and religious coping with trauma, stress, anxiety and grief (Levant et al., 2004; Pargament, 1977; Park, 2005; Seligman, 2001). They could also develop new coping methods that would address the special challenges that may be raised by terrorism in the name of religion. For example, psychologists could help increase public awareness, as well as the awareness of decision makers, security personnel, and media representatives, of the psychological manipulations used by terrorists in order to magnify the fears of populations and increase their support of the terrorists' cause (Ditzler, 2004), and by emphasizing the discrepancy that is often found between the actual damage caused by terrorists versus the power they claim to have.

Second, psychologists should be the leaders in discouraging prejudice, discrimination, and hate crimes toward individuals who belong to the same religion as the terrorists—for example, by discouraging anti-Islamic and anti-Middle Eastern hate crime incidents and the erosion of civil liberties in the United States, which seemed to increase after the September 11, 2001, terrorist attacks on New York and Washington DC (Levant et al., 2004; Wuthnow, 2004). It is extremely important to emphasize that the war against terrorism is not a religious war against Islam, and that most Muslims are not fundamentalists and most fundamentalists are not terrorists (Lewis, 2003). Psychologists should develop research-based interventions that aim at the reduction of prejudice and discrimination in this particular context.

The fact that the 21st century has started with religions demonstrating their destructive potential in facilitating conflicts, war and terrorism all over the world (e.g., Juergensmeyer, 2003; Kimball, 2002; Silberman et al., 2005) is not going to make it a unique century. Hopefully, through the collaborative efforts of researchers, political and religious leaders, and community members, this century will become a special and memorable one by revealing the unique potential of religions to facilitate conflict resolution and to create cultures of peace (Silberman, 2002, 2003b).

ACKNOWLEDGMENTS

I wish to thank Jonathan Fox for his helpful comments on previous versions of this chapter and Miriam Frankel, Eliezer and Nechama Silberman, Aviad Shragai, and Naomi Struch for their encouragement and support.

REFERENCES

Adams, D. (2000). Toward a global movement for a culture of peace. *Peace and Conflict: Journal of Peace Psychology, 6, 259–266.*

Ain, S. (2004, October, 22). Rabbis divided over dividing land. *The Jewish Week*, pp. 36–37.

Allport, G. W. (1966). The religious context of prejudice. *Journal for the Scientific Study of Religion, 5, 447–457.*

Appleby, R. S. (2000). *The ambivalence of the sacred: Religion, violence and reconciliation.* Lanham, MD: Rowman & Littlefield.

Bandura, A. (2004). The role of selective moral disengagement in terrorism and counterterrorism. In F. M. Moghaddam & A. J. Marsella (Eds.), *Understanding terrorism: Psychological roots, consequences, and interventions* (pp. 121–150). Washington, DC: American Psychological Association.

Bar-Tal, D. (1990). *Group beliefs: A conception for analyzing group structure, processes, and behavior.* New York: Springer-Verlag.

Bar-Tal, D. (2000). *Shared beliefs in society: Social psychological analysis.* Thousand Oaks, CA: Sage.

Batson, C. D., Schoenrade, P., & Ventis, W. L. (1993). *Religion and the individual.* New York: Oxford University Press.

Baumeister, R. F. (2002). Religion and psychology: Introduction to the special issue. *Psychological Inquiry, 13*(3), 165–167.

Beck, A. T. (1999). *Prisoners of hate: The cognitive basis of anger, hostility, and violence.* New York: HarperCollins.

Beit-Hallahmi, B., & Argyle, M. (1997). *The psychology of religious behavior, belief and experience.* New York: Routledge.

Benard, C. (2004). Five pillars of democracy: How the West can promote an Islamic reformation. *RAND Review, 8*(1), 10–13.

Bunker, B. B. (2000). Managing conflict through large-group methods. In M. Deutsch & P. T. Coleman (Eds.), *The handbook of conflict resolution: Theory and practice* (pp. 546–567). San Francisco: Jossey-Bass.

Bergen, P. L. (2002). *Holy war inc.: Inside the secret world of Osama Bin Laden.* New York: Touchstone.

Bodansky, Y. (2000). *Islamic anti-Semitism as a political instrument.* Tel Aviv, Israel: Tammuz.

Bush, Kerry Debate Domestic Policies. (Transcript, 2004a, October 14). Retrieved June 6, 2005, from www.cnn.com/2004/ALLPOLITICS/10/14/debate.transcript3/index.html.

Bush, Kerry Debate Domestic Policies. (Transcript, 2004b, October 14). Retrieved June 6, 2005, from www.cnn.com/2004/ALLPOLITICS/10/13/debate.transcript/index.html.

Carroll, J. (2001). *Constantine's sword: The church and the Jews—a history.* Boston: Houghton Mifflin.

Carroll, J. (2002, March 19). *After Constantine's sword: Past, present and future of Christian–Jewish relations.* Presentation at the Jewish Theological Seminary, New York, NY.

Coleman, P. T. (2000). Intractable conflict. In M. Deutsch & P. T. Coleman (Eds.), *The handbook of conflict resolution: Theory and practice* (pp. 428–450). San Francisco: Jossey-Bass.

Cox, H., Sharma, A., Abe, M., Sachedina, A., Oberoi, H., & Idel, M. (1994). World religions and conflict resolutions. In D. Johnston & C. Sampson (Eds.), *Religion, the missing dimension of statecraft* (pp. 266–282). New York: Oxford University Press.

de Rivera, J. (2004). Assessing cultures of peace. *Peace and Conflict: Journal of Peace Psychology, 10*(2), 95–100.

Deutsch, M. (2000). Cooperation and competition. In M. Deutsch & P. T. Coleman (Eds.), *The handbook of conflict resolution: Theory and practice* (pp. 21–40). San Francisco: Jossey-Bass.

Diener, E., Dineen, J., Endersen, K., Beaman, A. L., & Fraser, S. C. (1975). Effects of altered responsibility, cognitive set, and modeling on physical aggression and deindividuation. *Journal of Personality and Social Psychology, 31,* 328–337.

Ditzler, T. F. (2004). Malevolent minds: The teleology of terrorism. In F. M. Moghaddam & A. J. Marsella (Eds.), *Understanding terrorism: Psychological roots, consequences, and interventions* (pp. 187–206). Washington, DC: American Psychological Association.

Durkheim, E. (1933). *The division of labor in society.* New York: Macmillan.

Durkheim, E. (1954). *The elementary forms of religious life* (J. W. Swain, Trans.). Glencoe, IL: Free Press. (Original work published 1912)

Dweck, C. S. (1999). *Self theories: Their role in motivation, personality and development.* Philadelphia: Psychology Press.

Eidelson, R. J., & Eidelson, J. I. (2003). Dangerous ideas: Five beliefs that propel groups toward conflict. *American Psychologist, 58*(3), 182–192.

Election Analysis: The Religious Vote. (2000, November 10). Retrieved October 28, 2004, from www.pbs.org/wnet/religionandethics/week411/election.html.

Emmons, R. A. (1999). Religion in the psychology of personality: An introduction. *Journal of Personality, 67*(6), 873–888.

Emmons, R. A. (2005). Striving for the sacred: Personal goals, life meaning and religion. *Journal of Social Issues, 61*(4).

Emmons, R. A., & Paloutzian, R. F. (2003). The psychology of religion. *Annual Review of Psychology, 54,* 377–402.

Epstein, S. (1985). The implications of cognitive-experiential self theory for research in social psychology and personality. *Journal of the Theory of Social Behavior, 15*(3), 283–310.

Evans, B. F. (1979). Campaign for human development: Church involvement in social change. *Review of Religious Research, 20,* 262–278.

Firestone, R. (1999). *Jihad: The origin of holy war in Islam.* New York: Oxford University Press.

Fox, J. (1999). Do religious institutions support violence or the status quo? *Studies in Conflict and Terrorism, 22*(2) 119–139.

Fox, J. (2000). Is Islam more conflict prone than other religions?: A cross-sectional study of ethnoreligious conflict. *Nationalism and Ethnic Politics, 6*(2), 1–23.

Fox, J. (2001). Religion as an overlooked element of international relations. *International Studies Review, 3*(3), 53–73.

Fox, J. (2004). The rise of religious nationalism and conflict: Ethnic conflict and revolutionary wars, 1945–2001. *Journal of Peace Research, 41*(6), 715–731.

Gaertner, S. L., Dovidio, J. F., Nier, J. A., Ward, C. M., & Banker, B. S. (1999). Across cultural divides: The value of a superordinate identity. In D. A. Prentice & D. T. Miller (Eds.), *Cultural divides: Understanding and overcoming group conflicts* (pp. 173–212). New York: Russell Sage Foundation.

Ganor, B. (2001). *The foundations of deterrence in the war against terror.* Paper presented at the International Policy Institute for Counter-Terrorism, the Interdisciplinary Center, Herzlia, Israel.

Ganor, B. (2002). Terror as a psychological warfare. Retrieved September 5, 2004, from www.ict.il/articles/articledet.cfm?articleid=443.

Garfinkel, R. (2004). What worked?: Evaluating interfaith dialogue programs. *Special Report* (Vol. 123, pp. 1–12. Washington, DC: United States Institute of Peace.

Geertz, C. (1973). *The interpretation of culture.* New York: Basic Books.

Gibbs, N. (2004, June 21). The faith factor. *Time,* pp. 26–33.

Glock, C. Y. (1973). *Religion in sociological perspective: Essays in the empirical study of religion.* Belmont, CA: Wadsworth.

Goodstein, L., & Yardley, W. (2004, November 5). Faith groups: President benefits from efforts to build a coalition of religious voters. *New York Times,* p. A22.

Gopin, M. (2000). *Between Eden and Armageddon: The future of world religions, violence, and peacemaking.* New York: Oxford University Press.

Gopin, M. (2002). *Holy war, holy peace.* New York: Oxford University Press.

Hardin, C., & Higgins, E. T. (1996). Shared reality: How social verification makes the subjective objective. In R. M. Sorrentino & E. T. Higgins (Eds.), *Handbook of motivation and cognition: Vol. 3. The interpersonal context* (pp. 28–84). New York: Guilford Press.

Helmick, R. G. (2001). Does religion fuel or heal in conflicts? In R. G. Helmick & R. L. Peterson (Eds.), *Forgiveness and reconciliation: Religion, public policy and conflict transformation* (pp. 81–95). Philadelphia: Templeton Foundation Press.

Helmick, R. G., & Petersen, R. L. (Eds.). (2001). *Forgiveness and reconciliation: Religion, public policy and conflict transformation*. Philadelphia: Templeton Foundation Press.

Higgins, E. T. (2000). Social cognition: Learning about what matters in the social world. *European Journal of Social Psychology, 30*, 3–39.

Hoffman, B. (1993). *Holy terror: The implications of terrorism motivated by a religious imperative (RAND Research Paper P-7834)*. Santa Monica, CA: RAND Corporation.

Hoffman, B. (1998). *Inside terrorism*. New York: Columbia University Press.

Hunsberger, B., & Jackson, L. M. (2005). Religion, meaning and prejudice. *Journal of Social Issues, 61*(4).

Huntington, S. P. (2003). *The clash of civilizations and the remaking of the world*. New York: Simon & Schuster.

James, W. (1982). *The varieties of religious experience*. New York: Penguin Books. (Original work published 1902)

Johnston, D. M. (2001). Religion and peacemaking. In R. G. Helmick & R. L. Peterson (Eds.), *Forgiveness and reconciliation: Religion, public policy and conflict transformation* (pp. 117–128). Philadelphia: Templeton Foundation Press.

Johnston, D. M., & Sampson, C. (Eds.). (1994)). *Religion, the missing dimension in statecraft*. New York: Oxford University Press.

Juergensmeyer, M. (2003). *Terror in the mind of God: The global rise of religious violence*. Berkeley, CA: University of California Press.

Kearney, M. (1984). *World view*. Novato, CA: Chandler & Sharp.

Kelman, H. C. (1990). Applying a human needs perspective to the practice of conflict resolution: The Israeli–Palestinian case. In J. W. Burton (Ed.), *Conflict: Human needs theory* (pp. 283–297). New York: St. Martin's Press.

Kelman, H. C. (1997). Social-psychological dimensions of international conflict. In I. W. Zartman & J. L. Rasmussen (Eds.), *Peacemaking in international conflict: Methods and techniques* (pp. 191–237). Washington, DC: United States Institute of Peace Press.

Kelman, H. C. (1999). The interdependence of Israel and Palestinian national identities: The role of the other in existential conflicts. *Journal of Social Issues, 55*, 581–600.

Kimball, C. (2002). *When religion becomes evil*. San Francisco: HarperCollins.

Kirkpatrick, D. D. (2004, June 4). Bush campaign seeks help from congregations. Retrieved October 24, 2004, from www.nytimes.com/2004/06/03/politics/campaign/03CHURCH.html.

Kressel, K. (2000). Mediation. In M. Deutsch & P. T. Coleman (Eds.), (2000). *The handbook of conflict resolution: Theory and practice* (pp. 522–545). San Francisco: Jossey-Bass.

Kuhn, T. S. (1962). *The structure of scientific revolutions*. Chicago: University of Chicago Press.

Kushner, H. S. (1989). *When bad things happen to good people*. New York: Avon Books.

Levant, R. F., Barbanel, L., & DeLeon, P. H. (2004). Psychology's response to terrorism. In F. M. Moghaddam & A. J. Marsella (Eds.), *Understanding terrorism: Psychological roots, consequences, and interventions* (pp. 265–282). Washington, DC: American Psychological Association.

Levitt, M. (2003). Hamas blood money. Retrieved September, 6, 2003, from www.ict.org.il/articles/articledet.cfm?articleid=481.

Lewis, B. (2003). *The crisis of Islam: Holy war and unholy terror*. New York: Modern Library.

Lincoln, B. (Ed.). (1985). *Religion, rebellion, revolution: An interdisciplinary and cross-cultural collection of essays*. New York: St. Martin's Press.

Lustick, I. S. (1993). *Unsettled states, disputed lands: Britain and Ireland, France and Algeria, Israel and the West Bank–Gaza*. Ithaca, NY: Cornell University Press.

Martin, J. P. (2005). The three monotheistic world religions and international human rights. *Journal of Social Issues, 61*(4).

Marty, M. E., & Appleby, R. S. (Eds.). (1991). *Fundamentalisms observed*. Chicago: University of Chicago Press.

Marx, K. (1964). In T. B. Bottomore & M. Rubel (Eds.), *Selected writings in sociology and social philosophy*. Baltimore: Penguin Book. (Original work published 1848)

Maton, K. I., Dodgen, D., Sto. Domingo, M. R., & Larson, D. B. (2005). Religion as a meaning system: Policy implications for the new millennium. *Journal of Social Issues, 61*(4).

McIntosh, D. N. (1995). Religion as a schema, with implications for the relation between religion and coping. *The International Journal for the Psychology of Religion, 5*, 1–16.

Midlarsky, M. I. (1998). Democracy and Islam: Implications for civilizational conflict and the democratic peace. *International Studies Quarterly, 42*(3), 458–511.

Miller, W. R., & Thoresen, C. E. (2003). Spirituality, religion and health: An emerging research field. *American Psychologist, 58*(1), 24–35.

Moghaddam, F. M. (2005). The staircase to terrorism: A psychological exploration. American Psychologist, *60*(2), 161–169.

Moghaddam, F. M., & Marsella, A. J. (Eds.). (2004). *Understanding terrorism: Psychological roots, consequences, and interventions*. Washington, DC: American Psychological Association.

Montville, J. V. (2001). Religion and peace making. In R. G. Helmick & R. L. Peterson (Eds.), *Forgiveness and reconciliation: Religion, public policy and conflict transformation* (pp. 97–116). Philadelphia: Templeton Foundation Press.

Moscovici, S. (1988). Notes toward a description of social representations. *European Journal of Social Psychology, 18*, 211–250.

Myers, D. G. (2000). The funds, friends, and faith of happy people. *American Psychologist, 55*(1), 56–67.

Nelson, L. D. (1988). Disaffiliation, desacralization, and political values. In D. G. Bromley (Ed.), *Falling from the faith: Causes and consequences of religious apostasy* (pp. 122–139). Newbury Park, CA: Sage.

Nepstad, S. E. (2004). Religion, violence, and peacemaking. *Journal for the Scientific Study of Religion, 43*(3), 297–301.

Oman, D., & Thoresen, C. E. (2003). Spiritual modeling: A key to spiritual and religious growth? *The International Journal for the Psychology of Religion, 13*(3), 149–165.

Paloutzian, R. F., & Silberman, I. (2003). Religion and the meaning of social behavior: Concepts and issues. In P. Roelofsma, J. Corvelyn, & J. van Saane (Eds.), *One hundred years of psychology and religion* (pp. 155–167). Amsterdam, The Netherlands: VU University Press.

Pargament, K. I. (1997). *The psychology of religion and coping: Theory, research, practice*. New York: Guilford Press.

Pargament, K. I., Magyar, G. M., & Murray-Swank, N. (2005). The sacred and the search for significance: Religion as a unique process. *Journal of Social Issues, 61*(4).

Park, C. L. (2005). Religion as a meaning-making framework in coping with life stress. *Journal of Social Issues, 61*(4).

Park, C. L., & Folkman, S. (1997). Meaning in the context of stress and coping. *Review of General Psychology, 1*(2), 115–144.

Peres, Y. (1995). Religious adherence and political attitudes. In S. Deshen, C. S. Liebman, & M. Shokeid (Eds.), *Israeli Judaism: The sociology of religion in Israel*. New Brunswick, NJ: Transaction.

Poethig, K. (2002). Moveable peace: Engaging the transnational in Cambodia's Dhammayietra. *Journal for the Scientific Study of Religion, 41*(1), 19–28.

Powell, B. (2004, September 13). Struggle for the soul of Islam. *Time*, pp. 46–64.

Religion and the 2004 Presidential Election. (2004, June 16). Retrieved October 28, 2004, from usinfo.state.gov/dhr/Archive/2004/Jun/16-893025.html.

Religious Groups Mobilize Voters. (2004, September 30). Retrieved October 24, 2004, from www.cnn.com/2004/ALLPOLITICS/09/30/campaigning.churches.ap/index.html.

Roccas, S. (2005). Religion and value systems. *Journal of Social Issues, 61*(4).

Roccas, S., & Schwartz, S. H. (1997). Church–state relations and the association of religiosity with values: A study of Catholics in six countries. *Cross-Cultural Research, 31*(4), 356–375.

Ross, J. I. (1995). Psychocultural interpretation theory and peacemaking in ethnic conflicts. *Political Psychology, 16,* 523–544.

Ross, J. I. (1997). The relevance of culture for the study of political psychology and ethnic conflict. *Political Psychology, 18,* 299–326.

Rubin, B. (1994). Religion and international affairs. In D. Johnston & C. Sampson (Eds.), *Religion, the missing dimension in statecraft* (pp. 20–34). New York: Oxford University Press.

Rye, M. S., Pargament, K. I., Ali, M. A., Beck, G. L., Dorff, E. N., Hallisey, C., Narayanan, V., & Williams, J. G. (2000). Religious perspectives on forgiveness. In M. E. McCullough, K. I. Pargament, & C. E. Thoresen (Eds.), *Forgiveness: Theory, research and practice* (pp. 17–40). New York: Guilford Press.

Schwartz, S. H., & Huismans, S. (1995). Value priorities and religiosity in four Western religions. *Social Psychology Quarterly, 58,* 88–107.

Selengut, C. (2003). *Sacred fury: Understanding religious violence.* Walnut Creek, CA: Altamira Press.

Seligman, E. P. (2001). Amid the despair, there is hope. *Monitor on Psychology, 32*(10) 52–53.

Silberman, I. (1999). *Religiosity as a call for world change: Contradiction in terms or Messianism?* Unpublished doctoral dissertation, Columbia University, New York, NY.

Silberman, I. (2002, August). *Religion as a factor in international conflicts and their resolutions.* Symposium paper presented at the 110th annual convention of the American Psychological Association, Chicago.

Silberman, I. (2003a). Spiritual role modeling: The teaching of meaning systems. *The International Journal for the Psychology of Religion, 13*(3), 175–196.

Silberman, I. (2003b). *Religions as facilitators of world peace.* Paper presented at the Metanexus Conference on Works of Love: Scientific and Religious Perspectives on Altruism, Philadelphia, PA.

Silberman, I. (2004). Religion as a meaning system: Implications for pastoral care and guidance. In D. Herl & M. L. Berman (Eds.), *Building bridges over troubled waters: Enhancing pastoral care and guidance* (pp. 51–67). Lima, OH: Wyndham Hall Press.

Silberman, I. (2005a). Religion as a meaning-system: Implications for the new millennium. *Journal of Social Issues, 61*(4).

Silberman, I. (Ed.). (2005b). Religion as a meaning-system. *Journal of Social Issues* [special issue], *61*(4).

Silberman, I. (2005c). Religion as a meaning system: Implications for individual and societal well-being. *Psychology of Religion Newsletter: American Psychological Association Division 36, 30*(2), 1–9.

Silberman, I., Higgins, E. T., & Dweck, C. S. (2000). *The relation between religiosity and openness to change.* Paper presented at the 108th annual convention of the American Psychological Association, Washington, DC.

Silberman, I., Higgins, E. T., & Dweck, C. S. (2001). *Religion and well-being: World beliefs as mediators.* Paper presented at the 109th annual convention of the American Psychological Association, San Francisco, CA.

Silberman, I., Higgins, E. T., & Dweck, C. S. (2005). Religion and world change: Violence and terrorism versus peace. *Journal of Social Issues, 61*(4).

Smith, C. (1996). Correcting a curious neglect, or bringing religion back in. In C. Smith (Ed.), *Disruptive religion: The force of faith in social movement activism* (pp. 1–25). New York: Routledge.

Spilka, B., & Bridges, R. A. (1992). Religious perspectives on prevention: The role of theology. In K. I. Pargament, K. I. Maton, & R. E. Hess (Eds.), *Religion and prevention in mental health: Research, vision, and action* (pp. 19–36). New York: Haworth Press.

Staub, E. (1989). *The roots of evil: The origins of genocide and other group violence.* Cambridge, UK: Cambridge University Press.

Staub, E. (2004). Understanding and responding to group violence: Genocide, mass killing and terrorism. In F. M. Moghaddam & A. J. Marsella (Eds.), *Understanding terrorism: Psychological roots, consequences, and interventions* (pp. 151–168). Washington, DC: American Psychological Association.

Stern, J. (1999). *The ultimate terrorists*. Cambridge, MA: Harvard University Press.

Stern, J. (2003). *Terror in the name of God: Why religious militants kill*. New York: HarperCollins.

Sternberg, R. J. (2003). A duplex theory of hate: Development and application to terrorism, massacres, and genocide. *Review of General Psychology, 7*(3), 299–328.

Struch, N., & Schwartz, S. H. (1989). Intergroup aggression: Its predictors and distinctness from ingroup bias. *Journal of Personality and Social Psychology, 56*(3), 364–373.

Suskind, R. (2004, October 17). Without a doubt. Retrieved October 23, 2004, from www.nytimes.com/2004/10/17/magazine/17BUSH.html.

Terrorism Research Center. (1997). The basics: Combating terrorism. Retrieved September 20, 2004, from www.terrorism.com/modules.php?op=modload&name=News&file=article&sid=5671.

Thompson, L., & Fine, G. A. (1999). Socially shared cognition, affect, and behavior: A review and integration. *Personality and Social Psychology Review, 3*, 278–302.

Time. (2004, April 26). The lives and ideas of the world's most influential people. [Special Issue].

Triandis, H. C. (1996). The psychological measurement of cultural syndromes. *American Psychologist, 51*, 407–415.

Tsang, J., McCullough, M. E., & Hoyt, W. T. (2005). Psychometric and rationalization accounts of the religion-forgiveness discrepancy. *Journal of Social Issues, 61*(4).

Tumuly, K. (2004, June 21). Battling the bishops. *Time*, pp. 34–37.

U.S. Department of State. (2004, December 29). Foreign terrorist organizations. Retrieved January 13, 2005, from www.state.gov/s/ct/rls/fs/2004/3791.htm.

Van Biema, D. (2003, June 30). Missionaries under cover. *Time*, pp. 36–44.

Volkan, V. (1997). *Bloodlines: From ethnic pride to ethnic terrorism*. New York: Farrar, Strauss & Giroux.

Volkan, V. D., Julius, D. A., & Montville, J. V. (Eds.). (1990). *The psychodynamics of international relationships* (Vol. 1: Concepts and theories). Lexington: Lexington Books.

Walzer, M. (1982). *The revolution of the saints: A study in the origin of radical politics*. Cambridge, MA: Harvard University Press.

Wellman, J. K., & Tokuno, K. (2004). Is religious violence inevitable? *Journal for the Scientific Study of Religion, 43*(3), 291–296.

Woodward, K. I. (2004, May 28). A political sacrament. *The New York Times*, p. A21.

Wuthnow, R. (2003). Is there a place for "scientific" studies of religion? *The Chronicle Review*, B10–B11. Retrieved April 11, 2004, from www/psychwww.com/psyrelig/wuthnow.html.

Wuthnow, R. (2004). Presidential address 2003: The challenge of diversity. *Journal for the Scientific Study of Religion, 43*(2), 159–170.

Young, G. (1995, November 6). Rabin's assassination has parallels with Sadat's. Retrieved December 8, 2004 from www.cnn.com/WORLD/9511/rabin/11-06.

Zakaria, F. (2005, March 14). Where Bush was right. *Newsweek*, pp. 22–26.

Zimbardo, P. G. (2001). Opposing terrorism by understanding the human capacity for evil. *Monitor on Psychology, 32*(10), 48–50.

30

One Step toward Integration
and an Expansive Future

CRYSTAL L. PARK
RAYMOND F. PALOUTZIAN

It is appropriate now to step back from the details of the impressive body of research reported in this handbook, offer an assessment of the field, and point to some possible directions for its future. Given that the five integrative themes for the psychology of religion were introduced in Chapter 1, it is appropriate to use them here as the framework within which such an assessment is made. Doing this accomplishes the dual goals of providing a clear, meaningful framework within which all of the topics can be discussed, and of providing the first published test run of the utility of the five integrative themes themselves.

The five integrative themes we use to organize this material are the issue of paradigm, methods and theory, the question of meaning, the path of the psychology of religion, and the role of the psychology of religion. These five integrative themes create the most compelling framework of which we are aware, providing the language and the intellectual breadth needed for a broad assessment of the field. These themes cut across all of the material in the topical chapters of the book in that that material is either already stated in the terms of those integrative themes or is related to them. By examining the extant research within the framework of these themes, it is possible to identify trajectories in research that should be continued, areas of research in which it would be beneficial to change directions, ways in which a variety of methods not previously used to research a problem can be adapted to it, specific examples of how the concept of religion as a meaning system works as a language that can allow easy connections between topic areas, suggestions for how research in one area can feed research in other areas, and the religious and geographical scope (or lack of it) of the body of research collected so far. The vantage of this five-theme framework increases perspectives for expanding the work multi-

---

Chapters 1 and 30 form a collaborative unit, with the authors' names in alternate alphabetical order on each chapter.

religiously and transreligiously so that the psychology of religion might have a global reach, and provides insights into how this knowledge can be used at the individual, societal, and international levels.

Religion is present in and intrinsic to human phenomena worldwide. Religion is big and seemingly burdensome at times, and yet often is enormously powerful in human affairs. Finally, and most important for the purpose of a scientific understanding of religion, it has myriad specific aspects, many of which have shown a glimpse of themselves in the research reported in this book. Yet, to see the big picture, we need the tools necessary to enable us to stand back, look at all of the pieces, and then fit them together into an accurate whole. We believe that the five integrative themes facilitate this understanding. Therefore, in the following sections, we use this framework as a set of guidelines for how we can proceed to assemble the pieces into a whole configuration.

TAKE-HOME MESSAGES

Because the five-theme framework in the opening and closing chapters in this handbook presents a new way to conceptualize the broad band of material in the psychology of religion, there is an understandable question about the essential, take-home messages of each chapter. The primary message of Chapter 1 is elucidation of the five integrative themes themselves and an appreciation for their usefulness in helping us to have a dialogue about the substantive topics. With those ideas in mind, the primary message of Chapter 30 is that exciting new directions are evolving, and that these can be fruitfully discussed within the framework of the multilevel interdisciplinary paradigm and the model of religion as a meaning system; by doing so, the psychology of religion can make great contributions to the larger discipline of psychology, to allied sciences, and to human welfare.

In Chapter 1, the five integrative themes were introduced as the umbrella under which the approaches to research to date in the psychology of religion could be seen to fit together. In Chapter 30, they are the guides that help us to set the directions for future research and application of the material. Looking back at the research topics in the 28 substantive chapters in this book in light of the five integrative themes leaves us with a sense of how wide a scope of topics this combination of themes can accommodate. Thus, given the large, diverse, and multilevel research in the psychology of religion that has been documented in this book, we provide some intellectual, methodological, and strategic direction for its future.

Taken as a whole, the scholarship presented in this book represents a major step forward. This handbook itself is both part of and an expression of that step, because this is the first time that a discussion of such a wide range of research in the psychology of religion has been assembled under one cover in the history of the field. Let us see how a few ideas and lines of work might evolve in light of them.

MULTILEVEL INTERDISCIPLINARY PARADIGM

Whenever something as grand or comprehensive as an idea for a paradigm is promoted, it is appropriate to ask several questions of it. In this case, for example, it is helpful to clarify such issues as whether the multilevel interdisciplinary paradigm is descriptive or prescriptive, broad or narrow, and a general framework or a metatheory. The field's stance on each of these distinctions would undoubtedly evolve over time or even change abruptly from time to time, but at any one point scholars can communicate more accurately if they share a common perspective on these issues.

Descriptive or Prescriptive?

The two straightforward ways of identifying the time period of applicability of the multilevel interdisciplinary paradigm are to see it either as representative of the research that occurred between the publication of the *Annual Review of Psychology* chapters by Gorsuch (1988) and by Emmons and Paloutzian (2003), or to see it as a direction-setting concept for research in the future. During the 15 years between the two *Annual Review* chapters, the nature of the research in the psychology of religion changed dramatically. Those changes both reflected and fed the development of the concept of the multilevel interdisciplinary paradigm. However, the paradigm is far more prescriptive and direction setting than it is descriptive of past or current research. Although some of the research of the recent past (e.g., Silberman, 2005a) seems to fit this paradigm, Emmons and Paloutzian (2003) introduced it primarily to serve as an umbrella concept within which future research could flourish.

The paradigm will demonstrate its value to the field if it facilitates research in which studies once conducted along fairly narrow lines are tied to studies from different but related areas, such that new hypotheses emerge because of the blending of approaches combined with findings that speak to questions about the interfacing of ideas from different subdisciplines, disciplines, and levels of analysis. For example, research on the neuropsychology of religious experience (Newberg & Newberg, Chapter 11, this volume) can be juxtaposed with research on the phenomenology of religious, spiritual, and mystical experience (Hood, Chapter 19, this volume) to generate research at the boundaries of these two areas of knowledge. Further, it may be possible to integrate both of these topics with knowledge of religious cognition (Ozorak, Chapter 12, this volume) since such experiences would be mediated by an individual's information-processing system. If we then translate this combined knowledge and ideas into common terms that reflect what such experiences mean to people, such as religion as a meaning-system framework (Park, 2005 and Chapter 16, this volume; Silberman, 2005a), and add to this understanding the notion that meaning may depend on the culture and the specific religion (Hunsberger & Jackson, 2005), we move from a history of single-track lines of research to truly integrative research and theory. In this sense, therefore, the multilevel interdisciplinary paradigm can be seen as a way of proceeding rather than as a fixed model that predicts how findings should unfold.

Broad versus Narrow?

The notion of a paradigm can be understood in various ways, from relatively broad to relatively narrow in scope. In its more narrow, focused usage, a paradigm represents an explicit set of assumptions or rules that link together certain ideas, qualities, or facts into a cohesive pattern or model. Taken in this sense, a paradigm outlines what phenomena or information are of interest, how these data will be interpreted, and the manner in which the interpretations are evaluated and extended. The multilevel interdisciplinary paradigm reflects a broader framework that can accommodate more focused ideas and that suggests ways that the more specific aspects of theory building can evolve. The multilevel interdisciplinary paradigm represents a metamethodological stance that supports a multimodal approach to the psychology of religion. This approach argues that information from various disciplines and levels of analysis has something to contribute to our understanding of religious phenomena and that this information can be integrated into a larger, coherent whole. The specific mechanisms, assumptions, and processes that allow this linking of information have yet to be developed, but the time seems ripe for it.

General Framework or Metatheory?

The multilevel interdisciplinary paradigm is a framework within which theories of different scope can develop and cohere within a broad metatheory. Theories differ in their content and in their scope. For example, there are minitheories about memory and forgetting, and overall theories designed to explain all of human functioning, such as the recent developments in psychoanalysis (Corveleyn & Luyten, Chapter 5, this volume). There are midlevel theories about a particular range of human behaviors, such as attachment theory, models of single aspects of personality, such as Emmons's (1999, 2000) notion of spiritual intelligence, and social-cognitive models of the perception of various aspects of other people, such as attribution theory. Piedmont (Chapter 14, this volume) reviews a number of personality theories that are being used to examine religious qualities. One metatheory large enough to contain the midlevel theories and the minimodels in the life sciences, including psychology and the psychology of religion, is evolutionary theory (Kirkpatrick, 2005, and Chapter 6, this volume).

Of course, these midlevel theories and minimodels differ in some ways, if for no other reason than because they are attempts to explain different things, perhaps at different levels of analysis. However, they are not necessarily incompatible with each other. More synthesis is possible among these ideas than psychologists commonly believe. As long as the rules of logic and evidence are followed in the process of examining the compatibility of ideas, and so long as decisions about the fit or nonfit between ideas is based upon the data and the robust ideas are carried forward, time should show their synthesis and integrity. To this end, we can profit much from using a multimethod approach.

METHODS–THEORY–APPLICATION FEEDBACK LOOP

The call for pluralism in methods and theory has been made with a view toward a collaborative system of research that would see efforts to study religion from the inside (e.g., phenomenological approaches) and the outside (e.g., experimental manipulation) as complements that service the larger goal of a comprehensive, complete understanding. A number of pitfalls and correctives are fairly obvious: appreciate rather than reject contradictory findings, value and relate one's own work to findings that come from alternative approaches, test an idea with multiple methods and a variety of participant categories, design studies that simultaneously test competing ideas or minimodels. In addition to these fairly straightforward ways of proceeding, there are at least two obvious needs for research in the psychology of religion.

The Need for Meaning-Sensitive Measures

Because religion takes so many forms, it is doubtful that a measure of religiousness developed within the context of one religion will have the same meaning for people from a markedly different religion. The measures available today are far better in statistical properties than in the past (Hill, Chapter 3, this volume; Hill & Hood, 1999), but they reflect the context in which most psychology of religion research during its first century has been conducted, a Western Judeo-Christian context. But the manifestations of religion globally go far beyond this one (relatively speaking) category of traditions. Psychological research on non-Western religions is recent and sparse (Sheridan & North, 2004), although some research has begun (Hunsberger, 2005; Roccas, 2005). An immense volume of it is needed if our scientific theories about religion are to be comprehensive regarding religion as a common human phenomenon.

In order for this to happen, it is necessary to create measures of religious behavior and experience that yield scores that are both accurate representations of the meaning of the religion to its participants and comparable as representations of equivalent concepts in other religions. This is a tall order for many different methods. For example, a questionnaire measure of intrinsic and extrinsic religious orientation developed in the English language (Allport & Ross, 1967; also see Hill & Hood, 1999) is difficult to translate, in terms of weight and connotation of meaning, on an item-by-item basis into Polish (Socha, 1999) or Persian (Ghorbani, Watson, Ghramaleki, Morris, & Hood, 2002). Also, the religious dimensions measured by a scale in one culture may not exist with the same meaning or to the same degree in another culture. This would mean that direct culture-to-culture comparison on those dimensions is not possible. In fact, partly in response to problems of this sort encountered in attempts to adapt the intrinsic–extrinsic religious orientation measures for participants in Belgium, Hutsebaut and his colleagues (Duriez, Fontaine, & Hutsebaut, 2000; Hutsebaut, 1996) developed the Post-Critical Belief Scale to more validly assess religious meanings in Belgian subjects. This problem is probably deeper than simply one of language. For example, religious traditions, affiliations, or denominations may differ in the emphasis or meaning or value of various aspects of religion. Cohen, Hall, Koenig, and Meador (2005) found that social religious motivations were more valued by Catholics and Jews than by participants from U.S. Protestant denominations.

For test scores from different cultures, languages, and religious groups to be validly comparable, it is not sufficient to merely translate the scale. One must also ensure that the mathematical weight of the items and the totals reflect functionally equivalent meanings to functionally equivalent degrees. This would require extensive effort. We shudder at the thought that in order to do valid research that can compare psychological aspects of religion across religions, languages, and cultures, it would be necessary to revert back to a measurement paradigm (Gorsuch, 1988). However, refinements in measures at this level of precision would represent the best of an empirical research tradition stretching far enough to reach religion worldwide. The need is clear to do whatever measurement development is necessary to serve the larger hypothesis-testing and theory-building enterprise, while avoiding the *measurement trap* (Kirkpatrick, 2005).

The Need for Meaning and Diversity of Religions: Going Global

One way to understand the diversity of human religions and its recently recognized counterpart, spirituality, is to identify the critical psychological dimensions in which they differ. For example, some religions place the emphasis on collectivity (e.g., Judaism, Roman Catholicism), whereas others place the emphasis on individualism (e.g., U.S. spirituality, evangelical Protestantism) (Cohen et al., 2005). Much of Judaism, for example, is collectivist. Jews are taught that they share a historical link, an ethnic link, and a common destiny and that it is a commitment to the community and a continuation of the traditions that is paramount. The collective performance of rituals, much of it in public and, in orthodoxy, regulating virtually every aspect of daily life, serves as a social-psychological force to bind the people together with common behavior patterns and a common identity. Prayer, sin, and repentance are both personal and communal. Both Judaism as a whole and an individual's personal feelings about it, matter. It may be because of this that within the collectivist nature of Judaism, different construals of personal faith, including the nature of God, are accepted and perhaps even encouraged. Faith in one God is the core of Judaism, but Judaism teaches that God is beyond human comprehension, and there are thus many different interpretations of the nature of God in Jewish theology. In contrast, some expressions of Christianity are individualistic in pronounced ways. One instance of this appears in Evangelical Christianity, wherein beliefs such as "God is interested in saving the individual," "Sin is individual," and "One's own spiritual life is what matters" are held. Such beliefs lead to behaviors such as invoking God to heal the disease of one's own loved one or oneself. The individual accepts and gives assent to the faith. It is the *content* of the particular faith that matters. This simple distinction between religion as communal versus individualistic may have profound effects on the meaning of religion for its participants, their self-identity, the form in which they would face trials, to whom they might go for help, what asking God for help might mean to them, and their perceived need to make their religion seem attractive to others.

Issues such as the collectivist–individualist dimension are important in our efforts to expand the scope of psychology of religion research from its narrow beginnings to understanding religion globally and cross-culturally. The importance of this cannot be overstated. To illustrate how differently concepts like religion, psychology of religion, science, theory, psychological understanding, and research can be understood, even among psychologists of religion with PhDs from Western universities, examine the dialogue between Sebastian Murken (University of Trier, Germany) and Ashiq Ali Shah (International Islamic University, Malaysia) (Kahlili, Murken, Reich, Shah, & Vahabzadeh, 2002; Murken & Shah, 2002). One mind understands the psychology of religion as a science and as open to various points of view with no prescribed requirement for being religious; the science of the psychology of religion does not prescribe or proscribe religion in general or any specific religion. The other mind understands one particular "religious psychology" as true, derived from Scriptures believed to be God's direct revelation and containing the inherently valid, immutable, unchanging, binding principles of human functioning and well-being. In their extreme forms, these two ways of thinking are incompatible and the potential for conflict rather than dialogue between them is great. The only way to change this is to engage in mutually beneficial collaborative research that answers questions the parties have in common. For this to happen, a highly meaning-sensitive approach combined with knowledge of the belief system, religious practices, and way of life of the research partners is essential.

RELIGION AS A MEANING SYSTEM

Like Spilka, Hood, Hunsberger, and Gorsuch (2003) and Silberman (2005a), we are convinced that a meaning-based approach to the psychology of religion allows for the joining together of many seemingly distinct and disparate areas of research. We propose that future research should carry this meaning-system approach a step further and use it as a means of integrating an even wider circle of material. Many of the chapters in this volume explicitly invoke meaning and are also interconnected with other topics in the handbook. For example, the chapter on struggle and doubt (Exline & Rose, Chapter 17, this volume) concerns the strains individuals experience when their meanings are challenged, such as when their view of God is inconsistent with their present experience. Further, this meaning-related material connects with the topics of other chapters, such as emotions, coping, mental and physical health, and cognitive interpretations of experience. Indeed, the utility of the multilevel interdisciplinary paradigm becomes apparent in putting the material on struggle and doubt into such a larger context.

Altemeyer and Hunsberger's work on fundamentalism (Chapter 21, this volume; see also Hunsberger & Jackson, 2005) provides another example of the centrality of meaning and the usefulness of a meaning-centered approach in integrating the topic at hand with other subdisciplines—in this case by addressing the size, reach, and permeability of the individual's schemas. Because religious fundamentalism is defined as possessing a strict set of beliefs with rigid boundaries, the meanings of beliefs as contained in these restrictive schemas are typically judged dichotomously as either all or none, good or bad, and so on. Therefore, studies that use cognitive-psychological methodologies may be able to illustrate aspects of fundamentalism in an experimental context. For example, research might reveal a pronounced psychological reactance to information assigned a meaning contrary to one's beliefs, tying fundamentalism to research in emotion and personality.

The meaning-system approach appears to hold great promise for integrating various phenomena that have been studied within the psychology of religion, but only a few researchers have begun to take full advantage of these integrative possibilities (Silberman, 2005a). Future work should explicitly focus on the ways that meaning informs all aspects of religious experience, from beliefs and motivations and cognitive processing to coping with and resolving stressful life experiences. The critical contribution of the meaning approach is that it encourages researchers to view their topics of study through a phenomenological lens (i.e., to start with the interior experience and understanding of the perspective of the individual). From that base, any topic can be explored, and many, if not most, topics can be integrated. Future research should extend the use of the meaning-system framework. This extension can be accomplished by making explicit the meaning-related aspects of many topics within the psychology of religion and being more deliberate in conceptualizing and assessing meaning-related constructs (see Park, 2005 and Chapter 16, this volume, and Silberman, 2005a, for research recommendations).

Of course, the meaning-system approach is not without limitations. For one, the role of emotions may get short shrift in this framework. While many researchers promote the view that emotions are largely mediated by cognitions (e.g., Lazarus, 1993), it is true that human beings may be more ruled by their passions than by their intellects. A broad perspective on meaning can encompass both emotions and cognitions by emphasizing the centrality of goals in individuals' meaning systems and the perceptions of the extent to which people's experiences are congruent with these goals, which is what generates emotion (happiness and contentment, anger, frustration, sadness) (Lazarus, 1993). Therefore, researchers must be careful not to yield to the temptation of applying a purely cognitive framework to phenomena within the psychology of religion.

WIDENING AND INTEGRATING THE RESEARCH PATH

This is a very exciting time to be a researcher in the field of psychology of religion. While the goals of science remain the same (description, prediction, explanation, and control), the possibilities within this area of science have opened up dramatically in only a few short years. In particular, many areas that were previously not considered appropriate or relevant have opened up, ranging from genetics to terrorism. At the same time, broad-based theories have developed, begging to be tested by empirical research. Meanwhile, psychologists of religion have begun to exploit many methodologies with tremendous potential to further this research.

While research examining the psychology of religion has sprouted in many directions, there are renewed possibilities for integration of these diverse topics. Thus, rather than developing an increasingly fragmented psychology of religion consisting of independent subareas of knowledge that do not inform one another, it may be that through a multilevel and interdisciplinary approach our understanding will become deeper even as it also takes in broader and broader swaths of knowledge. As noted above, meaning systems offer one framework from which to examine many phenomena. The evolutionary psychology theory, which incorporates attachment theory, described by Kirkpatrick (Chapter 6, this volume), may also be used to examine functional and adaptive aspects of religiousness. The movement appears to be toward increased theory-driven research, a trend that we applaud and encourage.

As an example of these possibilities, consider the work described by Newberg and Newberg (Chapter 11, this volume). Neurobiological perspectives on religion tie together research on multiple levels, from the cellular and neurotransmitter levels to that of behavior and personality. The research findings cited by Newberg and Newberg and the findings of other scholars who work at the same levels of analysis are not only multilevel but also fit with and can inform evolutionary psychology and depth psychology approaches.

The beginning work on the neurobiological substrates of religion is concerned with religious experience, an observation that has a historical parallel. A hundred years ago when experimental psychology began, the early introspectionists also focused on learning about perceptual experience. We may hypothesize, therefore, that the neurobiological-level work on religion will expand in a manner parallel to the development of general psychology as a whole and both borrow from and make significant contributions to a number of other subdisciplines.

For example, recent findings in neuroimaging have revealed that intensive imaginal experiencing (imagination!) can leave memory traces that are indistinguishable from actual experience (Gonsalves et al., 2004). Although these findings are not based explicitly on religious imagination, the implications are clear. If neural evidence indicates that vivid imagining can lead to false memories, then it is possible that vivid imagining of religious symbols (often strongly promoted by a religion, and often strongly sought after by religious adherents) can lead to permanent "memory" traces in the brain that are just as "real" to the individual as if they were put there by an actual engagement with that religious symbol. Although nobody (to our knowledge) has ever seen God, religions encourage people to be "conscious of God's presence," imagine that they are "talking with Jesus," know that they will see their deceased loved ones in heaven, "hear" God's voice, and so forth. If such processes lead to permanent "memory" traces, then they also form part of the core of the nonveridical, self-validating nature of a religious meaning system itself. Adding together the findings that vivid imaging can lead to false memories, evidence for distinctive cognitive neural patterns for religious experience (Azari, Missimer, & Seitz, in press; Azari et al., 2001), and the argument that the subjective meaning attributed to even fairly ambiguous spiritual experiences is dependent upon perceptual set and the social context in which the interpretation is made (Paloutzian, Fikes, & Hutsebaut, 2002), and the implications are far reaching and fit well with the argument of religion as a meaning system and with the multilevel interdisciplinary paradigm.

Expanding and Integrating Areas of Inquiry

Thus, it is clear that the field is expanding its domain of inquiry. As we noted earlier, psychologists of religion have increasingly taken on topics that were heretofore unexamined with an eye toward their religious relevance. Many of these topics promise to further both the depth and the breadth of the psychology of religion. For example, the work on fundamentalism presents a way of connecting it with both spiritual transformation and personality research. Because higher levels of fundamentalism are related to increased tendencies to proselytize (for those groups that teach it), the consequence may be that those so converted tend to be more strict about their beliefs and their application to their behavior, and, as a consequence, may be increasingly religiously conservative over time, with a parallel decrease in keeping an open mind (Altemeyer & Hunsberger, Chapter 21, this volume).

Another area of integration involves an aspect of global life meaning involving religious beliefs, such as those regarding the roles and meanings of God, human nature, suffering, bearing witness, servanthood, and evil, which may be usefully understood from a clinical psychology perspective as being more or less functional (or even dysfunctional). These beliefs in part determine the emotions that people experience, and, in the long run, their coping styles and mental health. For example, the belief in the desirability of living in partnership with God, colloquially expressed in the United States in sayings such as "God is my copilot," leads to higher use of collaborative coping and generally higher levels of positive emotion and physical and psychological well-being (see Pargament, 1997, for a review). Those who do not believe in God or believe in a God who does not participate directly in human affairs will use less collaborative coping and more self-directive coping, which is less adaptive (see Pargament, 1997, for a review). When an individual's beliefs, whatever the content, are contrary to his or her perceptions of current experience, he or she may experience significant struggle and distress (Exline & Rose, Chapter 17, and Park, 2005 and Chapter 16, this volume). Such struggle may give rise to religious transformation or even conversion (Paloutzian, Chapter 18, this volume). The extent of comfort or struggle that people's beliefs and experiences engender have important implications for both mental and physical health (Miller & Kelley, Chapter 24, and Oman & Thoresen, Chapter 24, this volume).

Improving and Expanding Methodologies

Regarding research methodology, many important advances have been made, while others appear to be on the horizon, and the incorporation of these newer methodologies into the broadening areas of inquiry will lead to a much richer psychology of religion in the future.

As we noted in Chapter 1, researchers have become increasingly aware of the limitations of studying primarily white Christian college students, especially because the particulars of religion vary dramatically among different groups, affiliations, ages, origins, and so on. Studies of medical populations, the elderly, minority groups, and others have begun to appear with increasing frequency.

As Hill (Chapter 3, this volume) notes, measurement tools have also advanced in leaps and bounds. While most research in the field remains, by necessity, based on questionnaires, the questionnaires used increasingly reflect more functionally based and more finely delineated religious concepts and measures rather than global ones (Hill & Pargament, 2003; Hill, Chapter 3, this volume). In addition, studies have begun to examine physiological and behavioral measures with increased frequency. Particularly in the realm of religion and health, many studies assess health behaviors such as physician visits and immunizations and "hard" or objective outcomes such as blood pressure, days of hospitalization, and mortality (e.g., Contrada et al., 2004).

New and creative methods of gathering data are being employed with this subject matter as well (Hood & Belzen, Chapter 4, this volume). Some researchers have turned to large longitudinal and epidemiological databases to examine shifts in religious behaviors over time (e.g., McCullough, Tsang, & Brion, 2003) or influences of religion on health and mortality (Oman & Thoresen, Chapter 25, this volume). Some researchers have turned to the World Wide Web to gather information (e.g., Peterson & Seligman, 2003), while others are employing techniques such as momentary assessment (e.g., Keefe et al., 2001; Pargament & Mahoney, 2005) and brain imaging (Newberg & Newberg, Chapter 11, this volume).

In addition to broadening data collection strategies, psychologists have also begun to employ ever-more sophisticated approaches to data analysis. For example, psychologists have recently applied growth curve analyses to understanding individual differences in the course of spirituality over time (e.g., Brennan & Mroczek, 2002), and hierarchical linear modeling techniques, which allow within-subject analysis, to examine relationships between daily spiritual experience and daily pain (Keefe et al., 2001). These varied and diverse approaches to capturing and understanding religious beliefs, feelings, and behaviors provide a heretofore undreamt-of richness and opportunity.

Returning to the goals of the science of the psychology of religion, it is important to note a development in both theory and methodology, that of attending to the concept of mediation (George, Ellison, & Larson, 2002). That is, researchers have begun to search not only for relationships, but for the links or mechanisms that are responsible for the relationships identified. In other words, it is not enough to know that religion is related to, for example, physical health or mortality. Rather than simply noting these relationships and making assumptions or speculating, researchers are endeavoring to understand not only to what variables religion is related but *how* these relationships come about. That is, we want not only to predict, but to understand; we not only want to know *what* but also *how*.

PSYCHOLOGY OF RELIGION IN THE SCIENCE OF PSYCHOLOGY

We are at a transition point from a narrow linear history (i.e., the psychology of mostly Protestant Christianity in the United Kingdom and the United States) to a future of an expansive psychology of religion that is global in scope. This expansiveness could include extending the research to multiple religions and spiritualities, cross- and multiculturally, and geographically worldwide. Theory and research methods would have to evolve with

these extensions. The multilevel interdisciplinary paradigm and religion as a meaning system will serve as good conceptual guides to link research done at different levels, from
different disciplines, and within diverse religions and cultures.

Traps to Avoid

The repeated cry for a definition of religion that captures what it "really" is, as if it were
possible to say in words what it is in essence, is unlikely to be satisfied. Some reasons for
this are addressed in Chapter 1. Why should psychologists of religion think that they
would ever be able to state a definition of religion that is true, final, and accurate? Doing
this would require that religion by its own nature be static. But it is not static. It takes on
myriad forms, has an indefinite number of meanings to people, promotes every imaginable and even contradictory behavior, depends heavily upon the imaginative capacities as
well as the unique cognitive structures within each human being, and appears to be infi-
nitely plastic. When we add to this the knowledge that the very process of imagining can
create false memories that are stored in the brain at a neurobiological level, and realize
that religion relies heavily on such mechanisms of neuroplasticity, it is no wonder that
just as the nature of religion shifts from person to person and from time to time in the human mind, our efforts at defining it must do so as well.

Kirkpatrick (2005) has pointed out three errors for us to avoid, each a trap that extends from the complexity and psychological bases of religion itself. He advises us to
avoid the a priori *definitional trap* because religion is not a static entity and because the
process of research requires that we let definitions evolve with it. Good definitions are
"working definitions," not statements of what religion's essence "really" is. We are also
advised to avoid the *evaluative trap* because it has long interfered with the scientific integrity of the field and because both "good religion" and "bad religion" are the consequence
of the same psychological processes that make religion what it is. Religion is therefore
neither "good" nor "bad," but rather "both" and "neither." Finally, and obvious in light
of a proper understanding of the purposes and limits of science, we are advised to avoid
the *veridicality trap*. Scientific psychology may yield knowledge about the nature of religion in the human mind, but it has nothing to say about the truth or falsity of religious
claims and is logically orthogonal to them.

Of Application and Control

Moving beyond the goals of description, prediction, and understanding, we stated earlier
that one of the goals of the psychology of religion as a discipline is *control*. Although
widely accepted as a goal of science at large, stating control as a goal for the psychology
of religion may make some people uncomfortable. However, the ultimate payoff of science, including our endeavors within the psychology of religion, is to make a difference,
to use the knowledge gained for some purpose (ideally, a positive purpose!). Perhaps as
an alternative to the term *control*, the word *application* may create less unease. Only very
recently have clinicians devoted attention to how religious issues may be involved in the
therapeutic enterprise, but the development of psychospiritual and psychoreligious interventions has increased at a rapid rate (Shafranske, Chapter 27, this volume). The increased attention to issues of religion within clinical psychology has also raised questions
about ethics and therapist competence, issues that will clearly become more prominent in
future discussions of religion-based interventions. In addition to applications for clinical

psychology, some researchers have broached the issues of religion in healthcare and the practical and ethical issues that it introduces (Koenig, 2002). It should be noted that some dissent has been voiced regarding the appropriateness of "using" religion in the service of goals such as health or healing (e.g., Shuman & Meador, 2002).

There are areas for which the term *regulation* may be appropriate as a level of contribution for the psychology of religion that lies between the less direct *application* and the more direct *control*. For example, in the United States, a person is free to hold any religious belief that he or she wishes to hold; beliefs may not be defined, promoted, or inhibited by the government. However, a person is not free to display any religious practice no matter what the consequence. Behaviors, including religious behaviors, may be freely performed so long as they do not hurt someone else or otherwise violate the law. Therefore, for example, a parent is free to withhold medical treatment from him- or herself on grounds of religion, but that same parent is not free to withhold life-saving medical treatment from his or her young child on grounds of the *parent's* religion (e.g., see Bottoms, Shaver, Goodman, & Qin, 1995). The parents have the freedom to practice their own religion on themselves, but they do not have total freedom to extend its practice *onto* their children. Such freedom stops at the point of risk to the health and welfare of the child. This is an area to which psychology of religion can contribute, in the service of protecting the right of people to hold any religious beliefs while applying the knowledge from the field to help to regulate religious behaviors when that is appropriate and necessary for the health and well-being of others. Again, some scholars have cogently argued that religion in the service of health or well-being is theologically inappropriate (e.g., Shuman & Meador, 2002).

Why Study This?

From time to time the question "Should psychologists study religion?" comes up. Each time a discussion evolves in which those who argue the "pro" side say that psychologists should study religion because it is unique (a theoretical reason) and because it is important (a practical reason). Those taking the "anti" side reply that although religion is important for practical reasons, much religion can be explained by the same principles that explain many other behaviors and that therefore it may not be unique, and therefore not be as essential to study from the point of view of the basic science of psychology, as the "pros" say.

A fine incarnation of this discussion was edited by Baumeister (2002). It included three target articles that argued the "pro" side, 12 commentary articles whose responses to the target articles ranged from "maybe a little" to "no, anti." We wish to address the crux of the "no, anti" point of view, stated so clearly and plainly by Funder (2002). First, many aspects of religion are nonunique and can be explained by the same principles that explain any other behavior. This is nothing new, it is in agreement with the view of Funder, and we would be surprised if it were otherwise. Second, however, the research in this field and the arguments stated in the first and last chapters of the book are compelling that some aspects of religion are unique and require unique ideas to explain them. There is no need to repeat these arguments. We add only the following comment with an applied focus.

Even if the theoretical and research arguments for the psychology of religion were not compelling, and we think they are, it would be naïve in the extreme to think we can afford the luxury of *not* doing research on religion now. Only a fool would think religion is to be overlooked among topics studied by psychologists in today's world. Regardless of one's personal inclinations about religion, we would be wise to focus as much research effort as possible on this topic. It is perhaps the most important topic that could be studied by any psychologist, given what is happening socially and politically in the world. To neglect a thorough psychological study of religion during the next generation seems foolhardy in the extreme. Every day we see the manifestations of religion in the real world. It is to the betterment of this world that we hope this field contributes.

ACKNOWLEDGMENTS

We thank the authors in this handbook for providing a number of good suggestions for the preparation of these chapters, and Adam Cohen, Ralph Hood, Jr., and Ralph Piedmont for helpful critical comments on the rough drafts.

REFERENCES

Allport, G. W., & Ross, J. M. (1967). Personal religious orientation and prejudice. *Journal of Personality and Social Psychology, 5*, 432–443.

Azari, N. P., Missimer, J., & Seitz, R. J. (in press). Religious experience and emotion: Evidence for distinctive cognitive neural patterns. *The International Journal for the Psychology of Religion*.

Azari, N. P., Nickel, J., Wunderlich, G., Niedeggen, M., Hefter, H., Tellmann, L., Herzog, H., Stoerig, P., Birnbacher, D., & Seitz, R. J. (2001). Neural correlates of religious experience. *European Journal of Neuroscience, 13*, 1649–1652.

Baumeister, R. F. (Ed.). (2002). Religion and psychology [Special issue]. *Psychological Inquiry, 13*(3).

Bottoms, B. L., Shaver, P. R., Goodman, G. S., & Qin, J. (1995). In the name of God: A profile of religion-related child abuse. *Journal of Social Issues, 51*, 85–111.

Brennan, M., & Mroczek, D. K. (2002). Examining spirituality over time: Latent growth curve and individual growth curve analyses. *Journal of Religious Gerontology, 14*, 11–29.

Cohen, A. B., Hall, D. E., Koenig, H. G., & Meador, K. (2005). Social versus individual motivation: Implications for normative definitions of religious orientation. *Personality and Social Psychology Review, 9*, 48–61.

Contrada, R. J., Goyal, T. M., Cather, C., Rafalson, L., Idler, E. L., & Krause, T. (2004). Psychosocial factors in outcomes of heart surgery: The impact of religious involvement and depressive symptoms. *Health Psychology, 23*, 227–238.

Duriez, B., Fontaine, J. R. J., & Hutsebaut, D. (2000). A further elaboration of the Post-Critical Belief Scale: Evidence for the existence of four different approaches to religion in Flanders–Belgium. *Psychologica Belgica, 40*, 153–181.

Emmons, R. A. (1999). *The psychology of ultimate concerns: Motivation and spirituality in personality*. New York: Guilford Press.

Emmons, R. A. (2000). Is spirituality an intelligence?: Motivation, cognition, and the psychology of ultimate concern. *The International Journal for the Psychology of Religion, 10*, 3–26.

Emmons, R. A., & Paloutzian, R. F. (2003). The psychology of religion. *Annual Review of Psychology, 54*, 377–402.

Funder, D. C. (2002). Why study religion? *Psychological Inquiry, 13*, 213–214.

George, L. K., Ellison, C. G., & Larson, D. B. (2002). Explaining the relationships between religious involvement and health. *Psychological Inquiry, 13*, 190–200.

Ghorbani, N., Watson, P. J., Ghramaleki, A. F., Morris, R. J., & Hood, R. W. (2002). Muslim–Christian Religious Orientation Scales: Distinctions, correlations, and cross-cultural analysis in Iran and the United States. *The International Journal for the Psychology of Religion*, 12(2), 69–91.

Gonsalves, B., Reber, P. J., Gitelman, D. R., Parrish, T. B., Mesulam, M.-M., & Paller, K. A. (2004). Neural evidence that vivid imagining can lead to false remembering. *Psychological Science*, 15(10), 655–660.

Gorsuch, R. L. (1988). Psychology of religion. *Annual Review of Psychology*, 39, 201–221.

Hill, P. C., & Hood, R. W., Jr. (1999). *Measures of religiosity*. Birmingham, AL: Religious Education Press.

Hill, P. C., & Pargament, K. I. (2003). Advances in the conceptualization and measurement of religion and spirituality: Implications for physical and mental health research. *American Psychologist*, 58, 64–74.

Hunsberger, B., & Jackson, L. M. (2005). Religion, meaning and prejudice. *Journal of Social Issues*, 61(4).

Hutsebaut, D. (1996). Post-critical belief: A new approach to the religious attitude problem. *Journal of Empirical Theology*, 9(2), 48–66.

Kahlili, S., Murken, S., Reich, K. H., Shah, A. A., & Vahabzadeh, A. (2001). Religion and mental health in cultural perspective: Observations and reflections after the First International Congress on Religion and Mental Health, Tehran, *16–19 April 2001. The International Journal for the Psychology of Religion*, 12(4), 217–237.

Keefe, F. J., Affleck, G., Lefebvre, J., Underwood, L., Caldwell, D. S., Drew, J., Egert, J., Gibson, J., & Pargament, K. I. (2001). Living with rheumatoid arthritis: The role of daily spirituality and daily religious and spiritual coping. *Journal of Pain*, 2, 101–110.

Kirkpatrick, L. A. (2005). *Attachment, evolution, and the psychology of religion*. New York: Guilford Press.

Koenig, H. G. (2002). *Spirituality in patient care: Why, how, when, and what*. Philadelphia: Templeton Foundation Press.

Lazarus, R. S. (1993). Coping theory and research: Past, present, and future. *Psychosomatic Medicine*, 55, 234–247.

McCullough, M. E., Tsang, J., & Brion, S. (2003). Personality traits in adolescence as predictors of religiousness in early adulthood: Findings from the Terman Longitudinal Study. *Personality and Social Psychology Bulletin*, 29, 980–991.

Murken, S., & Shah, A. A. (2002). Naturalistic and Islamic approaches to psychology, psychotherapy, and religion: Metaphysical assumptions and methodology—a discussion. *The International Journal for the Psychology of Religion*, 12(4), 239–254.

Paloutzian, R. F., Fikes, T., & Hutsebaut, D. (2002). A social cognition interpretation of neurotheological events. In R. Joseph (Ed.), *Neurotheology: Brain, science, spirituality, religious experience* (pp. 215–222). San Jose, CA: University Press California.

Pargament, K. I. (1997). *The psychology of religion and coping*. New York: Guilford Press.

Pargament, K. I., & Mahoney, A. (Eds.). (2005). Sacred matters: Sanctification as a vital topic for the psychology of religion [Special issue]. *The International Journal for the Psychology of Religion*, 15(3).

Park, C. L. (2005). Religion as a meaning-making framework in coping with life stress. *Journal of Social Issues*, 61(4).

Peterson, C., & Seligman, M. E. P. (2003). Character strengths before and after September 11. *Psychological Science*, 14, 381–384.

Roccas, S. (2005). Religion and value systems. *Journal of Social Issues*, 61(4).

Sheridan, L. P., & North, A. C. (2004). Representations of Islam and Muslims in psychological publications. *The International Journal for the Psychology of Religion*, 14, 149–159.

Shuman, J. J., & Meador, K. G. (2002). *Heal thyself: Spirituality, medicine, and the distortion of Christianity*. New York: Oxford University Press.

Silberman, I. (Ed.). (2005a). Religion as meaning system. *Journal of Social Issues* [special issue], *61*(4).

Silberman, I. (2005b). Religion as a meaning system: Implications for the new millennium. *Journal of Social Issues*, *61*(4).

Socha, P. M. (1999). Ways religious orientations work: A Polish replication of measurement of religious orientations. *The International Journal for the Psychology of Religion*, *9*(3), 209–228.

Spilka, B., Hood, R. W., Jr., Hunsberger, B., & Gorsuch, R. (2003). *The psychology of religion: An empirical approach* (3rd ed.). New York: Guilford Press.

Author Index

Subject Index

"f" following a page number indicates a figure; "n" following a page number indicates a note; "t" following a page number indicates a table.